Handbook of Research on Personal Autonomy Technologies and Disability Informatics

Javier Pereira
University of A Coruña, Spain

Medical Information Science Reference

MEDICAL INFORMATION SCIENCE REFERENCE

Hershey · New York

Director of Editorial Content:	Kristin Klinger
Director of Book Publications:	Julia Mosemann
Acquisitions Editor:	Lindsay Johnston
Development Editor:	Julia Mosemann
Publishing Assistant:	Milan Vracarich, Jr.
Typesetter:	Milan Vracarich, Jr.
Production Editor:	Jamie Snavely
Cover Design:	Lisa Tosheff

Published in the United States of America by
Medical Information Science Reference (an imprint of IGI Global)
701 E. Chocolate Avenue
Hershey PA 17033
Tel: 717-533-8845
Fax: 717-533-8661
E-mail: cust@igi-global.com
Web site: http://www.igi-global.com

Library of Congress Cataloging-in-Publication Data

Handbook of research on personal autonomy technologies and disability informatics / Javier Pereira, editor.
p. ; cm.
Includes bibliographical references and index.
Summary: "This book offers a comprehensive description of the needs that must be considered by IT engineers when designing technical assistance tools that can be used by disabled persons according to their specific motoric, visual, auditive, or psychic needs"--Provided by publisher.
ISBN 978-1-60566-206-0 (hardcover) -- ISBN 978-1-60566-207-7 (eISBN) 1. Assistive computer technology--Handbooks, manuals, etc. 2. Self-help devices for people with disabilities--Handbooks, manuals, etc. I. Pereira, Javier, 1972-
[DNLM: 1. Self-Help Devices. 2. Communication Aids for Disabled. 3. Disabled Persons--rehabilitation. 4. Equipment Design. 5. Man-Machine Systems. 6. Needs Assessment. 7. User-Computer Interface. WB 320 H2364 2011]
HV1569.5.H3645 2011
681'.761--dc22
2010024445

British Cataloguing in Publication Data
A Cataloguing in Publication record for this book is available from the British Library.

All work contributed to this book is new, previously-unpublished material. The views expressed in this book are those of the authors, but not necessarily of the publisher.

Table of Contents

Section 3
Internet Accessibility

Section 4
Computer Access

Detailed Table of Contents

The potential impact of new assistive technologies to help elderly stay in their own homes for longer, age well and independently is a crucial challenge to improve their quality of life and independence. It is important to draw attention to the characteristics of the elderly and their situation regarding the increase in life expectancy and aging-related aspects, increasing the risk of disability and dependence.

This chapter reports on data collected through interviews with adults who use aided communication. In these interviews, the adults highlight the complex factors that influence their use of aided communication and their aspirations and expectations of aided communication. They discuss the limitations and the potential of new technologies and explore how these developments impact on their participation in meaningful social interactions.

Smart ICT systems, essentially based on multisensory approach, are becoming of great interest in the field of perceptive impairments. In this chapter examples of multisensory systems supporting daily activities of visually impaired people are addressed. The proposed architectures adopt low cost sensors, dedicated signal processing and smart algorithms. The latter approach, which moves the design focus from expensive hardware to smart paradigms, allows for boosting the system performances especially in terms of reliability and redundancy of the information to be provided to the user.

Preface

BACKGROUND

"There is no true progress if technology is not within range of everybody" Henry Ford

Human beings are active by nature and involve in significant activities and occupations that allow them to satisfy their needs according to their interests and desires.

This definition is valid as long as there exists a correct interaction between the corporal factors (structures and functions), the features of the individual (activities), and the environmental elements (participation), as defined in the social model of the International Classification of Functioning, Disability, and Health (CIF). Contextual factors are so important for personal development that their diminished integration can lead to the restriction of the person's social participation.

Day after day, people with functional diversity face environmental obstacles, barriers, and difficulties that complicate their normal interaction and participation in activities that are important to them.

Between 10 and 20% of the world population suffer from some type of disability, i.e. approximately 600 million people. Almost 43% of them subsist on less than $1 a day, and 70% of them reside in developing countries. These numbers give an idea of the inequality that is common to this population group.

Undoubtedly, the "technological revolution" has allowed the development of new devices and products that have optimized our systems of information, socialization, and communications. But this revolution has also contributed to the increase of the above inequality and has led to what is now known as the "digital breach", which separates those that can normally use technology and those than cannot.

In order to end this situation, technological development must consider not only the demands of the activity but also contextual factors and person-specific features and needs. It is in this context that "support technology" has appeared and known its largest growth in 30 years. This denomination is used to refer to all devices, services, strategies, and practices that were created and applied to mitigate the difficulties of disabled people.

People with functional diversity use support technology in a wide range of areas, such as daily life, education, work, free time, and activities of social participation. Support technology can be a fundamental tool to guarantee their participation, integration, and equality of opportunities, but only if real interaction exists between the human being and the technology. The features of the device, the identification of significant activities, and the perspective of the user must intercommunicate and respond to their specific context.

The efficiency and efficacy of support technology depend on its ability to adapt to the needs and desires of the user, respond to the purposes it was designed for, and integrate with the user's personal environment.

"Technology is not a purpose in itself, but a means between the knowledge society and global development".

BOOK ORGANIZATION

Recent years have shown remarkable progress in the development of assistive technologies, especially in the field of Information and Communications Technologies (ICT). This situation has facilitated their incorporation as basic resources for promoting personal autonomy. The aim of the 1st chapter, entitled "*Assistive Technologies, Tools, and Resources for the Access and Use of Information and Communication Technologies by People with Disabilities*", is to provide information about assistive technology, and specifically those directly related to ICT.

A growing number of individuals with severe physical disabilities do not have access to communication or environmental interaction. The 2nd chapter, "*Nascent Access Technologies for Individuals with Severe Motor Impairments*", introduces three emerging access technologies for individuals with severe disabilities: near-infrared spectroscopy, electroencephalographic measurement of visually evoked potentials, and infrared thermographic imaging of the face. We present the physiological underpinnings of each technology, the necessary instrumentation, and the relevant scientific evidence to date.

The 3rd chapter, "*Elderly People, Disability, Dependence, and New Technologies*", shows the potential impact of new assistive technologies to help the elderly stay in their own home, allowing them to improve their quality of life and independence. It is important to draw attention to the characteristics of the elderly and their situation regarding the increase in life expectancy and aging-related aspects such as disability and dependence.

The 4th chapter, "*Augmentative and Alternative Communication Devices: The Voices of Adult Users*", reports on data collected through interviews with adults who use aided communication. In these interviews, the adults highlight the complex factors that influence their use of aided communication and their aspirations and expectations of aided communication. They discuss the limitations and the potential of new technologies and explore how these developments have an impact on their participation in meaningful social interactions.

Smart ICT systems, essentially based on multisensory approach, are becoming of great interest in the field of perceptive impairments. The 5th chapter, "*Innovative Smart Sensing Solutions for the Visually Impaired*", addresses examples of multisensory systems that support the daily activities of visually impaired people. The proposed architectures adopt low cost sensors, dedicated signal processing, and smart algorithms. The latter approach, which moves the design focus from expensive hardware to smart paradigms, allows for boosting system performances especially in terms of reliability and redundancy of the information to be provided to the user.

The Etiology of Persistent Developmental Stuttering (PDS) is still a largely unknown subject despite centuries of research and modern neuroimaging techniques. A new etiological model of PDS is presented and discussed in the 6th chapter, "*An Advanced Concept of Altered Auditory Feedback as a Prosthesis-Therapy for Stuttering Founded on a Non-Speech Etiologic Paradigm*". Two major asseverations are that PDS is a non-innate and a non-speech based disorder. The implications of the model have guided the design of a new adaptive AAF device.

It has been demonstrated that rhythmic sensory stimulation facilitates locomotive function in patients with Parkinson's disease. In the 7th chapter, "*The Role of Sensory Rhythmic Stimulation on Motor*

Rehabilitation in Parkinson's Disease (PD)", we review the current knowledge on the use of sensory stimulation as a tool to improve motor performance in parkinsonian patients with a focus on gait. The different sensory modalities (auditory, visual, and somatosensory) are considered and some methodological principles reported in the scientific literature to better administrate stimulation are taken into account.

Transcranial magnetic stimulation (TMS) is a procedure in which electrical activity in the brain is influenced by a pulsed magnetic field. The early clinical uses of TMS were restricted to the field of neurology, where it was used to examine conduction in the central and peripheral nervous system by stimulating neurons. More recently, TMS and repetitive TMS (rTMS) have been used to investigate aspects of cortical processing, including sensory and cognitive functions. The 8th chapter, "*Transcranial Magnetic Stimulation (TMS) as a Tool for Neurorehabilitation in Parkinson's Disease*", introduces the basic principles of the technique and reviews some works on the therapeutic use of rTMS on Parkinson's disease.

The 9th chapter, "*A Feedback Controlled FES in Rehabilitation*", shows how a feedback control functional electrical stimulation (FES) system was proposed to prevent quadriceps weakness and drop-foot of the hemiplegia during gait training. The proposed knee locker device with closed-loop FES system is capable of providing a hemiplegic patient with regular walking restoration after appropriate gait training.

The 10th chapter, "*Human-Centered Metal Hydride Actuator Systems for Rehabilitation and Assistive Technology*", reviews the motivation for the development of some of the leading artificial muscle-like actuators, outlines a new and unique actuator using metal hydride materials, and describes its applications for joint rehabilitation, prevention of disuse syndrome, transfer assistance, and seat lift for wheelchair in quality-of-life technology.

Many disabled users consider the Web to be their primary source for information, employment, and entertainment. However, there are millions of people who have disabilities that affect their use of the Web. To understand the needs of disabled users is to understand the needs of everyone. The 11th chapter, "*Web Accessibility: Current Trends*", first examines the intersection between accessibility, disability, and technology; it then presents current practical trends towards achieving Web accessibility; finally, it discusses future trends.

The 12th chapter, "*Catering for Personal Autonomy with E-Mentoring Supported by Recommendations*", presents a technology solution based on a recommender system. In order to support the needs of people with intellectual disabilities towards their work integration and independent life, we addressed two challenges: i) facilitating the mentoring work for human mentors, and ii) reproducing some of this support and offering it dynamically when specific actions of the users are detected in the environment.

The 13th chapter, "*Blind User Interfacing: Requirements, Models, and a Framework*", presents the requirements for blind user interfacing, the changes to be made to the human-computer interface models, and a framework that improves the development of dual user interfaces. The framework includes a set of guidelines for interface design, a toolkit for the low effort implementation of dual user interfaces, and a programming library for speech and Braille. A case study of the development of one such dual interface application is also presented.

The 14th chapter, "*Sensors in Assistive Technology*", reports on the development of an eyeglass-type infrared-controlled computer interface for the disabled. The system is designed for individuals with spinal cord injuries and disabled people whose movements are severely restricted. The infrared transmitting module can be easily mounted on eyeglasses or artificial limbs.

Brain-computer interface (BCI) technologies translate brain activity into action and thus allow the user to control devices directly without motor activity. The 15th chapter, "*Non-Manual Control Devices: Direct Brain-Computer Interaction*", consists in a review of basic principles and methodologies underlying BCI operation, and a discussion between two practical examples: BCI-based control of a humanoid robot for physical manipulation of objects, and BCI-based interaction with the popular global navigation programme Google Earth.

Wireless sensor networks and systems are the most powerful technologies applied to control and supervising systems. The 16th chapter, "*Wireless Sensor Networks and Systems*", is focused on their use for disabled and elderly people. It will show a study about the four main wireless technologies used for this purpose and a survey with the benefits when they are applied. It demonstrates that Zigbee is the most often used technology, but that in some cases WLAN is the best technology.

Scanning keyboards are a type of Augmentative and Alternative Communication (AAC) devices used by many individuals with speech and motor disorders in their day-to-day communication. A scanning keyboard refers to an on-screen keyboard operated with a scanning input method. User models, in conjunction with automatic design space exploration methods, provide efficient ways to design and evaluate scanning keyboards. A review of the related works reported in the literature, including their limitations and scope for further research, is presented in the 17th chapter, "*Model-Based Approaches for Scanning Keyboard Design: Present State and Future Directions*".

The 18th chapter, "*Projects from the Orange Foundation in Favor of People with Obstacles to Communication*", takes a look at the most important projects carried out by the Orange Foundation in order simplify communication for people with disabilities. It tries to demonstrate how, by using different technologies and playing with them, those people can get a better communication experience.

The 19th chapter, "*Occupational Therapists' Perceptions about the Non-Use of Recommended Assistive Technology (AT)*", presents findings from a study which aims at obtaining occupational therapists' perceptions about the non-use of assistive technology (AT). Therapists identified the client-, AT- , and intervention-focused factors found to influence AT use. Overall, results support the need for therapists to use a client-centered approach during the provision of AT in order to facilitate optimal use by clients.

Many systems and devices have been developed in order to improve the quality of life of the disabled and elderly people. The 20th chapter, "*Sensors and their Application for Disabled and Elderly People*", introduces a classification of the sensors, their main circuits, their basic principles, and the most well known sensor applications for the disabled and elderly. It is very useful in facilitating the development of sensors in this area.

A modern society must offer individuals the possibility to access all resources available, especially elderly and disabled people. The progress of remote ICT has led to spectacular advances such as Telegerontology, a system that not only includes the basic principles of accessibility and usability, but also those of gerontology attention, i.e., the capacity to assess the patient before the intervention. This new branch is introduced in the 21st chapter, "*Telegerontology: A New Technological Resource for Elderly Support*".

The 22nd chapter, "*Experiences Using Information and Communication Technologies with Elderly People*", describes an experiment conducted with new technologies in the Red Cross Elderly Day Care Centre of A Coruña, using the In-TIC software and a specific methodology for intervention with elderly individuals. The implementation of these types of experiences may improve accessibility to ICTs for the elderly and help to encourage their social integration and occupational performance.

The 23rd chapter, "*Experiences Using Information and Communication Technologies with Children Affected by Cerebral Palsy*", shows the experience of using information and communication technologies in a centre specialized in Cerebral Palsy. Specifically, the intervention was carried out with In-TIC software, developed by the IMEDIR Centre (University of A Coruna). The participants in this experience are people with cerebral palsy who attend the ASPACE Center and have potential abilities to benefit from the application of the new technologies.

RELEVANCE AND CONCLUSION

This book is addressed to people who are related to support technologies and the promotion of the personal autonomy of persons with functional diversity. Professional experts, students, and teachers will be able to extend their knowledge on this matter by receiving a general vision on the latest advances in research and learning from the experiences of people who believe in the power of new technologies to raise the level of independence and autonomy of the disabled to their highest level.

It is our wish that this book may be useful to all readers, but in particular persons with functional diversity, who constitute the essence of our work and dedication.

The impact of technology in our modern world is undoubtedly positive. If technology is put at the disposal of persons with functional diversity, the possibilities of application become almost infinite.

According to the World Health Organization (WHO), health must be defined as a state of complete physical, mental, and social well-being, rather as the mere absence of illnesses; people with functional diversity suffer from physical, cognitive, sensorial, and/or social limitations in the activities that constitute the daily life of all human being, i.e. Basic Daily Life Activities, Instrumental Daily Life Activities, Education, Work, Free Time, and Sleep.

There are various frameworks, models, and conceptualizations regarding technologies that increase personal autonomy, but Information and Communications Technologies that are developed for and by the persons implied really contribute to improve their personal autonomy, independence, and quality of life.

This book is based on the contributions of people who describe their experiences with technologies, products, services, and research, and allow us to compare, analyze, and summarize a wide range of technological applications for people with functional diversity.

Acknowledgment

The editors would like to acknowledge the help of all the people involved with collation and review process of the book, without whose support, the project could not have been satisfactorily completed. A further special note of thanks also goes to the Orange Foundation, whose contributions during the past years have been invaluable.

It is also due to thank the reviewing team which members have provided constructive and comprehensive reviews to each chapter proposal.

In closing, we wish to thank all of the authors for their insights and excellent contributions to this book. We also want to thank the resources and support of the staff of RNASA-LAB (Artificial Neural Network and Adaptive Systems Laboratory) as well as the TIC department (Department of Information and Communication Technologies), both of them included at the University of A Coruña.

Finally, the editor, Javier Pereira Loureiro, wants to thank his wife Silvia for her love and patience, as well as he would like to dedicate this work to his first daughter, Alicia.

Javier Pereira
Editor

Section 1
Assistive Technologies

Chapter 1
Assistive Technologies, Tools and Resources for the Access and Use of Information and Communication Technologies by People with Disabilities

Betania Groba
University of A Coruña, Spain

Thais Pousada
University of A Coruña, Spain

Laura Nieto
University of A Coruña, Spain

ABSTRACT

A person with disabilities can present difficulties in occupational performance. It is necessary to develop a set of resources, technological or otherwise, to offset these difficulties, and contribute to the integration of people with functional diversity in society. These resources are called support products or technology support, but do not eliminate the deficits, they can eliminate the limitation of the performance of persons with disabilities. Moreover, the Information Communication and Technologies (ICT) were formed as an alternative to personal empowerment of people with disabilities. To access and use of these new technologies are used to support specific products. In the market there is a diversity and variety of assistive technology, so it is necessary the classification and analysis of various products before the person can use it. The purpose of this chapter is to provide information about assistive technology, and specifically those directly related to ICT.

DOI: 10.4018/978-1-60566-206-0.ch001

INTRODUCTION

As individuals and members of a social community, people need to carry out a series of activities in order to maintain their habits and roles, as well as balance in different areas of performance.

On occasions, people may have either temporary or permanent disabilities that affect their abilities, as a result of one or more alterations in their functions and/or bodily structures (World Health Organization, 2001).

Spanish Law 39/2006 on the Promotion of Personal Autonomy and Attention for Persons in a Situation of Dependency defines the concept of autonomy as the ability to control, confront and adopt, on one's own initiative, personal decisions regarding how to live according to one's own standards and preferences, as well as to carry out the basic activities of daily life.

Two conclusions may be derived from this definition: the individual is an agent of their own personal actions (self-governance), and gradually acquires autonomy through their personal development.

Focusing on this meaning, functional deficit does not imply, in itself, any reduction in the person's degree of autonomy. This concept goes beyond bodily structures or functions, and belongs to the intellectual sphere of the individual, constituting the capacity for decision, awareness of oneself, and self-governance (ASEM Federation, 2008).

However, the presence of functional deficits may lead to limitations in a person's activity if they do not have the suitable resources available to overcome this situation. Finally, if society is not prepared to include persons with some type of limitation in its activities, due to the presence of a deficit, and does not develop or apply the necessary instruments to ensure their participation in a situation of equal opportunities, then a situation known as restriction in participation may occur (World Health Organization, 2001).

As a result of the appearance of this social restriction, the individual experiences a major reduction in their level of personal autonomy, understood as the ability to make decisions. In other words, the person has sufficient self-governance to choose or decide what they want to do (when, how, where, with whom), but the obstacles or impositions of the environment (whether these are physical, social, cultural, spiritual, virtual, temporal or even personal) constitute a genuine impediment to the full development and participation of the person.

Faced with this situation, there is a need to develop a series of resources – technological or otherwise – that make it possible to compensate for these difficulties, reduce the distance between exclusion and participation, and contribute towards the integration of persons with functional diversity into society as capable and self-governing citizens.

And so, from the second half of the twentieth century onwards, there has been a genuine technological revolution, leading to the development of different devices, tools, resources and solutions aimed at achieving this objective.

The term "Assistive Technology" was proposed in the Technology-Related Assistance for Individuals with Disabilities Act of 1988, although the concept, under a series of guises or none in particular, long predates this legislation (Sherer, 2001).

In order to achieve more independent functionality and to compensate limitations in activity caused by some type of deficit in bodily structures and/or functions, people with functional diversity require different types of assistance. This support is necessary in different personal spaces and surroundings, such as the home, school, workplace or leisure areas in the community.

A wide range of resources exists for promoting personal autonomy, and may involve assistance from a third person (a family member acting as a carer, or a paid personal assistant), a guide dog, or assistive technology (Sherer, 2001).

In recent years, we have witnessed remarkable progress in the development of assistive technologies, above all in the field of Information and Communications Technologies (ICT). This situation has facilitated their incorporation as basic resources for promoting personal autonomy.

Assistive devices are tools used to encourage independence in the functioning of persons with some type of physical limitation (Sherer, 2001). However, in order to ensure that assistive technologies comply with this main objective, it is essential to promote the resources, disseminate the strategies used to provide them, and to publicise the different methods for information and consultation.

The International Classification of Functioning, Disability and Health (World Health Organization, 2001) represents a change in the concept of health and disability, and recognises the necessity and right to medical, rehabilitative, educational and preventative interventions. It also highlights the limitations that hinder participation in activities, with special emphasis on public education, social reform and legislation, initiatives in terms of architectural design, and equal opportunities.

The objectives of this chapter are:

- To provide specific information on Assistive Technologies and in particular those related to ICT.
- To examine the classifications and the products that assist in the access and use of the ICT most frequently used by persons with functional diversity.
- To analyse which is the most appropriate procedure for the prescription of assistive technology, and which factors are involved in the abandonment of the use of this technology by persons with functional diversity.

BACKGROUND

The main theme of this chapter is assistive technology, tools and resources for persons with functional diversity. Specifically, assistive technology associated with ICT forms a part of the belief that people with functional diversity have the same rights to access information as the rest of the population. The General Assembly of the United Nations, in its Universal Declaration of Human Rights from 1948 (United Nations General Assembly, 1948), approved and announced this right in Article 19 and Article 27:

- Article 19. "Everyone has the right to freedom of opinion and expression; this right includes freedom to hold opinions without interference and to seek, receive and impart information and ideas through any media and regardless of frontiers."
- Article 27. "Everyone has the right freely to participate in the cultural life of the community, to enjoy the arts and to share in scientific advancement and its benefits."

Also, Article 9 of the International Convention of the United Nations on the rights of persons with disabilities (United Nations Organization, 2006) states that the public powers must:

- f) Promote other appropriate forms of assistance and support to persons with disabilities to ensure their access to information;
- g) Promote access for persons with disabilities to new information and communications technologies and systems, including the Internet;
- h) Promote the design, development, production and distribution of accessible information and communications technologies and systems at an early stage, so that these technologies and systems become accessible at minimum cost.

A review of the literature provides an insight into the different concepts and classifications currently applied in relation to assistive technology, ICT and persons with functional diversity.

Definitions

Assistive Technology (Cook and Hussey, 1995): Any item, partial or total piece of equipment or any system that may be acquired commercially or adapted to a person, which is used to enhance or improve the functional capacities of individuals with disabilities, or to modify or establish behaviours.

Assistive Devices, UNE standard EN ISO 9999: 2007 (European Commitee for Standardization, 2007): Any product (including devices, equipment, instruments, technologies and software) that is specially manufactured or available on the market to prevent, compensate for, control, mitigate or neutralise deficiencies, limitations to activity and restrictions to participation.

As we will see, a wide range of assistive technology is available on the market, which may hinder the process of evaluating and choosing the most appropriate device based on the specific abilities and needs of a user, delaying the process of establishing a connection between persons and technology.

Different Types of Classification

Taking into account the latest developments and their wide possibilities, assistive technology is highly diverse and extensive. Assistive devices or products range from prostheses or orthoses to systems for accessing computers (IMSERSO, 2009), including a series of devices that facilitate activities as basic as washing, dressing or feeding, or other more complex types such as driving vehicles or playing sports.

In the report entitled "Access to assistive technologies in the European Union", it is estimated that there are more than 20,000 assistive devices currently available on the European market. In turn, in 2001, M. Sherer proposed an even higher number, estimating the number of different types of assistive technologies to be around 26,000 (Sherer, 2001).

This diversity means that it is extremely complex and time consuming to provide information that is up to date, appropriate and accessible to the end users, persons with functional diversity.

As a result, faced with the quantity and variety of existing devices, it is necessary to establish a uniform system of classification or categorisation that makes it easy to carry out searches, and to unify terms at international level.

In order to achieve this objective, different types of classification have been proposed based on different criteria. The main categories that are currently available are listed below:

- Standard classification. UNE – ISO 9999 standard (2007): This is the most widely known, publicised and applied. The assistive devices are classified according to their functions, and will be explored in detail in the following paragraphs.
- Classification according to technological level: in this case, the assistive devices are categorised as Hi-Tech, Mid-Tech or Lo-Tech, or No-Tech when they have no technological level. Many of the assistive devices used for accessing computers that are dealt with in this chapter belong to the first two categories.
- Classification according to complexity (Basil et. al, 1998):
  - Basic technical aids: easy to manufacture, and low cost.
  - Simple mechanical, electrical or electronic aids, with a low technological level: these are more complex devices than the former category, but still easy to use.
  - Complex electronic aids: these are assistive devices that offer extensive

possibilities for communication, providing they are suitably adapted to each user.

- Alcantud's functional classification (Alcantud, 2000): This divides assistive devices into different groups. In this case we have underlined those that are connected with the main theme of this chapter:
    - Systems for habituation, learning and entertainment.
    - Alternative and augmentative systems for accessing information from the environment.
    - Technology for accessing computers.
    - Alternative and augmentative communication systems.
    - Technologies for personal mobility.
    - Technologies for manipulation and control of the environment.
    - Rehabilitation technologies.
    - Assistive technologies.
    - Technologies for sport, leisure and free time.
    - Technologies for daily life.
- Classification according to areas of execution (Cook and Hussey, 1995): These authors propose dividing assistive products into the following categories:
    - Augmentative and alternative communication systems.
    - Technologies for personal mobility.
    - Technologies for manipulation and control of the environment.
    - Sensory aids for persons with visual, auditory or tactile disabilities.
- In 1999, King proposed an interesting classification for the concepts dealt with in this chapter. In this case, assistive technology was divided into the following categories:
    - Augmentative and alternative communication.
    - Computer access systems.
    - Systems to help with listening and seeing.
    - Environmental control.
    - Adapted games and leisure.
    - Aids for posture and position.
    - Mobility and assisted mobility.
    - Prostheses.
    - Robots for rehabilitation.
    - Integration of technology in the home, school, community and workplace.
- Others: Other classifications exist that propose differentiating assistive technologies according to the following criteria (Díez, 2006):
    - Hard versus Soft technologies.
    - Devices versus Tools.
    - Commercial versus Personalised technologies.

Factors to be Taken into Account for the Prescription and Use of Assistive Technology (Sherer, 2001)

Faced with this wide variety of assistive technology, it is not only essential to determine the specific needs of the end user, but also to develop tools that make it possible to obtain tangible results on the advantages of one device over another.

It may be the case that a person with functional diversity has decided to use a specific assistive device but does not find it useful in their environment, considers it difficult to use, or that its instructions are too complicated.

In this case, we should analyse the factors that may lead to a decrease in the use of assistive technologies by persons with functional disability. The level of abandonment in the use of these devices may reach levels of close to 30%. Different studies have demonstrated the low level of use of assistive products, restriction in their use due to the influence of the context, and their abandonment (Philips and Zao, 1993; Riemer-Reis, 2000; Pape, Kim and Weiner, 2002; Verza et al, 2006), including the use of assistive devices for accessing ICT.

The factors underlying the abandonment of assistive technologies are directly associated with

Table 1. Factors to be taken into account for the prescription and use of assistive technology (Sherer, 2001)

Factors associated with the user	Factors associated with the supplier	External factors
Demographic Characteristics	Role performance and expectations	Legislation
Temperament and personality	Technological service delivery	Larger society
Coping and adaptation	Technological education	Public policy
Pain experience	Counselling and partnership skills	Prevailing cultural practices and perspectives
Technology readiness, comfort and satisfaction	Systems change and program implementation	
Knowledge and education	Professional certification and quality assurance	

the environment and the individual characteristics of each person (Martine and Connolly, 2008), although this situation may also be influenced by the attitude and lack of knowledge of the team of professionals involved, regarding the benefits of their application (Huntinger, Johanson & Stoneburner, 1996). This last factor has a direct influence on making incorrect choices for assistive technology, without focusing on the specific needs of the users or the changes they may bring about for them.

In the light of this high level of abandonment, it was considered necessary to create different models to evaluate assistive technology. These instruments can be divided into two main blocks (Díez, E. 2006), which are detailed below:

- General methods: The integral evaluation of all of the fundamental elements involved in taking decisions on the use of assistive technology. As an example, this group includes the following instruments:
  - Human activity assistive technology (Cook and Polgar, 2007): This has been developed to analyse the individual characteristics of a disabled person carrying out an activity in a given context, especially when the use of assistive technology forms a part of this context.
  - Matching Person and Technology – MPT (Sherer, 2004): This is a global tool, with a series of questionnaires that make it possible to evaluate the person's expectations and preferences, their background prior to the use of assistive technologies, their family, their environment and economic factors.
  - Student, Environment, Task and Tools – SETT (Zabala, 1995, 1996): This is a tool that helps gather and organize information that can be used to guide collaborative decisions about services that foster the educational success of students with disabilities.
  - Wisconsin Assistive Technology Initiative – WATI (WATI, 1998): Its main aim is to provide a comprehensive framework for the process of evaluating the use of assistive technologies, aimed at children with disabilities at school age.
- Specific tools: these focus on evaluating specific abilities using objective methods, in order to guide the process of selecting the most appropriate assistive technology for the user's abilities. This group includes the following tools, associated with evaluating the necessary abilities to use computers:

- ◦ Assessment of Computer Task Performance (Dumont and Vincent, 2002): This makes it possible to evaluate the functional ability of a person to access a computer, regardless of the type of assistive device they use.
- ◦ COMPASS (Koester et al., 2003): This makes it possible to evaluate two areas: access to the computer and the use of augmentative communication. With regard to the ability to access computers, the evaluation is based on comparing the use of three different assistive devices, also making it possible to verify the efficacy of an intervention.
- ◦ Evaluware (AbleData Information Center, 2004): This tool focuses more on evaluating the abilities of children. It makes it possible to identify the most appropriate assistive technology based on four areas: motor skills, visual abilities, auditory abilities and other related abilities. The evaluation process involves using examples with games.
- ◦ ETAO Tool (Díez et al., 2008): This consists of a functional evaluation for tasks involving computer access, which makes it possible to identify the most appropriate assistive devices and the use of augmentative communication. This is the only technological evaluation tool that has been integrally created and designed in Spain, by the team of the Institute for Integration in the Community (INICO).

Assistive Technologies for Accessing Computers

'Hi-Tech' assistive devices have a very important role in the lives of many people with major limitations to their activity, by providing a means of accessing and controlling devices they use in their daily life. (Shone et al., 2002).

ICT can be used as a way of reducing distances between the person and their environment, in this case applying the term 'assistive technologies' (Díez, 2006). The use of assistive technology as a means of increasing, maintaining or improving the functional abilities of users has been discussed in different studies (Alcantud and Soto, 2003; Cook and Hussey, 1995; Sherer, 2001).

The ISO 9999:2007 standard is the most widely used and stable classifications at international level for assistive products that are specially designed or available on the market for the people with disabilities. These standards use the terminology of the International Classification of Functioning, Disability and Health (ICF) (WHO, 2001).

This standard (European Committee for Standardization, 2007) has a hierarchical structure, divided into classes, subclasses and divisions. At one level, the classification establishes:

- Assistive products for personalised medical treatment.
- Assistive products for the teaching/learning of skills.
- Orthoses and prostheses.
- Assistive products for personal care and protection.
- Assistive products for personal mobility.
- Assistive products for domestic activities.
- Furnishings and adaptations for homes and other premises.
- Assistive products for communication and information.
- Assistive products for the manipulation of objects and devices.
- Assistive products for improving the environment, tools and machinery.
- Assistive products for leisure.

If we focus on the classification at two levels, based on the theme of this chapter, Assistive products for communication and information, we obtain the following result:

- Assistive products for seeing
- Assistive products for hearing
- Assistive products for vocal production
- Assistive products for manual drawing and writing
- Assistive products for calculations
- Assistive products for working with audiovisual information and video
- Assistive products for face to face communication
- Assistive products for telephoning
- Assistive products for alarms, indications and signalling
- Assistive products for reading
- Computers and terminals
- Input devices for computers
- Output devices for computers

In the third level of classification, "Input Devices for Computers", the classification to be taken into account is the following:

- **Keyboards.** This category also includes Braille keyboards and accessories for making telephone calls. The existing keyboard models on the market have different functions that permit access and more intuitive use by persons with disabilities. Examples of these input systems are:
    - Keyboard emulator: this allows the person to emulate all of the keyboard functions, and by pressing a previously configured key it provides them with access and simplifies the features of the keyboard.
    - Flexiboard: a conceptual keyboard with 128 squares that are programmed according to the needs of the people who use them. They function with any operating system, and are connected directly to the keyboard port. Different templates can be created that are placed on top of the board, and it is also possible to configure the size of the squares and the sensitivity for pressing the keys (see Figure 1).
    - Desktop keyboard: a keyboard that is 4 times larger than a conventional keyboard. The keys are divided into colours, which simplifies the functions of the keyboard at cognitive level. They also have larger sized numbers, making them easier to use for people with visual difficulties (see Figure 2).
    - Artmedia virtual keyboard: this virtual keyboard can be used with the Windows operating system with a mouse. It has a predictive system that helps with writing and reduces the

Figure 1. Flexiboard: template with options to promote personal autonomy

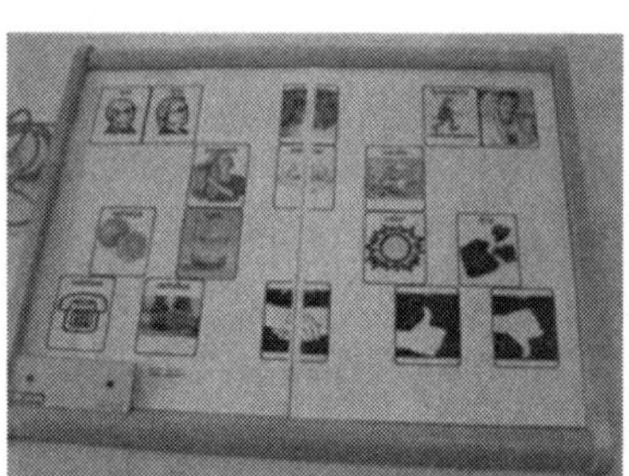

Figure 2. Keyboard with keys larger size and with colors that make it easier

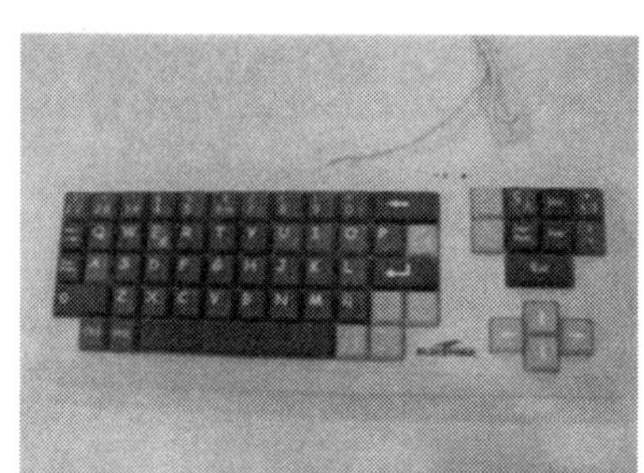

number of times it has to be pressed (see Figure 3).

  - Ergonomic keyboard for two hands: this keyboard is specially designed to reduce the number of movements and pressure required to press the keys, making them easier to use for people with physical limitations. They also have spaces to rest the wrists, which also reduces the range of movement used in shoulders and elbows.

- **Mouse.** Trackballs, optical pens, joysticks connected to the mouse port and mouse emulators are some of the assistive products included in this category.
  - Mouse emulators: emulators make it possible to work on a flat surface, and to move the pointer in all directions using a joystick, emulating all of the basic functions: clicking, double clicking, dragging and releasing. They also make it possible to download the mouse functions to external switches. In some models the mouse speed can be configured, and they have housings that facilitate the precision of fine motor movements to press the keys (see Figures 4 and 5).
  - Mouse emulators using buttons: this type of emulator allows users to control the cursor with buttons for the different directions and functions. Others provide control using external switches for each function (see Figure 6).
  - Head mouse: these allow the cursor to be controlled by small head movements, and their functions can be configured. For example, leaving the cursor over an icon for a given period of time will produce a click or a double click. They normally use an infrared

Figure 3. Virtual keyboard for Windows operating system

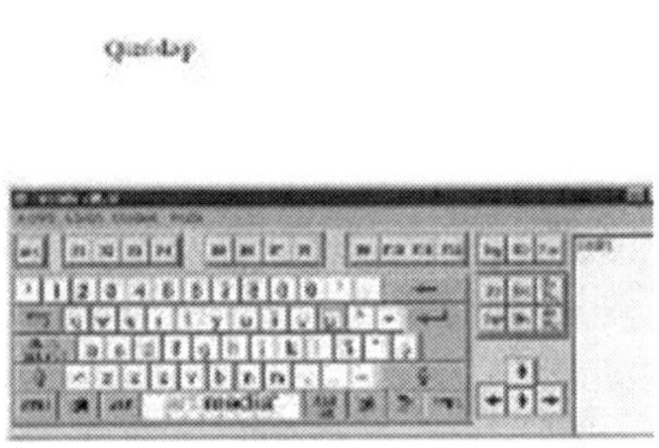

Figure 4. Mouse emulator

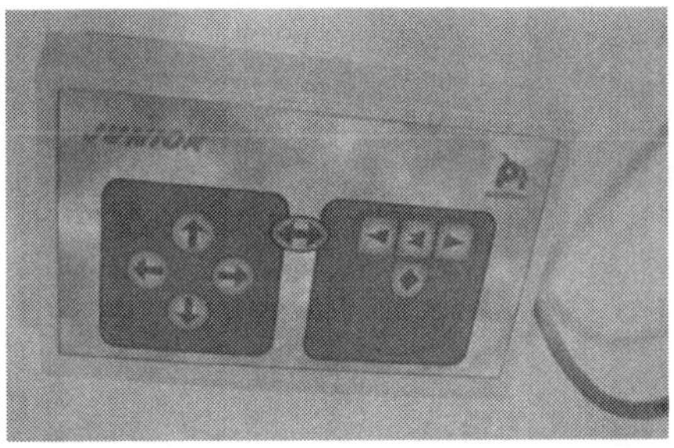

Figure 5. Joystick with buttons that emulate the functions of a mouse

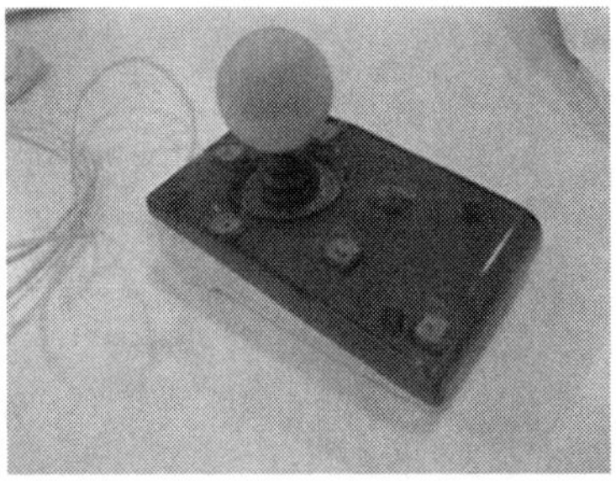

Figure 6. Mouse emulator with buttons

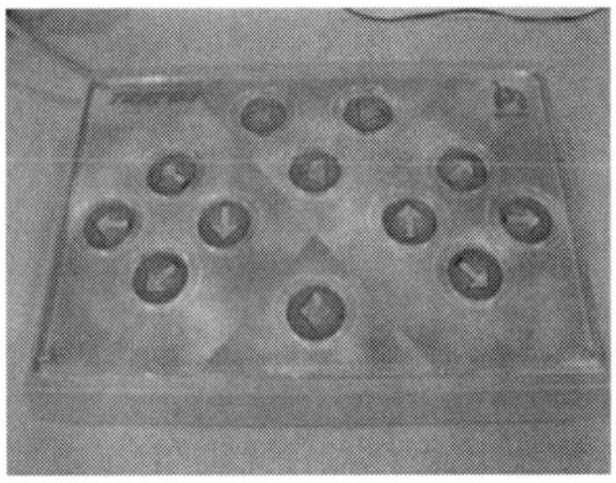

system that detects the signal, either from stickers on the user's forehead, glasses or straps around the head.

  - Mouse emulator controlled by scanning: this type of device makes it possible to control he functions and directions of the mouse cursor using a switch-activated scanning method (which highlights different groups of keys with a light, until the user selects a group and reaches the required key). The scanning speed can be configured to make access easier (see Figure 7).
  - Touch screen: today, touch screens are one of the most interesting alternatives for persons with voluntary movement, as it allows them to directly access icons by emulating the functions of a mouse (see Figure 8).
  - Eye controlled mouse: this tool makes it possible to control a PC by eye movements, after calibrating the user's visual precision and movement. It includes a system for monitoring eye movement, which allows the user to move the mouse cursor by looking towards the required position. In order to select the function, all the user has to do is continue looking at the position for a given time, or to blink.
  - Trackball: these types of mice provide greater precision, as they are larger than a conventional mouse and can even be controlled using external switches (see Figure 9).
  - Mouth or lip-operated mouse: in this case, only the mouth or lips need to be used to control the cursor. The functions are activated by breathing or blowing, depending on the option that is configured.
- Joysticks: including buttons or switches with similar functions. A conventional joystick can be adapted to emulate mouse functions, by combining it with specific software for this type of use.
- Alternative input devices: Scanners, voice recognition units, concept boards and data gloves. Other examples of alternative input devices include voice recognition systems that allow text to be edited with voice commands, optical card readers or graphic tablets.

Figure 7. Box for connecting external switches

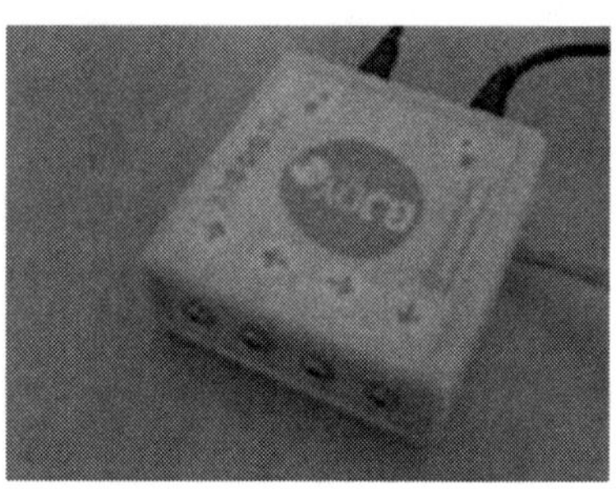

Figure 8. Touch screen

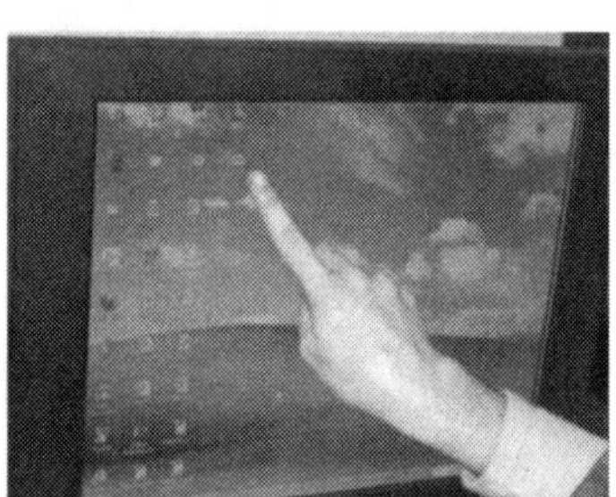

Figure 9. Trackball

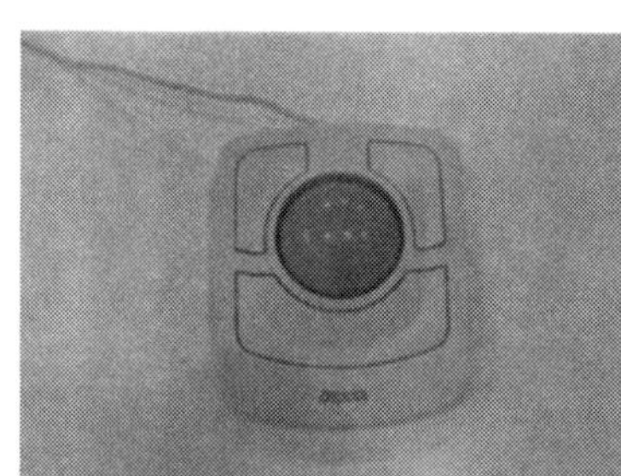

- Input accessories: Devices that connect the input systems of a computer, such as word libraries and lists of independent words, connection boxes, cables and tablets.
- Switches: an indirect access system that allows persons with physical difficulties to use them by emulating a specific mouse function. It allows PCs to be controlled by using them with other devices, such as a scanning system (see Figure 10).
- Input software: virtual on-screen keyboards and digital fingerprint readers. An example of this software is The Grid 2, a computer programme for computer access and communication. Using virtual keyboards, it offers a simplified and personalised environment for the user, so that they can open different applications and use them with a single click on the virtual keyboard buttons (see Figure 11).

The categories of *Computers and terminals* and *Computer output devices*, despite being associated with the theme of this chapter, do not meet the requirements of favouring the access and use of ICT, and so they will not be covered in detail.

At European level, in 2003 an International Alliance of Suppliers of Information in Assistive Technologies was created. Its main objective is to establish cooperation structured between centres for information and consultancy on technical aids. The European Assistive Technology Information Network (EASTIN), has the following specific aims (Minusval, 2009):

- To provide adequate and complete information on assistive technology for persons with functional diversity, in order to provide them with an active role in their choice.
- Increasing cooperation between information suppliers, in order to share it at worldwide level.

Countries such as the USA, Canada, the UK or Brazil form a part of this alliance.

In Spain, this role is represented by the State Centre for Personal Autonomy and Technical Assistance (CEAPAT, 2009) of the Institute of the Elderly and Social Services (IMSERSO) of the Ministry of Education, Social Policy and Sport. This centre applied the ISO 9999:2007 Classification to produce the Catalogue of Assistive Products (previously known as the Catalogue of Technical Aids), although at first it was only available in printed format that was published every year. Finally, in 2009 the CEAPAT launched a new digital version of the Catalogue of Assistive Products. The classification is based on the purpose of the assistive products, according to the ISO 9999:2007 standard.

Figure 10. Switches

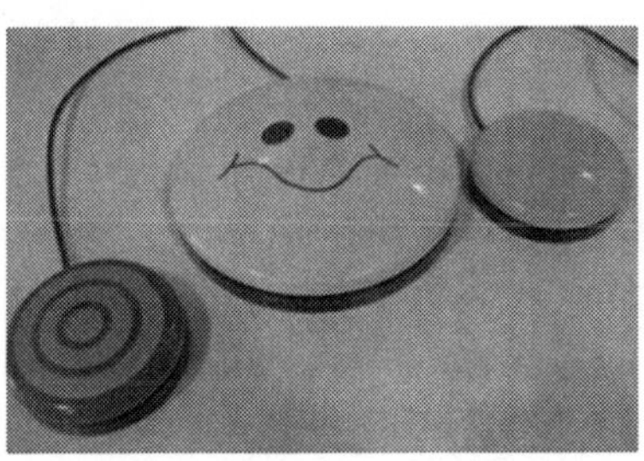

Figure 11. Virtual keyboard using the free software In-TIC

FUTURE TRENDS

Abandonment of Assistive Devices

A good match of person and technology requires attention to aspects of the environments in which the technology will be used, the needs and preferences of the user, and the functions and features of the technology (Sherer and Craddock, 2002).

29.3% of devices are completely abandoned (Philips and Zhao, 1993).

Ebner, 2004, has indicated the existence of levels of abandonment as high as 80%.

The highest level of abandonment is seen with "high technology" (Riemer-Reiss, 2000) and in technologies for mobility (Philips and Zhao, 1993).

The highest level of abandonment occurs during the first year and after 5 years of use.

The conclusions of the European Conference on Accessibility and Design for All (2008) stated that there was "a need to adopt advanced and pioneering initiatives in order to promote research and innovation in the development of goods, services and equipment, installations and environments based on the principles of design for all."

This decalogue goes on to state: "the information and knowledge society will only be complete project when all persons are able to take part and take advantage of the potential offered by new technologies now and in the future."

CONCLUSION

The number of users of assistive products is on the rise, as well as satisfaction with the use of innovative products that are adapted to different situations (Minusval, 2009). Cost-profit analyses have revealed the benefits of making good use of these products and technologies.

The solution to the digital divide does not only lie in incorporating technologies, regardless of how closely adapted and suited they are to the users, as they also have received training in digital literacy, which allows them to take full advantage of assistive technology (Cabero, 2004).

In 2006, the Organising Committee and Scientific Committee of the Tecnoneet Forum (Rodriguez et al., 2006) proposed a "Decalogue for Digital Inclusion". This proposal came about as a result of evidence regarding the difficulties that existed in obtaining appropriate technological resources, and making use of them in a sensible way with persons with functional disability, and the need to eliminate or reduce the digital divide. Considering their importance with regard to the main theme of this chapter, and as a conclusion, the main statements of this Decalogue are listed below (Soto and Fernández, 2005):

- Duration: quality of the concepts and quality of the materials.
- Accessibility: Use of products and services that are susceptible to being adapted to each specific need.
- Re-utilisation: Exhausting the useful life of the resources.
- Savings: Gaining space, time and resources.
- Harmlessness: The products must not be toxic.
- Sufficiency: Making public good references that are clearly visible and accessible to all.
- Gratification: The goods and services must be essentially gratifying.
- Collaboration: Sharing is gratifying and improves efficiency.
- Equity: Fair distribution, responsible consumption.
- Efficiency: Low cost, high level of service.

It is clear that everyone is involved in the whirlwind of advances associated with ICT and the Information Society. It is impossible not to form a part of this phenomenon, as the social context in which we operate influences us completely. Being able to access the resources, tools and possibilities that provide us with a virtual context is a right, and it is impossible to deny that these possibilities may offer alternatives that are capable of reducing limitations or otherwise favouring the social participation of persons with functional diversity, enhancing their abilities and making it possible for them to control their own actions.

REFERENCES

Alcantud, F. (2000). Nuevas Tecnologías, viejas esperanzas. In Soto, F. J., & López, J. A. (Eds.), *Nuevas tecnologías, viejas esperanzas: las nuevas tecnologías en el ámbito de la discapacidad y las necesidades educativas especiales* (pp. 257–262). Murcia: Consejería de Educación y Universidades.

Alcantud, F., & Soto, F. J. (2003). *Tecnologías de ayuda en personas con trastornos de comunicación*. Valencia: Nau Llibres.

Basil, (1998). *Sistemas de signos y ayudas técnicas para la comunicación aumentativa y la escritura*. Barcelona: Masson.

Cabero, J. (2004). Reflexiones sobre la brecha digital y la educación. In Soto, F.J. & Rodríguez, J. (Coords.), *Tecnología, educación y diversidad* (pp. 23-42). Murcia: Conserjería de Educación y Cultura.

Centro Estatal de Autonomía Personal y Ayudas Técnicas (CEAPAT). (2009). *Catálogo de productos de apoyo*. Retrieved September 2009, from http://www.catalogo-ceapat.org/acercade

Cook, A. M., & Hussey, S. M. (1995). *Assistive Technologies: principles and practice*. St. Louis: Musby, Inc.

Cook & Polgar. (2007). *Assistive Techonology. Principles and practice (Hardcover)*. St. Louis, MI: Mosby Elsevier.

Díez, E. (2006). Evaluación para el uso de tecnologías de ayuda en personas con discapacidad. In Verdugo Alonso, M. A. & Jordán de Urríes Vega, F. B. (Coord.). *Rompiendo inercias. Claves para avanzar. VI Jornadas Científicas de Investigación sobre Personas con Discapacidad* (pp. 297-305). Salamanca: Amarú.

Díez, E. (2008). Tecnologías que ayudan: Mitos y realidades. [RAMPA]. *Revista de Atención Integral y Medicina Familiar para la Atención Primaria, 4*, 14–19.

Dumont, C., Vicent, C., & Mazer, B. (2002). Development of a Standardized Instrument to Assess Computer Task Performance. *The American Journal of Occupational Therapy., 56*, 60–68. doi:10.5014/ajot.56.1.60

European Committee for Standardization. (2007). [*Assistive Products for persons with Disability. Classification and Terminology. Geneva, Switzerland:* BSI.]. *International Standard EN ISO, 9999*, 2007.

European Conference EDeAN (European Design for all e-Accessibility Network). (2008). *Conclusiones del encuentro: Decálogo de León por la accesibilidad.* León: Ministerio de Educación, Política Social y Deporte.

Federation, A. S. E. M. (2008). *Guía de las enfermedades neuromusculares. Información y apoyo a las familias*. Jaen: Formación Alcalá.

Huntinger, P., Johanson, J., & Stoneburner, R. (1996). Assistive technology applications in educational programs of children with multiple disabilities: a case study report on the state of the practice. *Journal of Special Education Technology, 13*(1), 16–35.

Instituto de Migraciones y Servicios Sociales (IMSERSO). (2009). Productos de Apoyo. Dossier. *Revista Minusval, 173*, 9–29.

Koester, H. H., LoPresti, E., Ashlock, G., McMillan, W., Moore, P., & Simpson, R. (2003 March). Compass: Software for Computer Skills Assessment. Paper presented at the *Proceedings of CSUN 2003 International Conference on Technology and Persons with Disabilities*. Los Angeles, CA.

Martine, M. S., & Connolly, I. (2008). Roles of aided communication: perspectives of adults who use AAC. *Disability and Rehabilitation. Assistive Technology*, *3*(5), 260–273. doi:10.1080/17483100802338499

Pape, T. L.-B., Kim, J., & Weiner, B. (2002). The shaping of individual meanings assigned to assistive technology: a review of personal factors. *Disability and Rehabilitation*, *24*, 5–20. doi:10.1080/09638280110066235

Philips, B., & Zhao, H. (1993). Predictors of assistive technology abandonment. *Assistive Technology*, *5*, 36–45. doi:10.1080/10400435.1993.10132205

Rieme-Reis, M. L., & Wacker, R. R. (2000). Factors Associated with assistive technology discontinuance among individuals with disabilities. *Journal of Rehabilitation*, *66*, 44–50.

Rodríguez Vázquez, J., Sánchez Montoya, R., & Soto Pérez, F. J. (Coords.) (2006). *Las tecnologías en la Escuela Inclusiva: nuevos escenarios, nuevas oportunidades. (Actas del Congreso Tecnoneet-ciiee 2006)*. Murcia: Consejería de Educación y Cultura/Real Patronato sobre Discapacidad.

Sherer, M. J. (2001). *Assistive Technnology: Matchin Device and consumer for successful rehabilitation*. Washington, DC: American Psychological Association.

Sherer, M. J. (2004). *Matching person and assistive technology process and accompanying assessment instruments* (Rev. Ed.). Webster, NY: Institute for Matching Person & Technology.

Sherer, M. J., & Craddock, G. (2002). Matching person and technology (MPT) assessment process. *Technology and Disability*, *14*, 125–131.

Shone, S. M., Ryan, S., Rigby, P. J., & Jutai, J. W. (2002). Toward a comprehensive evaluation of the impact of electronics aids to daily living: evaluation of consumer satisfaction. *Disability and Rehabilitation*, *24*(1-3), 115–125. doi:10.1080/09638280110066794

The AbleData Information Center. (2004). *AbleData: your source for assistive technology information. Evaluware Software.* Retrieved October 2009, from http://www.abledata.com/abledata.cfm?pageid=113583&top=0&productid=114098&trail=0

United Nations General Assembly. (1948). Universal Declaration of Human Rights. Retrieved September 2009, from http://www.un.org/es/documents/udhr/

United Nations Organization. (2006). *Convention on the Rights of Persons with Disabilities*. New York: Headquarters of the United Nations.

Verza, R., Carvalho, M., Battagia, M., & Uccelli, M. (2006). An interdisciplinary approach to evaluating the need for assistive technology reduces equipment abandonment. *Multiple Sclerosis*, *12*, 88–93. doi:10.1191/1352458506ms1233oa

Wisconsin Assistive Technology Initiative (WATI). (1998). *Assessing students' needs for assistive technology: a resource manual for school district teams*. Amherst, WI: WATI.

World Health Organization. (2001). *International Classification of Functioning, Disability and Health*. Geneva: World Health Organization.

Zabala, J. S. (1995). *The SETT framework: critical areas to consider when making informed assistive technology decisions*. Houston, TX: Region IV Education Service Center.

Zabala, J. S. (1996). Setting the stage for success: Building success through effective use of assistive technology. *Proceedings of the Southeast Augmentative Communication Conference* (pp. 129-187). Birmingham, AL: United Cerebral Palsy of Greater Birmingham.

KEY TERMS AND DEFINITIONS

Assistive Technologies/Assistive Device/Assistive Products: Any product (including devices, equipment, instruments, technologies and software) that is specially manufactured or available on the market to prevent, compensate for, control, mitigate or neutralise deficiencies, limitations to activity and restrictions to participation.

ICT/ICTs: Information and Communication Technologies. A set of technologies, components and techniques related to the media and the processing and transmission of information.

Disability/Disabilities: Part of the multi-aspects of the interaction between the individual and social environmental context in which it operates. Therefore a disabled person is a person who has impairment, activity limitation or participation restriction (World Health Organization).

Personal Autonomy: The ability to control, manage and take his own initiative, personal decisions about how to live according to the rules and preferences, and to develop the basic activities of daily living.

Chapter 2
Nascent Access Technologies for Individuals with Severe Motor Impairments

Sarah Power
University of Toronto, Canada

Saba Moghimi
University of Toronto, Canada

Brian Nhan
University of Toronto, Canada

Tom Chau
University of Toronto, Canada

ABSTRACT

As the number of individuals without physical access to communication or environmental interaction escalates, there are increasing efforts to uncover novel and unconventional access pathways. In this chapter, we introduce three emerging access technologies for individuals with severe disabilities: near-infrared spectroscopy, electroencephalographic measurement of visually-evoked potentials and infrared thermographic imaging of the face. The first two technologies harness activity directly from the brain while the third exploits spontaneous temperature changes in the face. For each technology, we discuss the physiological underpinnings, the requisite instrumentation, the scientific evidence to date and the future outlook.

INTRODUCTION

Personal autonomy in the context of physical chronic illness can be conceptualized as the correspondence between the desired and actual life of an individual (Mars et al., 2008). To achieve this correspondence, Mars et al. (2008) asserts that individuals need to "develop principles expressing what their lives to be like" (p. 345) through daily interactions, choice-making and experiences.

DOI: 10.4018/978-1-60566-206-0.ch002

However, many individuals do not have physical access, due for example to an environment that does not support the functional capability of the individual. A lack of access severely limits one's daily interactions, choice-making and social experiences and thus impinges upon personal autonomy. To restore a level of correspondence, a common approach in rehabilitation is to augment the opportunities for interpersonal connection through an access solution.

An access solution provides a means of interacting meaningfully with one's milieu (people and objects within the environment) when functional speech or movements are not available, due for example to severe motor impairments. Often times access solutions are technology-mediated. In such case, the technical components of an access solution include an access technology and a user interface technology (Tai et al., 2008) as depicted in Figure 1. The access technology comprises of (a) an access pathway, that is, the input devices by which an expression of functional intent (e.g., a movement or physiological change) is translated into an electrical signal, and (b) a signal-processing unit that analyzes (e.g., filtering and pattern classification) the input signal and generates a corresponding control signal. The control signal in turn operates a user interface, which may be an iconic display for an electronic communication aid, a front panel for an environmental control unit, or an on-screen keyboard running on a computer.

The objective of this chapter is to introduce the reader to three nascent access technologies for individuals with severe disabilities, namely, near-infrared spectroscopy, electroencephalographic measurement of visually-evoked potentials and facial infrared thermography. While these pathways are in the pre-clinical research stages, existing scientific evidence supports their continued development into viable body-machine interfaces.

BACKGROUND

A Growing Population without Access

The incidence of severe and multiple disabilities (concomitant profound sensory, physical and speech impairments) among children has been increasing globally (Tudehope et al., 1995). This upward trend is expected to continue into the foreseeable future due to improved early identification of disabilities (Rumeau-Rouquette et al., 1997), increased life expectancy of medically fragile

Figure 1. Components of a technology-mediated access solution

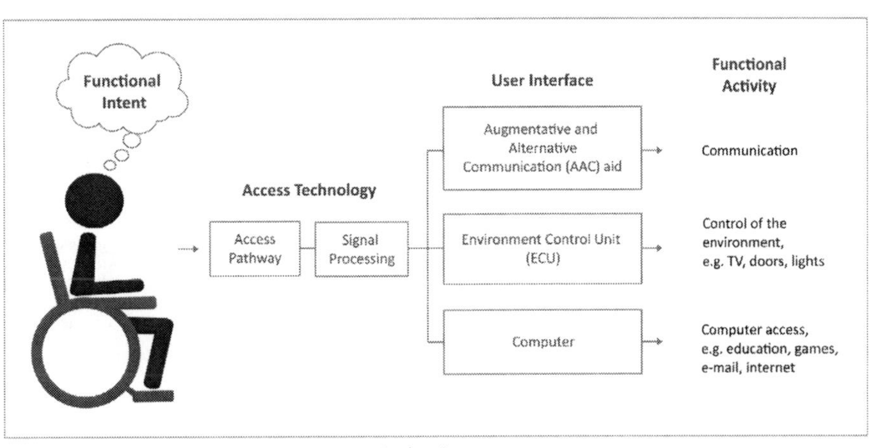

children with multiple disabilities (Jeppesen et al., 2003; Eagle et al., 2002) and higher survival rates of very low birth-weight, premature infants, the majority of whom develop disabilities (Goldson, 1996). According to United Cerebral Palsy (www.ucp.org), there are annually 5,000 new cases of children born in Canada and the USA with severe physical involvement.

An elusive challenge in the education and care of this population is the identification of a reliable access solution (Beukelman et al., 2000). Most of the individuals described above do not have functional speech, nor any repeatable volitional movements or overt physical responses. As a result, there is no obvious channel through which they may interact with teachers, caregivers, family members and peers.

No Access: The Consequences

When an individual is without any physical access to the world, he or she is denied any decision-making prerogative, and is powerless in directing his or her own care. The negative impacts are dire, including near certainty of social exclusion (Rabiee et al., 2005), the development of learned helplessness and a profound loss of independence. Families of individuals with severe disabilities who are nonverbal report heightened levels of distress and diminished ability to cope. Health care professionals often perceive an inability to provide adequate care for a patient who does not communicate via conventional means (Hemsley et al., 2007). As well, these individuals are two to six times more likely to experience physical, mental and sexual abuse (Sobsey, 1994). Unsurprisingly, the establishment of a reliable access pathway has been associated with an improved quality of life and the ability to live in the community (Bach, 1993).

The Opportunity for Innovation

The vast majority of alternate access pathways available today rely on microswitch technology, where the challenge of communication is reduced to a problem of intentionally activating a single switch. With graphical software and reliable muscle function, individuals may act on many possible pre-recorded or synthesized messages. These messages can be presented in a sequential manner to the user who in turn, activates the switch to select the desired message. While the microswitch can be a liberating mechanical access pathway for individuals who retain some extant movement (Lancioni et al., 2006), its suitability may be limited when the only available movement is effortful, non-repeatable or buried amid involuntary muscle activations.

Recognizing this limitation, many scientists have attempted to directly harness intention-bearing physiological signals via superficial measurement of the brain's electrical activity (Lotte et al., 2007) or electrodes invasively implanted on the surface of the brain or deep within (Patil et al., 2004). Despite some encouraging results with patients who otherwise would have no access, these interfaces have not been widely adopted, possibly because they do not exploit spontaneous thought but require extensive user training to consciously modulate specific neural rhythms. Furthermore, invasive neural implants have a very limited lifespan at present (Hochberg et al., 2006).

Scope

In this chapter, we introduce three nascent access technologies. The first two technologies, namely, near-infrared spectroscopy and electroencephalographic measurement of visually-evoked potentials, harness hemodynamic and evoked electrical activity directly from the brain, respectively. For the sake of brevity, we will refer to the latter simply as "visually-evoked potentials". The final technology is the infrared themographic imaging of the face, for which we'll use the compact terminology "facial thermography". All three technologies would be suitable for individuals with no extant physical movement below the neck according to the access technology taxonomy (Tai et al., 2008). For each technology, we discuss the physiological mechanisms that bring about detectable change in the measured signal, the instrumentation required, the existing scientific evidence that supports its continued development as an access solution, and the challenges and opportunities that lie ahead.

PHYSIOLOGICAL FOUNDATIONS

We begin by outlining the physiological mechanisms the give rise to measurable changes associated with expressions of functional intention. Our discussion here and in subsequent sections will be organized according to the three access technologies of interest.

Near-Infrared Spectroscopy

Near-infrared spectroscopy (NIRS) is an optical imaging technology that is used to non-invasively assess functional brain activity. Like functional magnetic resonance imaging (fMRI), NIRS measures the neural hemodynamic response, which is related to functional activity through a mechanism called neurovascular coupling (Villringer & Chance, 1997). Cerebral metabolism relies on a constant supply of oxygen, which is maintained by cerebral blood flow (CBF) through the brain's complex vascular system. During mental activity, the increased metabolic demand of the neural tissue is accompanied by a subsequent increase in regional CBF and oxygen delivery that exceeds the increase in local oxygen consumption. The result is typically an increase in the concentration of oxygenated hemoglobin (oxy-Hb) in the tissue, with a corresponding decrease in the concentration of deoxygenated haemoglobin (deoxy-Hb). Note, however, that other trends have been reported (Xie et al., 2001; Villringer & Drnagl, 1995). While the BOLD (blood oxygen level dependent) signal used in fMRI is based on variations in the levels of deoxy-Hb, NIRS can be used to detect changes in both oxy- and deoxy-Hb.

Visually-Evoked Potentials

The human brain's response to visual input changes with the nature of the stimulus (Kuba et al., 2007). Some characteristics of the stimuli are naturally embedded in the evoked brain activity and can be extracted from the corresponding electroencephalographic signal (Moratti et la., 2007; McKeefry et al., 2001). In turn, the extracted stimulus characteristics can be used to identify the target at which the subject is looking (Guo et al., 2008; Wang et al., 2006), and eventually decode an individual's choice through a brain computer interface (BCI). Since visually-evoked potentials (VEPs) are based on the brain's natural responses, eliciting and harnessing VEPs requires little to no user training (Cheng et al., 2002; Wang et al., 2008). As a result, VEPs are an appealing means of communication for individuals with severe disabilities.

Here, we will discuss steady-state and stimulus-onset visually evoked potentials, both of which have been successfully used as a BCI. Steady-state visually evoked potentials (SSVEP) are periodic responses caused by exposure to repetitive visual stimulus with frequencies higher than 6Hz (Kelly et al., 2005). These periodic responses, observed in EEG, oscillate at the same frequency as the stimulus which in turn causes an increase in the power spectrum amplitude at the stimulus frequency. Although the optimal topography of the SSVEPs has to be evaluated for each human subject (Müller-Putz et al., 2008), studies show that the magnitude of this response is usually more significant in the occipital region of the brain (Morgan et al., 1996). Investigators have attempted to elicit SSVEPs using a variety of different stimuli, including for example, pattern reversal of a checker-board (Lalor et al., 2005) and flashing lights. A comparison between different stimuli sources can be found in (Wu et al., 2008).

The physiological mechanism underlying SSVEP is still under investigation. Morrati et al. (2007) devised a set of experiments identifying the phase alignment of the ongoing background EEG as a primary source for SSVEP generation, and Pastor et al. (2003) found that the amplitude of the SSVEPs are closely related to an increase in synaptic activity.

The stimulus-onset visually evoked response is another natural response of the human brain which has been recently exploited for BCI. This response is time-locked to the onset of changes in the visual stimuli (Guo et al., 2008). Following the onset of some change (e.g., initiation of motion or flickering) in the visual stimuli, three consecutive peaks known as P1, N2 and P2 are observed in the EEG response of the brain. These dominant peaks have different magnitudes based on the characteristics of the visual stimuli (Kuba et al., 2007) and the recording sight (Makeig et al., 2002). These visually evoked responses have a latency of less than 200 ms from the onset of the stimuli (Kuba et al., 2007), and are caused by phase-resetting of electroencephalographic processes (Makeig et al., 2002).

Facial Thermography

Descending from the brain, we now consider thermal activity in the face. The human body is constantly generating heat through digestion, metabolism, and muscle movement. Core body temperature remains relatively constant at a typical internal set point between 35° C and 37° C. Maintenance of core temperature is achieved through homeostatic processes controlled by neuronal negative-feedback loops in the hypothalamus (Jones, 1998). Specialized sensory neurons called thermoreceptors in the hypothalamus constantly monitor temperature in the blood to initiate proper control responses. Temperature drops are mediated through vasoconstriction of the blood vessels along with shivering. Temperature increases on the other hand are mediated through vasodilation, sweating and in extreme cases, reduction in metabolic rate (Stanfield & Germann, 2007). Collectively, the aforementioned processes can be referred to as physiological thermoregulation. In contrast, emotional thermoregulation is not homeostatic in nature. Emotional thermoregulation involves emotional sweating, dilation of vessels and diversion of blood flow in response to different stimuli (e.g., in fight or flight responses) (Shastri et al., 2009; Pavlidis et al., 2007). In either form of thermoregulation, essentially all heat transfer to and from the body occurs at the skin surface. Heat from the core and blood is transferred to the skin surface through conductive and convective transfer modes which is measurable by some technological transduction. As a result, the skin surface is often cooler in temperature as compared to tissues closer to core (e.g., oral cavity, auditory canal) and to expired air (Murthy et al., 2004). In the application of thermal infrared imaging as a movement-based access technology, these temperature differences could be used to detect eye blinks, mouth openings or breathing alterations. In the application of thermal infrared imaging as a physiological signal-based access technology, one would endeavour to measure and quantify emotional thermoregulation.

Studies of human thermal signals have shown that healthy persons tend to exhibit contralaterally symmetric thermal signatures. Uematsu (1986) found that the average temperature difference in corresponding areas of interest on either side of the body is in the order of 0.2^o C. More recently, studies focusing on facial skin temperature (FST) distributions have suggested a connection between changes in FST and emotional state (e.g., Pavlidis et al., 2007 ; Pavlidis & Levine, 2002 ; Levine et al., 2001 ; Pollina et al., 2006 ; Shastri et al., 2009). The fluctuation of temperature in various facial areas is primarily due to changes in blood flow rate and perfusion. During mental stress, there is an increase in blood flow to the brain. This is accompanied by an increase in blood flow to the frontal vasculature in the center of the forehead at and just above the corrugator muscle. The increased blood flow and perfusion results in increased heat dissipation to the skin surface of the aforementioned areas. Hence temperature increases in the forehead region have been observed in conjunction with mental stress activities (Pavlidis et al., 2007). Changes in FST signatures have also been reported in anxious and stressed emotional states. These increases seem to be related to increased sympathetic activation in preparation for fight or flight responses (Shastri et al., 2009).

INSTRUMENTATION

With an appreciation of the physiological underpinnings of the access pathways under study, we now describe the instrumentation required to detect these physiological changes.

Near-Infrared Spectroscopy

NIRS was first reported as an experimental technique for continuously monitoring biological chromophores by Jobsis (1977). An NIRS device typically consists of one or more near infrared light sources and a detector that collects the light after it has interacted with the biological tissue. The near infrared spectrum provides an optical window (approximately 700-900nm) within which the absorption coefficient of water is low, making the biological tissue relatively transparent to the light. In this range, photons can be effectively transmitted through the cranium, reaching sufficient depth to allow investigation of cerebral cortical metabolism. When the photons enter the tissue, they are either absorbed - primarily by oxy-Hb and deoxy-Hb, the dominant chromophores for the NIR spectrum - or they undergo scattering at extra- and intra-cellular boundaries of the different layers of the head (e.g. scalp, skull, cerebrospinal fluid, cortex, etc.). The scattered photons follow a relatively predictable crescent-shaped path back to the surface and exit the head centimetres away from the entry point. Changes in the concentrations of oxy-Hb and deoxy-Hb in the neural tissue, which correlate with brain activity, affect the tissue characteristics and thus alter the amount of light that is absorbed and scattered. By monitoring changes in the intensity of returned light, it is possible to make inferences about the corresponding changes in the concentrations of oxy-Hb and deoxy-Hb, and in turn, ascertain the level of functional activity in the neural tissue.

Visually-Evoked Potentials

VEPs are monitored using electroencephalographic (EEG) recordings which measure electric potentials of the brain through electrodes positioned on the scalp surface. The voltages detected on the scalp surface have very small amplitudes (a few micro-volts), and are magnified using differential amplifiers. Using modern differential amplifiers, reliable EEG signals can be recorded with scalp electrode impedances as high as 40kΩ (Ferree et al., 2001). SSVEPs can be recorded from the occipital region. In particular, the O1 and O2 leads according to the international 10-20 EEG system are commonly used for this purpose (Cheng et al., 2002; Gao et al., 2003). Flickering stimuli can be presented using different displays such as light emitting diodes (LEDs), cathode ray tubes (CRTs) and liquid crystal displays (LCDs). A comparison between different stimuli sources can be found in (Wu et al., 2008). Stimulus-onset VEPs are also monitored using EEG recording devices. These VEPs are mostly detected by electrodes placed on extrastriate temporo-occipital and associate parietal cortical regions (Kuba et al., 2007; Guo et al. 2008; Lee et al., 2008).

Facial Thermography

Thermal infrared imaging cameras provide images that are spatial two-dimensional (2-D) maps of the 3-D temperature distribution of a surface (Jones & Plassmann, 2002). These thermal infrared images of temperature are obtained non-invasively by way of specialized lenses focusing thermal infrared radiation, emitted by all surfaces above absolute zero, onto thermal detector arrays (Jones & Plassmann, 2002). Thermal detector arrays can be classified into four general categories based on their underlying operating principles (Jones, 1998; Levine, 1993):

- Ferroelectric arrays - measure temperature dependent polarization charge;
- Microbolometers – measure changes in electrical resistance due to heating caused by incident thermal infrared radiation;
- Photovoltaic arrays - detect voltage variations with incident radiation level;
- Quantum-well infrared photodetectors (QWIP) - detect optical transition of photocarriers, i.e., as a photocurrent.

Thermal detectors are sensitive to thermal radiation in the infrared wavelength band of the electromagnetic spectrum, i.e., approximately 1.1 to 15.0 μm (Holst, 2000). Within this range, specifically 2.0 to 14.0 μm, human skin possesses an essentially constant emissivity of 0.98±0.01, invariant to skin colour (Steketee, 1973). Thus, human skin behaves very similar to a black body (i.e., no reflected radiation is present) where thermal radiation originating from the epidermis depends only on surface temperature and is independent of race (Jones, 1998; Steketee, 1973).

EVIDENCE

In this section, we present the scientific evidence supporting further exploration of each of the access technologies introduced above.

Near-Infrared Spectroscopy

Though NIRS has been used extensively in various other applications to assess functional brain activity (Franceschini, Fantini, Toronov, Filiaci & Gratton, 2000; Huppert, Hoge, Franceschini & Boas, 2005; Huppert, Hoge, Diamond, Franceschini & Boss, 2006; Jasdzewsky, Strangman, Wagner, Kwong, Poldrack & Boas, 2003; Kuboyama, Nabetani, Shibuya, Machida & Ogaki, 2004; Boas, Strangman, Culver, Hogel, Jasdzewsky, Rosen & Mandeville, 2003; Strangman, Culver, Thompson & Boas, 2002; Mehagnoul-Schipper, van der Kallen, Colier, van der Sluijs, van Erning, Thijssen, Oeseburg, Hoefnagels & Jansen, 2002; Herrmann, Walter, Ehlis & Fallgatter, 2006; Quaresima, Ferrari, Torricelli, Spinelli, Pifferi & Cubeddu, 2005; Boecker, Buecheler, Schroeter & Gauggel, 2007; Herrmann, Plichta, Ehlis & Fallgatter, 2005; Herrmann, Ehlis & Fallgatter, 2003; Yang, Zhou, Liu, Ruan, Gong, Luo & Lu, 2007; Tanida, Sakatani, Takano & Tagai, 2004; Tanida, Katsuyama & Sakatani, 2007; Herrmann, Walter, Schreppel, Ehlis, Pauli, Lesch & Fallgatter, 2007), its potential as a basis for personal autonomy technologies has only recently been explored. In this application, the goal is to develop a switch that a user can operate by consciously controlling functional activity in a pre-defined region of the brain. When the user desires to activate the switch, he or she would simply perform some mental task known to elicit activity in the region under interrogation. NIRS would be used to detect this activity, and the resultant signals would be used to control an assistive device, like a communication aid or environmental control unit.

In recent years several research groups have investigated the potential of using NIRS in the development of BCI technologies. The initial studies involved able-bodied participants and focused on conscious modulation of activity in the motor cortex due to performing various left- and/or right-hand motor imagery tasks (Coyle, Ward, Markham & McDarby, 2004; Coyle, Ward & Markham, 2007; Sitaram, Hoshi & Guan, 2005; Sitaram, Zhang, Guan, Thulasidas, Hoshi, Ishikawa, Shimizu & Birbaumer, 2007). Because motor cortical activation due to overt motor tasks had been successfully investigated in other NIRS studies (Franceschini et al., 2000; Huppert et al., 2005; Huppert et al., 2006; Jasdzewsky et al., 2003; Kuboyama et al., 2004; Boas et al., 2003; Strangman et al., 2002; Mehagnoul-Schipper et al., 2002), and because motor imagery is often used in the control of EEG-based (electroencephalography) BCIs (Pfurtscheller, Neuper, Schlögl & Lugger, 1998; Pfurtscheller, Neuper, Guger, Harkam, Ramoser, Schlögl, Obermaier & Pregenzer, 2000), this was a logical starting point. Coyle et al. (2007) conducted a three-participant study to measure activation due to a motor imagery task at positions C3 and C4 over the left and right motor cortices, respectively. Using a relatively straightforward analysis technique based on signal amplitude thresholding, they observed an average accuracy of 80% across subjects in a simple online target selection task. Taking this a step further, Sitaram et al. (2007) attempted to differentiate cortical activation (again at positions C3 and C4) due to left and right covert finger tapping in five able-bodied volunteers. Applying a common pattern recognition algorithm (namely, Hidden Markov Models) offline, they were able to classify the tasks as left-hand or right-hand imagery with an average accuracy of 89.1%. These studies demonstrate that NIRS can be used to detect motor cortical activity that is consciously generated by mental imagery of hand movement, and moreover, that left- and right-hand motor imagery can be differentiated, in able-bodied individuals. This could potentially allow for 2-dimensional cursor control, rather than just single-switch operation.

Other recent studies investigating NIRS for use in BCIs have focused on deriving control signals from the prefrontal cortex (PFC) (Ayaz, Izzetoglu, Bunce, Heiman-Patterson & Onaral, 2007; Bauernfeind, Leeb, Wriessnegger & Pfurtscheller, 2008; Naito, Michioka, Ozawa, Ito, Kiguchi & Kanazawa, 2007; Ogata, Mukai & Yagi, 2007; Utsugi, Obata, Sato, Katsura, Sagara, Maki & Koizumi, 2007). Monitoring the PFC is desirable over the motor cortex because it circumvents the issue of motion and attenuation due to hair, which can significantly affect performance and signal quality (Coyle et al., 2007). Also, because the PFC can be activated by different higher cognitive tasks, e.g. mental arithmetic, even individuals with only their cognitive abilities intact will be able to operate the device. A motor cortex-based system may not be as widely accessible; for those either with lesions in the motor cortex or who are many years post-cerebral insult, conscious modulation of motor cortical activity may be difficult.

Naito et al. (2007) carried out single-channel NIRS measurement over the left forehead to detect prefrontal cortical activation due to mental arithmetic or mental singing in 23 individuals with amyotrophic lateral sclerosis (ALS). At the time of writing, this is the only study investigating the potential of NIRS for use in BCIs that was conducted on individuals from the target population. Using two-dimensional linear discriminant analysis, they achieved an average detection rate of 80%. Bauernfeind et al. (2008) further demonstrated the ability of NIRS to detect the hemodynamic response to mental arithmetic tasks. They observed relatively stable and reproducible task responses in a group of 13 able-bodied participants. However, their observation during mental activation of a decrease in [HbO_2] and an increase in [HHb] is in contrast to the typical hemodynamic responses previously reported. Ayaz et al. (2007) also focused on the prefrontal cortex, investigating the response to various conditions of an N-back working memory test in eight able-bodied adults. In agreement with previous fMRI studies (Braver,

Cohen, Nystrom, Jonides, Smith & Noll, 1997), they discovered a positive relationship between increasing workload and the oxygenation observed in the dorsolateral prefrontal cortex.

While the aforementioned studies of the prefrontal cortex were based on offline analysis, in Utsugi et al. (2007), 14 able-bodied subjects attempted to freely control a model electric train by starting and stopping mental tasks that required high levels of mental concentration, short-term memory and recall ability (namely, various calculation and verbal tasks). The movement of the train provided a source of perceptual feedback of the user's hemodynamic response. Biofeedback has been noted as an essential component of BCIs (Coyle et al., 2004). Only qualitative results were reported, but the study suggested that all subjects, who had no previous training, were able to control the train with some degree of success, with three of the subjects achieving complete control.

Visually-Evoked Potentials

SSVEPs have been successfully used in BCIs for games (Lalor et al., 2005), cursor control (Trejo et al., 2006; Maggi et al., 2006), and spelling (Friman et al., 2007). Different techniques have also been investigated for improving choice detection using SSVEP (Kluge et al., 2007; Müller-Putz et al., 2005). The Shangkai Gao group at Tsinghua University has made many contributions in SSVEP-based BCI systems (Cheng et al., 2002; Gao et al., 2003; Wang et al., 2006; Jia et al., 2007). A review of the current stage of research in SSVEP-based BCIs has been recently published (Wang et al., 2008).

As stimulus-onset VEPs are time-locked to certain changes in the visual stimuli, multiple objects with changes happening at different time instances can be displayed to the user, and the object the user is looking at can be identified according to the timing of stimulus-onset VEPs. This sequential exposure can be used to identify user's choice in a BCI. Flash and motion-onset visually evoked potentials are two stimulus-onset visually evoked responses previously explored as a BCI.

Motion-onset visually evoked potentials (MVEPs) are elicited when an object at which the human eye is looking, starts to move (Makeig et al., 2002; McKeefry et al., 2001). Following the onset of the stimulus motion, the P1, N2 and P2 peaks appear in the EEG response of the brain. The use of MVEPs as a BCI has been recently proposed by Guo et al. (2008). In their study, 15 participants were exposed to a virtual keyboard composed of four buttons. A moving red vertical line appeared on each of these buttons at separate time instances. The participant was required to attend to a certain button. The offline analysis of the recorded MVEPs achieved over 90% accuracy in detecting the attended button when data from only three trials were averaged. To the best of our knowledge, the MVEP has not yet been tested in a real-time BCI.

When an object displayed to the human eye starts to flicker, flash-onset visually evoked potentials (FVEPs) appear in the EEG response. FVEPs have also been used for brain computer interfacing. Lee et al. (2008) tested FVEPs for generating a sequence of digits in real time. In their study, five volunteers were required to generate a pre-defined sequence of digits by gazing at intended numbers on a virtual keyboard with twelve buttons. Each of the digits in the keyboard switched between ON and OFF states. The duration of each state was chosen randomly between 116.7 and 350 ms to ensure temporal independence between flickering sequences. Two of the participants who had prior experience using the system achieved an information transfer rate (ITR) of 45.73 bits/min while the remaining participants operated at 25.06 bits/min. The mean accuracy of target detection was 92.18%.

VEPs have also been previously explored as a means of communication for individuals with disabilities. Sutter (1992) used an 8×8 array of 64 rectangles displayed on a CRT monitor to elicit evoked EEG responses in 70 able-bodied participants and 20 individuals with severe disabilities including amyotrophic lateral sclerosis (ALS) and cerebral palsy (CP). The virtual keys in the stimulus array underwent transient changes such as red/green flickering, a stimulus behavior which was found to evoke significant EEG responses in subjects. The transient changes in the keys were modulated in time according to a pseudo-random binary sequence so that the generated responses were nearly uncorrelated. The able-bodied participants achieved a response time ranging between 1 and 3 seconds. The recordings from the target population were contaminated with electromyographic (EMG) artifacts, and the performance was inadequate due to recording difficulties. To overcome these issues, the system was tested by an individual with ALS who volunteered to have four platinum electrodes implanted in the epidural space. Using this system, the individual was able to activate a speech synthesizer, and a universal remote control to access audio and video equipment. The participant achieved communication rates of 10 to 12 words/min prior to his death due to reasons unrelated to the project. Wang et al. (2006) tested an SSVEP-based BCI system for a group of sixteen able-bodied individuals, and eleven persons with spinal cord injury (ranging from C4 to C7). The optimal channel for SSVEP monitoring was chosen among 13 EEG recording sites on the scalp by independent component analysis prior to the actual experiments. For the able-bodied participants, the task was to control a keypad displayed on a CRT monitor which was composed of a matrix of 13 frequency-coded flickering choices. In this case, the participants were operating the system in a dimly lit room free of distractions, and were able to achieve an average ITR of 43 bits/min. For the participants with spinal cord injury, the task was to control a TV with a trainable remote controller in a doctor's office which was prone to distractions. In this control task, ten of the eleven participants were able to operate the remote with an average ITR of 21 bits/min.

Facial Thermography

To date, thermal infrared imaging has only been employed in a movement-based access application. Researchers utilized the temperature difference between internal and external tissues to detect voluntary mouth openings in both able-bodied and target populations (Memarian et al., 2009). Physiological signal-based access applications of thermal infrared imaging have yet to be explored. However, the potential to quantify an individual's intentions from natural changes in FST distribution has been demonstrated through various event-related emotion and polygraphy studies. In these studies, relationships were found between FST changes and emotional arousal (e.g., Nozawa & Tacano, 2009; Merla & Romani, 2007), anxiety (Pollina et al., 2006), fear (Levine et al., 2001), joy (Nakanishi & Imai-Matsumura, 2008), stress (Shastri et al., 2009) and pain (Merla et al., 2004). These studies suggest that cognitive processing of affect altering stimuli manifests on the skin surface through some form of emotional thermoregulation; of which is measurable with thermal infrared imaging. Foundations for a physiological signal-based thermal infrared imaging access pathway have been established through the quantification of baseline characteristics of FST signals (Nhan & Chau, 2009). With a defined baseline state, one can envision an intervention using thermal infrared imaging to measure FST distributions, compare changes against a known baseline state and classify into different affect/response categories.

FUTURE TRENDS

Having reviewed the current state-of-the-art revolving around the three emerging access technologies, we wrap up the chapter with a consideration of their future opportunities and foreseeable challenges.

Near-Infrared Spectroscopy

NIRS offers a number of advantages in the development of BCIs for individuals with no reliable motor control. It "promises flexibility of use, portability, metabolic specificity, good spatial resolution, localized information, high sensitivity in detecting small substance concentrations, and affordability" (Sitaram et al., 2007, pp. 1416). Furthermore, the thought processes required to consciously modulate the signals are relatively simple since the signals more directly reflect cognitive function than their more conventionally used EEG counterparts (Coyle et al., 2004).

However, despite its advantages, NIRS also has some inherent challenges from the perspective of personal autonomy technologies. One significant challenge (though not unique to NIRS) is that the brain region of interest, from which the control signals are derived, will inevitably become activated not only through intentional performance of the designated mental task, but also through other task-irrelevant thoughts and mental processes, and responses to external stimuli, occurring when the user is not actively trying to exert control. This "non-command brain activity" could cause unwanted activation of the device, and, if too frequent, these false positive activations could result in frustration on the part of the user. Before an NIRS-based BCI becomes suitable for practical applications, this challenge must be overcome, possibly either through the use of sophisticated signal processing schemes, or through taking advantage of the information provided by the fusion of different control sources (e.g. hemodynamic response from multiple brain regions rather than a single region; fusion of the hemodynamic response with other physiological signals like EEG, heart rate, or electrodermal activity). Training users to more accurately control their brain activity in the region of interest, using biofeedback, may also be of benefit.

Another significant challenge is the relatively poor temporal resolution of the hemodynamic response, which has been reported to peak at approximately 5-8 seconds after the onset of mental activity (Benaron, 2000). A BCI based on this signal would have a delay between when the user initiates activation of the device, and when the device ultimately responds. The latency of the hemodynamic response would significantly limit the maximum information transfer rate of the system. However, there are potential solutions to this problem. Advanced signal processing techniques, or even fusion of different control sources, as previously mentioned, could potentially allow reliable detection of mental activity earlier, before the hemodynamic response peaks. Also, though not as well understood as the hemodynamic response, NIRS can be used to detect another type of brain signal – a fast signal (Wolf, Wolf, Choi, Gupta, Safonova, Paunescu, Michalos & Gratton, 2002; Wolf, Wolf, Choi, Toronov, Paunescu, Michalos & Gratton, 2003; Gratton & Fabiani, 2003) that is reported to appear milliseconds after stimulation. Though faster, this signal is more difficult to detect than the slow hemodynamic signal because it is small in magnitude and can be dominated by other physiological signals (Sitaram et al., 2007). When the associated problems have been sufficiently overcome, this fast signal could potentially improve the temporal resolution of NIRS-based BCI technologies.

As noted by Matthews et al. (2008), the power of NIRS signals is dominated by both physical and physiological noise - introduced by subject movement, heart rate, respiration, and other physiological trends like the Mayer wave - making functional activity very difficult to identify without significant pre-processing. Many different noise removal methods (e.g. Weiner filtering, Savitzky-Golay smoothing, adaptive FIR filtering) have been employed in clinical NIRS research, but have yet to be applied to NIRS-BCI development. The reader is referred to Matthews et al. (2008) for a list of the most common noise removal techniques used in functional NIRS. The incorporation of some of these techniques into a

NIRS-BCI system could significantly improve performance.

Though studies to date suggest the great potential of NIRS as a basis for BCI technologies, the research is still in its preliminary stages with a relatively small number of published clinical studies. Furthermore, the majority of studies has involved offline analysis techniques, and has been performed on able-bodied participants. It is not clear how the results obtained with healthy individuals will compare with those from the target population. Much more extensive work will be necessary to overcome the inherent challenges discussed above and realize the full potential of this modality.

Visually-Evoked Potentials

Like NIRS, visually-evoked potentials have tremendous promise as an access technology but are not without inherent drawbacks. To our best knowledge, all of the real-time BCI technologies tested using the SSVEP use low frequency stimuli (below 25Hz). Exposure to low frequency oscillations tends to fatigue the eyes and thus preclude its usage as a long term communication device for persons with disabilities. Exposure to oscillating visual stimuli may also lead to photoepileptic seizures (Fisher et al., 2005). Photosensitivity is more common in persons with epilepsy but is not limited to this population (Fisher et al., 2005). In addition, each individual may be sensitive to a different frequency range, color and light intensity which make prospective diagnosis very challenging. In a study of 170 persons with photosensitivity, Harding et al. (1999) illustrated that sensitivity to stimuli is much higher in the 15-25 frequency band.

Investigating SSVEPs in response to high frequency visual stimuli may result in a potential access solution for persons with disabilities. Wang et al (2005) showed that for frequencies up to 43 Hz, the SSVEP is detectable. This high frequency solution would overcome both the fatigue issue and the risk of seizures. Furthermore, recent findings have shown that using SSVEPs does not require gaze shifting (Allison et al., 2008; Kelly et al., 2005). Therefore, a user can be exposed to overlapping stimuli and make a choice simply by shifting covert attention rather than gaze direction.

In current stimulus-onset-based BCIs, the communication speed decreases with increasing number of choices in the BCI, which is due to the sequential exposure to the stimuli. Since all the choices are displayed sequentially, the decision cannot be made until all of choices have been presented. For instance, the minimum exposure to visual stimuli used in MVEPs recording is found to be 200 ms (Kuba et al., 2007). However, the time lag between successive decisions accumulates as the number of choices increases. The time lag is further prolonged when it is necessary to average over multiple trials to achieve high signal-to-noise ratios.

On the upside, MVEPs magnitudes are resistant to changes in luminance and contrast (Kuba et al., 2007). Therefore, stimuli with lower brightness levels which are more pleasant and less fatiguing to the eyes can still elicit detectable changes in the brain response. As a result, MVEPs have the potential to be used as a long-term BCI. The real-time application of the MVEPs as a BCI, however, has yet to be evaluated.

Facial Thermography

The non-contact, non-invasive nature of this technology makes it an attractive option in cases where contact sensors are undesirable and risks of contamination should be minimized. As well, its relative portability and operational invariance to environmental and lighting conditions overcomes some of the limitations of conventional computer vision-based access technologies. In physiological signal-based access applications, abstract training and validation necessary to gain control of body signals may be circumvented by focusing efforts on measuring and quantifying the natural evolution of FST changes.

However, a thermal infrared imaging-based access technology would be more expensive than traditional (i.e., motion or switch) access interventions. Though costs have steadily decreased, thermal infrared imaging cameras are still considered as specialty equipment with typical price tags in the tens of thousands. That being said, for an individual with little to no volitional motor control who must rely on some physiological signal-based access technology, thermal infrared imaging provides many potential advantages to other more invasive approaches. In fact, individuals possessing little residual movement are best suited for a thermal infrared-based access technology. Minimal movement from the user would help to alleviate issues with loss of focus and tracking of the facial regions of interest. This would allow the access technology to operate with a very simple tracking algorithm (or no tracking at all if the individual is completely devoid of movement) which would reduce processing time. In such cases, the possibility for real-time applications becomes more realistic.

CONCLUSION

Personal autonomy in the context of chronic physical disability relates to the correspondence between desired and actual health and well-being. For individuals with severe disabilities who currently do not have physical access to communication or environmental control, the development of personal autonomy can be facilitated through physiological access technologies. Near-infrared spectroscopy and electroencephalographic measurement of visually-evoked potentials are two promising access technologies that non-invasively tap into brain function while facial infrared thermography exploits spontaneous emotional responses manifested in facial thermal temperature changes. However, each technology has its limitations, for example, low temporal resolution of NIRS, risk of ocular fatigue and seizures with SSVEP and exuberant cost of thermal cameras. At the present time, there is a paucity of clinical studies invoking these access technologies with individuals with disabilities. Nonetheless, the existing evidence from device development and psychophysical studies, do establish a solid scientific basis for further development of these nascent access technologies for the purpose of augmenting personal autonomy.

REFERENCES

Allison, B. Z., McFarland, D. J., Schalk, G., Zheng, S. D., Jackson, M. M., & Wolpaw, J. R. (2008). Towards an independent brain-computer interface using steady state visual evoked potentials. *Clinical Neurophysiology*, *119*(2), 399–408. doi:10.1016/j.clinph.2007.09.121

Ayaz, H., Izzetoglu, M., Bunce, S., Heiman-Patterson, T., & Onaral, B. (2007). Detecting cognitive activity related hemodynamic signal for brain computer interface using functional near infrared spectroscopy. *3rd International IEEE EMBS Conference on Neural Engineering* (pp. 342-345). IEEE Press.

Bach, J. R. (1993). Communication status and survival with ventilatory support. *American Journal of Physical Medicine & Rehabilitation*, *72*(6), 343–349. doi:10.1097/00002060-199312000-00002

Bauernfeind, G., Leeb, R., Wriessnegger, S. C., & Pfurtscheller, G. (2008). Development, set-up and first results for a one-channel near-infrared spectroscopy system. *Biomedical Engineering*, *53*, 36–43.

Beukelman, D. R., Yorkston, K. M., & Reichel, J. (2000). *AAC for adults with acquired neurologic disorders*. Baltimore, MD: Brookes Publishing Company.

Boas, D. A., Strangman, G., Culver, J. P., Hogel, R. D., Jasdzewsky, R. A., & Rosen, B. R. (2003). Can the cerebral metabolic rate of oxygen be estimated with near-infrared spectroscopy? *Physics in Medicine and Biology*, *48*, 2405–2418. doi:10.1088/0031-9155/48/15/311

Boecker, M., Buecheler, M. M., Schroeter, M. L., & Gauggel, S. (2007). Prefrontal brain activation during stop-signal response inhibition: An event-related functional near-infrared spectroscopy study. *Behavioural Brain Research*, *176*(2), 259–266. doi:10.1016/j.bbr.2006.10.009

Braver, T., S., Cohen, J., D., Nystrom, L., E., Jonides, J., Smith, E., E., & Noll, D.C. (1997). A parametric study of prefrontal cortex involvement in human working memory. *NeuroImage*, *5*(1), 49–62. doi:10.1006/nimg.1996.0247

Cheng, M., Gao, X., Gao, S., & Xu, D. (2002). Design and implementation of a brain-computer interface with high transfer rates. *IEEE Transactions on Bio-Medical Engineering*, *49*(10), 1181–1186. doi:10.1109/TBME.2002.803536

Coyle, S., Ward, T., Markham, C., & McDarby, G. (2004). On the suitability of near-infrared (NIR) systems for next-generation brain-computer interfaces. *Physiological Measurement*, *25*, 815–822. doi:10.1088/0967-3334/25/4/003

Coyle, S. M., Ward, T. E., & Markham, C. M. (2007). Brain–computer interface using a simplified functional near-infrared spectroscopy system. *Journal of Neural Engineering*, *4*, 219–226. doi:10.1088/1741-2560/4/3/007

Eagle, M., Baudouin, S. V., Chandler, C., Giddings, D. R., Bullock, R., & Bushby, K. (2002). Survival in Duchenne muscular dystrophy: improvements in life expectancy since 1967 and the impact of home nocturnal ventilation. *Neuromuscular Disorders*, *12*(10), 926–929. doi:10.1016/S0960-8966(02)00140-2

Ferree, T. C., Luu, P., Russell, G. S., & Tucker, D. M. (2001). Scalp electrode impedance, infection risk, and EEG data quality. *Clinical Neurophysiology*, *112*(3), 536–544. doi:10.1016/S1388-2457(00)00533-2

Fisher, R. S., Harding, G., Erba, G., Barkley, G. L., & Wilkins, A. (2005). Photic- and pattern-induced seizures: A review for the epilepsy foundation of america working group. *Epilepsia*, *46*(9), 1426–1441. doi:10.1111/j.1528-1167.2005.31405.x

Franceschini, M. A., Fantini, S., Toronov, V., Filiaci, M. E., & Gratton, E. (1999). Cerebral hemodynamics measured by near-infrared spectroscopy at rest and during motor activation. In A. Ganjbakhche (Ed.), *Proceedings of Inter-Institute Workshop on In Vivo Optical Imaging at the NIH* (pp.73-80). Washington DC: Optical Society of America

Friman, O., Lüth, T., Volosyak, I., & Gräser, A. (2007). Spelling with steady-state visual evoked potentials. *3rd International IEEE EMBS Conference on Neural Engineering:* (Vol. 54, pp. 354-357).

Gao, X., Xu, D., Cheng, M., & Gao, S. (2003). A BCI-based environmental controller for the motion-disabled. *IEEE Transactions on Neural Systems and Rehabilitation Engineering*, *11*(2), 137–140. doi:10.1109/TNSRE.2003.814449

Goldson, E. (1996). The micropremie: infants with birth weight less than 800 grams. *Infants and Young Children*, *8*(3), 1–10. doi:10.1097/00001163-199601000-00003

Gratton, G., & Fabiani, M. (2003). The event-related optical signal (EROS) in visual cortex: Replicability, consistency, localization, and resolution. *Psychophysiology*, *40*(4), 561–571. doi:10.1111/1469-8986.00058

Guo, F., Hong, B., Gao, X., & Gao, S. (2008). A brain-computer interface using motion-onset visual evoked potential. *Journal of Neural Engineering*, *5*(4), 477–485. doi:10.1088/1741-2560/5/4/011

Harding, G. F. A., & Harding, P. F. (1999). Televised material and photosensitive epilepsy. *Epilepsia*, *40*(9SUPPL. 4), 65–69. doi:10.1111/j.1528-1157.1999.tb00909.x

Hartmann, M., & Kluge, T. (2007). Phase coherent detection of steady-state evoked potentials: Theory and performance analysis. *3rd International IEEE EMBS Conference on Neural Engineering: Vol. 54* (pp. 179-183).

Hemsley, B., Balandin, S., & Togher, L. (2007). Older unpaid carers' experiences supporting adults with cerebral palsy and complex communication needs in hospital. *Journal of Developmental and Physical Disabilities*, *19*(2), 115–124. doi:10.1007/s10882-007-9040-1

Herrmann, M. J., Ehlis, A. C., & Fallgatter, A. J. (2003a). Frontal activation during a verbal-fluency task as measured by near-infrared spectroscopy. *Brain Research Bulletin*, *61*(1), 51–56. doi:10.1016/S0361-9230(03)00066-2

Herrmann, M. J., Ehlis, A. C., & Fallgatter, A. J. (2003b). Prefrontal activation through task requirements of emotional induction measured with NIRS. *Biological Psychology*, *64*(3), 255–263. doi:10.1016/S0301-0511(03)00095-4

Herrmann, M. J., Plichta, M. M., Ehlis, A. C., & Fallgatter, A. J. (2005). Optical topography during a go-NoGo task assessed with multi-channel near-infrared spectroscopy. *Behavioural Brain Research*, *160*(1), 135–140. doi:10.1016/j.bbr.2004.11.032

Herrmann, M. J., Walter, A., Ehlis, A. C., & Fallgatter, A. J. (2006). Cerebral oxygenation changes in the prefrontal cortex: Effects of age and gender. *Neurobiology of Aging*, *27*(6), 888–894. doi:10.1016/j.neurobiolaging.2005.04.013

Herrmann, M. J., Walter, A., Schreppel, T., Ehlis, A. C., Pauli, P., & Lesch, K. (2007). D4 receptor gene variation modulates activation of prefrontal cortex during working memory. *The European Journal of Neuroscience*, *26*(10), 2713–2718. doi:10.1111/j.1460-9568.2007.05921.x

Hochberg, L. R., Serruya, M. D., Friehs, G. M., Mukand, J. A., Saleh, M., & Caplan, A. H. (2006). Neuronal ensemble control of prosthetic devices by a human with tetraplegia. *Nature*, *442*, 164–171. doi:10.1038/nature04970

Holst, G. C. (Ed.). (2000). *Common sense approach to thermal imaging.* Bellingham, Washington: The International Society for Optical Engineering: JCD Publishing.

Huppert, T. J., Hoge, R. D., Diamond, S. G., Franceschini, M. A., & Boss, D. A. (2006). A comparison of BOLD, ASL, and NIRS hemodynamic responses to motor stimuli in adult humans. *NeuroImage*, *29*, 368–382. doi:10.1016/j.neuroimage.2005.08.065

Huppert, T. J., Hoge, R. D., Franceschini, M. A., & Boas, D. A. (2005). A spatial-temporal comparison of fMRI and NIRS hemodynamic responses to motor stimuli in adult humans. *Proceedings of SPIE, 5693*, 191-202. In B. Chance, R. R. Alfano, B. J. Tromberg, M. Tamura, & E. M. Sevick-Muraca (Eds.), *Proceedings of the SPIE: Vol. 5693: Optical Tomography and Spectroscopy of Tissue VI* (pp. 191-202). Bellingham, WA: SPIE.

Jasdzewsky, G., Strangman, G., Wagner, J., Kwong, K. K., Poldrack, R. A., & Boas, D. A. (2003). Differences in the hemodynamic response to event-related motor and visual paradigms as measured by near-infrared spectroscopy. *NeuroImage*, *20*, 479–488. doi:10.1016/S1053-8119(03)00311-2

Jeppesen, J., Green, A., Steffensen, B. F., & Rahbek, J. (2003). The Duchenne muscular dystrophy population in Denmark, 1977-2001: prevalence, incidence and survival in relation to the introduction of ventilator use. *Neuromuscular Disorders*, *13*(10), 804–812. doi:10.1016/S0960-8966(03)00162-7

Jia, C., Xu, H., Hong, B., Gao, X., Zhang, Z., & Gao, S. (2007). A human computer interface using SSVEP-based BCI technology (LNCS 4565, pp. 113-119).

Jobsis, F. (1977). Noninvasive, infrared monitoring of cerebral and myocardial oxygen sufficiency and circulatory parameters. *Science*, *198*(4324), 1264–1267. doi:10.1126/science.929199

Jones, B., & Plassmann, P. (2002). Digital infrared thermal imaging of human skin. *IEEE Engineering in Medicine and Biology Magazine*, *21*, 41–48. doi:10.1109/MEMB.2002.1175137

Jones, B. F. (1998). A reappraisal of the use of infrared thermal image analysis in medicine. *IEEE Transactions on Medical Imaging*, *17*(6), 1019–1027. doi:10.1109/42.746635

Kelly, S. P., Lalor, E. C., Finucane, C., McDarby, G., & Reilly, R. B. (2005). Visual spatial attention control in an independent brain-computer interface. *IEEE Transactions on Bio-Medical Engineering*, *55*(9), 1588–1596. doi:10.1109/TBME.2005.851510

Kuba, M., Kubová, Z., Kremlacek, J., & Langrova, J. (2007). Motion-onset VEPs: Characteristics, methods, and diagnostic use. *Vision Research*, *47*(2), 189–202. doi:10.1016/j.visres.2006.09.020

Kuboyama, N., Nabetani, T., Shibuya, K., Machida, K., & Ogaki, T. (2004). The effect of maximal finger tapping on cerebral activation. *Journal of Physiological Anthropology and Applied Human Science*, *23*(4), 105–110. doi:10.2114/jpa.23.105

Lalor, E. C., Kelly, S. P., Finucane, C., Burke, R., Smith, R., & Reilly, R. B. (2005). Steady-state VEP-based brain-computer interface control in an immersive 3D gaming environment. *EURASIP Journal on Applied Signal Processing*, *19*, 174–181.

Lancioni, G., O'Reilly, M. F., Singh, N. N., Sigafoos, J., Oliva, D., Baccani, S., & Groeneweg, J. (2006). Microswitch clusters promote adaptive responses and reduce finger mouthing in a boy with multiple disabilities. *Behavior Modification*, *30*(6), 892–900. doi:10.1177/0145445505283416

Lee, P., Hsieh, J., Wu, C., Shyu, K., Chen, S., & Yeh, T. (2006). The brain computer interface using flash visual evoked potential and independent component analysis. *Annals of Biomedical Engineering*, *34*(10), 1641–1654. doi:10.1007/s10439-006-9175-8

Lee, P., Hsieh, J., Wu, C., Shyu, K., & Wu, Y. (2008). Brain computer interface using flash onset and offset visual evoked potentials. *Clinical Neurophysiology*, *119*(3), 605–616. doi:10.1016/j.clinph.2007.11.013

Levine, B. (1993). Quantum-well infrared photodetectors. *Journal of Applied Physics*, *74*(8), 1–81. doi:10.1063/1.354252

Levine, J. A., Pavlidis, I., & Cooper, M. (2001). The face of fear. *Lancet*, *357*(9270), 1757–1757. doi:10.1016/S0140-6736(00)04936-9

Lotte, F., Congedo, M., Lécuyer, A., Lamarche, F., & Arnaldi, B. (2007). A review of classification algorithms for EEG-based brain-computer interfaces. *Journal of Neural Engineering*, *4*(2), 1–13. doi:10.1088/1741-2560/4/2/R01

Maggi, L., Parini, S., Piccini, L., Panfili, G., & Andreoni, G. (2006). A four command BCI system based on the SSVEP protocol. *Annual International Conference of the IEEE Engineering in Medicine and Biology Society*: *Vol. 1.* (pp. 1264-1267).

Makeig, S., Westerfield, M., Jung, T., Enghoff, S., Townsend, J., & Courchesne, E. (2002). Dynamic brain sources of visual evoked responses. *Science*, *295*(5555), 690–694. doi:10.1126/science.1066168

Mars, G. M. J., Kempen, G. I. J. M., Widdershoven, G. A. M., Janssen, P. P. M., & van Eijk, J. T. M. (2009). Conceptualizing autonomy in the context of chronic physical illness: relating philosophical theories to social scientific perspectives. *Health*, *12*(3), 333–348.

Martinez, P., Bakardjian, H., & Cichocki, C. (2007). Fully online multicommand brain-computer interface with visual neurofeedback using SSVEP paradigm. *Computational Intelligence and Neuroscience*, (94561): 13–13.

Matthews, F., & Pearlmutter, B., A., Ward, T. E., Soraghan, C. & Markham, C. (2008, January). Hemodynamics for brain-computer interfaces. *IEEE Signal Processing Magazine*, *25*(1), 87–94. doi:10.1109/MSP.2008.4408445

McKeefry, D. J. (2001). Visual evoked potentials elicited by chromatic motion onset. *Vision Research*, *41*(15), 2005–2025. doi:10.1016/S0042-6989(01)00080-3

Mehagnoul-Schipper, D. J., van der Kallen, B. F. W., Colier, W. N. J. M., van der Sluijs, M. C., van Erning, L. J. T. O., & Thijssen, H. O. M. (2002). Simultaneous measurements of cerebral oxygenation changes during brain activation by near & hyphen; infrared spectroscopy and functional magnetic resonance imaging in healthy young and elderly subjects. *Human Brain Mapping*, *16*(1), 14–23. doi:10.1002/hbm.10026

Memarian, N., Venetsanopoulos, A., & Chau, T. (2009). Infrared thermography as an access pathway for individuals with severe motor impairments. *Journal of Neuroengineering and Rehabilitation*, *6*(11), 1–8.

Merla, A., Ciuffolo, F., D'Attilio, M., Tecco, S., Festa, F., Michele, G. D., et al. (2004). Functional infrared imaging in the diagnosis of the myofascial pain. *26th Annual International Conference of the IEEE EMBS* (pp. 1188-1191). IEEE Press.

Merla, A., & Romani, G. L. (2007). Thermal signatures of emotional arousal: A functional infrared imaging study. *29th Annual International Conference of the IEEE EMBS* (pp. 247-249). IEEE Press.

Moratti, S., Clementz, B. A., Gao, Y., Ortiz, T., & Keil, A. (2007). Neural mechanisms of evoked oscillations: Stability and interaction with transient events. *Human Brain Mapping*, *28*(12), 1318–1333. doi:10.1002/hbm.20342

Morgan, S. T., Hansen, J. C., & Hillyard, S. A. (1996). Selective attention to stimulus location modulates the steady-state visual evoked potential. *Journal Proceedings of the National Academy of Sciences of the United States of America*, *93*(10), 4770–4774. doi:10.1073/pnas.93.10.4770

Muller-Putz, G. R., Eder, E., Wriessnegger, S. C., & Pfurtscheller, G. (2008). Comparison of DFT and lock-in amplifier features and search for optimal electrode positions in SSVEP-based BCI. *Journal of Neuroscience Methods*, *168*(1), 174–181. doi:10.1016/j.jneumeth.2007.09.024

Muller-Putz, G. R., Scherer, R., Branuneis, C., & Pfurtscheller, G. (2005). Steady-state visual evoked potential (SSVEP)-based communication: Impact of harmonic frequency components. *Journal of Neural Engineering*, *2*(4), 123–130. doi:10.1088/1741-2560/2/4/008

Murthy, R., Pavlidis, I., & Tsiamyrtzis, P. (2004). Touchless monitoring of breathing function. *26th Annual International Conference of the IEEE EMBS* (pp. 1196-1199). IEEE Press.

Naito, M., Michioka, Y., Ozawa, K., Ito, Y., Kiguchi, M., & Kanazawa, T. (2007). A communication means for totally locked-in ALS patients based on changes in cerebral blood volume measured with near-infrared light. *IEICE Transactions on Information and Systems. E (Norwalk, Conn.)*, *90-D*(7), 1028–1037.

Nakanishi, R., & Imai-Matsumura, K. (2008). Facial skin temperature decreases in infants with joyful expression. *Infant Behavior and Development*, *31*, 137–144. doi:10.1016/j.infbeh.2007.09.001

Nhan, B. R., & Chau, T. (2009). Infrared thermal imaging as a physiological access pathway: a study of the baseline characteristics of facial skin temperatures. *Physiological Measurement*, *30*(23-N), 35.

Nozawa, A., & Tacano, M. (2009). Correlation analysis on alpha attenuation and nasal skin temperature. *Journal of Statistical Mechanics*, *P01007*, 1–10.

Ogata, H., Mukai, T., & Yagi, T. (2007). A study on the frontal cortex in cognitive tasks using near-infrared spectroscopy. *Proceedings of the 29th Annual International Conference of the IEEE EMBS Cite Internationale, Lyon, France* (pp. 4731-4734). IEEE Press.

Pastor, M. A., Artieda, J., Arbizu, J., Valencia, M., & Masdeu, J. C. (2003). Human cerebral activation during steady-state visual-evoked responses. *The Journal of Neuroscience*, *23*(37), 11621–11627.

Patil, P. G., Carmena, J. M., Nicolelis, M. A. L., & Turner, D. A. (2004). Ensemble recordings of human subcortical neurons as a source of motor control signals for a brain-machine interface. *Neurosurgery*, *55*(1), 27–35.

Pavlidis, I., Dowdall, J., Sun, N., Puri, C., Fei, J., & Garbey, M. (2007). Interacting with human physiology. *Computer Vision and Image Understanding*, *108*(1-2), 150–170. doi:10.1016/j.cviu.2006.11.018

Pavlidis, I., & Levine, J. (2002). Thermal facial screening for deception detection. In *Proceedings of the Second Joint EMBS/BMES Conference* (pp. 1143-1144). IEEE Press.

Pfurtcheller, G., Neuper, C., Guger, C., Harkam, W., Ramoser, H., & Schlögl, A. (2000). Current trends in Graz Brain-Computer Interface (BCI) Research. *IEEE Transactions on Rehabilitation Engineering*, *8*(2), 216–219. doi:10.1109/86.847821

Pfurtscheller, G., Neuper, C., Schlögl, A., & Lugger, K. (1998). Separability of EEG signals recorded during right and left motor imagery using adaptive autoregressive parameters. *IEEE Transactions on Rehabilitation Engineering*, *6*(3), 316–325. doi:10.1109/86.712230

Pollina, D. A., Dollins, A. B., Senter, S. M., Brown, T. E., Pavlidis, I., & Levine, J. A. (2006). Facial skin surface temperature changes during a concealed information test. *Annals of Biomedical Engineering*, *34*(7), 1182–1189. doi:10.1007/s10439-006-9143-3

Quaresima, V., Ferrari, M., Torricelli, A., Spinelli, L., Pifferi, A., & Cubeddu, R. (2005). Bilateral prefrontal cortex oxygenation responses to a verbal fluency task: A multichannel time-resolved near-infrared topography study. *Journal of Biomedical Optics*, *10*(1), 1–12. doi:10.1117/1.1851512

Rabiee, P., Sloper, P., & Beresford, B. (2005). Desired outcomes for children and young people with complex health care needs, and children who do not use speech for communication. *Health & Social Care in the Community*, *13*(5), 478–487. doi:10.1111/j.1365-2524.2005.00578.x

Rumeau-Rouquette, C., Grandjean, H., Cans, C., du Mazaubrun, C., & Verrier, A. (1997). Prevalencc and timc trends of disabilities in school-age children. *International Journal of Epidemiology*, *26*(1), 137–145. doi:10.1093/ije/26.1.137

Shastri, D., Merla, A., Tsiamyrtzis, P., & Pavlidis, I. (2009). Imaging facial signs of neurophysiological responses. *IEEE Transactions on Bio-Medical Engineering, 56*(2), 477–484. doi:10.1109/TBME.2008.2003265

Sobsey, D. (1994). *Violence and abuse in the lives of people with disabilities*. Baltimore, MD: Paul H. Brookes Publishing Company.

Stanfield, C. L., & Germann, W. J. (2007). *Principles of human physiology*. San Francisco, CA: Pearson Benjamin Cummings.

Steketee, J. (1973). Spectral emissivity of the skin and pericardium. *Physics in Medicine and Biology, 18*(5), 686–694. doi:10.1088/0031-9155/18/5/307

Sutter, E.E. (1992). The brain response interface: communication through visually-induced electrical brain responses. *Journal of Microcomputer Applications, (15)*, 31–45.

Trejo, L. J., Rosipal, R., & Matthews, B. (2006). Brain-computer interfaces for 1-D and 2-D cursor control: Designs using volitional control of the EEG spectrum or steady-state visual evoked potentials. *IEEE Transactions on Neural Systems and Rehabilitation Engineering, 14*(2), 225–229. doi:10.1109/TNSRE.2006.875578

Tudehope, D. I., Burns, Y. R., Gray, P. H., Mohay, H. A., O' Callaghan, M. J., & Rogers, Y. M. (1995). Changing patterns of survival and outcome at 4 years of children who weighted 500-999 g at birth. *Journal of Paediatrics and Child Health, 31*(5), 451–456. doi:10.1111/j.1440-1754.1995.tb00856.x

Uematsu, S. (1986). Symmetry of skin temperature comparing one side of the body to the other. *Thermology, 1*, 4–7.

Wang, Y., Gao, X., Hong, B., Jia, C., & Gao, S. (2008). Brain-computer interfaces based on visual evoked potentials. *IEEE Engineering in Medicine and Biology Magazine, 27*(5), 64–71. doi:10.1109/MEMB.2008.923958

Wang, Y., Wang, R., Gao X., & Gao, S. (2005). Brain-computer interface based on the high-frequency steady-state visual evoked potential. *Processing of Neural Interface and Control,* 37-39.

Wang, Y., Wang, R., Gao, X., Hong, B., & Gao, S. (2006). A practical VEP-based brain-computer interface. *IEEE Transactions on Neural Systems and Rehabilitation Engineering, 14*(2), 234–239. doi:10.1109/TNSRE.2006.875576

Wu, Z., Lai, Y., Xia, Y., Wu, D., & Yao, D. (2008). Stimulator selection in SSVEP-based BCI. *Medical Engineering & Physics, 30*(8), 1079–1088. doi:10.1016/j.medengphy.2008.01.004

KEY TERMS AND DEFINITIONS

Access Pathway: The actual sensors or input devices by which an expression of functional intent (e.g., a movement or physiological change) is transduced into an electrical signal.

Access Technology: A technology that captures an expression of functional intent (e.g., physical movement or physiological change) from the user via sensors, and processes the ensuing electrical signal into a control signal that drives some user interface (e.g., AAC, ECU or computer). The access technology encompasses an access pathway and a signal processing block.

Augmentative and Alternative Communication (AAC): Refers to the strategies and approaches to enhance or substitute speech or writing and range from no-tech solutions such as hand gestures, to low-tech alternatives such as paper-based picture boards, all the way to high-tech devices such as electronic, multi-input tablets with synthesized voice output.

Environmental Control Unit (ECU): Typically an interface technology that accepts one or more user control signals (through an access technology) as input commands to operate electrical (e.g., lights, electric door-openers) or electronic appliances (e.g., television) in one's living environment.

SSVEP: Steady state visually-evoked potential. The measurable brain potential that naturally occurs in response to the observation of a persistent oscillating visual stimulus. The measured potential possesses a distinct spectral component at the frequency of the stimulus oscillation.

Stimulus Onset Visually-Evoked Potential: A measurable brain potential that is time-locked to the instant of change in the visual stimulus. The change may be associated with the initiation of motion or flickering, in which case the potential is respectively named the motion onset visually-evoked potential (MVEP) and flash onset visually-evoked potential (FVEP).

Chapter 3
Elderly People, Disability, Dependence and New Technologies

José C. Millán-Calenti
University of A Coruña, Spain

Ana Maseda
University of A Coruña, Spain

ABSTRACT

The potential impact of new assistive technologies to help people stay in their own homes for longer, age well and independently is a crucial challenge for future empowerment of the elderly. The main goals of this chapter are to draw attention to the characteristics of the elderly population and their situation regarding the increase in life expectancy and aging-related aspects, increasing the risk of disability and dependence. Notably, the role of information and communication technologies as supportive tools can help the elderly to improve their quality of life and independence. Services adapted to this population, e.g., tele-health, domotics or robotics, are examined in the text. We also look at the most relevant future opportunities and challenges to society towards new products and services.

INTRODUCTION

The change in health conditions, related to the increase in quality of life has generated an important social change. One of its key elements is the increase in the proportion of elderly people in the total population. These elderly people enjoy perfect perceived health in general but in many cases, they will develop diseases that that lead to disability.

Dependence is directly connected to disability and has been defined by the Council of Europe as "that situation in which people, due to a physical, psychical or intellectual autonomy loss need significant assistance or help to be able to manage themselves in their daily activities". Put simply,

DOI: 10.4018/978-1-60566-206-0.ch003

it is the need for technical or personal help in carrying out an activity.

Facing this situation, in which more and more people reach old age with the risk of presenting a lack of functional capacity and the need of a third person as a carer, it is necessary to look for new attention alternatives. The combination of aging, disease and disability places a considerable burden on the capacity of individuals to live independently. Adaptation to the environment and the provision of technical aids should facilitate mental autonomy and physical independence, given that new information and communication technologies are a key element in the present society.

This chapter focuses on new Information and Communication Technologies (ICT) as a new tool offering applications and services to society and, more specifically, to elderly people with dependence. From the tele-alarm devices to the most advanced robots, there is a wide range of technological resources that are being developed by different research groups and which have their application in the field of the elderly as the reader will find through the different sections of this chapter.

BACKGROUND

Situation of the Elderly Population

One of the clearest achievements of human development has been the increase of life expectancy that at present reaches the age of 80 in developed societies. However, it has not always been like this; back in 1900, life expectancy for Spanish people was no more than 40. A drastic change in people's life conditions and particularly in their health conditions has been necessary to reach the current situation. Advances in prevention and health promotion together with those referred to as the therapeutic diagnosis and intervention techniques have succeeded in decreasing mortality in all life stages, hence facilitating people to reach ages inconceivable one century ago.

According to the Eurostat (European Statistic Agency), the increase in life expectancy will continue, which, together with the decrease in fertility, will lead a further increase in the mean age of the population. The population above 60 who constituted 17% in 1960 has increased up to 21% in 1997 and is predicted to reach 30% in 2030.

However, this change in health conditions, related to the increase in quality of life has also generated an important social change. One of its key elements is the increase in the proportion of elderly people in the total population. These elderly people enjoy perfect perceived health in general but in many cases will develop diseases that lead to disability.

Disability and the Elderly

Disability is the external sign of health problems. It is necessary to know the affected population in order to carry out the suitable support measures and look for a more fair society where those less integrated will be the beneficiaries of more resources. Nowadays, disability is one of the biggest worries in developed society. The different levels of public administration are trying to establish the real dimension of this problem not only for the elderly, but also for people of all ages.

Knowing the prevalence of disability will allow us to know one of the well-being indicators relating to the concept of "quality of life", which is a basic element in the search for an egalitarian society where all people will have the same opportunities. In particular, when referring to young people suffering congenital problems or accident sequelae, or to elderly people needing long-term care.

Since the situation in most developed countries (Western Europe and North America) is quite similar, we will take the case of Spain as an example of this phenomenon.

In Spain, the INE (Spanish Statistic Agency), in collaboration with the IMSERSO, carried out the first Survey on Disabilities, Deficiencies and Handicaps back in 1986. This survey allowed for calculating the Life Expectancy in Health for the first time in Spain. This experience was followed in 1999 with the survey on Disabilities, Deficiencies and Health (EDDES) that collected data from 79 000 homes and 220 000 people. As well as identifying the number of people with disability, it also ascertained its severity and origin, thus identifying the risk factors and life habits that affect the general well-being of the population.

According to this survey, 3 525 222 out of 39 247 010 Spanish people declared having same kind of disability; that is, 8.98% of those interviewed. Disability proved to be associated with age and the female gender, the most common case being difficulty in leaving the house and doing the housework. We must highlight that these data show a higher percentage of disability in the rural environment than in the urban environment.

Many times, we will find the co-disability phenomenon, i.e., several concomitant disabilities, and the fact that the severity of the disability will be determined not only by the person's characteristics but also by the relationship between the individual's capacity and the environment requirements. Intervention in this case can be made on two levels: improving the individual's capacity or reducing the environment demands.

The disability can progress according to its prognosis from recoverable situations, improvable with restrictions, stable without improving perspectives or with health deterioration. Age clearly affects both the evolution and the perception of improvement.

Disabilities have their origin in deficiency; thus, for sensorial disabilities, the origin will be problems mainly in the vision and hearing organs; systemic problems will affect minor proportion. In elderly people, communication disabilities will have their origin in cerebrovascular accidents, injuries, other speaking disorders (aphasia, dysarthria, dysphonia, dysphemia) or dementias. Disabilities for mobility have their main origin in osteoarticular deficiencies, mainly mechanical and motor alterations in the head, spine and extremities. Mental disabilities are caused by dementias and other mental deficiencies such as autism, schizophrenia, phobias, psychotic problems or personality disorders.

Alternatively, deficiencies can have their origin in other areas such as: intrauterine development (congenital), problems during the labour, traffic accidents, domestic accidents, industrial or leisure accidents, common illnesses (the most frequent cause), professional accidents or aspects related with morpho-functional aging.

Dependence and the Elderly

Dependence is directly connected with disability, and has been defined by the Council of Europe as "that situation in which people, due to a physical, psychical or intellectual autonomy loss need significant assistance or help to be able to manage themselves in their daily activities". Put simply, it is the need for technical or personal help in carrying out an activity.

Dependence is a worldwide phenomenon affecting all individuals but in a different way. We must refer to it specifying the affected area and activity. Thus, for example, we would refer to a person with crutch dependence for mobility. When measuring dependence, we should not follow the scales measuring concept as not all of them include the same items and one person can be dependent without establishing such dependence in according to the scale.

Dependence has to be measured based on the activity and the scale, and it is not always in direct connection with the welfare load. We can think of a person in a coma as a low welfare load and a person suffering a dementia as a heavy welfare load, especially if the illness is associated with behavioural and psychological disorders.

We must not confuse the terms dependence and autonomy; dependence refers to the help provided by a third person and autonomy, particularly intellectual autonomy, is the abstract ability to manage their own life and self-determination.

The dependence assessment allows classification of the individuals into isogroups and establishes the degree of dependence. It also allows the evaluation of staff, caring, intervention and the carrying out of data analysis. For example, we could establish three big groups regarding users' classification: not dependent, autonomous, dependent and greatly dependent, complex or psycho geriatrics. Based on these groups, we could calculate the financing costs related to consumption of resources and/or plan the socio sanitary policies.

According to official data (Dependence White Book), there are more than 1 125 000 dependent people in Spain, and in most cases, they do not receive the correct support from the public sector. This creates an important caring deficit with the resulting loss in quality of life.

ICT Support

Facing this situation, in which more and more people reach old age with the risk of presenting a lack of functional capacity and the need of a third person as a carer, it is necessary to look for new attention alternatives. These alternatives, through the environment adaptation and the provision of technical aids should facilitate the mental autonomy and physical independence of the person, given that new information and communication technologies are a key element in the present society.

The increasing number of elderly people has the effect of creating demand for more healthcare provision and ICT, being used within both the environment of the physical and the cognitive patient. Internet is an element that should be considered in order to provide different services to the user's home such as interactive videoconferences, agendas, domotic control, establishment of biomedical parameters and much more. The aforementioned, together with the increasingly accessible hardware development will no doubt contribute to a more fair society where disability will not be a handicap that decreases the possibilities of the individual in front of others.

TECHNOLOGY AS A SUPPORTIVE TOOL

ICT play an essential role in supporting daily life in today's digital society. They are used at work, in day-to-day relationships, in dealing with public services as well as in culture, entertainment, leisure and when participating in community and political dialogue. E-inclusion policy promotes the use of ICT to overcome social exclusion, and improve economic performance, employment opportunities, quality of life, social participation and cohesion. According to the European Commission's communication, we must go "Towards an accessible information Society" and acknowledges that ICT is "crucial in today's society and economy and they can greatly improve personal autonomy and quality of life, particularly for people with disabilities or elderly".

ICT supportive tools address the issues of social inclusion and homecare of the elderly suffering from disabilities and/or dependence, a rapidly increasing population group. Those people need support of caregivers and are at risk of social exclusion, yet this problem, if not well addressed by ICT technology, would lead to a social and economical pressure to stay at home as long as possible. Care services offered by smart home solutions and/or robotic systems can significantly improve the care and the carer's interaction with their assistive system. Thus, technology presents an opportunity to improve quality of life, a means of dealing with disability and a chance to enhance independence (Bagley & Williams, 1998).

The European Initiative "Ambient Assisted Living" (AAL) emerges as the name of a new European technology and innovation funding programme focused on the aim of establishing a real connection between elderly people and technology. The programme is intended to address the needs of the aging population, to reduce innovation barriers of forthcoming promising markets, but also to lower future social security costs. AAL aims - by the use of intelligent products and the provision of remote services including care services – at extending the time older people can live in their home environment by increasing their autonomy and assisting them in carrying out their daily living activities.

Technology helps elderly to keep in touch with families and friends, ensures more safety at home, assisting and facilitating them in health care (Czaja, 1996, in Mikkonen Vayrynen, Ikonen, & Heikkala, 2002), bringing new stimuli into their lives and providing more access to information (Mikkonen et al., 2002). Other studies confirm the role of technology in increasing social interaction and pride (Kautzamann, 1990), self-esteem (Lustbader, 1997), life satisfaction (Sherer, 1996), and perceived autonomy (McConatha, McConatha, & Dermigny, 1994). Moreover, ICT give elderly people the possibility to share their experiences in social networks, perhaps with others who have the same diseases or disabilities who can provide suggestions and emotional support, but could not possibly move from their home or live alone (Charness & Schaie, 2003).

To increase the use of ICT among elderly people, their acceptance to use it is very important. The percentage of elderly people using computers is constantly increasing (Burdick & Kwon, 2004). Elderly people who want to use computers need to acquire computer skills, i.e., learning an unfamiliar mechanism (Blit-Cohen & Litwin, 2004). Most elderly people initially show anxiety about using computers (Whitcomb, 1990). Once having gained experience in using computers, they show a less negative attitude towards them (Dyck & Smither, 1996) and elderly people who are more computer savvy are more satisfied with their lives (Karavidas, Lim, & Katsikas, 2005). This satisfaction is derived from higher self-efficacy and lower computer anxiety as users learn more about computers. Implicit benefits of having computer knowledge, such as being more independent, keeping up to date (about health matters) and maintaining a social network, result in higher life satisfaction. If we focus on those topics more fitting to this population, in 2004, the SeniorNet organization conducted a survey on its members' interests when using the Internet and reported that 'searching for health information' was only seconded by 'sending emails or photos' (http://www.seniornet.org).

Apart from this use, technology gives society a new opportunity for providing care services to the population with dependence. The great demand for medical and social care of the elderly in most developed countries and the costs involved could motivate a drive for telecare applications for this target group. One barrier to this development is the perceived negative attitude among elderly persons towards the use of modern technology. This is solved when the "tele-receptive" individuals understand that due to the offered tele-services they will be able to stay at home for longer. The Spanish Centre of Sociological Research has conducted a survey to find the preferences of elderly people regarding staying in their own home or being cared for at a "residential home care centre". This survey shows that more than 70% of the people surveyed prefer to stay in their own home, avoiding nursing homes for as long as possible. If they do need help, they still prefer to stay in their own homes adapting them to their needs. The same study shows that according to the age of the person surveyed, for more than 80% of the people aged over 65, the preferred option is their own home rather than nursing homes and assisted living centres.

Because the elderly evidently want to take care of themselves as long as possible, housing has to be adapted to their changing abilities. Support is also necessary for caregivers of people with dependence, since elderly people at home have an increasing need for help from their family and professional caregivers. Familial caregivers feel powerless to help and support their care-recipients so that they carry a heavy burden. Both the person being cared for and the carer have a reduction in their quality of life and need increasing support which is where ICT may play an important role. Supportive technologies can cover the demand for knowledge, education, adequate advice and training skills in caring for disabled persons for both professionals and family carers,. For both families and professionals, training sessions are difficult to implement because of the high cost. Here, ICT (e.g. domotics and/or robotics) can be an important aid to increase the safety and autonomy of the elderly and/or their families. These new technologies will be more easily accepted by seniors if they are user-friendly and affordable. Based on this, when a technology is developed, it must follow a "universal design", also called "design for all", which is rooted in the concept of "universal accessibility". This refers to the global requirement for access to information by individuals with different abilities, requirements and preferences in a variety of contexts. Biological, cognitive, psychological, social and economic factors connected with later phases of life may form a barrier for the adoption of ICT. For example, failing eyesight, declining abilities to learn and to remember new materials, reducing contact with environments that feature new technologies, and limited financial means, may hinder ICT-adoption.

People with disabilities are dependent on, or function best with, adaptation to the environment, which enable them to function optimally and perform daily activities. However, many of these adaptations would not be necessary if universal design was applied to environments as a standard.

Tele-Health Technologies

Tele-health technologies can be employed to diagnose and monitor chronic illnesses, such as heart failure, respiratory diseases and diabetes (Burdick & Kwon, 2004). Data collected through common (blood pressure, temperature, heart rate sensors) and specialized (electrocardiograms, heart and lung sounds, blood oxygen levels) systems is transmitted to monitoring stations or directly to caregivers. As a composite of all these aspects referring to gerontology and technology, the term gerontechnology was introduced (Graafmans, Taipale, & Charness, 1997).

There are specific technologies providing various aids for the tasks and activities of daily living (taking medication, daily schedule, social contacts), interventions (cognitive stimulation, nutritional education), and automatic detection of potentially dangerous/critical situations (falls or panic attacks). The interface tailored to the patients' remaining skills and services is set up and implemented, including testing by patients, families and professionals.

Well functioning tele-medical equipment could, from the doctors' perspective, be seen as a valuable tool to facilitate remote consultations and medical treatments of patients not possible to treat by other means (Tsuchiya, 1998). Experts expect that, by 2030 a large proportion of the screening processes will be taken care of by ICT. A patient could, for instance, fill out a survey on the internet in order to get an immediate diagnosis.

It must be highlighted that health information services need to be customized to the specific needs of this very target group both in their content and in their mode of presentation. When technological facilities are offered to the elderly, it is very important to develop user-adaptive web browser interfaces to enable people, who suffer from a reduction of cognitive or functional skills, to access the internet or the systems. We must also consider developing supportive programs using advanced visualisation and interaction interfaces with highly preventive, therapeutic value that will allow elderly people to enjoy new ways of leisure and entertainment while improving cognitive, functional and social skills.

Intelligent Houses: Domotics

Recent statistics show a trend of rapid growth in the number of people with physical disabilities and aged people who need external help in their everyday movement tasks (Saito, 2000). Smart houses are considered a good alternative for the independent life of older persons and persons with disabilities. These adapted houses offer an optimistic view that the quality of life for these people can be significantly improved by means of various modern technologies, in particular, through intelligent houses (Warren & Craft, 1999). At home, several risks could result from disabilities such as cognitive deficits, e.g. lack of memory or judgement loss. The most obvious risks are fires, wounds, burns, cuts, food and medication poisoning or falls. Bad hygiene and malnutrition could also occur. Primarily, the decision of whether to maintain the elderly at home depends on the control of these risks with smart houses offering a good solution.

Smart houses differ from each other in the types and arrangements of the installed devices and can be classified into the following groups:

- smart house for people with functional disabilities;
- smart house for elderly people;
- smart house for people with vision impairment;
- smart house for hearing impaired people;
- smart house for people with cognitive impairment.

These intelligent houses include useful functionalities such as: automatic kitchen equipment; light and door controllers; indoor temperature controllers; water temperature controllers; home security devices. They can also include typical electromechanical devices for movement assistance including powered wheelchairs, specialized lifting devices (for transfer of the user between the bed and the wheelchair), and specialized standing-up devices for powered wheelchairs, bath lifts, walking and lifting aids. Another very useful functionality is the inclusion of electronic medical records for monitoring medical parameters of elderly people.

Intelligent devices, Internet-enabled appliances, motion sensors, video systems, even sensors embedded in clothing, jewellery, and furniture combined with predictive modelling and related algorithms can be used to effectively monitor the health and daily activities of older people living at their own homes 24 h a day, 365 days a year. Such solutions will have strong positive emotional impact on the patients, improving their quality of life, giving them privacy, safety and the feeling of living in an ordinary house, not in a hospital.

Rehabilitation and Supportive Robots

Apart from domotics and smart homes, we must highlight the development of robotics in the field of gerontology and geriatrics. Most of the rehabilitation robots are designed to assist disabled individuals in their everyday needs, such as eating, drinking and object replacement. Research into the field of mobile service robots designed to care for people with dependence at home is in its infancy. Here, we will detail just some of these:

The ROBOTS@HOME (http://www.robots-at-home.org) provides an open mobile platform for the widespread introduction of robots into the homes of all, also providing a multi-modal sensor for learning and mapping of the rooms and classifying the main items of furniture, stating a safe and robust navigation method that finally sets the case for using the platform in homes everywhere.

The COGNIRON robot (http://www.cogniron.org) is designed to serve humans (not primary elderly or cognitively impaired persons) as a companion in their daily life. Besides the necessary functions for sensing, moving and acting, such a robot will exhibit the cognitive capacities enabling it to focus its attention, to understand the spatial and dynamic structure of its environment and to interact with it, to exhibit a social behaviour and communicate with other agents and with humans at the appropriate level of abstraction according to context.

The commercially available US service robot CareBot (http://www.geckosystems.com) was developed with the scenario of assisting elderly people in mind.

The CMU Pittsburg NurseBot project (http://www.cs.cmu.edu/~nursebot/), focused on robotic assistance for the elderly, has produced a robotic platform to test several ideas for such a companion, including, but not limited to, intelligent reminding functions, tele-presence applications, surveillance, simple social interaction and help for physically impaired people.

The RoboCare (http://robocare.istc.cnr.it) is a multi-agent system which generates user services for human assistance.

Care-O-Bot (http://www.care-o-bot.de/english) is a mobile service robot which has the capability to interact with and assist humans in typical housekeeping tasks.

FUTURE TRENDS

Assistive technology is an area of fast growing and continuous research and study. With the increasing demands from society and especially from elderly people with disability, it must continuously increase its findings. Technological tools using ICT are becoming necessary to keep social and health costs for this population down, while at the same time, helping to favour the social inclusion of people with disability.

Health care providers are challenged to develop new models of care delivery for this unique population. These areas of research include ubiquitous computing (e.g., home monitoring systems), health care technologies (e.g., telehealth), robotics (e.g., Nursebot), and automated systems (e.g., cruise control). Finally, we consider the opportunities and challenges to the research of human factors as the field to continue addressing the questions of optimizing technology for older adult users.

Patients welcome medical monitoring as they know the new opportunities offered by ICT applied to the social and medical field. It is important to promote the independence of people by improving the consistency of services adapted to elderly and disabled people.

Based on this, more diagnosis will be carried out using video and tele-links to hospital based specialists giving patients more equitable access to care, less waiting and travelling; and clinicians more appropriate referrals, improved use of resources, better provision of information and advice about health, social care, etc. over the phone, TV, Internet at home. The provision of alarm services linked to a central call response team will be especially relevant, decreasing care costs and improving safety and protection.

In the near future, we must highlight the importance of establishing national/ international laws regulating this assistive technology addressed to elderly and disabled people, and also the establishment of standards to be applied and the corresponding ethical rules to consider.

Given the expected wide number of elderly dependent people in the future, an important task for public policy will be to limit the negative effects of non-adoption of ICT by future elderly (i.e. social exclusion) and to stimulate the positive effects (which, on an aggregate scale might provide a solution for the financial problems related to the greying of the population).

CONCLUSION

Improving the quality of life for the elderly and/or disabled people is becoming an essential task for society today. An important aspect for all people having the need to be supported in their daily-life-activities is still to be integrated into social life despite their existing disabilities.

ICT supportive technologies such as tele-health are helping to cover the increasing demands on the health care system as the population ages.

For the immediate future, we must focus our research on reaching the objective "home care before institutional care" of the elderly while disability and dependence allow it, reducing medical and social costs for in-house care.

REFERENCES

Bagley, S. P., & Williams, T. F. (1988). Technology and aging: the new frontier. *Frontiers in Aging Series*, *6*, 19–25.

Blit-Cohen, E., & Litwin, H. (2004). Elder participation in cyberspace: A qualitative analysis of Israeli retirees. *Journal of Aging Studies*, *18*, 385–398. doi:10.1016/j.jaging.2004.06.007

Burdick, D. C., & Kwon, S. (2004). *Gerotechnology: Research and Practice in Technology and Aging*. New York: Springer Publishing Company.

Charness, N., & Schaie, C. W. (2003). *Impact of Technology on Successful Aging*. New York: Springer Publishing Company.

Czaja, S. J. (1996). Interface design for older adults. In Ozok, A. F. (Ed.), *Advances in a lied ergonomics* (pp. 262–265). Istanbul, West Lafayette: USA Publishing.

Dyck, J. L., & Smither, J. A. (1996). Older Adults' Acquisition of Word Processing: The Contribution of Cognitive Abilities and Computer Anxiety. *Computers in Human Behavior*, *12*(1), 107–119. doi:10.1016/0747-5632(95)00022-4

Graafmans, J., Taipale, V., & Charness, N. (1997). *Gerontechnology: A Sustainable Investment of the Future*. Amsterdam, The Netherlands: IOS.

Karavidas, M., Lim, N. K., & Katsikas, S. L. (2005). The effects of computers on older adults. *Computers in Human Behavior*, *21*, 697–711. doi:10.1016/j.chb.2004.03.012

Kautzamann, L. N. (1990). Introducing computers to the elderly. *Physical & Occupational Therapy in Geriatrics*, *9*(1), 27–36.

Lustbader, W. (1997). On bringing older people into the computer age. *Generations (San Francisco, Calif.)*, *21*(3), 30–32.

McConatha, D., McConatha, J. T., & Dermigny, R. (1994). The use of interactive computer services to enhance the quality of life for long-term care residents. *The Gerontologist*, *34*, 553–556.

Mikkonen, M., Vayrynen, S., Ikonen, V., & Heikkala, M. O. (2002). User and Concept Studies as Tools in Developing Mobile Communication Services for the Elderly. *Personal and Ubiquitous Computing*, *6*, 113–124. doi:10.1007/s007790200010

Saito, M. (2000). Expanding welfare concept and assistive technology. *Proceedings of the IEEK Annual Fall Conference*, 156-161.

Sherer, M. (1996). The impact of using personal computers of the lives of nursing residents. *Physical & Occupational Therapy in Geriatrics*, *14*, 13–31.

Tsuchiya, H. (1998). Telemedicine using a desktop conference system (Phoenix) in Kyushu, Japan. *Telemedicine Journal*, *4*, 43–48.

Warren, S., & Craft, R. (1999). Designing smart health care technology into the home of the future. In S. M. Blanchard, E. C. Eckstein, J. M. Fouke, R. M. Nerem, & A. P. Yoganathan (Eds.), *Proceedings of The First Joint BMES/EMBS Conference: Vol. 2. Serving Humanity, Advancing Technology* (p. 677). MA, USA: IEEE Service Center.

Whitcomb, R. G. (1990). Computer Games for the Elderly. In R. E. Anderson, & C. D. Martin (Eds.), *CQL '90: Proceedings of the conference on Computers and the quality of life* (pp. 112-115). New York: ACM.

KEY TERMS AND DEFINITIONS

Dependence: A state in which persons, by reason of lack or loss of physical, psychological or intellectual autonomy, require significant assistance or help in carrying out the usual day-to-day activities.

Design for All/ Universal Design: The design of goods, services and environments to make them usable by people with different needs and abilities to the greatest extent possible.

Disability: Any restriction or lack (resulting from an impairment) of ability to perform an activity in the manner or within the range considered normal for a human being.

E-Health: Concept strongly connected to the use and development of the Internet and even more, Internet-mediated access to health care services, products, and capabilities. It includes the integration of telehealth technologies with the Internet; it reflects the development whereby the health consumer has in different ways an almost unlimited access to interactive health information and consultations via the Internet.

Gerontechnology: Interdisciplinary field of research and application involving gerontology and technology; using technology to prevent, delay, or compensate for the perceptual, cognitive, and physical declines of aging.

Tele-Health: Reflects a further broadening of the concepts of telemedicine /telecare to also include health information and activities accessible at a distance to the general public.

Tele-Presence: The experience of presence at a remote site via the use of information and communication technologies and virtual reality.

Chapter 4
Augmentative and Alternative Communication Devices:
The Voices of Adult Users

Martine Smith
Trinity College Dublin, Ireland

Janice Murray
Manchester Metropolitan University, UK

ABSTRACT

Over the last 30 years, significant advances have been made in the technology supporting augmentative and alternative communication devices. However, technology often brings with it as many problems as solutions. This chapter reports on data collected in interviews with adults who use aided communication. In these interviews, they discuss aspects of their communication world and the opportunities and barriers they face. The chapter highlights some of the diversity of individuals who use, or who choose not to use, aided communication. It also considers the complexity of factors that may critically influence communication experiences and discusses some of these factors within the framework of the International Classification of Functioning, Disability and Health (ICF).

INTRODUCTION

Over the last number of decades, technological developments have increased exponentially, impacting on all aspects of life. Within the field of disability and rehabilitation, the positive impact of these developments has been great. For individuals with communication impairments, new opportunities afforded by technological advances have been revolutionary. However, the value of technology lies not so much in its latent potential, but in its implementation as a solution to specific problems. The initial excitement about the potential of technology is now maturing to an evaluation of the impact of these developments in a rehabilitation context. Attention has shifted

DOI: 10.4018/978-1-60566-206-0.ch004

from the tools to an emphasis on the end goal of intervention and rehabilitation – successful communication. The objective in this chapter is to share the insights of adults with significant physical disabilities, who are finding their own models for integrating aided communication into their communication world. The data within the chapter are drawn from interviews with adults who use communication aids. As is clear from the interview data, these adults consider not only the benefits of aided communication, but also note why they do not always use their communication aids. Their insights into both the power and the pitfalls of aided communication remind us of the complexity of communication. They also highlight the crucial importance of support networks if communication is to work well and allow aided communicators to be fully integrated into the social world in which they live.

BACKGROUND

Many individuals with severe congenital physical impairments do not develop sufficient motor control to allow them to use speech that is sufficiently functionally intelligible to meet their communication needs. Often these difficulties are associated with an underlying diagnosis of cerebral palsy, where not only speech, but also many aspects of motor control are affected. Other impairments including sensory and cognitive difficulties may co-occur, creating a profile of multiple disabilities. If speech is not functional for most communication purposes, augmentative or alternative communication modes may be harnessed to supplement or support natural speech abilities. Some of these modes may be 'unaided', that is, draw on the physical resources of the communicator and require no additional supports or props. Examples of unaided communication modes are facial expression, manual signing, gesture and eye gaze. By contrast, aided communication refers to the use of communication supports or props that are external to the individual, including communication boards and voice output devices (Smith & Connolly, 2008). The remainder of this chapter will focus primarily on aided communication systems. The use of aided communication also implies a system of access to the aided mode. Access refers to the method by which an individual selects the specific symbol or symbol element (e.g., a letter of the alphabet). While some individuals may be able to access a target symbol directly, using perhaps a finger or an optical head pointer, others may rely on using switches to scan and select particular symbols. In general, the goal is to achieve an effective marriage of an individual's motor, perceptual, sensory, cognitive and linguistic abilities with a communication system, including a physical means of accessing that system. The physical access also incorporates issues such as seating, mounting or placement of the communication aid and mounting of any switches that may be needed. As individuals grow, develop and acquire new skills, changes may be needed to any of these components – the communication aid, the access system, the switch, the mount or the seating support. In addition, system developments such as changes in communication software or support technologies inevitably mean that models of specific communication aids change in regular cycles over a period of a short number of years.

The impact of advances in speech synthesis and computer technology in the field of Augmentative and Alternative Communication (AAC) emerged largely in the 1980s and has steadily increased its influence since that time (Beukelman & Mirenda, 1998) Individuals who were first introduced to speech output technology at that time are now adults, with up to twenty years' experience of using communication aids. Over that time span, most have experienced several changes of aid type, as well as of seating, switch technology and communication software. Often such changes are not driven by their own desire for innovation, but more by market developments, changes in their own motor skills, sometimes changes in their cognitive and linguistic skills and often by the sheer inevitability of wear and tear, leading to a need to replace existing systems with the closest possible match available. Unlike natural speakers who continue to expand and develop their linguistic skills across the lifespan but retain a core language system that is stable, aided communicators have to juggle often unwanted, yet technologically driven, demands of learning new ways of accessing, navigating and operating an expressive communication system. Each change brings with it new learning demands, often affecting not only the aided communicator, but also their circle of communication partners.

Aided Communication in a Multimodal Context

Individuals who have severe speech and physical impairments face many challenges. In developing effective communication skills that can be interpreted easily by their communication partners, all communicators rely on both aided and unaided modes of communication, using gestures, facial expression and body movements to enhance, support or replace speech as a mode of communication. One aspect of communication that is recognized in the general population as indicating competence is the ability to selectively harness different communication modes according to the specific demands of particular communication situations and communication messages. For individuals with both speech and physical impairments, all modes of communication may be compromised. Building an effective total communication system may mean harnessing typical communication modes (e.g., eyegaze and facial expression) in exceptional ways, as well as incorporating more unusual communication modes such as manual signs, picture communication symbols or synthetic speech output to fulfill functions achieved otherwise with natural speech. The configuration of specific modes within a total communication system is both dynamic and unique to each individual and often varies across different communication partners and contexts. For example, if a communication partner cannot read, an alphabet board may have to be set aside in favor of more extensive use of eye-gaze; in noisy environments, speech synthesis may be waived in favor of visually-based communication modes. Ideally, individuals develop a wide repertoire of communication modes, allowing them flexibility of choice of communication mode. Within this dynamic system, aided and unaided communication modes exist on a continuum (Beukelman & Mirenda, 1998).

Aided communication modes can be further subdivided into low-tech and high-tech devices. Low-tech options such as picture or symbol communication charts require no integrated circuitry (Wasson, Arvidson, & Lloyd, 1997) unlike high-tech modes such as computer-based speech generating devices. There are many advantages to such low-tech communication devices, including their reliability, low cost, durability and portability (Murphy, 2004; Smith & Connolly, 2008; Wasson et al., 1997). However, such systems often have a restricted vocabulary base, often limited to fewer than 200 lexical items. Communication using these forms also can rely heavily on partner co-construction of the message, with associated risks of misinterpretation or over-interpretation. Distance communication is particularly problematic using low-tech forms of communication, as there is no audio output. Over the past several decades, more sophisticated high-tech possibilities for encoding and formulating communication have emerged. These developments have been derived from technological advances in many areas including computer science and speech synthesis. Highly sophisticated communication devices are now available that offer the potential to access potentially unlimited vocabulary, to communicate across space, and to prepare messages in advance, whilst also offering opportunities for immediate and spontaneous participation in conversations.

Despite the advances in technology that have supported the development of such sophisticated systems, it remains difficult to integrate aided communication effectively into a total communication system, with unaided modes reported as dominant in much of the research literature (Clarke, McConachie, Price, & Wood, 2001; Falkman, Sandberg, & Hjelmquist, 2002; Harris, 1982; Light, Collier, & Parnes, 1985b; Murphy, Marková, Collins, & Moodie, 1996; Smith & Connolly, 2008). Some of the barriers to effective use of aided communication are further discussed later in this chapter.

The International Classification of Functioning, Disability and Health (ICF)

The International Classification of Functioning, Disability and Health (ICF; World Health Organization, (2001) provides a framework for representing disability as a shared, universal human experience, rather than a pathological state restricted to a small defined group. This paradigm shift has promoted a new emphasis away from a narrow focus on impairment at the level of the individual, to a broader view encompassing and highlighting participation in social and societal activities. Within the ICF, human functioning is conceptualized and categorized in two major parts: Functioning and Disability and Contextual Factors. Functioning and disability is further subclassified into (a) Body Structure and Function and (b) Activities and Participation. Contextual Factors also consists of two components, Environmental Factors and Personal Factors. Within this framework, disability is characterized as the outcome of complex relationships between an individual's health condition (i.e., their attributes in terms of body function and structure, and the activities and participation opportunities available to them), their personal factors (gender, age motivation, interests), and environmental factors (services and supports, personal relationships, etc.).

Over recent years, the ICF has been increasingly used as a general framework for evaluating the effectiveness of particular interventions, including interventions for individuals developing aided communication (Raghavendra, Bornman, Granlund, & Bjorck-Akesson, 2007). These developments have fostered increased attention to environmental factors, such as the social context of participation and communication functioning for people who use aided communication. Social networks, isolation (Milner & Kelly, 2009) and loneliness (Balandin, Berg, & Waller, 2006; Ballin & Balandin, 2007b) have been highlighted as core contextual considerations impacting on the communication experiences of people who use aided communication. Increasingly, studies have drawn on the experiences of adults with many years' experience using aided communication to reflect on the impact of interventions on real communication outcomes (Ballin, Balandin, Togher, & Stancliffe, 2009; Hemsley, Balandin, & Togher, 2008). Milner and Kelly (2009) challenge the meaning of 'inclusion' for many people with disabilities. Their focus group discussions with adults with disabilities highlighted the loneliness and isolation of many of the participants, and their sense of being involved in but not part of their local community. These understandings challenge us to broaden our focus in intervention and in our evaluation of the impact of interventions.

Use of Assistive Technology

As noted above, a recurrent theme in relation to many different forms of assistive technology is the question of 'under-utilization' of the technology. This is a concern that has been raised also in relation to aided communication technology (e.g., Allaire, Gressard, Blackman, & Hostler, 1991; Johnson, Inglebret, Jones, & Ray, 2006; McCall, Markova, Murphy, Moodie, & Collins, 1997). Many factors have been cited in explanation of this apparent 'under-use' of technology. For example, Murphy et al (1996) suggested four primary factors limiting the use of devices: (1) lack of training in device use, for both the adults with speech impairments and their communication partners; (2) lack of accessibility of devices, with access often requiring support from a communication partner for set-up or problem-solving; (3) vocabulary restrictions, necessarily limiting the value of using a communication device; and (4) restricted availability, with many devices available for use only in specific locations or at specific times. Some of these themes have emerged in related research. For example, Smith and Connolly (2008) interviewed eighteen adults who use aided communication and found that while most (14) had the device available to them most of the time, three participants reported that the device was kept either at home or in a particular centre, necessarily limiting its use.

Pape, Kim and Weiner (2002) reviewed a wide range of research to explore the personal factors affecting integration of AT, including communication devices. These authors suggested that the meanings assigned to aided communication devices can create barriers to maximizing their use. Personal factors that influence these meanings include: (i) tolerance for communication breakdowns; (2) a desire to belong to a peer group; and (3) a sense of conversation control. In interviews with seventeen school children who use AAC, Clark and colleagues (Clarke et al., 2001) found that while almost two-thirds of the children acknowledged that their devices were useful to them, most nonetheless felt they were uncool or boring, did not fit their self-image, and did not yield the desired benefit in terms of interaction control. Factors such as social acceptability may be particularly relevant at certain points across the lifespan, most particularly in adolescence, when peer image is particularly crucial. In the sections that follow, the views of adults with many years' experience of aided communication are explored. The insights of these adults draw from interview data collected in both Ireland and the United Kingdom (UK). Eighteen adults participated in questionnaire-based structured interviews in Ireland with the first author, while a further twenty adults were interviewed by Murray in the UK. Although the interviews followed different structures in both contexts, many similar themes and topics emerged during the course of all the interviews. These comments have been collated for the purposes of this chapter. The adults who participated ranged in age from 18 to 45, and males outnumbered females by almost 2:1.

In addition to the differences in data collection across both cohorts, there are also differences in the service structure of the UK and Ireland. Nonetheless, as was evident from the interview data, there are shared experiences of service limitations, including highly fragmented, fragile and varied services for adults with communication impairments. In both contexts, adults are frequently expected to assume responsibility for managing their own communication needs, including seeking appropriate supports, even where such supports are either extremely limited or, in some cases non-existent.

A SUM OF ITS PARTS: REFLECTIONS FROM ADULTS WHO USE ATYPICAL COMMUNICATION MODES IN CONVERSATION

Many different themes emerged in the interviews with the participating adults, and aspects of some of these findings have been reported elsewhere (Smith & Connolly, 2008). In this chapter we focus on four core themes. The first relates to what could be termed the body structure and function level of the ICF. In other words, specific impairment factors associated with the physical resources of the individuals interviewed, as well as the physical limitations of the communication devices impacted on participants' willingness and ability to use aided communication. A second theme relates more to activity limitations and participation in social contexts. Within this theme, we focus primarily on communication partner factors. The third theme discussed relates to the broader societal context and the barriers to and facilitators of effective use of aided communication. Finally, we consider some of the individual personal factors that were considered important by the participants. All the extracted comments from interviews below are presented verbatim, as communicated by the adults who participated. Comments are presented in italic font, supported occasionally with a gloss or supplementary information in brackets after the comment.

Before discussing some of the challenges faced by adults using aided communication, it is important to acknowledge the high value assigned by many of the interview participants to their aided communication systems. Many commented on the status high-tech devices provided, with comments such as 'people see me, not wheelchair'. One participant commented that this machine is 'the best thing ever', while another recalled his relief on getting his first communication aid, commenting 'I did feel thank you God! I can say what I think and I did feel person again'. Some participants also welcomed the added benefits of having access to environmental control. However, despite these positive aspects, there were also limitations associated with device use that emerged.

Theme 1: Body, Structure and Function: Health Condition Factors and Aided Communication

All of the adults interviewed acknowledged that there were factors associated with communication devices and their operation that limited the extent to which they could be used. For example, some participants could only reliably access their device from specific positions, such as seated in a chair. In addition, some commented on limitations related to their own physical health and resilience, such as when they were tired, which impacted on their stamina and endurance in using aided communication. Although Raghavendra et al (2007) list aided communication system characteristics under the heading of Activity rather than Body Function and Structure, in this chapter we include aided communication components as an extension of the body function and structure of the individual.

Device Function and Structure Considerations

Poor reliability of aided communication devices was a recurrent concern among participants, with comments such as 'frequent breakdown; keeps breaking down; broken' cited as specific reasons for not using a device (see Table 1). Other technical problems also caused difficulty. These included poor key durability ('if I use it often it gets stuck'); problems with independently operating the device (hard to turn it on) and with access ('would like to use it when lying down'). Technical restrictions were a common source of frustration, with one participant commenting 'Sorry, I can't chat at the moment we're outside. There's too much glare on my screen, I will speak to you when we get inside' (referring to the screen not being visible in bright light). Battery power and durability also caused some frustration (see Table 1). Some limitations that were mentioned related to difficulties simultaneously balancing communication, mobility and access needs. Others arose because of screen or voice output quality.

Body Function and Structure Considerations

Participants noted that their own physical abilities and skills impacted on the extent of their device use. Fatigue, ill health, poor positioning or changes in position affected their ability to access their aided communication as well as their levels of stamina for communication (see Table 2). Many people who use aided communication experience changes in their physical abilities across their lifespan, so that access that works effectively at one point may need significant revision over time.

Table 1. Limitations of devices

Poor reliability	Constant breakdown frequent breakdown keeps breaking down broken I want … a (unintelligible) device that doesn't crash or throw a hissy fit at the touch of a button (laughs) There have been so so so so many times over the last 2 years that my laptop let me down. It was away been fixed last October, and I had a holiday and I had not a communication device
Context restrictions	can't be used in sun in wet weather, hard to use I'd like to be able to speak outdoors in daylight I cannot use my device outside Rain kills it
Battery limitations	it does go dead battery every few months shopping – battery can be low (so I don't use the device) (I want) Good battery, or an additional battery, which will allow me to use the aid for a day without recharging
Lack of independent access	Ability for new plug in charger also USB devices for myself independently Hard to turn it on
Combining multiple functions/ needs	(I want) a robust desk and also wheelchair mounting system where when using the aid in my wheel-chair I can still see over the top to drive I would like to see the key guard thing I talked about changed (talking about the difficulty of ac-cessing a dynamic screen rather than a static keyboard) In powered chair – cannot be used simultaneously
Limited voice quality	In my next communication aid I want the voice of my choice, a voice that can be easily heard in a crowd, or in a big room Cinema too noisy (so can't use the device) In the pub, too noisy (so can't use the device) (need) louder volume

Often these changes are triggered only through periods of extensive difficulty with the existing access system. Some individuals recognized that their skills also limited their effectiveness in using a device. These skill limitations sit somewhat between the categories of Body Function and Structure and Activity Limitations, as specific aided communication components present specific cognitive, sensory, motor and linguistic demands. This ambiguity highlights the limits of any model of analysis where integration of skills, abilities, potential and limitations require on-going consideration. However, device features are considered here under the broad heading of Body Function and Structure.

Theme 2: Activity Limitations and Participation Factors

The introduction of an aided communication mode has implications not only for the person using it, but also for their communication and conversational partners. Many of the adults interviewed commented on the reactions of communication partners and the impact of these reactions on their own willingness and effectiveness in communicating. Smith and Connolly (2008) asked interview participants what influenced their use of aided communication the most. In response to this question, participants responded *who I am talking to* almost twice as frequently as any other parameter (what I am talking about; how you feel; where I am; what is 'in' the device).

Table 2. Limitations of body structure and function affecting device use

Fatigue or illness factors	You cannot be always working on a computer all day When tired (I don't use it) My spas (spasticity) is up (I don't use it) I sick (I don't use it)
Position changes	Out of chair (I can't use it) In bed – position (so I can't use it) Would like to use it when lying down Not when eating I am in car, bed, bathroom, swimming pool (cannot use it)
Access changes	On transport it is too bumpy for good access I cannot use a talker by just its screen because I need a key G (keyguard) and you cannot program them with 1 on
Skill limitations	Do not know how to trouble shoot problems You are able to transfer text from a PC onto a Lightwriter, but I don't know how to Would like to be better at reading I want to go to a PC based where I can use a joystick When I understand it more, I'll use it more

Partners affected device use in a number of different ways. For example, some of the adults noted that very familiar partners often did not need the communication device in order to have effective communicate interaction. When asked about times they would never use their communication device, participants suggested:

- 'Never use the device with people who are familiar/ friends and who may understand me'
- 'With family, social occasions'
- 'At home with my mother because she is used to me'.

Equally however, participants reported that they were unlikely to use their aided communication with people who were unfamiliar, given the demands of coping with aided communication interactions. Some commented on specific partner behaviors, others on the social acceptability of aided communication, when asked about times they would never use aided communication:

- 'When someone is waiting for me to finish what I am saying - it's hard enough sometimes to have a conversation'
- 'In stressful situations, when I have to hurry'
- 'If the person has difficulties like me they cannot read the chart'
- 'Staff do not know the device'
- 'People jump'
- 'People not take the time'
- 'If I am out socially, my computer is the last thing I would want'
- 'Sometimes very hard especially on the phone where they can not see what you are using'
- 'People don't give me the time to talk'
- 'I really hate people looking at me like I'm dumb'

Theme 3: Contextual Factors and Aided Communication: Environmental Factors

Barriers and facilitators outlined by the participants in the interviews can be viewed in terms of three different levels of influence. Within the communication dyad, partner factors were important in either facilitating or compromising satisfying communication interactions. Within the broader environmental context, the structural supports available to participants also affected the ease with which they could access, use and develop their skills in aided communication. Finally, at a societal level the extent of social networks available to participants both defined and reflected the extent of their inclusion in their community and hence their ability to participate effectively within that community.

At the level of the communication dyad, time emerged as a recurrent issue for participants. Aided communication is slow relative to natural speech (Kraat, 1987), even for expert device users. Having conversations with people who use aided communication is time-consuming and for many of those interviewed, partners' lack of time, or their awareness that it will take more time, made it difficult. They commented 'people don't take enough time'; 'the person has not time'; 'people stay when I am talking to them'; 'getting the person to stop work and sit down'. In this respect, time seemed to operate as both a barrier and a facilitator for participants. Time pressure acted as a significant barrier to entering into dialogue, but successfully persuading potential partners to take the time to stop and engage in conversations created opportunities for authentic conversations, mirroring the findings of Ballin and Balandin (2007) from their interviews with older people with cerebral palsy.

At a broader level, participants also recognized their own need for structural supports in order to develop and maintain the skills necessary to use aided communication effectively. In both the UK and Ireland, services for adults with physical impairments are less developed than those for children up to the age of 18. There is greater variability in service supports that can be accessed and often services are fragmented and difficult to access. For example, sixteen of the 18 adults interviewed by Smith and Connolly (2008) relied on themselves or family members for programming devices, and only nine had access to a speech and language therapist or specialist team for maintenance queries. Six participants had no one they could readily contact if a problem occurred with their communication aid. Given their experiences with reliability of devices, the lack of structural supports for trouble-shooting problems was particularly problematic. One participant had been without a communication device for twelve weeks due to delays in repair; another had been without her device the entire duration of her holiday because it was away for repair. When asked what would facilitate greater use of aided communication, one participant suggested 'having someone who knows how to set it up'. Another commented 'no (one) work with me'. These comments highlight the lack of essential structural supports that make it possible to use a communication device effectively.

Participants interviewed by Murray relied heavily on device suppliers with all 20 participants citing suppliers as an important support and only seven having access to a speech and language therapist for support. One participant commented 'I do feel most times it is discrimination because I need to fight more about life more and people think government give us anything we need and I do get angry sometimes about some groups because they do say they want us to go more in life but sometime they do stop changes themselves…'. Another commented on awareness of aided communication devices more generally and the implications for funding: 'I think the more that people know about how AAC (augmentative and alternative communication) can change somebody's life more that it may get better to get funding'.

Ballin and Balandin (2007) highlighted the risk of isolation and loneliness for older people with cerebral palsy, particularly those with communication difficulties. Although the question of loneliness was not specifically addressed in the interviews reported here, some participants commented on the lack of communication partners available to them. For example, when asked what would facilitate greater use of aided communication for them, one commented have people to listen to me, while another suggested people stay

Table 3. Personal factors: aspirations for the future

Travel	I love to go to China Start – I start airport
Occupation	I would like to get back into a paid job To be a secretary And we do forget sometimes we can work anywhere we don't need to work on communication aids because we have them ourselves Ultimately I want to be fully occupied teaching inclusive creative dance practice to people in my part of the country and developing my present work showing dances how to include people with disabilities in all aspects of dance
Personal development	I like writing stories so would like to write a book My plans for the future are firstly to write my first full length book about what dance means to me To get something from my working H-O-B-hobby

when I am talking to them and yet another felt getting Personal Assistant would support more communication opportunities.

Theme 4: Personal Factors

Raghavendra and colleagues (2007) list gender, age, habits, motivation and interest and acceptance of augmentative and alternative communication as important personal factors to consider. As noted above, the participants in these interviews ranged in age from 18 to 45 and males outnumbered females by a ratio of almost 2:1. Given the voluntary nature of participation in the interviews, it seems likely that both cohorts discussed here represent a particularly motivated and interested group of individuals who use aided communication. It is therefore not surprising that they were particularly vocal about the benefits of using aided communication. As one participant commented 'Using a talker changed my life'. Another participant echoed this view of aided technology as life-changing, offering a sense of hope and opportunity that had been missing: 'Until I was 31 I had little help with communication. I used some signs and facial expressions but only people who knew me well could understand me. It was very frustrating and isolating. After attending a special school and then a special college where about the only useful thing I learned were going to the pub...day centre for fourteen years. I was almost bored to death and had little hope for my future'. Having access to aided communication opened new possibilities for some of the participants, leading to aspirations for future travel, work and personal development, as captured in some of the comments in Table 3.

Participants also recognized the challenges implicit in developing the skills necessary to become an expert aided communicator. Several of their comments speak to the theme of personal persistence and resilience; other comments highlight the importance they assign to becoming autonomous and in control of all aspects of the aided communication system, especially programming of high-tech devices (see Table 4).

In sum, the adults interviewed here acknowledge the complexity and multidimensionality of the factors influencing their use of aided communication. Some of these factors are intrinsic to the individuals, reflecting their own physical, cognitive and linguistic abilities as well as their personal interests, motivation and experiences. Others are external, relating more to the social and service supports made available to them. These multiple influences interact in ways that are unique to each aided communicator. As noted by Ragavendra et al., (2007), the ICF offers a useful framework for evaluating these complex interrelationships, so that intervention plans can

Table 4. Personal factors identified as important to aided communication

Persistence	It's going to be hard work I would say at first you will find it very very hard but keep going People will understand you (if you keep practising using it) I would say that to keep going as it opens a world of communicate
Resilience	Never let anybody tell you that you'll never be able to do something Get more confidence, because if nervous I forget how to spell words
Autonomy and control	Get a Pathfinder and learn how to programming it yourself. I don't think it's good other people just knowing how to programming it Play around with the icons (to learn to programme it) Gives me privacy to be on my own and independent to say what I want

be developed that respect this complexity, and intervention effectiveness can be evaluated in terms of their authentic impact on health and well-being, rather than specific skill development. It is also clear that the adults interviewed here are uniquely positioned to share insights into what it means to use aided communication. It may also be abundantly clear from what appears to be on offer to them that technology enables and restricts their function and participation in ways that may not be considered by those able to communicate through natural speech or other more conventional methods. Some of their comments point to the need for technical solutions. It seems so little to ask that one should be able to enjoy the sunshine and have a conversation at the same time and yet this simple pleasure remains elusive for many of the participants here. Other changes, such as the attitudes of society to aided communication or the time pressures on communication partners probably require more complex, collaborative solutions. Finally, personal resilience, drive and persistence are always likely to feature in determining the ultimate success or outcome of intervention with aided communication. These latter factors are rarely addressed in the literature.

FUTURE TRENDS

As the ICF has been more widely applied in planning and evaluating interventions, the shift in emphasis from disability to participation and from the individual to the environment has accelerated. Despite these positive developments, many aspects of the ICF remain under-specified and difficult to apply, as demonstrated here, in relation to communication and specifically aided communication (Raghavendra et al, 2007). As noted in this chapter, the position of aided communication components within the overall framework remains ambiguous and open to discussion and future research exploration. It is hoped that within these developments, the voices of aided communicators will play a significant role. Their unique insights and experiences should inform not only future device developments but also the evaluation of intervention programs.

Among the anticipated developments, the question of reliability of high-tech communication devices is one that remains of critical importance. Many aided communicators face an intractable dilemma. Effectively integrating aided communication into their communication network implies developing a reliance on the aided component, yet their experience has demonstrated that many devices are inherently unreliable. In order to address this dilemma, reliable external supports are needed. These personal circles of support should incorporate service organizations or agencies, manufacturers and suppliers of communication devices as well as personal acquaintances and family members. Furthermore, there is a need for longer-term planning so that this circle remains available, flexible and adaptable across the lifespan. No natural speaker would expect to have to remain silent for twelve weeks for routine voice problems yet this is the reality for some aided communicators. Addressing these issues will require creative and committed collaboration across many different service perspectives.

CONCLUSION

The technological developments over the past two decades have opened up extraordinary opportunities for people with severe speech and communication difficulties and yet profoundly simple communication experiences remain elusive for many people who use aided communication. In order for the full potential of the existing developments to be realized fully, the lens we apply both to planning and evaluating interventions needs to be sufficiently broad to capture all the levels incorporated in the ICF, considering both the individual and the environment, while also remaining sufficiently narrow to ensure that the unique personal attributes of each individual are fully recognized and reflected.

ACKNOWLEDGMENT

The authors would like to acknowledge with gratitude the willingness of the interviewees to share of their time and their insights into the experience of living and using aided communication and the assistance from Isobel Connolly in collecting interview data.

REFERENCES

Allaire, J., Gressard, R., Blackman, J., & Hostler, S. (1991). Children with severe speech impairments: caregiver survey of AAC use. *Augmentative and Alternative Communication*, *7*, 248–255. doi:10.1080/07434619112331275983

Balandin, S., Berg, N., & Waller, A. (2006). Assessing the loneliness of older people with cerebral palsy. *Disability and Rehabilitation*, *28*(8), 469–479. doi:10.1080/09638280500211759

Ballin, L., & Balandin, S. (2007). An exploration of loneliness: Communication and the social networks of older people with cerebral palsy. *Journal of Intellectual & Developmental Disability*, *32*(4), 315–326. doi:10.1080/13668250701689256

Ballin, L., Balandin, S., Togher, L., & Stancliffe, R. J. (2009). Learning to use augmentative and alternative communication (AAC): is there a mentoring role for adults experienced in using AAC? *Journal of Intellectual & Developmental Disability*, *34*(1), 89–91. doi:10.1080/13668250802676038

Beukelman, D., & Mirenda, P. (1998). *Augmentative and Alternative Communication: Management of severe communication disorders in children and adults* (2nd ed.). Baltimore, MD: Paul H. Brookes Publishing.

Clarke, M., McConachie, H., Price, K., & Wood, P. (2001). Views of young people using augmentative and alternative communication systems. *International Journal of Language & Communication Disorders*, *36*(1), 107–115. doi:10.1080/13682820150217590

Falkman, K. W., Sandberg, A. D., & Hjelmquist, E. (2002). Preferred communication modes: prelinguistic and linguistic communication in non-speaking preschool children with cerebral palsy. *International Journal of Language & Communication Disorders*, *37*(1), 59–68. doi:10.1080/13682820110096661

Harris, D. (1982). Communicative interaction processes involving nonvocal physically handicapped children. *Topics in Language Disorders*, *2*, 21–37. doi:10.1097/00011363-198203000-00005

Hemsley, B., Balandin, S., & Togher, L. (2008). 'I've got something to say': interaction in a focus group of adults with cerebral palsy and complex communication needs. *Augmentative and Alternative Communication, 24*(2), 110–122. doi:10.1080/07434610701830579

Johnson, J., Inglebret, E., Jones, C., & Ray, J. (2006). Perspectives of Speech Language Pathologists regarding success versus abandonment of AAC. *Augmentative and Alternative Communication, 22*(2), 85–99. doi:10.1080/07434610500483588

Kraat, A. (1987). *Communication interaction between aided and natural speakers: An IPCAS study report* (2nd ed.). Madison, Wisconsin: University of Wisconsin-Madison, Trace Research & Development Centre.

Light, J., Collier, B., & Parnes, P. (1985b). Communicative interaction between young nonspeaking physically disabled children and their primary caregivers: Modes of communication. *Augmentative and Alternative Communication, 1*, 125–133. doi:10.1080/07434618512331273621

McCall, F., Markova, I., Murphy, J., Moodie, E., & Collins, S. (1997). Perspectives on AAC systems by the users and by their communication partners. *European Journal of Disorders of Communication, 32*, 235–256.

Milner, P., & Kelly, B. (2009). Community participation and inclusion: people with disabilities defining their place. *Disability & Society, 24*(1), 47–62. doi:10.1080/09687590802535410

Murphy, J. (2004). "I prefer contact this close": Perceptions of AAC by people with Motor Neuron Disease and their communication partners. *Augmentative and Alternative Communication, 20*(4), 259–271. doi:10.1080/07434610400005663

Murphy, J., Marková, I., Collins, S., & Moodie, E. (1996). AAC systems: obstacles to effective use. *European Journal of Disorders of Communication, 31*(31-44.).

Pape, T. L.-B., Kim, J., & Weiner, B. (2002). The shaping of individual meanings assigned to assistive technology: a review of personal factors. *Disability and Rehabilitation, 24*(1-3), 5–20. doi:10.1080/09638280110066235

Raghavendra, P., Bornman, J., Granlund, M., & Bjorck-Akesson, E. (2007). The World Health Organization's International Classification of Functioning, Disability and Health: implications for clinical and research practice in the field of augmentative and alternative communication. *Augmentative and Alternative Communication, 23*(4), 349–361. doi:10.1080/07434610701650928

Smith, M. M., & Connolly, I. (2008). Roles of aided communication: perspectives of adults who use AAC. *Disability and Rehabilitation. Assistive Technology, 3*(5), 260–273. doi:10.1080/17483100802338499

Wasson, C., Arvidson, H., & Lloyd, L. (1997). Low Technology. In Lloyd, L., Fuller, D., & Arvidson, H. (Eds.), *Augmentative and Alternative Communication: A handbook of principles and practices* (*Vol. 1*, pp. 127–136). Boston: Allyn and Bacon.

World Health Organization. (2001). *International classification of functioning, disability and health*. Geneva: World Health Organisation.

KEY TERMS AND DEFINITIONS

Access: Physical means by which an individual selects a particular symbol or element of a message.

Aided Communication: Communication in which the expression of the intended message relies in part at least, on some physical form external to the communicator, such as a communication aid, a graphic symbol, a picture, or an object.

Communication Device: Any physical object or device used to represent communication forms, ranging from simple object or picture sets to computer based technology incorporating synthetic speech output

Communication Mode: The medium or channel through which communicative intent is expressed. Typical communication modes include natural speech, facial expression and gesture. Exceptional communication modes include the use of graphic symbols or synthetic speech. Communication generally draws on multiple modes, such as vocalization, speech, gesture and symbols, and is referred to as multimodal.

ICF: The International Classification of Disability, Health and Functioning, a framework for representing disability as a shared, universal human experience, published by the World Health Organisation.

Chapter 5
Innovative Smart Sensing Solutions for the Visually Impaired

Bruno Andò
University of Catania, Italy

Salvatore Baglio
University of Catania, Italy

Salvatore La Malfa
University of Catania, Italy

Vincenzo Marletta
University of Catania, Italy

ABSTRACT

Although several aids have been developed to help people with visual impairment in the accomplishment of daily activities, indoor and outdoor navigation remains a critical task when considered both as a technological and a social issue. The development of new technological approaches (such as the use of smart multi-sensor architecture) allowing for the perception of the neighboring environment and providing the user with an optimized form and degree of information are activities focused by researchers working on the field. In the chapter some systems currently being developed at the D.I.E.E.S. in Catania are briefly discussed, highlighting the efforts dedicated to develop smart methodologies for the optimization of the information the user is provided with. In particular, the attention will be focused on the PYRUS system, which adopts a multi-sensor architecture and quite complex smart post-processing to provide the user with information useful to perform urban mobility tasks, and orientation and mobility aid based on a multi-sensor network of ultrasound transducers to localize the user in the environment and to guide him/her in a safe way through the environment.

DOI: 10.4018/978-1-60566-206-0.ch005

INTRODUCTION

Since the sixties, with the rapid growth in electronic and sensing technology, a new research area dealing with the healthcare and the development of innovative and intelligent products supporting older and impaired people has appeared, progressively earning interest from universities, research centers and industries and creating a thriving market. In the last decade the research aimed to enhance the quality of life of older and impaired people has increased at an unprecedented rate. The ferment in this area has affected not only healthcare research centers and universities (just as the large number of scientific papers shows) but industries and politics too. In confirmation of this, the European Community is financing many research activities dealing with Ambient Assisted Living (AAL) with the objective to enhance the quality of life of older people through the use of Information and Communication Technologies, ICT (The AAL Joint Program web site).

Substantial interest has always been attracted by the challenge of developing effective devices or systems able to support visually impaired people performing daily activities. Several methodologies and electronic aids have been proposed over the years, a useful classification of them can be conducted on the basis of the task performed, from specific tasks (color sensing, light sensing, temperature sensing, etc) to complex tasks (clear path indicators, orientation and mobility etc.) or on the basis of the employed approach (Committee on Vision, 1986): sensory enhancement, sensory supplementation, sensory substitution. In particular, sensory enhancement aims to partially recover the functionality of depressed receptors, while the use of devices giving supplementary information for the accomplishment of a particular task is known as sensory supplementation. As an example, magnifiers are common devices performing a vision enhancement task for low-vision disabilities, while the use of smart image processing techniques represents a valuable solution for image enhancement (Peli, Goldstein, Young, Trempe and Buzney, 1991; Peli, Lee, Trempe, and Buzney, 1994). Advanced methodologies such as Stochastic Resonance (SR) are intriguing solutions to improve the sensitivity of depressed receptors (Moss, Ward and Sannita, 2004). Sensory substitution, in general, means replacement of one sensory input (vision, hearing, touch, taste or smell) by another. Research in this area aims at providing some equivalent of vision via hearing or touch etc. or vice versa (Meijer, 1992).

Although several aids have been developed to help people with visual impairments in the accomplishment of daily activities to the purpose of developing more effective aids a deeper understanding of needs and abilities of the visually impaired must be gained. Disability is one of the most relevant causes of social marginalization and blindness is the worst disability in the world. Actually, there are about 330 million people with some form of impairment in the world; among them about 160 million people are visually impaired (The World Health Organization web site). For such people the possibility to autonomously access public sites and available information is a fundamental need. Anyway, structural and technological barriers often limit the site accessibility thus causing marginalization and precluding blind people from the possibility to share environments and available informative stimuli with other people. This limitation creates serious discouragement in visually impaired people and can dramatically compromise their possibility to gain adequate cultural stimuli and skills for suitable social inclusion. Rather than asking a visually impaired to live in already structured environments it should be desirable to create environments-for-all, including visually impaired or other people with disabilities. In this sense, the idea of enriching environments with adequate sensing solutions (e.g. networked sensors) could be a convenient way to boost site accessibility for people with disability.

In particular, indoor and outdoor navigation remains a critical task when considered both as a technological and a social issue. In fact, a critical task for blind pedestrians is often travelling from a starting place to a destination (the mobility task) on their own. Independent travel is an important goal sought by most visually impaired and blind people.

The very first aid for blind people was the long cane (1950) which allows detection of obstacles very close to the user and requires an instantaneous reaction when an obstacle is encountered. This aid can provide the visually impaired with a lot of useful information about their surroundings. Subsequently a huge number of electronic devices were developed, mostly using the transmission of an energy wave (usually ultrasonic or infrared) and the reception of echoes from objects, or CCD cameras (Committee on vision, 1986; Darling, Goodrich and Wiley, 1977; Farmer, 1978; Foulke, 1982; Loughborough, 1979; Raymond and Leibowitz, 1985; Simon, 1984; Warren, Anooshian and Bollinger, 1973). The Mowat Sensor, The Russell Pathsounder, The Binaural Sonic Aid (Sonicguide), the C-5 Laser Cane, the GuideCane and other complex navigation systems, are examples of electronic aids (Airasian, 1973; Bailey, Hall, Kekelis and Raasch, 1984; Benjamin, Ali and Schepis 1973; Blenkhorn and Evans, 1997; Borenstein and Ulrich, 1997; Bousbia-Salah, Larbi and Bedda, 2004; Garaj, Jirawimut, Ptasinski, Cecelja and Balachandran, 2003; Jirawimut, Ptasinski, Garaj, Cecelja and Balachandran, 2003; Kay, 1974; Nye, 1973; Petrie, Johnson, Strothotte, Raab, Michel, Reichert and Schalt, 1997; Pressey, 1977; Russell, 1965).

Many reasons have hindered the widespread use of electronic aids: from consumer diffidence to the unsatisfactory degree and way the information is provided to the user. Other not negligible reasons are the cost, the auditory cues (natural echoes must not be masked), training difficulties, cosmetics, scaling limitations and lack of performance measures (Brambring, 1985; Foulke, 1971). Great efforts and lots of industrial research are hence required to boost performance of electronic aids in order to provide autonomy similar to that of sighted people, especially in unfamiliar surroundings. An important point is the degree and redundancy of information that is required to develop a specific task. Efforts must be made by physicians and engineers to define the degree and redundancy of information to be provided to the end-user. Sometimes a simplified form of the original information would be very useful to the user.

Studies about visually impaired person navigation have demonstrated that the most important traveling aids for the visually impaired person are still the white cane and the guide dog. They are multifunctional, reliable and also tell others that the person is visually impaired. Therefore, instead of trying to develop devices replacing primary traveling aids, one should develop complementary systems (to be used along with the cane or the dog) which are reliable, efficient, easy-to-use and providing an optimized redundancy of information (Andò, 2006; Andò and Savalli, 2008). The most suitable form of information depends on the environmental characteristics and the abilities and skills of the end-user (Brambring, 1985; Darling et al., 1977). As an example, in the case of aids for the blind natural sounds (echoes) must not be masked by an auditory interface. The degree and form of information can seriously affect the security level provided to the user.

The assessment of aiding devices is a key point to be addressed. Direct and indirect performance measurements are adopted to assess the performance of systems developed by providing information such as the number of obstacles avoided or the stress status of a visually impaired person while performing a mobility task (Airasian, 1973; Bailey et al., 1984; Genensky et al., 1979).

The development of new technological approaches (such as the use of smart multi-sensor architecture) allowing for the perception of the neighboring environment and providing the user with an optimized form and degree of information are activities focused by researchers working on the field. Until 1990, a huge number of obstacle detection systems, based on Ultrasound Sensors, InfraRed detectors or lasers were developed (Kay, 1964 and 1966; Nye, 1973).

In the 1990s the focus was moved from obstacle detection to orientation and location tasks. Remarkable efforts have been dedicated to the development of indoor navigation systems based on digital tags, active badges, accelerometers, temperature and photodiodes to transmit some form of remote signal once the user gets into the range of the device which then delivers an audible message either as a tone or speech (Bentzen et al., 1995; Blenkhorn et al., 1997; Kawakubo, Chansavang, Tanaka, Iwasaki, Sasaki, Hirota, Hosaka and Ando, 2006). Anyway, such approaches suffer from the discontinuous information provided to the user apart from high installation costs due to a large number of signs to be placed in the environment.

Solutions based on inertial sensors to measure the distance traveled by the blind suffer from a cumulative position error and drift, which can be partially overcome by a footswitch (when the footswitch is closed the velocity and acceleration are equal to zero and this can be used to apply a correction) (Bousbia-Salah, 2004).

A recent solution is based on the use of a Wi-Fi LAN (Ji, Biaz, Pandey and Agrawal, 2006) determining user location on the basis of distance estimations performed by computing the received signal strength. This solution, which makes use of an already existing network, suffers from a huge number of noise sources which affect the system accuracy.

Navigation systems for outdoor environments mainly use GPS systems (Global Positioning Systems), GIS (Geographic Information Systems) and digital maps to locate users in the environment and provide them with automatic navigation instructions in the form of synthesized voice messages or other possible forms of coding. The kind of information the user is provided with changes greatly according to the application (incoming obstacles, hazards, services and environmental features). The most notable projects in this field are MoBIC and GPS Talk (Petrie et al. 1997). The main drawbacks of these systems are the poor accuracy of commercially available GPS systems, the loss of GPS signals, multi-path effects occurring when the GPS signal is reflected off by objects such as tall buildings before it reaches the receiver, thus introducing positioning errors, and the GIS databases which do not accommodate dynamic changes in environments. Furthermore, the use of these systems is highly demanding and the navigation instruction system is not sufficiently flexible. Differential DGPS has been used for many years to increase GPS positioning accuracy, but there is no single DGPS system that is accessible from anywhere on Earth. Other solutions adopt low-cost inertial systems to compensate for GPS imprecision and signal loss. By using inputs from accelerometers and gyroscopes, the inertial system is able to calculate the distance walked by the user and his changes in direction. Using these two pieces of information combined to map data enables the orientation aid to follow a user's path along street segments even if a GPS signal loss occurs (Jirawimut, Prakoonwit, Cecelja, Balachandran, 2003). Again, drift and cumulative position error over the user's displacement make this solution relatively inefficient. To fix drift and cumulative error issues some indoor points of interest can be geo-referenced, thus enabling a reset of the inertial system cumulative error when the orientation aid detects one of these points of interest, or a vision system can be integrated with the GPS device (Jirawimut, Ptasinski, Garaj, Cecelja, Balachandran, 2003). A relevant example is a system for remote sighted guidance of visually impaired pedestrians, which uses a remote vision facility and a GPS system allowing the user to remotely access a sighted guidance service (Garaj et al., 2003).

In order to make electronic aids comparable with traditional aids, electronic aids must produce a suitable amount of information which has to be notified to the user in a proper way without masking natural sounds (echoes): while adopting the electronic aid the user must be sufficiently free to catch the environment and must receive the proper amount of information on the basis of his/her needs, skills and abilities.

Researchers at the Dipartimento di Ingegneria Elettrica, Elettronica e dei Sistemi (DIEES) of the University of Catania are actively involved in developing new methodologies and multi-sensorial architectures to assist visually impaired people, which act as a kind of sensory supplementation (Andò, Graziani and Pitrone, 2001; Andò, 2003, 2005, 2006; Andò, Graziani, Lombardo and Pitrone, 2004; Andò and Pitrone, 2005; Andò and Ascia, 2007; Andò, Giannone and Pitrone, 2007; Andò and Savalli, 2008; Andò, Baglio, Marletta and Pitrone, 2009; Andò, Baglio, Marletta and Savalli, 2009; Andò, Baglio, La Malfa and Pitrone, 2009). The activity at the DIEES laboratory aims to develop low-cost electronic aids for the visually impaired, including devices for colour classification, light classification, stress monitoring, obstacle detection, orientation and mobility tasks (surroundings recognition, dangerous event recognition, landmark recognition, etc.). The technology adopted uses low-cost sensors, such as ultrasonic sensors, inertial sensors, IR sensors and CCD cameras, and suitable smart algorithms for signal processing usually running on dedicated micro-controllers. Based on the target to be reached, different smart processing techniques are adopted, which mainly define the degree and redundancy of information. The use of multi-sensor architectures, smart paradigms for signal processing and stand alone architectures, are key points in the strategy adopted making it possible to overcome the limitations of existing technologies. Activities aiming to measure the performance of the proposed devices (by a direct and indirect methodology) are also being carried out.

EXAMPLES OF ASSISTIVE DEVICES FOR BLIND PEOPLE

In this chapter some systems currently being developed at the D.I.E.E.S. in Catania are briefly discussed, highlighting efforts dedicated to develop smart methodologies for the optimization of the information the user is provided with. In particular, the attention will be focused on the following systems:

- **The PYRUS system:** a multi-sensor architecture which uses a smart post-processing to provide the user with information useful to perform urban mobility tasks. The proposed prototype can be easily connected to a suitable tactile user interface to provide the user with information about the status of the surroundings. A degree of ready-to-go (or alert) directly related to the possibility to perform the task in a safe way is given.
- **An orientation and mobility aid:** based on a multi-sensor network of ultrasound transducers to localize the user in the environment and to guide him/her in a safe way through the environment. This system can be useful to access public sites (e.g. museums, schools, theatres, gardens, etc.). As a first task the user must be notified with the presence of critical events (stairs presence or other dangerous events). Moreover, the user will be assisted during the exploration of restricted areas within the structure.

THE PYRUS SYSTEM

In this section, a new multisensor architecture adopting smart signal processing to help blind people performing urban mobility tasks is discussed (Andò, 2008). Essentially the system consists in a detection section including the conditioning circuitry, a microcontroller based

Figure 1. Schematization of the multisensor architecture supporting mobility tasks in urban environment

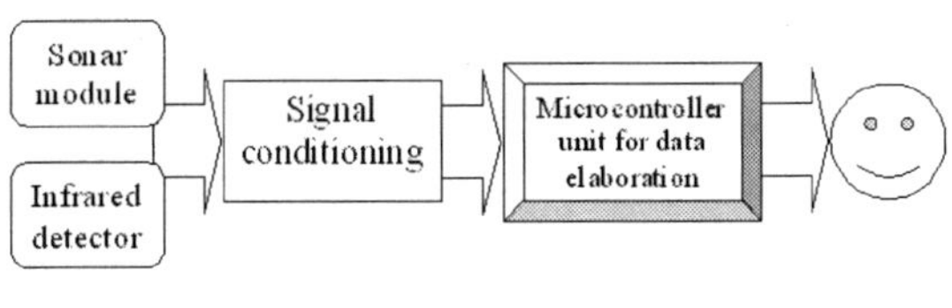

processing unit for signal elaboration and a user interface notifying the user with information useful to perform urban mobility tasks. In particular, three working modes are available for user choice to perform human detection, walking in crowded aereas and road crossing. The user can select the desired working mode and if receiving either a continuous flow of information (which can be suitable in the crowded walking mode) or on request information (which can be (desired) useful in the human detection mode and in the road crossing mode). Information produced by suitable data fusion paradigms is provided to the user in the form of attention levels which assume different meanings on the basis of the action to be performed. In the prototype developed attention levels are represented by a 5 led array included in the sensor probe.

An overview of the device architecture. The sensing probe, as schematized in Figure 1, consists of a multisensor architecture including a sonar module and an infrared motion sensor. The sonar module is used to provide information about both target distance and velocity by two successive measures. The sonar device uses a 49.4 kHz pulse train generated by internal quartz. After a brief settling time, which follows its powering up the device waits for an initial signal and then emits 16 pulses. Echo reflected by the target is detected and made available to estimate the flight time, which is directly related to the target distance. Init generation and time flight estimation are managed by the microcontroller, which cyclically performs such kind of measurements. Moreover, two consecutive distance measurements make it possible to calculate relative object velocity.

Although the sonar can work in a dual echo mode, a single echo mode was chosen for the sake of reliability. The passive infrared sensor detects changes in infrared radiation due to the presence of a person which is different in temperature from the surroundings. As this sensor detects temperature variations, it is well suited to detect the motion of people by their body temperature. With this sensor, even slight people motions will be easily detected within approximately 2 meters and hence it can be adopted for human detection. This sensor contains an amplifier circuit, a comparator circuit and output through on/off switching which enables connection directly to the microcontroller unit. Signals from the sonar module and the infrared sensor are conveyed to the microcontroller unit belonging to the family of 8-bit Intelligent Controller Units (ICU), by ST-Microelectronics. This device was chosen due to its flexible I/O configuration, smart timer management and the possibility to implement smart processing paradigms. It includes integrated on-chip peripherals that allow maximization of system reliability, and decreased system costs in order to minimize the number of external components.

A real view of the packaged prototype (the sensor module and the processing unit) is reported in Figure 2 together with the alert led array in the sensor module.

Another led matrix interface is mounted on the front side of the processing unit for the sake of debugging. During the operation of the device the developer can use the led matrix to obtain information about target distance and velocity. It is important to note that this information is not available for the blind user who is only notified about the level of alert related to the task being performed.

The developed algorithms performing sensors management and signal elaboration are discussed in the next section. Despite the possibility to

Figure 2. A real view of the developed prototype. A led matrix interface for the developer is included on the front side of the processing unit while another 5 led array user interface (in the enlargement) is available on the multisensor probe

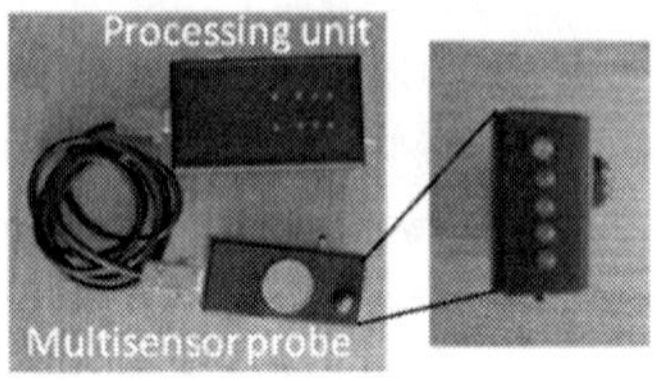

use any type of interface (acoustic, vibratory or tactile) during the preliminary development phase the led array interface was chosen for the sake of simplicity and efficiency. During the preliminary test of the prototype an expert joined the user to communicate the attention level (visible by the led interface) to him. Only 5 levels of alert are used and so optimizing the degree of information and avoiding complex training. The presence of the expert who joins the user makes these preliminary tests possible without having their execution determined by the user ability to properly associate the codified information with the actual attention level.

Algorithms for sensors management and data fusion. In order to obtain distance and velocity information from the sonar module and indications on human presence from the infrared detector a suitable algorithm was implemented in the microcontroller. The algorithm structure is schematized in Figure 3. At first, the sonar module is initialized and two timers are used to perform flight time estimation cyclically, T_f. Successively, a signal from the infrared device is acquired and all the data are sent to the data fusion paradigm.

Distance, *d*, is estimated by the following expression (Doebelin, 1985):

Figure 3. A schematization of the algorithm managing the sonar module to perform distance estimation. The data acquisition step acquires a signal from the infrared device. After two measurement cycles, obtained measurements are processed by the data fusion paradigm

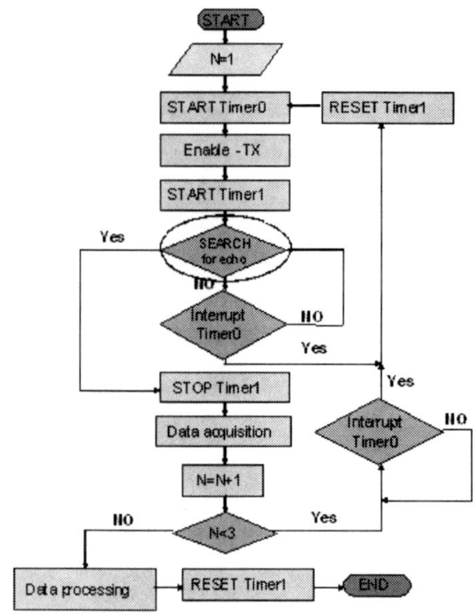

$$d = \frac{T_f v_{sound}}{2} \tag{1}$$

where v_{sound} is the sound velocity, and

$$T_f = \frac{N_{counts}}{f_{clock1}} \tag{2}$$

where N_{counts} is the number of pulses counted in the time interval between init event and echo event, and f_{clock1} is the frequency of *Timer1*.

A suitable experimental set-up was realized to characterize the sonar module as a distance sensor (Doebelin, 1985) and several measurements were performed.

Preliminary results obtained during the device characterization have shown an uncertainty of approximately 10 cm.

By using two successive distance measurements, d_1 and d_2, the object velocity is also estimated, according to the following expression:

$$v = (d_2 - d_1) f_{clock0} \tag{3}$$

where f_{clock0} is the frequency of *Timer0*.

An uncertainty of 1.75m/s for the velocity estimation has been obtained propagating the uncertainty on distance measurements (ISO, 1997).

Data coming from the sensing section (sensors and signal processing) are then used by three different algorithms to assist the blind user in human detection mode, crowded walking and road crossing. Each algorithm performs dedicated data fusion between information given by the sensors and provides a level of alert. On the basis of the alert level notified, the blind user must decide how to react to reduce risks associated to that particular action.

A test and trials approach was used to refine rule sets for the different working modes on the basis of the user feedback. In particular, this approach was precious to improve the way to codify the information provided from the sensing devices and to set thresholds for velocity and distance.

Figure 4 schematizes the rules used in the crowded walking algorithm (a) and the road crossing algorithm (b), respectively. Data coming from the infrared detector (notifying for the presence of people in the detecting regions of the device) and information on target distance and relative velocity between the user and the target are used.

Suitable distance and velocity thresholds have been fixed on the basis of real experiments performed during the device characterization. The crowded walking algorithms aim to reduce the need for user movement to avoid obstacles, except when a high speed target or an inanimate object is detected on the user path. The road crossing algorithm privileges the user safety due to the critical action to be performed and leaves the user free to cross only if long distance and low speed objects are detected.

Figure 4. Rules implementing the data fusion algorithms for (a) the crowded walking mode and (b) the road crossing mode; d_i and v_i are suitable thresholds estimated on the basis of experiments performed with the device, H is the status given by the infrared detector: H=0 states for "no human detected", H=1 states for "human detected"

Data fusion algorithms

(a) Crowded walking algorithm

	$DV \leq 0$	$0 < Dv \leq v_1$	$Dv > v_1$
$d \leq d_1$	5	4	5
$d_1 < d \leq d_2$ & H=1	5	2	4
$d_1 < d \leq d_2$ & H=0	5	5	5
$d > d_2$	3	1	3

As an example, levels of alert can be interpreted as follows: 1=free to go, 2=move slowly, 3=reduce speed, 4=stop, 5= move to avoid collision.

(b) Road crossing algorithm

	$Dv \leq v_2$	$Dv > v_2$
H=1	5	5
$d < d_3$ & H=0	3	4
$d > d_3$ & H=0	1	3

As an example, levels of alert can be interpreted as follows: 1=free to go, 3=sign and go, 4=stop, 5=people detected, try again.

In the case of human presence (which can occur in case of people waiting to cross) a new acquisition is requested. Examples on how the user can interpret alert levels are given at the bottom of figure 4.

Preliminary results and conclusions. Preliminary results obtained during a large number of performance tests demonstrate good reliability of the developed architecture.

After the device characterization several tests have been carried out in an outdoor environment to assess the device performances, especially during walking and road crossing tasks. Direct measurements evaluating indexes strictly related to the task to be accomplished by the device (such as people and obstacle avoidance, decision to cross the road) have been performed. These measurements include also expert judgments, self-reports on the quality of performance, estimates of personal satisfaction.

Experiments were conducted both by experts and blind people in a supervised mode. In particular, an expert joined the blind involved in device testing to communicate the attention level provided by the device (and visible by the led array) to him.

Although the prototype was tested in a supervised mode, a simple 5 dot tactile interface can be used to provide the information to the blind user.

This kind of interface will not require a stressful training and allows for fast decision and reaction. During this experiment, the efficiency of the strategy adopted in terms of the quality and the degree of information provided to the blind user is (would be) estimated. Actually the supervisor communicates the level of alert given by the device to the user and the latter must only decide the action to be performed at that level of alert. To avoid hazards in performing tests in an unstructured environment, these tests were performed in a safe area.

Work in progress will focus on the optimization of the data fusion algorithm which could exploit the facility of the microcontroller adopted to implement a Fuzzy data-fusion paradigm instead of a set of crisp rules. Moreover, other options could be included, for example allowing the user to choose the degree and the redundancy of the information provided by the device.

The device, when marketed, would be a really inexpensive mobility help, which uses low cost sensors and the power of a microcontroller based architecture for smart signal processing.

AN ORIENTATION AND MOBILITY AID

Independent indoor and outdoor travelling remains an important goal sought by most visually impaired and blind people. Complying with these needs, in the latter years researchers of DIEES have proposed contributions to support visually impaired exploring an unfamiliar structured environment (Andò et al. 2008, 2009a, 2009b). The proposed solutions exploit multisensory systems (ultrasound sensors, RF-ID and inertial sensors) and smart signal processing techniques to provide people with visual impairments with an optimized degree of information about the presence of services and hazards. The use of systems which are easily reconfigurable and continuously interacting with the users would terrifically improve their perception of the environment, their context awareness, their autonomy and self-esteem.

In this section a navigation system based on a multi-sensor network of ultrasound transducers to localize the user in the environment and to guide him/her in a safe way through the environment is described. This system can be useful to access public sites (e.g. museums, theatres, gardens, etc.) aiming to notify the presences of services and hazards and assisting the user in the exploration of restricted areas within the structure. It must be specified here that the developed system must coexist with other forms of mobility aids (e.g. tactile paths, white canes).

Two real scenarios can be considered: the users are free to move in the environment or the users are supposed to follow a well defined path (e.g. tactile path). In the first case the system will assist the users during their travelling providing them with information about hazards or incoming obstacles/services. In the second scenario the system can be used to manage missing paths or emergencies.

An overview of the proposed strategy. The proposed system performs a continuous monitoring of the user position inside the environment thus providing him/her with information on the presence of services and managing emergency events, e.g. fires or any other user needs. In the present form, the system is not supposed to drive the user through the environment itself; a new version including a routing algorithm is already under development. Moreover, the system proposed here has been designed to provide some information about the presence of static obstacles (intrinsically belonging to the environment) leaving the detection of dynamic obstacles (i.e. moving objects, people, or any other object which does not belong to the environment itself) for the visually impaired user himself. Future releases will also cope with dynamic obstacles.

Essentially the multi-sensor orientation system consists of a CAN-BUS network of ultrasound sensor nodes, a user module implementing the communication with the sensor nodes and a software tools implementing setting, monitoring and assisting tasks.

A schematic representation of the system is given in Figure 5 for two different scenarios: an indoor environment (a) and a structured outdoor environment (b), respectively. The implemented methodology exploits a trilateration approach to localize the user in the environment and a smart algorithm to perceive events to be notified to the user. In particular the localization of the user is performed by detecting his/her distance from a number of fixed "sensing nodes" distributed in the environment. The user is equipped with a device housing the sensing and the communication systems. Data gained from the sensor network are then passed to suitable tools running on a PC station (server). The tools developed here make communication with the sensor network, the environment setting (environment maps including services and obstacles), the monitoring of the users position and the user assistance during travelling possible. In particular, a Warning&Services Algorithm (W&SA) provides the user with information on upcoming services or hazards on the basis of available data about the environment (maps, obstacles, services, etc.). The user is notified with short audio messages provided through a Bluetooth headphone.

Figure 5. A schematization of the localization system for two different scenarios: (a) an indoor environment and (b) a structured outdoor environment

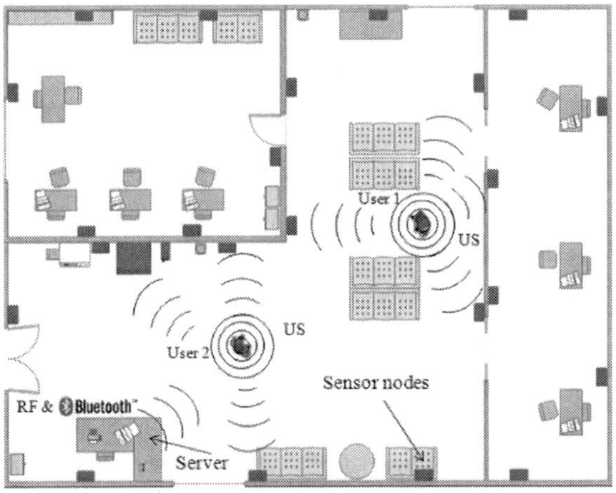

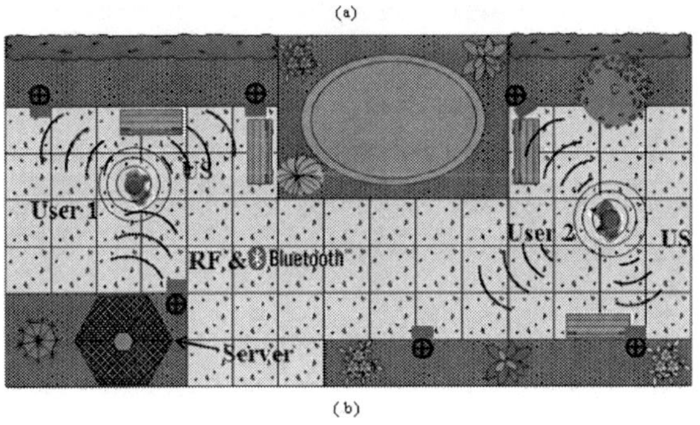

Actually, the system caters for fixing the degree of assistance to be provided to the users on the basis of their needs, ability and skills: (e.g. only services notification, or both services and obstacles notification, distance of notification, etc.) and is oriented to provide visually impaired people exploring an unfamiliar environment with context awareness.

System peculiarities are the continuous monitoring of the user position, the system re-configurability and an adaptive degree of assistance to the user needs, which could fix some drawbacks of traditional systems.

Hardware and Software tools. Figures 6 and 7 give a schematization of the hardware and software tools implementing the orientation system and its functionalities, respectively. As already mentioned the system adopts the widely used CAN-BUS network to connect sensors nodes. The choice to use this type of bus is due to its features (easy to set-up, low response time, decentralized control and monitoring, affordable, reliability, robustness,

Figure 6. (© [2009] IEEE) Schematization of the Hardware tools implementing the orientation system

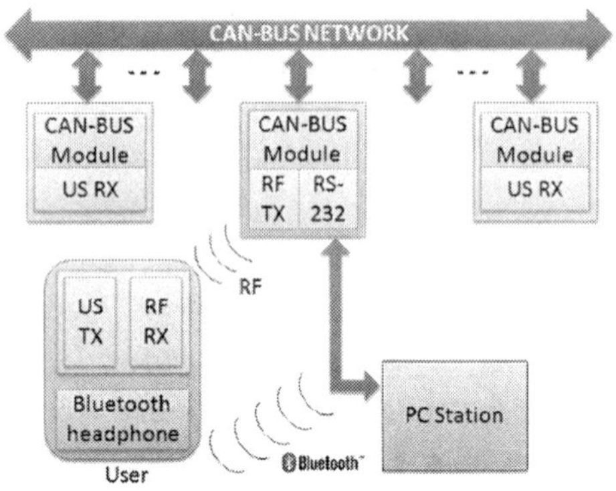

upgradeability etc.) which make it suitable for the aimed tasks.

Essentially each sensor node consists of two modules: an ultrasound (US) receiver module (including a microcontroller) working at a frequency of 40±3 kHz and a CAN-BUS module implementing the communication protocol. The network is connected to a dedicated PC station by a Server Node implementing the RS-232 protocol allowing the communication between the network and the PC station and for the synchronization of the measuring ultrasound system by an RF transmitter module. Moreover, to compensate possible variations of temperature influencing the US module operation, a NTC resistor has been included.

The visually impaired user is equipped with a battery operated module using an RF receiver to receive the synchronization signal from the server module, a microcontroller and an ultrasound transmitter with a working frequency of 40±3 kHz. The audio feedback was implemented through a Bluetooth headphone.

The procedure which makes it possible to determine user localization can be summarized by the following steps:

1. *Synchronization and system start-up.* To correctly estimate the user distance from the

Figure 7. (© [2009] IEEE) Schematization of the software tools implementing the system functionalities

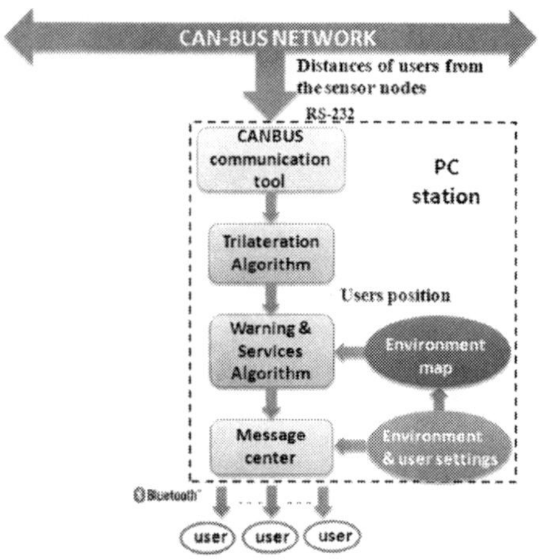

sensor nodes, the US transmitter and receivers (sensor nodes) must be synchronized. To such aim the server node sends a synchronization signal to the user module (via RF) and to the sensor nodes (via CAN-BUS).
2. *Time-of-flight estimation.* When a sensor node receives the ultrasound echo the on board microcontroller computes the time-of-flight and then estimates the distance from the user. The estimated distance value is then transferred to the server node (via CAN-BUS).
3. *Data collection and user localization.* The server node collects data coming from all nodes and transfers the whole data set to the PC station. A suitable software tool localizes the position of the user in the environment by a trilateration algorithm.
4. *User assistance.* The estimated user position is compared with obstacles and services position and eventually an audio message is sent via the Bluetooth headphone to notify such event to the user.

Two main LabView® based software tools running on the PC have been implemented. The first tool (the CAN-BUS communication tool in Figure 7) manages the communication between the PC station and the CAN-BUS network through the server node. This tool collects distances from the server node and organizes data in a matrix where each row represents the distances of one user from the sensor nodes.

The second tool enables to set the environment characteristics and the user settings. Moreover, it provides for the calculation (via the trilateration algorithm) and monitoring of the user position, detecting upcoming events via the W&SA algorithm and supplying the information to the user via a Bluetooth audio feedback.

Figure 8a shows the interface used to define the maps of the environment, the number of sensors nodes and their position, the position and the type of services and obstacles (both represented as rectangles). The interface makes it also possible to define the degree of assistance to be provided to the user via the audio feedback (e.g. services and/or obstacles).

A second interface (the monitoring interface) permits continuous monitoring of the user position. Figure 8b shows an example of a very simple map of the monitored environment (including services and obstacles defined through the environment setting interface) in which a single user (the circle) is moving and a number of obstacles and services have been defined. Small squares represent the sensor nodes. Some other information (useful during the test phase) such as the estimated distance between the users and the sensor nodes, the position of the users, the type of service and the audio message delivered are also evincible.

As stated before, in order to estimate the user position a trilateration algorithm (TA) (Borenstein, Everett and Feng, 1996) working with the data matrix coming from the communication tool has been implemented. A preliminary characterization of the orientation system, performed by meshing a typical environment in cells and collecting about 200 measurements in each point of the grid, revealed an uncertainty around 0.5 cm in the estimation of the user position. The estimated user position is then passed to the W&SA which evaluates hazards, services and obstacles close to the user and determines the appropriate audio message to be delivered, taking into account the users preferences. The results show reliable performances of the developed localization system in terms of both repeatability and uncertainty making the system suitable for the proposed task.

Figure 8. (© [2009] IEEE) The user interface for the environment and user performances setting (a) and the monitoring interface showing an environment where a user (the circle) is moving (b)

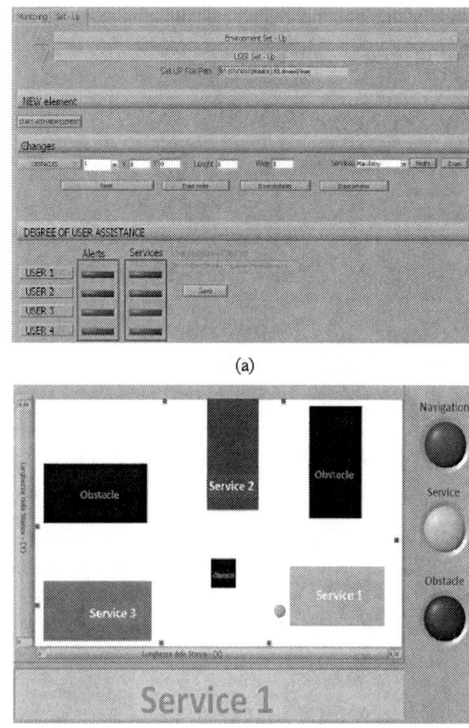

(b)

Summarizing, the proposed multi-sensor system appears to be suitable to operate as an orientation support for visually impaired and be used concurrently with the traditional systems. The main advantages of the system are the continuous monitoring of users' position inside the environment, the optimized redundancy of information for the notification of services or hazards to the user, the hardware and software re-configurability of the system thus allowing an easy adaptability to new environments and the configurable level of assistance to be provided to the user on the basis of his/her needs, ability and skills.

REFERENCES

Airasian, P. W. (1973). Evaluation of the binaural sensory aid. *AFB Research Bulletin*, *26*, 51–71.

Andò, B. (2003). Electronic sensory systems for the visually impaired. *IEEE Mag. Instrum. Meas.*, *6*(2), 62–67. doi:10.1109/MIM.2003.1200287

Andò, B. (2005). An environmental sensor providing home light classification to blind people. *IEEE IMTC*, *2*, 1438–1442.

Andò, B. (2006). Sensors that provide security for people with depressed receptors. *IEEE Mag. Instrum. Meas.*, *9*(2), 58–63.

Andò, B. (2008). A Smart Multisensor Approach to Assist Blind People in Specific Urban Navigation Tasks. *IEEE Transactions on Neural Systems and Rehabilitation Engineering*, *16*(6). doi:10.1109/TNSRE.2008.2003374

Andò, B., & Ascia, A. (2007). Navigation Aids for the Visually Impaired: From Artificial Codification to Natural Sensing. *IEEE Mag. Instrum. Meas.*, *10*(3), 44–51. doi:10.1109/MIM.2007.4284258

Andò, B., Baglio, S., La Malfa, S., Marletta, V., & Savalli, N. (2009). A Distributed Sensor Network Approach for Orientation Tasks. In *Proceedings of the IEEE IMTC 2009.*

Andò, B., Baglio, S., La Malfa, S., & Pitrone, N. (2009). A remote monitoring system to improve educational activities of visually impaired students. In *Proceedings of the XIX IMEKO World Congress.*

Andò, B., Baglio, S., Marletta, V., & Pitrone, N. (2009). A Mixed Inertial & RF-ID Orientation Tool For The Visually Impaired. In *Proceedings of the IEEE SSD 2009.*

Andò, B., Giannone, P., & Pitrone, N. (2007). A multi-sensor architecture to assist visually impaired people performing educational activities. *IEEE SSD*, *2007*, 1–4.

Ando, B., Graziani, S., Lombardo, C. O., & Pitrone, N. (2004). Development of a smart clear path indicator. *IEEE IMTC*, *1*, 492–497.

Andò, B., & Pitrone, N. (2005). A new vision supplementation strategy to perform step detection. *SSD*, *4*, 1–5.

Andò, B., & Savalli, N. (2008). CANBUS Networked Sensors Use in Orientation Tools for the Visually Impaired Wired versus Wireless Technology. *IEEE Instrumentation & Measurement Magazine*, *11*(1), 49–52. doi:10.1109/IMM.2008.4449015

Bailey, I. L., Hall, A. T., Kekelis, L. S., Raasch, T. W., Goodrich, G. D., & Morrissette, D. (1984). Telescope use by low vision patients: A survey. *American Journal of Optometry and Physiological Optics*, *61*(10), 79.

Benjamin, J. M., Ali, N. A., & Schepis, A. F. (1973). A Laser Cane for the Blind. *Proceedings of the San Diego Biomedical Symposium*, *12*, 53–57.

Bentzen, B. L., & Mitchell, P. A. (1995). Audible Signage as a Wayfinding Aid – Verbal Landmark versus Talking Signs. *Journal of Visual Impairment & Blindness*, *89*(6), 494–505.

Blenkhorn, P., & Evans, D. G. (1997). A system for enabling blind people to identify landmarks: the sound buoy. *IEEE Transactions on Rehabilitation Engineering*, *5*, 276–278. doi:10.1109/86.623019

Borenstein, J., Everett, H. R., & Feng, L. (1996). *Where am I? Sensors and methods for mobile robot positioning*. The University of Michigan.

Borenstein, J., & Ulrich, I. (1997). The GuideCane - A Computerized Travel Aid for the Active Guidance of Blind Pedestrians. *IEEE International Conference on Robotics and Automation* (pp. 1283-1288). Albuquerque, NM, April.

Bousbia-Salah, M., Larbi, A., & Bedda, M. (2004). An interface card for measuring distance travelled by blind pedestrians. *AVT, 38*, 68–74.

Brambring, M. (1985). Perceptual and Cognitive Processes of Blind Pedestrians. *Presentation to Symposium on Spatial Cognition*, University of Louisville.

Committee on Vision. (1986). *Electronic Travel Aids: New Directions for Research.* Washington, D.C.: National Academy Press.

Darling, N. C., Goodrich, G. L., & Wiley, J. K. (1977). A follow-up study of electronic travel aid users. *Bulletin of Prosthetics Research, 10*(27), 82–91.

Doebelin, E. O. (1985). *Measurement Systems* (3rd ed.). McGraw-Hill Book Company.

Farmer, L. W. (1978). Mobility devices. *Bulletin of Prosthetics Research*, (Fall): 47–118.

Foulke, E. (1971). The perceptual basis for mobility. *Amer. Found. for the Blind Research Bulletin, 23*, 1–8.

Foulke, E. (1982). A Reading Braille. In Schiff, W., & Foulke, E. (Eds.), *Tactile Perception: A Source Book.* New York: Cambridge University Press.

Garaj, V., Jirawimut, R., Ptasinski, P., Cecelja, F., & Balachandran, W. (2003). A system for remote sighted guidance of visually impaired pedestrians. *British Journal of Visual Impairment, 21*(2), 55–63. doi:10.1177/026461960302100204

Genensky, S. M., Berry, S. H., Bikson, T. H., & Bikson, T. K. (1979). *Visual Environmental Adaptation Problems of the Partially Sighted: Final Report.* Santa Monica, Calif.: Center for the Partially Sighted.

ISO(1997). Guide to the expression of Uncertainty in Measurement.

Ji, Y., Biaz, S., Pandey, S., & Agrawal, P. (2006). Dynamic Indoor Localization Using Wireless Ethernet: The ARIADNE System. In T. Braun et al. (Eds.) *Wired/Wireless Internet Communications* (LNCS 3970, pp. 299-310).

Jirawimut, R., Prakoonwit, S. Cecelja, F. Balachandran. W. (2003). Visual Odometer for Pedestrian Navigation. *IEEE Trans. On Instrumentation and Measurements, 52*(4).

Jirawimut, R., Ptasinski, P., Garaj, V., Cecelja, F., & Balachandran, W. (2003). A Method for Dead Reckoning Parameter Correction in Pedestrian Navigation System. *IEEE Transactions on Instrumentation and Measurement, 52*(1), 209–215. doi:10.1109/TIM.2002.807986

Kawakubo, S., Chansavang, A., Tanaka, S., Iwasaki, T., Sasaki, K., Hirota, T., et al. (2006). Wireless network system for indoor human positioning. *1st International Symposium on Wireless Pervasive Computing.*

Kay, L. (1964). *An ultrasonic sensing probe as a mobility aid for the blind. Ultrasonics.* April/June.

Kay, L. (1966). Ultrasonic spectacles for the blind. *The Journal of the Acoustical Society of America, 40*(6), 1564. doi:10.1121/1.1910269

Kay, L. (1974). A Sonar Aid to Enhance Spatial Perception of the Blind: Engineering Design and Evaluation. *Radio and Electronic Engineer, 44*(11), 605–627. doi:10.1049/ree.1974.0148

Loughborough, W. (1979). Talking lights. *Journal of Visual Impairment and Blindness.*

Meijer, P. B. L. (1992). An Experimental System for Auditory Image Representations. *IEEE Transactions on Bio-Medical Engineering, 39*(2), 112–121. Retrieved from http://www.seeingwithsound.com. doi:10.1109/10.121642

Moss, F., Ward, L., & Sannita, W. G. (2004). Stochastic resonance and sensory information processing: a tutorial and review of application. *Clinical Neurophysiology*, *115*, 267–281. doi:10.1016/j.clinph.2003.09.014

Nye, P. W. (1973). *A Preliminary Evaluation of the Bionic Instruments-Veterans Administration C-5 Laser Cane. National Research Council.* Washington, D.C.: National Academy of Sciences.

Peli, E., Goldstein, R. B., Young, G. M., Trempe, C. L., & Buzney, S. M. (1991). Image enhancement for the visually impaired: simulations and experimental results. *Investigative Ophthalmology & Visual Science*, *32*, 2337–2350.

Peli, E., Lee, E., Trempe, C. L., & Buzney, S. (1994). Image enhancement for the visually impaired: the effects of enhancement on face recognition. *Journal of the Optical Society of America. A, Optics, Image Science, and Vision*, *11*, 1929–1939. doi:10.1364/JOSAA.11.001929

Petrie, H., Johnson, V., Strothotte, T., Raab, A., Michel, R., Reichert, L., & Schalt, A. (1997). Mobic: An aid to increase the independent mobility of blind travellers. *British Journal of Visual Impairment*, *15*(2), 63–66. doi:10.1177/026461969701500205

Pressey, N. (1977). Mowat sensor. *Focus (San Francisco, Calif.)*, *11-3*, 35–39.

Raymond, J., & Leibowitz, H. W. (1985). Viewing distance and the sustained detection of high spatial frequency gratings. *Vision Research*, *25*, 1655–1659. doi:10.1016/0042-6989(85)90137-3

Russell, L. (1965). Travel path sounder. In *Proceedings of Rotterdam Mobility Research Conference*. New York: American Foundation for the Blind.

Simon, E. P. (1984). A report on electronic travel aid users: Three to five years later. *Journal of Visual Impairment & Blindness*, *78*, 478–480.

The Ambient Assisted Living (AAL) Joint Programme. (n.d.). Retrieved from http://www.aal-europe.eu

The World Health Organization. (2009). Retrieved from http://www.who.int

Warren, D. H., Anooshian, L. J., & Bollinger, J. B. (1973). Early vs. late blindness: The role of early vision in spatial behavior. *American Foundation for the Blind Research Bulletin*, *26*, 151–170.

KEY TERMS AND DEFINITIONS

AAL: the Ambient Assisted Living is a program implemented by funding authorities of 20 European Member States having the objective to enhance the quality of life of older people.

Adaptive Assistance: the level of assistance provided to the user by taking his/her needs, ability and skills into account.

Data Fusion: techniques that combine data from multiple sources in order to achieve inferences.

ETA: an Electronic Travel Aid is a form of assistive technology having the purpose of enhancing mobility for the blind pedestrian.

Orientation and Mobility Tasks: tasks to be accomplished in daily life, in indoor and outdoor environments.

Sensors Network: a network consisting of spatially distributed autonomous devices using sensors to cooperatively monitor physical or environmental conditions.

Sensory Supplementation: the use of devices giving supplementary information for the accomplishment of a particular task.

Smart Signal Processing: signal processing adopting a high level algorithm.

Section 2
Rehabilitation Engineering

Chapter 6
An Advanced Concept of Altered Auditory Feedback as a Prosthesis-Therapy for Stuttering Founded on a Non-Speech Etiologic Paradigm

Manuel Prado-Velasco
University of Seville, Spain

Carlos Fernández-Peruchena
University of Seville, Spain

ABSTRACT

Persistent Developmental Stuttering affects 1-2% of the world adult population. Its etiology is still unknown, although modern neuroimaging techniques have shown a new and exciting perspective of earlier ideas and hypotheses. However, it is now clear that a new approach to understand the true nature of the disorder is needed. We present a new etiological model of persistent developmental stuttering based on a deep analysis of earlier models and on the stuttering phenomenology, described in basic, clinical, and even ethnographic sources. One of the more stimulating conclusions has been the suggestion that stuttering is a non-speech based disorder, in opposition to the accepted belief. The implications of this model have guided the design of a new adaptive AAF device for prosthetic and therapeutic functions. It is supported by a wearable multimodal intelligent system, which evolves from a preliminary proposal presented in (Prado & Roa, 2007).

DOI: 10.4018/978-1-60566-206-0.ch006

INTRODUCTION

Persistent Developmental Stuttering (PDS) is a disorder that affects 1 – 2% of world adult population. It is disorder recognized from the first civilizations and recurrently cited by Greek and other classic authors. Unfortunately, the complexity and associated strange behaviors guided the research on the etiology through strange and superficial roads since the starting of orthodox medicine. References to several of these hypotheses can help to understand this asseveration.

Hippocrates hypothesized that body humors were perturbed in these subjects, and thus prescribed the delivery of sticking blistering substances to the tongue (4th century BC). That causal model could be justified in that period, but it is more difficult to understand the prescription of surgical resections of tongue's chunks with the aim of avoiding the hypothetical spasms that cause the speech blocks, at half of 19th century, in Germany, England and France. That is, a century after the explosion of advances in the mechanistic vision of life that led the definition of physiology (Bobrick, 1996).

Modern treatments and causal explicative models acquired a more scientific methodology at 20th century. Current causal models defend an integrative conception of stuttering. The origin of this perspective is usually assigned to the demands and capacities model of Starkweather (C. W. Starkweather, 1987). That model is based on the diagnosogenic theory of Johnson (Johnson, 1942), and it considers some type of innate inability of child to respond to external demands. Therefore, this model combines environmental (external) factors with biological (internal) factors. The tendency to join different types of factors has continued up to now, justifying the definition of developmental stuttering as a consequence of bio-psycho-social elements (Rodríguez Carrillo, 2002). In our opinion this definition does not throw light in its etiology either helps to design therapies or prosthetic systems.

In agreement with the integrative causal models of PDS, current therapies combine logopedic (direct) treatments with psychological (indirect) ones. Studies show a high rate of relapse in adults (nearly 100%) (Craig, 1998; Hayhow, Cray, & Enderby, 2002). The scenario is even more complex for children because the difficulty to set apart the spontaneous recovery (Rogere J. Ingham & Bothe, 2001). However, there is a lack of significant and longitudinal studies.

The consequences of the failure of biomedicine for understanding and treating PDS include the deficit of speech language professionals (SLPs) specialized in PDS, and the proliferation of a high number of stuttering therapies, which are frequently selected as a function of the subjective preferences of professionals (Limongi, et al., 2005). There is also a serious and relevant reaction among PDS subjects featured by the negation of the PDS as a disorder (Loriente Zamora, 2006).

Stuttering is a disability with a very variable gradation and strong social and personal consequences. This disorder impedes that PDS subjects can communicate ideas in the manner they wish. An important characteristic of PDS is the emergence of blocking qualia at the same time that words appear to the consciousness. This leads to an exhausting fight for avoiding or overcoming these words, producing anxiety and fear. The true problem of PDS subjects is not the dysfluency perceived by the listener, but the collateral reactions and suffering that corrupt the communication and damage the person life.

PDS subjects try to hide the disorder because the exclusion and ignorance of societies regarding this disability. Governmental actions for assisting this population are just emerging, like the "Spanish Cabinet Council Agreement on October 21 of 2005 to remove the stuttering as an exclusion cause in the calls for accessing to public administration". However, there is still a lack of legal norms that build a proper framework for this disability.

It is well established that people who stutter improves their fluency when singing or talking in unison. This fact was attributed to the influence of speech signals on the speaker (Ward, 2006). AAF devices are an artificial approach to simulate such exogenous speech signals, according some researchers. Among AAF techniques, the most popular ones are Delayed Auditory Feedback (DAF), Frequency Altered Feedback (FAF) and Masked Auditory Feedback (MAF).

The application of altered auditory feedback to improve speech communication has been ongoing for decades, although the mean in which such devices inhibit stuttering remains undetermined (Kehoe, 2008). Initial stuttering treatments began in the late twenties, and they were focused on accepting stuttering, reducing stutterers' speech-related fears and anxieties, and helping stutterers to communicate better despite stuttering. AAF prosthetic devices improve the fluency of persons who stutter, changing how stutterers hear their voices (singing, choral speaking, masking, delayed or frequency altered feedback) (Reitzes & Snyder, 2006; Ryan, 2005).

It has been reported the enhancement of speech naturalness with AAF devices (without a reduced speech rate) (R.J. Ingham, Moglia, Frank, Ingham, & Cordes, 1997; Kalinowski, Guntupalli, Stuart, & Saltuklaroglu, 2004).

Early altered auditory feedback devices were large and thus confined to the laboratory or therapy room, but advances in electronics have permitted increasingly the development of wearable devices, including self-contained ear-level AAF devices.

This work presents our recent advances in the development of an assistive and therapeutic system based on embedded computing for treating the stuttering. This system is supported by a novel causal model about PDS. The model is mathematically implemented and linked to the subject by means of a technology that allows validating and refining the underlying hypotheses. A first and brief description about the system was presented in (Prado & Roa, 2007).

The study has two major goals. Firstly, a description of a causal model of persistent developmental stuttering able to explain the phenomenology of the disorder, considering the last findings on image neuronal patterns (Watkins, Smith, Davis, & Howell, 2008), as well as the more recent neuronal approaches to this problem (Alm, 2005; Dodge, 2009; Watkins, et al., 2008), together with a review of relevant causal models from 16th century.

Our studies point to the stuttering as a disorder produced by an operant conditioning of the inhibition reactive system, mediated by the amygdala, which is able to induce an involuntary block of complex motor supervised sequential tasks. This hypothesis shares some concepts with several causal models that are reviewed, but it claims singular differences with all of them. These differences simplify the explanatory framework that is necessary to understand the stuttering phenomenology. Moreover, it extends the concept of persistent stuttering to other supervised sequential tasks, like writing, sign language communication, or playing an instrument, in agreement with some few observational studies (Snyder, 2006).

Secondly, starting from this model, a wearable embedded computing system, founded on an adaptive altered auditory feedback (A-AAF), has been conceived. This chapter presents a description of the system, emphasizing new advances with respect to an earlier proposal (Prado & Roa, 2007), and the project stages.

FOUNDATION OF A NON-SPEECH ETIOLOGY

According to the International Classification of Diseases, 9th revision, Clinical Modification (ICD-9-CM) from the World Health Organization (WHO) the stuttering *is a disturbance in the normal fluency and time patterning of speech that is inappropriate for the individual's age. This disturbance is characterized by frequent repetitions or prolongations of sounds or syllables. Various other types of speech dysfluencies may also be involved including interjections, broken words, audible or silent blocking, circumlocutions, words produced with an excess of physical tension, and monosyllabic whole word repetitions. Stuttering may occur as a developmental condition in childhood or as an acquired disorder which may be associated with BRAIN INFARCTIONS and other BRAIN DISEASES. (From DSM-IV, 1994).* We address only the persistent developmental stuttering, whose phenomenology is well-known, it starts during the childhood and it develops during the evolution of the subject. This is the most usual type of stuttering.

Certainly, the above definition from WHO is unfortunate, since it is limited to the description of a perturbed pattern as it is perceived by an external listener and it neglects the internal perception of the stutterer. Another serious deficiency is to mix simplistically PDS with other types of stuttering disorders, like those acquired after an accident. Indeed, and in agreement with (Büchel & Sommer, 2004), the term stuttering refers to the symptom, despite it is frequently used to refer to both the disorder and symptom. PDS is an idiopathic stuttering with a well-known evolution since the childhood, whereas neurogenic or acquired stuttering is directly related to a brain damage, as for example stroke or head trauma. Phenomenology of PDS is also different from acquired stuttering, although a better analysis exceeds the scope of this chapter. It can be reviewed in (Büchel & Sommer, 2004; Craig, 2000; Loriente Zamora, 2006).

A Review of Current Causal Models

We have selected a model's taxonomy based on the nature of the causal mechanism underlying the disorder. The models are not developed with detail because this task has been successfully performed in other works (Andrews, et al., 1983; Büchel & Sommer, 2004; Craig, 2000; Hahn, 1956; Loriente Zamora, 2006) and it exceeds our objectives. We focus the review on the evolution of the models' foundations from scientific revolution in 16th century until now, with the goal of extracting clues that help us to understand better them and the phenomenology that they try to embrace. Hypotheses have fallen on three major types: *organic*, *psychological* and *linguistic - semiotic*.

The Figure 1 shows a conceptual tree with the most relevant explicative models of stuttering starting in the 16th century and organized according to the nature of their causal mechanisms (etiology). Directed edges reflect secondary influences between models or groups of models. The edge's color is equal to the color of the starting block, and indicates the type of influence that is carried. For example, the Starkweather's model is a logopedics-based model, but it uses concepts from the Wendell Johnson's model and the group of linguistic models, as shown. Three markers have been used along the tree to point those models or group of models that put emphasis in the *fear emotion*, those which have reached a *singular relevance*, and finally, those characterized by some *key concepts* according to our causal model (following Section).

The ***linguistic – semiotic*** type claims that persistent development stuttering is caused by a deficit in linguistic abilities of subjects. This hypothesis was based on a significant increment of stuttering in conceptual words with respect to function words and on the worse scores of stuttering children in grammatical and listening tasks according to several authors (Bloodstein, 1981; Santacreu & Fernandez-Zúñiga, 1991). This research hypothesis started in 30's (Bluemel, 1931) and it is already active, as proved a recent article that seems to support the hypothesis (Bloodstein, 2006).

The EXPLAN theory is a very recent model based on the assumption that language (PLAN) and motor (EX) processes constitute the basis of speech control (Peter Howell, 2002). Stuttering emerges when an element in the speech sequence is delayed due to the difficulty of linguistic system to generate it, thus the speech-motor system cannot continue the process. Howell explains classical

Figure 1. Conceptual tree with the most relevant causal models and hypotheses concerning PDS from 16th century

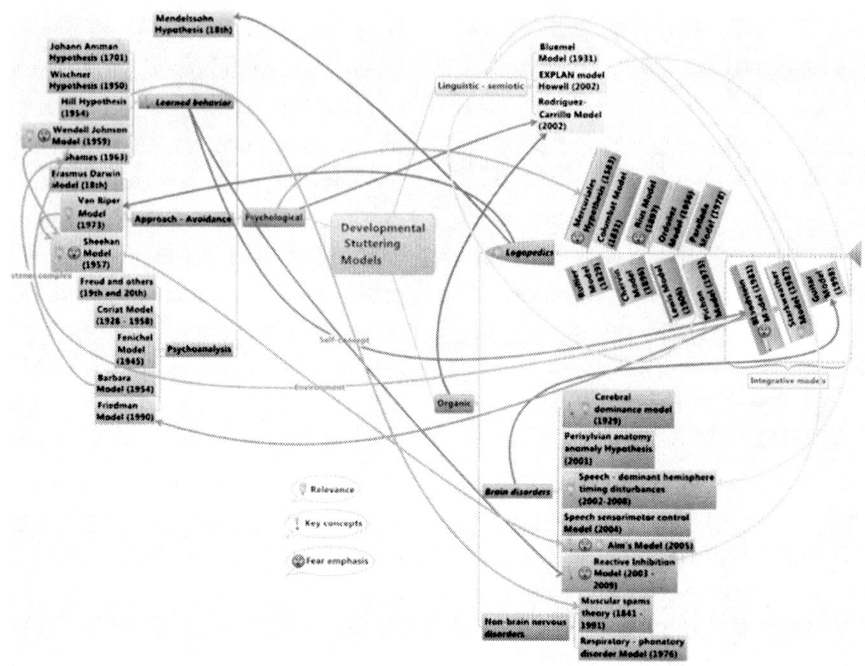

PDS speech features assuming this assumption. The importance of this model is due to its relationship with current organic hypotheses based on neuroimaging. Another interesting aspect of EXPLAN is the attempt to provide explanation of the PDS subject behavior to AAF. According to the independence between planning and execution in EXPLAN, the improvement of fluency produced by AAF is not associated to the feedback monitoring loop, but to the reduction in the speech rate associated with a change in rate control. A secondary mechanism proposed by Howell is the increase of the sensitivity to alerts (alerts due to fluency failures) of the timekeeper, due to the addition of load imposed by AAF, which compels the timekeeper to remove the excess of alerts that induce its saturation in a PDS subject (Peter Howell, 2002).

The demands and capacities model of Starkweather considers the delay to acquire linguistic capacities a major cause that promotes the developmental stuttering, starting a strong tendency to integrate external (environmental) with internal (innate or biological) factors (C. W. Starkweather, 1987). It is considered the origin of current integrative conception of stuttering. More details of this model are exposed in the organic models (see Figure 1).

There are important doubts regarding the linguistic nature of the disorder. A recent study based on a qualitative exploration examining verbal-descriptive data from structured interviews on 23 male children who stutter against 23 fluent male peers, indicated that stuttering children have a bad conception regarding their own communicative abilities, appointing to a low self-esteem in this area (Bajaj, Hodson, & Westby, 2005). This result suggests that stuttering itself could cause the more frequent grammatical errors in these children as a consequence of their low self-esteem in linguistic area. Other authors claim that stutterers and fluent people have the same linguistic capacities, in opposition to previous results (Rodríguez Carrillo, 2002).

In 80's decade this model evolves to suggest that stuttering is a semiotic disturb. This concept extends the communication disability to the whole communicative task, including vocal and kinesic elements (Rodríguez Carrillo, 2002). Vocal elements include linguistic and paralinguistic issues. Paralinguistic alterations include distortion in rhythm, pauses, and intonation. Kinesics complements paralinguistic behaviors, and embraces respiration and gestural movements. It is a matter of fact that vocal and kinesics is altered in stutterers, supporting the semiotic hypothesis and the current holistic vision of the disorder. However, this model fails to explain what causes that semiotic disorder. The model from Rodríguez Carrillo claims a holistic biopsicosocial perspective, connecting the three types of hypotheses as shown in Figure 1.

The models based on ***psychological hypotheses*** define an important line of research in 20th century. However they started in 16th century with the hypothesis of Mercurialis (1530 – 1606), which assumes the fear as one of the two causes of stuttering (Charles Van Riper, 1973). The other cause was the brain hyperactivity. Accordingly, he mixes two different types of therapeutic approaches: organic and behavioral. It has been linked to organics hypotheses in Figure 1 according to the weight given to these ones. He suggested not treating children under 7 years and to use the Avicena's method (deep breath) instead of previous surgical aggressive methods (Bobrick, 1996).

Three major groups of hypotheses have been developed within the psychological foundation: *learned behavior*, *approach-avoidance conflict*, and *psychoanalysis*. The *learned behavior* concept was first mentioned in 1701 by the Swiss physician Johann Amman (Bobrick, 1996). The *approach-avoidance conflict* emerged in the 18th century from Erasmus Darwin, father of the Charles Darwin's uncle and severe stutterer (Bobrick, 1996). It is interesting to remark that the advances in the comprehension of life by scientific mechanistic and chemical approaches in the 18th century concurred with the explosion of psychologist explanation of stuttering. Other psychological-type hypothesis of that century that has been preserved in the popular wisdom was proposed by Moses Mendelssohn, which assumed that stuttering is caused by the *collision of too many ideas concurrently in the mind* (Bobrick, 1996). This concept underlies several speech therapies pertaining to the logopedics, as shown in Figure 1.

The third group of hypotheses, *psychoanalysis*, emerged mainly at the end of the 19th century, pushed by the abortion of surgical treatments associated with several organic proposals. The most of them pointed to strange hypotheses without any kind of solid basis: repression of sexual emotions, fixation of oral and anal stages, conflict between superego and ego, etc. Freud assumed that stuttering, tics, and asthma share a similar neurosis of organ fixation (García Mila, 1987).

The *learned behavior* group of models takes one of the most influential expressions with the diagnosogenic theory (Johnson, 1959). Wendell Johnson suggests that stuttering is caused by the intention of the child to avoid infantile dysfluencies that are normal during the development (Johnson, 1942). The reasons for this behavior could be, for example, a non-proper reaction of parents to these ones. The model claims that the disorder appears after the diagnostic by parents or others. The diagnosogenic theory is one of the most cited and studied psychologist models of stuttering. A key aspect of this theory, according to Johnson and subsequent researchers, are the environmental responses to spontaneous dysfluencies which could disappear without treatment (Rogere J. Ingham & Bothe, 2001; Salgado, 2005; Yairi & Ambrose, 1999). Therapies based on this model seek removing the fear and the strategies to avoid stuttering.

It is accepted that the diagnosogenic theory of Johnson is the starting of the modern conception of stuttering as a learned behavior. However, many speech therapists have misunderstood the true basis of the diagnosogenic theory. What Johnson's theory stated is not that labeling stuttering to a speaker that repeat sounds and syllables causes developmental stuttering, but chronic stutterers were taught (even by themselves) to become frightened or ashamed when they stuttered, inducing attempts to avoid stuttering and this way inducing a feedback that reinforces the stuttering. Key words in this feedback are the anticipatory, apprehensive and hypertonic avoidance reactions of the subjects (Gateley, 2003). As a consequence, the diagnosogenic theory is not opposed to the successful outcomes of the Lidcombe program of early stuttering intervention (M. Jones, et al., 2005). This program was performed in New Zeland with 47 randomized selected participants with 3 – 6 years old (once discarded 7 participants that did not complete the trial), and showed a difference in the mean proportion of syllables stuttered nine months after the beginning of 2.3% (95% confidence interval 0.8 to 3.9) between treatment and control arms. Therapy was based on verbal contingencies provided by parents to children for periods of free speech and stuttering, by conversational exchanges in the child's natural environment. A key aspect of the program is that indications of parents to children did not transmit any type of reject to them. However, the outcomes are very limited by size, time, and even methods to measure the improvement of fluency.

Diagnosogenic theory uses operant conditioning as a causal mechanism for stuttering (Gateley, 2003). Others authors have presented similar conditioning, supported by different environmental responses. This is the case of (Shames & Sherrick, 1963) who proposed the imposition of wishes and demands as the operant mechanism for conditioning (Demostenes complex), connecting this type of models to the Psychoanalytic model of Barbara (Barbara, 1954). The latter is described below.

The classic conditioning has also been claimed as a causal model for stuttering: traumatic stress associated to speech during the childhood could induce an altered fluency (Bloodstein, 1981). Experimental studies associating electric shocks with a signal of speech starting support this hypothesis (Hill, 1954). Some authors associated the stuttering associated with classic conditioning with muscular spasms in vocal cords (Schwartz, 1977), connecting to the group of organic hypotheses.

As it could be expected, other subsequent authors in 70's tried to integrate classic and operant conditioning giving a new paradigm or causal model. Other models derived from the concept of learned behavior, classic and operant, emerged in 20th century. It is interesting to mention the model of Wischner, which considers that the avoidance behavior of stutterer is due to the intention of eluding the original consequences of the initial dysfluencies, as guilt or shame, consolidating the avoidance behavior and even de avoided consequences (Wischner, 1950, 1952).

Van Riper has been one of the most cited researchers in stuttering. He developed a therapy that is currently applied by speech therapists and discussed among many authors (Charles Van Riper, 1949, 1973, 1982). Van Riper considers that origin of stuttering is a muscle disorder that induces delays or interruptions associated with the bad regulation of speech movements, although the persistence of the disorder and thus the developmental stuttering in adults was associated with the fight or avoidance. Therefore, he pointed to learned behavior as the main causal mechanism. This one fills the gap between the childhood stuttering and the persistent developmental stuttering. The kernel of the therapy based on this model is to learn stuttering without fight and avoidance. This therapy may be considered the pathfinder in the *stuttering modification approaches*.

The approach-avoidance conflict started by Erasmus Darwin in 18th was developed by Sheehan, which wrote: "*Stuttering is a result of approach-avoidance conflict, of opposed urges to speak and to hold back from speaking. The "holding back" may be due either to learned avoidances or to unconscious motives; the approach-avoidance formulation fits both"* (Reed, Tomkins, & Alexander, 1958; Sheehan & Voas, 1957). Sheehan based on earlier models of Miller (1951) and Donald and Miller (1951), who had formulated the nature of conflicts, especially those related to the concurrent approach and avoidance tendencies. He also took into account the theories of Johnson (Johnson, 1942) and Van Riper (Charles Van Riper, 1949), among others, who stressed the implication of non-avoidance and fear (mainly Johnson) in the disorder. He also signals to other researchers that discussed the stuttering in terms of performing two mutually opposed tasks simultaneously: talk and not to stutter. He tried to answer to two essential questions in the stutterer's behavior: what makes him stop and what makes him to continue. These lead to the two central hypotheses of the Sheehan model of stuttering (Reed, et al., 1958):

- *The conflict hypothesis.* The position of stutterer is just the equilibrium point of those opposed drivers, approach (talk) and avoidance (non to stutter).
- *The fear-reduction hypothesis.* Occurrence of stuttering reduces the fear that drives the avoidance, so that during the block it is possible release the blocked word.

This issues lead to therapies that reduce fear, since this is the origin of conflict according to Sheehan. Combined therapies with indirect (psychological) and direct (logopedic) treatments have been used with this objective.

Psychoanalytic theories are characterized by a crowd of frameworks, many of them separated and opposed. Following the selection of (Loriente Zamora, 2006) we distinguish three main models. According to the Coriat model, stuttering is a psycho-neurosis due to persistence of oral, sadistic, and anal elements (Wingate, 1988). A more detailed description of this "theory", supported by many published articles during 1928 – 1958, exceeds the scope of this work. Fenichel disagrees with Coriat considering that the "key conflict" is not an oral fixation but anal (Fenichel, 1945; Charles Van Riper, 1973). In opposition to those works, the model of Barbara (Barbara, 1954) focuses to the speech blocks and assumes more diverse conflicts that can be addressed by classical psychoanalytical sessions. The Demosthenes complex was his more known share to this field, justifying the stuttering as a mechanism by which the subject seeks more special attention.

We consider finally in the psychoanalytic group a variant of Bloodstein logopedics-based model focused to the psychological field, which was proposed by Friedman. She asseverates that PDS is a cognitive state induced by a lack of self-confidence of the person who stutter (S. Friedman, 1990).

Models based on *organic hypotheses* are classified in this work on two types: brain (encephalon) disorders and non-brain nervous disorders. However, in many cases organic causal models point to a diffuse flaw (nervous etiology, bad regulation of sound emission…) that originates the childhood stuttering that develops as adult persistent developmental stuttering if it does not disappear spontaneously. These models have been grouped in a set of logopedics-based models. They are not certainly complete causal models, but there are a high number of models and associated-therapies that have been developed in this way due to the lack of knowledge regarding the disorder.

Logopedic conceptions point to nervous system, breath affections, and even linguistic disabilities as the major and original causes that impede a fluent speech. Treatments are oriented to improve the speech abilities by training, better control of articulatory and emission techniques, and reduction of stress due to the increase of self-confidence.

The hypothesis of brain hyperactivity of Mercurialis (1530 – 1606) can be considered the first organic hypothesis from our review from the 16th century. This author was earlier presented, although he has classified in logopedics hypotheses (Figure 1) according to the prescription of using breathing techniques to improve fluency.

Antoine Rullier proposed in 1829 a model based on the Mendelssohn hypothesis, focused to the inability of phonation muscles to reach the necessary temporal resolution. Notwithstanding, one of the first precursors of classic logopedics was Columbat (1831), who prescribed breath exercises and rhythm speech by a basic metronome (Le Huche, 2000). The method was completed in a second stage with syllabication, which was one of the most used logopedics techniques in 20th century. A subsequent logopedics technique was presented in (Chervin, 1896), who pointed to four key signs to diagnostic PDS: childhood beginning, breath disruptions, intermittence, and total disappear when singing. The method of Chervin was widely adopted in Spain in the late 19th. The work of (Rius, 1897) continued with Chervin concepts but added the fear feeling as a particular feature of stutters that should be mitigated.

Logopedics approaches in 20th, such as that proposed in (George Andrew Lewis, 1906) share similar concepts with the abovementioned, with slight variants. For example, the basis of Lewis's model is the nervous weakness of the stutterer. Therefore, he combined breathing and syllabication with relaxation. Two classic authors should be mentioned because of their influence in Spain. A basic book for physicians and speech therapists in 20th century was (Ordoñez, 1956). He emphasizes that stuttering is a nervous disorder that must be corrected by syllabic reading. A more recent Spanish author considered that the nervous disorder was characterized by an acute interior stress that induces spasms and speech haste (Parellada, 1978). He promoted a variant of logopedics methods with emphasis on keeping fill the lungs and disguising the voice (Parellada, 1978). A common concept of logopedics methods is the projection of guilty to the stutterer if the therapy is unsuccessful, that is "therapies fail due to the lack of effort of subjects" (Loriente Zamora, 2006).

Despite the aforementioned problems and inconsistencies with regard to the linguistic disability in stutterers, this causal hypothesis has been used also as support to logopedics (Pichon & Borel-Maisonny, 1973). These authors assume that linguistic disability impedes that sentences are timely built, which induces disturbances in the respiratory rhythm, and other paralinguistic deficiencies, in agreement with logopedics-based speech therapy.

The demands and capacities model (C. W. Starkweather, 1987) combines the influence of the environmental responses of the diagnosogenic model, in terms of speech demands, with the speech abilities (motor, linguistic, cognitive) available to satisfy them. It considers that stuttering appears when demands exceed the abilities. This model starts the tendency to integrate external (environmental) factors with internal (biological) ones, and justifies the current integrated and holistic treatments (Salgado, 2005). Other more recent models delimitate better the type of biological limitations of the Starkweather model. For example, the model of Guitar takes into account the differences in neuronal patterns between fluent and stuttering subjects, to propose a neurobiological deficiency (Guitar, 1998).

Another integrative logopedics-based theory was proposed by Bloodstein (Bloodstein, 1981). The main difference with respect to the Starkweather model is the assumption that the slight neuromuscular dysfunctions associated with stuttering are induced by the environmental responses and subject's experiences, once the anticipation and fear are established in the subject. Bloodstein assigns an important role to the *self-concept as a stutterer*. This role is associated with a system of beliefs that is built by the child and promotes the subsequent dysfunctions. Moreover, Bloodstein and other subsequent authors (Rodríguez Morejón, 2003; Salgado, 2005) suggest that these dysfunctions can be reverted if the stuttering role is changed. This concept is strongly related to the causal model that we develop in the following Section.

Models of stuttering based on *brain disorders* are mainly of 20th century. Many of them are based on neuroimaging techniques. In opposition to other models that are referred in Figure 1 by the author's name, brain disorders' based models are referred by the causal mechanism because there are many authors working currently in each one. Notwithstanding, we have used the author's name when he is well identified and causal mechanisms are complex.

The cerebral dominance theory or model emerged as a consequence of several stuttering observations in left handed children that are required to shift to the right hand (Orton, 1927; Travis, 1978; Travis & Herren, 1929). It was considered a deficit of hemispheric dominance, which was assumed necessary for the proper hemispheric coordination (Hardyck & Petrinovich, 1977). Other authors met also a relationship between left-handedness and stuttering (Bryngelson & Clark, 1933). Experiments performed administering sodium amytal to 4 severe developmental stuttering subjects (Wada test), both in right and left carotids, showed that they have "bilateral control" of language (R. K. Jones, 1966). Other authors obtained results suggesting also problems with auditory control dominance (Curry & Gregory, 1969).

Several results in 50's and 60's pointed to some type of feedback disorder (auditory, bony, or kinesthetic) in the speech control mechanisms, as cause of stuttering (Goldiamond, Atkinson, & Bilger, 1962; Lee, 1951; May & Hackwood, 1968; Ronald L. Webster & Lubker, 1968). Many of these first and the subsequent works showed the strong influence of the delayed auditory feedback (DAF) and other altered auditory feedback (AAF) mechanisms, such as frequency auditory feedback (FAF), masking, or chorus reading on the fluency, disrupting this one in non-stutterers (Goldiamond, et al., 1962; Lee, 1951), and improving fluency in stutterers (Alm, 2005; Roger J. Ingham, Warner, Byrd, & Cotton, 2006; Kehoe, 2008; Andrew Stuart, Kalinowski, Saltuklaroglu, & Guntupalli, 2006). We include *masking* and *chorus reading* as types of AAF.

Although the degree of fluency achieved by AAF depends on each person who stutters, the improvement is a general feature that should be explained by any valid causal model. Stuttering reductions under AAF are important, but the most dramatic are those achieved with choral speech, which is highly robust (Kiefte & Armson, 2008). Choral speech has proved to keep its effectivity despite changes in speech rate, familiar and unfamiliar speeches, and even when accompanist's voice is temporally lagged (Kiefte & Armson, 2008). DAF and FAF present different effectiveness as a function of the stress, environment and long-term behavior (Kehoe, 2008).

It is interesting to emphasize that AAF, for example chorus reading, is able to produce not only stutter free (or reduced) speech, but also significant reduction in speech effort (Roger J. Ingham, et al., 2006) and natural sounding (Andrew Stuart, et al., 2006). These outcomes agree with the amelioration of neuronal abnormalities found in the prime work of Fox et al., where stuttering and fluent speech among PDS and non-PDS adults were compared by means of positron emission tomography (PET) (Fox, et al., 1996). Authors found an underactivation of the frontal-temporal system implicated in speech production (left-side) and an overactivation of the premotor cortex, operculum and insula, with right cerebral dominance, in PDS with respect to non-PDS subjects. Chorus reading remediated the neuronal pattern difference associated with speech tasks. The effect of DAF was explored on fluent subjects by means of functional magnetic resonance imaging (fMRI), concluding that bilateral superior temporal gyrus (STG), together with middle temporal gyrus and supramarginal gyrus, is correlated with the degree of DAF effect, suggesting that temporo-parietal regions act as a conscious self-monitoring system in speech production (Hashimoto & Sakai, 2003).

The Fox et al. study boosts a research line about stuttering based on neuroimaging (Brown, Ingham, Ingham, Laird, & Fox, 2005; Fox, 2003). Although current discoveries by neuroimaging agree with the theory of cerebral dominance or deficit of hemispheric dominance, mentioned previously (Orton, 1927; Travis, 1978; Travis & Herren, 1929), researchers do not agree concerning the causes and their nature (compensatory or primary).

One of the first models of stuttering based on neuroimaging was proposed in (Foundas, Bollich, Corey, Hurley, & Heilman, 2001). It suggests that persistent developmental stuttering is a consequence of the anomalous anatomy of speech-language areas. Authors found that right and left planum temporale were significant larger and the magnitude of the planar asymmetry was reduced in adults with PDS. In general, volumetric MRI images showed more gyral variants in perisylvian cortical areas in PDS adults than controls.

An alternative more developed model was subsequently proposed to account for cortical anatomy anomalies. This one suggests that stuttering is due to a flaw in the speech-dominant left hemisphere. It is supported by timing disturbances between areas involved in language preparation and execution in dominant hemisphere (based on magnetoencephalographic images), and by the difference of white matter connecting motor-speech areas with temporal and frontal areas, between PDS and fluent subjects (diffusion tensor imaging) (Sommer, Koch, Paulus, Weiller, & Buchel, 2002). As a consequence, authors suggest that the right hemisphere overactivation is a compensatory mechanism. A subsequent study based on fMRI showed that activation on the right frontal operculum (RFO) observed in PDS subjects was negatively correlated with the severity of stuttering (Preibisch, et al., 2003). The same negative correlation was detected during baseline task consisting on passive viewing of meaningless signs. Both outcomes point, according to authors, to compensatory instead of primary dysfunction. A second experiment involving covert semantic decision task also showed that RFO activation.

A more recent study assessed the effect of fluency shaping techniques in the neuronal patterns of PDS subjects (Neumann, et al., 2005). It showed a widespread activation in frontal speech and language regions, and in temporal areas of both hemispheres, after therapy. The differences among post-treatment left-side activations occurred close to the white matter area detected by Sommer et al., which was considered by the authors a suggestion that therapy is able to remodel brain neuronal networks near the dysfunction source. The results point to a flaw in the speech-dominant left hemisphere, according to authors.

A very recent and detailed study using functional MRI and diffusion tensor imaging agrees with this causal model, according to authors (Watkins, et al., 2008). They give explicit support to the linguistic – semiotic type model EXPLAN, previously cited (Peter Howell, 2002). Authors found some common differences during speech production between PDS and control groups that were not related to the type of auditory feedback. These ones could reflect an invariant and characteristic pattern of activity of the stuttering brain. They do not consider choral speech in their study, but only DAF and FAF. It is key to mention the overactivity observed in the midbrain, close to the substantia nigra pars campacta, caudal to the red nucleus and subthalamic nucleus (STN) and to the putative location of the pedunculopontine nucleus (PPN), in PDS subjects. These nuclei are integrated in the circuitry of basal ganglia, and present reciprocal connections PPN – cortex, STN – globus pallidus, and outputs from PPN to cortex, striatum and substantia nigra, among others. In addition, authors refer to a recent study that correlates negatively stuttering severity and activity in substantia nigra, both before and after therapies. Authors do not provide any suggestion regarding this finding, with the exception of the hypothesis that a flaw in cortico-striatal-thalamic loops could be associated with the cortical abnormalities, due to the relationship among basal ganglia, the outputs to premotor system, and the inhibition of motor programs (Watkins, et al., 2008). This flaw hypothesis is supported, according to authors, by the improvement in fluency that follows administration of dopamine antagonists, as risperidone, and the deterioration that follows with the administration of dopamine agonists, such as levodopa.

Neuroimaging results and the behavior of PDS subjects have led to propose that stuttering is mainly due to a problem in the sensorimotor control of speech (Max, Guenther, Gracco, Ghosh, & Wallace, 2004). This model is essentially different of the causal model based on timing disturbances above presented. It is considered that central nervous system (CNS) performs complex command-to-motor output transformations during the planning of movement by means of control schemes, as well as the feedforward and feedback mechanisms involved in sensorimotor control and learning.

Mach et al. propose two hypotheses for persistent developmental stuttering. The first one assumes an unstable or insufficiently activated internal representation of transformations associated with the conversion of commands in speech. The second one considers the possibility that the motor control uses afferent signals with considerable time lags. Authors base both hypotheses on data related to differences on speech and non-speech movements between stutterers and non-stutterers. However, perhaps the most solid basis is the combination of MEG, PET and fMRI data showing that own speech modulates auditory cortex in a different manner that external auditory stimuli.

The first hypothesis gives an explanation to AAF fluency enhancement based on the activation of the internal control models (so, improving the feedback controllers prediction), used to monitor efference copies of motor commands rather than through actual auditory afferent signals. Max et al. presented a mathematical model that provides the error signal during speech in certain situations. This model implements some aspects of their hypothesis, although it is still immature.

Alm presented a causal model of stuttering that puts emphasis in the tangled effect of AAF, including choral speech, on the fluency (Alm, 2005). Alm had the ability to extricate some psychodynamic interpretations of the PDS behavior by means of neuro-physiological analysis. For example, he opposed to the conclusion that PDS subjects reduce stress when stuttering appears, based on the lower heart rate and blood pressure in comparison with non-stuttering persons (WIlliams H. Perkins, 1996). Instead, he argues that reduction of heart rate is a common response in mammals associated to sudden fear where sympathetic and parasympathetic nervous systems are co-activated. This is a well-known physiological mechanism denoted as "freezing response".

According to his model, stuttering is caused by an impairment of the medial premotor system, located along the midline of the brain, whose main parts include basal ganglia and supplementary motor area (SMA) (Alm, 2005). Basal ganglia have an important role on motor dysfunction disorders such as Parkinson's disease, and SMA is a part of cortex with a role in providing go-signals messages for movement. The model is completed considering that speech control is shift to the lateral system (lateral premotor cortex and cerebellum) when timing is linked to external stimuli or when there is an increased level of conscious attention of speech, such during change of role, imitation, etc. This mechanism is able to support the fluency enhancement of PDS subjects in many situations, including AAF. The model associates stuttering to a freezing state, in which the brain amygdale, located in the medial temporal lobes near to basal ganglia, has a key role. This way, the model allows relating emotional state to stuttering degree, although in a complex and unknown way. The model relates "involuntary" movements and increased muscular tension associated with stuttering events to a type of dystonia, in agreement with the role of basal ganglia in automated sequential motor tasks, although clearly distinguishes stuttering from dystonia. It is one of the first models that mention the similitude among task-specific dystonia associated with basal ganglia in tasks like walking, writing, or playing, and point to the metaphoric expressions of them as "stammering with instruments", etc., used by Bluemel (1930) (Alm, 2005). Finally, the author discusses many of the phenomenology of PDS, for example the increment of basal ganglia type D2 dopamine receptors at 2-3 years is hypothesized an important cause of the high rate of childhood recovery in that age, in agreement with his model.

A last and important model of stuttering based on brain causes that is considered relevant in this review was published by Dodge in 2003 in a personal web page and updated two times since then, to best of our knowledge, until the present version (Dodge, 2009). Current version attends to recent research results aforementioned, like the white matter tracts differences between PDS subjects and fluent subjects. The model is based on the assumption that persistent developmental stuttering originates from increasingly conditioned reactions of the amygdala to developmental dysfluencies, which may be associated with several types of temporary or permanent speech-languages impairment in childhood. Therefore stuttering emerges as an inhibition of the speech-language motor system, which induces disruption or freezing when some components of the speech mechanisms return an impaired and unexpected response. Behaviors like loss of speech control, compensatory movements (e.g. tension of speech musculature), etc., are compensatory reactions. Summarizing, Dodge's model hypothesizes that stuttering is not a neurological flaw but an extreme reaction to fear and threat conditioning to initial and slight impairments. The model seems to suggest that initial speech errors are greater in PDS subjects, who have a higher vulnerability to inhibition. It assumes also that the extreme inhibitory reaction in PDS may come from a genetic predisposition.

Dodge discusses with detail how the model supports the complex behavior of the PDS, including therapy relapse, and AAF. It is worth to mention the citation to current studies that show how rapid inputs from the sensory thalamus connect directly with amygdala, bypassing the slower sensory cortex representation (Phelps & LeDoux, 2005). This fast circuit must have had an important role in survival, but it could lead to inappropriate activation and even conditioning. For example, auditory stimuli can reach the lateral nucleus of amygdale via thalamus, and promoting freezing through the output from central nucleus in amygdale to the central gray. The latter is a neuron group within the midbrain with a key role in defensive behavior. The midbrain overactivity observed in PDS subjects (Watkins, et al., 2008) agrees with this hypothesis.

Several explicative models of stuttering that point to *non-brain nervous disorders* have been developed since 16th century. Certainly, they have not too relevance in recent days, but the most important should be cited in order to complete the image shown in Figure 1. They provided a better perspective of classical wrongs and misinterpretations of the PDS behavior in popular and even professional environments nowadays.

Several ideas emerged in early 19th century regarding the possible impairment of the nerves that enervate tongue and larynx in PDS. These concepts lead to the theory of stuttering as an spasm in the glottis that migrates up to the tongue, causing lingual cramps (Bobrick, 1996). This hypothesis justified the interruption of neurological impulse from glottis by surgeries techniques: cutting out a triangular wedge across the tongue. This technique started in 1841 by Dieffenbach. Other surgeons joined to this "brilliant idea", adding some variants and creating three schools in German, France, and England. Therapies were retired after several deaths, without any fluency improvement. However, muscular spasms are considered the underlying mechanism of stuttering by some professionals nowadays (Santacreu

& Fernandez-Zúñiga, 1991). The different EMG pattern between PDS and fluent subjects is used to support this hypothesis.

A different organic model points to tha lack of coordination between respiratory and phonatory systems, with important developments from (W. Perkins, Rudas, Johnson, & Bell, 1976) and (Adams & Hayden, 1976). This assumption was supported by experimental works and was taken into account by several researchers (Charles Van Riper, 1982), although many methodological doubts emerge from a critical analysis (Santacreu & Fernandez-Zúñiga, 1991).

In summary, despite neuroimaging techniques are helping to know better the neuronal correlates of persons who stutter, the nature of stuttering remains elusive. Some authors claim the necessity of a *new view* (Fox, 2003). The complex perspective that shows Figure 1 have led to the sensation that persistent developmental stuttering has multiple causes. The idea of a multiplicity of causes is shared by many researchers, and it is written in popular sources like Wikipedia (http://en.wikipedia.org/wiki/Stuttering). However, integrative and multidimensional therapies for stuttering have not achieved significant improvements in PDS subjects (Blomgren, Roy, Callister, & Merrill, 2005).

A Non-Speech Etiology: Basis and Discussion

A careful analysis of the state of the art shows that no model is able to provide a clear and non-forced explanation of the well-known phenomenology of persistent developmental stuttering. One of the most entangled behaviors is associated with AAF. Recent brain disorders' models based on neuroimaging suggest several flaws as the underlying cause, but there are many doubts regarding the causal or compensatory (or indeed any other) nature of the neuronal patterns measured.

We present in this Section a novel model of stuttering that provides a more natural explanation of the phenomenology and agrees with neuroimaging and other experimental findings. This model cannot be developed with a great neurophysiologic detail in this Chapter, but the description should clarify the key mechanisms and justify a new etiological paradigm.

We have marked several models or group of models that are particularly relevant, according to our knowledge, in Figure 1. These are the models of Johnson (1959), Van Riper (1973), and Sheehan (1957) with psychological nature, the Starkweather's model (1987) with logopedics nature, and models of cerebral dominance (1929), dominant hemisphere timing disturbances (2002 -2008), and Alm (2005), with a nature founded on brain disorders. The relevance of these models is justified on their wide scientific diffusion, references, and use as basis of therapies. We are aware that this is not the case for the models of Alm (2005) and timing disturbances (2002-2008). However, we are placed all of them together because these two last models, published in relevant journals, collect the most important conclusions reached using modern neuroimaging data nowadays.

A second important mark of Figure 1 points to those models that take into account the fear as an emotion that plays a key role in stuttering. We strongly agree with the influence that this quale has in the development of stuttering. Several of the marked relevant models, as those of Johnson, Sheehan, and Alm, put emphasis on this feeling. It has been a factor considered also by other models, starting with the hypothesis of Mercuriales in 1583 (with logopedics basis and psychological influences), models of Rius (1987) and Bloodstein (1981) (logopedics nature), and the model of reactive inhibition of Dodge (2003 – 2009). The latter has not been published in a scientific journal, to best of our knowledge, but in our opinion it is very close of the true nature of the disorder.

A final mark is necessary before presenting and discussing our model. According to our research, several models in Figure 1 are characterized by some key concepts (besides the fear quale) that are strongly associated with the true causal mechanism of developmental stuttering. These are the group of models based on learned behavior (psychological nature), the model of Bloodstein (1981) (logopedics nature), and the models of cerebral dominance (1929), Alm (2005), and Reactive Inhibition from Dodge (2003 – 2009). Our agreement with those different key concepts is compatible with a single causal mechanism for stuttering.

We hypothesize that persistent developmental stuttering is consequence of the blocking of complex motor supervised sequential tasks, programmed in the parallel and unidirectional poly-synaptic loops through basal ganglia and several thalamic nuclei, by means of operant conditioning mediated by amygdala in response to fear emotions (fear conditioning).

The figure 2 shows a grossly simplified diagram of these motor loops, according to (Barker & Barasi, 1999; Edelman & Tononi, 2000; Jhou, 2005; Phelps & LeDoux, 2005; Takakusaki, Saitoh, Harada, & Kashiwayanagi, 2004). Despite the diagram is very incomplete, it tries to put emphasis on the long and non-reentrant pathways that go out the thalamocortical system, passing through the basal ganglia to return to the thalamocortical system.

Many studies point to the key role of these pathways in the control of several types of behavioral expressions. This role is related to the contribution of the basal ganglia and brainstem structures (substantia nigra pertains to basal ganglia and brainstem) to the automatic control of movements, with emphasis in the emotionally triggered motor behavior (Takakusaki, et al., 2004). However, many cells within the basal ganglia are not clearly sensory or motor in terms of their response properties. This way, it seems that this cortical appendage takes highly processed information to convert it into some type of motor programme (Barker & Barasi, 1999).

An important characteristic of these loops is that they are constituted by projections which form parallel pathways, in such a way that this architecture seems to support independent neuronal subroutines (Barker & Barasi, 1999; Edelman & Tononi, 2000). This concept is well known and the experimental evidence is solid.

As shown in Figure 2, the most important outflow from the basal ganglia is via GPi and Substantia Nigra reticulata (SNr) to the Thalamus (ventroanterior and ventrolateral nuclei), as well as to the brainstem, mainly to PPN. Polysynaptic loops return to the cortex via Thalamus projection. There are also important back-projections from SN to striatum (dopaminergic nigrostriatal tract) and from other nuclei of the brainstem to basal ganglia. The Substantia Nigra compacta (SNc) is a well-known region because its implication in Parkinson disease.

Basal ganglia are strongly involved in functions of amygdala. Indeed and anatomically, the centromedial nucleus of amygdala can be considered part of the basal ganglia. Figure 2 shows the lateral nucleus (LA) and the central nucleus (CE), which in turn projects mainly to the Periaqueductal Gray (PAG).

It is also shown that the stimuli (auditory or somatosensory) can reach the PAG via projections from thalamus to LA, without cortex processing (Phelps & LeDoux, 2005).

The existence of these fast pathways has deep implications on the mechanism underlying the fear conditioning and the associated freezing behaviors, which are usually associated to the PAG region.

There is an overwhelming evidence of the role of amygdala in conditioned freezing, and it is well-known the relevance of fear in that process. However, the knowledge about basal ganglia an amygdala functions in human is still poor. In spite of this, several recent discoveries can throw important clues with regard to the causal mechanisms of stuttering according to our model. Some researchers suggest the possibility that a region within the brainstem near to Median Raphe Nucleus (MRN) and Ventral Tegmental

Figure 2. Simplified parallel poly-synaptic pathways through basal ganglia and several thalamic nuclei, with emphasis on feedback to the thalamocortical system and the involvement of the amygdala and several zones of brainstem. The different neuroanatomic zones are marked by different colors

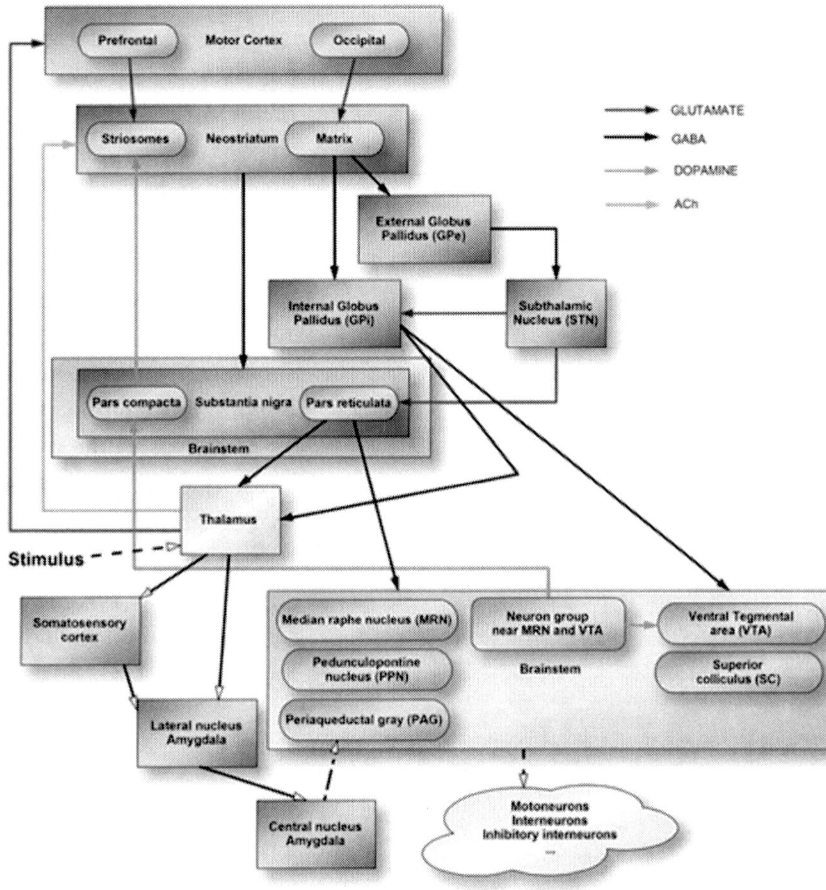

Area (VTA) regulates freezing via projections to the midbrain dopamine neurons (Jhou, 2005). That zone seems to integrate aversive information from multiple sources into a common pathway to inhibit dopamine neurons during learned aversive behaviors. Interestingly, the cited neuron group, within the medial portion of brainstem, has a strong dopaminergic projection to the SNc and VTA (Jhou, 2005). This is shown in Figure 2.

This brief description of some major underlying pathways and neuronal regions involved in stuttering, according to our model, allows developing some important derived issues that clarify the scope of the model. These are subsequently discussed.

- *Point 1.* PDS is not restricted to speech. It is a fear-mediated learned behavior associated with supervised sequential motor tasks (expressive communication), like speech, writing, sign language communication, or even playing an instrument. Fear is associated with the supervision (potential) by other subjects, particularly during the developmental childhood stage.
- *Point 2.* PDS is not due to any type of lack or innate disorder. Fear conditioning can

be modulated by a set of internal parameters of the subject, like the sensitivity to external threats or the synaptic plasticity involved in learning, and external conditions, like the reactions of parents, teachers, or other culture and social issues.

- *Point 3.* PDS is not associated with a particular behavioral subject profile in agreement with the previous point.
- *Point 4.* The variability of stuttering severity for a subject is due to two factors: the possibility of supervision and the subject's role. The first one induces reactive inhibition or freezing, which causes the emergence of blocks in complex sequential motor tasks. This is a learned process in a PDS subject (adult). The second one is related to the self-concept of the PDS subject. It is psychologically associated with a type of conscious state or experience, which in turn has a correlation with neuronal activity. The two factors are necessary to induce blocks and so stuttering.
- *Point 5.* Although the complex processes involved in the building of the semantic elements of a sentence (in any expressive communicative task), like words in speech or writing, do not pertain to the conscious experience, these final elements emerge to the consciousness. Similarly, the complex motor tasks involved in the communicative execution do not pertain to the conscious experience, with the exception of blocking quale in PDS subjects. It is interesting that these quale emerge together with the built word and compel these persons to avoid (or fight with) that word in order to produce the communicative expression. This mechanism was denoted by previous authors as anticipation and it is poorly known. It is the origin of the observed disturbance in vocal and kinesic elements.
- *Point 6.* Stuttering aid systems should work through the modulation of factors that control blocks: supervision and subject's role.
- *Point 7.* Current therapies for stuttering act similarly to stuttering aid systems, although they are oriented to achieve fluency at medium term instead of real time. The percentage of relapse in those therapies (near 100%) is due to the fact that fear-mediated learned behavior associated with expressive communication is kept. A long-term therapy should be able to modify the learned behavior, by means of synaptic depression in projections that cause inhibition of basal ganglia programmed motor tasks. However, as the subject role is a key factor in the induction of blocks, the ability of the subject to keep a different role, as occurs with some actors, professors, or professional speakers, can inhibit stuttering. Notwithstanding, the disorder persists in these persons.

The extension of PDS to other supervised sequential motor tasks claimed in point 1 implies a change in the paradigm of stuttering. It was firstly proposed in (Prado & Roa, 2007; Snyder, 2006). The earlier publication has also been presented recently in (Snyder, 2009). Snyder proposed the possibility of a new paradigm non-based on speech as a consequence of the interview with a student that stuttered both in speech and sign language. This student had analyzed the analogies between spoken and sign language stuttering in his Master Thesis for graduation (Whitebread, 2004). After some resistance to consider the validity of this phenomenon, Snyder reviewed the literature and found a list of studies from 1937 pointing to several cases and data regarding "some type of stuttering" in sign language. This manner, a study by Backus in 1938 found 0.4% of 13.691 students with deaf or hard hearing (HH) exhibiting stuttering either verbally or in sign. Other study by Silverman & Silverman in 1971 revealed stuttering signing in deaf or HH students, and showed that this behavior was more frequently associated with finger-spelling and often resulting in the repetition of a sign or initial letters of finger-spelling.

The study of Montgomery & Fiftch in 1988 involving 77 participant schools for hearing impaired students shown that 0.12% of the sampled population exhibited stuttering behavior in speech, sign, or during the simultaneous use of speech and sign (SimCom). The half of this stuttering population demonstrated stuttering-like behavior only in sign communication. The behaviors included blocking on sign production.

There are other studies that document blocking or stuttering in other expressive communications modalities such as piano, violin playing, and handwriting (Snyder, 2006). Although those studies present some distinctive features in these behaviors, they are not well-known, and thus diagnosis is difficult. As a study case, a subject with speech stuttering and "trumpet stuttering" reported that he felt exactly the same block qualia and avoidance behavior in both expressive communicative tasks (Snyder, 2006).

Those studies have been ignored or disregarded because of the preconception of stuttering as a speech pathology, but they provide support to the point 1 derived from our causal model. This manner, our model provides a single and common basis for stuttering in agreement with the Occam's razor.

It is relevant to emphasize that the semantic atoms of speech and other types of expressive communication, like playing music have different nature and they are related to different cortex neuronal activities patterns (Callan, et al., 2006), which disagrees with linguistic/semiotic hypotheses for PDS.

Despite the interest of the studies of (Snyder, 2006) and (Whitebread, 2004), they did not present a new causal model. They suggested a shift of paradigm based on the analysis of previous studies. Moreover, Snyder wrote that stuttering behaviors are symptomatic responses relative to their corresponding expressive modality, which in turn may be a response to errors in formulation, processing, and/or execution of expressive output in a central level, such as language. This manner Snyder keeps the idea that stuttering is based on some innate flaw, which disagrees with our hypothesis started in (Prado & Roa, 2007) and developed in this work.

Another important asseveration of point 1 is that fear is a key issue in the development of stuttering. Fear-conditioning has a well- known implication on operant conditioning and it has been pointed by a relevant group of causal models reviewed and presented in Figure 1.

Finally, the point 1 agrees with the concept of learned behavior, which underlies a group of psychological models of Figure 1 marked with the exclamation mark (key issue).

The absence of any innate flaw is asseverated in point 2. It is a key aspect of our model. However, we must answer some neuroimaging findings aforementioned. The bilateral activation of brain hemispheres, found experimentally in (R. K. Jones, 1966) using the Wada test in PDS subjects, and shown repeatedly by different neuroimaging techniques in many studies subsequent to the leading work (Fox, et al., 1996), seems to support the cerebral dominance model. It has been better developed afterwards to propose the existence of timing disturbances between areas involved in language preparation and execution, due to a flaw in the speech-dominant hemisphere (Sommer, et al., 2002). The difference of white matter connecting motor-speech areas with temporal and frontal areas between PDS and fluent subjects has been also used to support this model.

However, there are other explanations of these data. According to our model, the overactivation of several zones in right hemisphere should be caused by the anticipation and avoidance behaviors associated with the emergence of blocking qualia. This can be supported by studies that shown a correlation between conscious self-monitoring in speech production and temporo-parietal regions, using fMRI in DAF experiments with fluent subjects, as described in the previous Section (Hashimoto & Sakai, 2003). The negative correlation between the severity of stuttering and the overactivation of the RFO in PDS subjects shown in (Preibisch, et al., 2003) agrees with our hypothesis. Moreover, the RFO activation observed under covert semantic decision in (Preibisch, et al., 2003) is in agreement with the factors that control blocking, described in point 4. With the aim of clarifying this asseveration, it must be taken into account that it is not necessary a true supervision of the expressive communicative task to trigger stuttering, and thus the conscious anticipation and avoidance mechanisms. These factors are better discussed below.

The effect of fluency shaping techniques in left-side activations in PDS subjects was considered by (Neumann, et al., 2005) in agreement with the flaw in the speech-dominant hemisphere, but that interpretation could be erroneous. It should be expected that if a therapy is able to reduce stuttering, the neuronal activity associated to the conscious activity of avoidance should be modified.

In addition, the timing disturbance model does not provide any convincing explanation of the overactivity observed in the midbrain, close to SNc in PDS subjects (Watkins, et al., 2008). There is still a poor knowledge with regard to the effect, increase or decrease of dopamine release during aversive stimuli. However, the overactivity observed in the midbrain, close to SNc, and the effect of dopamine antagonists and agonists in PDS subjects are in agreement with the existence of a strong dopaminergic projection from a region within brainstem (near to MRN and VTA) that seems to integrate aversive information implicated in fear conditioning (Jhou, 2005). Therefore, the cited overactivity in midbrain is in agreement with our model of stuttering.

With respect to the reduction in white matter integrity underlying underactive areas in PDS subjects, it is well-known that the myelination process is active in human brain and it is modulated by experience, affecting the process of information by regulating velocity and synchrony between distant cortical regions (Fields, 2008). This manner, it could be expected that differences in white matter integrity were induced by differences in cortex pattern activations.

The model of hemisphere timing disturbances has been criticized in (William H. Perkins, 2001). The main argument of the author was the too slow cognitive function rates of Broca and Wernicke areas, which compels to discard them in the control of timing of high-speed phonatory and articulatory synchronization. According to (Rosenfield & Viswanath, 2002) this asseveration is not true, on the basis of the lack of knowledge concerning the manner that neurons process information in these areas. Moreover, the responding authors emphasize that there is not neuroscientific data indicating that we think at the rate that we talk, finishing with a brief mention to the hard problem of thought (Rosenfield & Viswanath, 2002).

The cognitive function rate mentioned by Perkins is related to the binding (cortical integration) problem, which points to the mechanisms that underlying the rapid integration of distributed and functionally specialized neuronal groups (Giulio Tononi & Edelman, 1998; Giullo Tononi, Sporns, & Edelman, 1992). Many studies shown that the integration of distributed differentiated neuronal regions through reentrant interactions in the thalamocortical system is required for conscious experience (Edelman & Tononi, 2000; Giulio Tononi & Edelman, 1998). In addition, it is required 100 - 150 ms to reach this binding, called unified neural process, which agrees with the psychological refractory period necessary to discriminate two sequential conscious states. This way, in our opinion, the criticism of Perkins is well founded, but it has a mistake. It must be hypothesized that the activity of Broca and Wernicke areas during speech occurs within a unified neural process.

Moreover, recent theories concerning neuronal dynamics suggest that degeneracy and redundancy has an influence greater than earlier was believed, in agreement with the theory of neural group selection (Edelman & Tononi, 2000). This agrees with the lack of histological differentiation in many regions and explains why the non-dominant hemisphere can perform functions of the dominant hemisphere, including language functions, especially but not solely in childhood. Our major conclusion is that the neuronal patterns differences observed is a consequence of a conscious experience related to the subject's role and strongly associated with the avoidance behavior. This is addressed with new details when discussing points 4 and 5.

The role that genetic factors play in the development of stuttering is another key issue that seems faced with the lack of an innate disorder that we claim. There are two major elements that contribute to this misleading concept. The first one is that sometimes PDS is confounded with others dysfluencies in cluttering, spastic dysphonia and even Tourette's disorder. The second one is due to the misinterpretation of linkage studies results. A recent study in the genetics of stuttering from (Suresh, et al., 2006) carried out with 100 families of European descent ascertained in the United States, Sweden, and Israel, can help us to clarify these elements. A synthesis of this work could be that the susceptibility locus for developmental stuttering is on chromosome 9 (LOD = 2.3 at 60 cM) if both persistent and recovered stuttering are considered, and on chromosome 15 (LOD = 1.95 at 23 cM) if only persistent stuttering is taken into account. However, when sex is considered in the population selection, evidence for linkage is on chromosome 7 (LOD = 2.99 at 153 cM) in the male-only subset, and on chromosome 21 (LOD = 4.5 at 34 cM) for female-only data set. When conditional linkage is analyzed, there is evidence for linkage on chromosome 12 (in agreement with previously reported signal in families ascertained in Pakistan), conditional on the evidence for linkage at chromosome 7. Moreover, there is also a region in chromosome 2 that increased the evidence for linkage conditional on either chromosome 9 (positive) or chromosome 7 (negative). Thus, chromosomes and loci associated to stuttering vary with the criterion used to select the population sample along six chromosomes. In addition, the evidence score (LOD) depended on the sample size. In our opinion, these data do not allow pointing to an innate disorder linked to genetic in stuttering.

In addition, even in the case that the genetic profile will be considered as a risk factor to stuttering, the plausible relationship genetic – stuttering predisposition does not involve an innate disorder.

The point 3 of our model derives from point 2 and it is supported by several review studies (Bloodstein, 1981; Loriente Zamora, 2006).

The point 4 derives directly from our model, and takes into account the behavior of the conscious experience as an array of "simpletons", which go in and out, as a consequence of demands of environment, providing variability to the self (Ornstein, 1991). This concept is well-accepted in evolutionary psychology and agrees with the neurophysiological hypotheses of the conscious experience as a "dynamic core" based on the aforementioned thalamocortical unified process (Edelman & Tononi, 2000; Giulio Tononi & Edelman, 1998). It is not possible to develop here completely this issue in connection with our model, notwithstanding we need to refer several key concepts.

The first one refers to the AAF phenomena described in the previous Section. Some works suggest that AAF promotes a conscious attention of speech, which in turns improves fluency by means of some mechanism. A relevant example was presented by the causal model of (Alm, 2005). It assumes that the conscious attention induces the shift of speech control from the medial premotor system to a hypothesized lateral system, which is not impaired, inducing thus the improving of fluency. However the Alm's model does not provide a clear explanation concerning the improvement of PDS subjects when talk without supervision or whisper. It uses the connection between basal ganglia and limbic system to propose that the cause is a low level of conflicting impulses (emotions or thoughts). In summary, although it is a very interesting model that emphasizes the key role of fear, basal ganglia and limbic system, it assumes an innate flaw and requires different and forced mechanisms to explain partly the phenomenology of stuttering.

In opposition, our model predicts the effect of AAF on stuttering severity on the basis of a change of the subject's role. The theory of dynamic core provides a very interesting physiological basis to this concept, since it relates the activity of the integrated and distributed neuronal regions in the thalamocortical system, to the activations of input and output ports, from and towards polysynaptic parallel loops, through cortical appendages like basal ganglia (Edelman & Tononi, 2000; Giulio Tononi & Edelman, 1998). Therefore, it is able to link conscious states (i.e. cortex neuronal patterns) associated with subject's roles to cognitive and motor tasks programs in those parallel pathways. With the proper conscious state (and thus subject's role), the possibility to be supervised activates the blocking mechanisms, mediated by operant conditioning, and causes stuttering.

The combination of the two factors of point 4 provides a more simple explanation of the stuttering phenomenology than other models. This includes also the elimination of stuttering in patients where some surgical operation modified strongly the cortex pattern activation, as occurred in the four patients of (R. K. Jones, 1966). A major difference with the other relevant models presented in Figure 1 is that it is not based on any innate flaw.

Moreover, the independence or lack of correlation among parallel and unidirectional polysynaptic pathways, through cortical appendages, justifies the specificity of the stuttering behaviors. That is, a subject can suffer only speech stuttering and not other type of expressive communication stuttering, in agreement with our current knowledge (Snyder, 2006).

The dynamic core hypothesis provides also a new perspective concerning the well-known emergence of blocking quale to the conscious experience of PDS subjects, referred in point 5. This quale would be acquired through the input ports associated to the cognitive-motor programmed tasks, linking the subject's role with learned blocking mechanisms, mediated by amygdala, in basal ganglia. This new point of view is very important according to the importance of the anticipation-avoidance mechanism in the stuttering behaviors, in agreement with many relevant models presented in the previous Section (see Figure 1).

The point 6 derives directly from point 4, and it provides an explanation for the effect of the many types of electronic devices for stuttering, including DAF, FAF, Metronome, Masked Auditory Feedback (MAF), etc. These devices modulate both supervision perception and modification of the subject's role in different ways, depending on the subject experiences. For example, the MAF device seems oriented to the modulation of the supervision perception, whereas FAF seems to act mainly on the role. Indeed, the change in the auditory feedback achieved by means of a simple cotton earplug can induce a role shift that improves greatly the fluency (non-published self-experience of the first author, which is stutterer).

The point 7 derives from the presented model and it is in agreement with the lack of effectiveness of therapies, which a percentage of relapses close to 100%. However, the achievement of a complete fluency by a PDS subject does not require unlearning the blocking mechanisms, but a good control of the subject's role. This issue explains why the stuttering severity uses to increase in familiar environments.

Finally, it is relevant to show that some of the conclusions of our model agree with other two important models previously addressed (Bloodstein, 1981; Dodge, 2009). These ones have flagged with two marks in Figure 1. The earlier is based on the self-concept as a stutterer, and hypothesizes that dysfunctions are induced by subject's experiences, in agreement with our model. The second one assumes that PDS is induced by conditioned reactions of amygdala and presents the mechanism of freezing as a key piece in the disorder, in agreement with us. However, it assumes the existence of some initial slight impairment and does not clarify the other regions or mechanisms that cooperate with amygdala in the stuttering development, despite discuss some cortical appendages that should be implied: "*"implicit" learning of the amygdala is accompanied by more situational ("explicit") and spatially cued learning of the hippocampus and associated rhinocortical areas, as well as by conditioned "implicit" learning in the basal ganglia (striatum) and the cerebellum.*" (Dodge, 2009).

Implications on Treatments and Wearable Prosthetic Devices

According to point 4 of our model of stuttering, the degree of fluency can be modulated by masking the speech or in general the expressive communication task, and by changing the subject's role. The first one seeks providing the subject the feeling: "there is not supervision of my communicative task", which avoids triggering the learned reactive inhibition. The second one is correlated with the dynamic core, which is implied in the activation of inputs /outputs associated with the parallel pathways programmed with that learned behaviour.

A stuttering aid device has as main goal the reduction of blocks to facilitate the communications, and it is not interested in keeping the fluency after its use. In such a case, an approach based on a role shift could be very efficient. Techniques like frequency altered frequency (FAF) or any other that helps the subject with this mission are adequate. It is interesting to note that these techniques should be dependent on the expressive communication. This conclusion should be validated in future works.

In opposition, the major objective of a therapy for stuttering should be the reduction of external (perceived by listener) and internal (qualia) blocks, in a long-term and context-independent manner. The ultimate objective is the cure. If our model is correct, then the only way to achieve this goal is to assure than parallel loops through cortical appendages that support the learned behaviour are not activated. Another possibility is that they could be modified. Aside from aggressive techniques that avoid the cortical integration associated with the stutterer's role (R. K. Jones, 1966), the modification of the synaptic weights related to those complex motor tasks by means of behavioral methods is an exciting possibility. Some clinical studies concerning AAF and other altered auditory feedback techniques (Kehoe, 2008), as well as works regarding the basic mechanisms associated with learning (Gruart, Munoz, & Delgado-Garcia, 2006; Sporns, Almassy, & Edelman, 2000) suggest that this possibility is feasible.

The development of a wearable device that combines stuttering aid with a therapeutic objective could be based on the selection of proper weights in supervision masking and role shifts techniques. The accommodative character of sensory system, particularly the auditory system (Sussman & Winkler, 2001), together with the effect that the environmental changes have in the stuttering severity (because its influence on role and supervision feeling), justify that the effect of AAF on fluency wears off in many subjects. This fact led us to design an adaptive AAF technique, based on the feedback of speech and other relevant biosignals, which was briefly presented by one of the authors in (Prado & Roa, 2007). The underlying methodology and the new advances are addressed in the following Section.

A relevant feature of the technology that we present is the ability to acquire and integrate speech and other biosignals used for feedback, into a personalized mathematical model, under a distributed architecture developed earlier (Prado, Roa, Reina-Tosina, Palma, & Milán, 2002). This approach allows validating several of the derived consequences of our causal model of stuttering. We will take into account definitions of neural complexity and other related measures proposed in (Giulio Tononi & Edelman, 1998), for analyzing quale, role's shift, and other mental states, in terms of neural dynamics.

ALTERED AUDITORY FEEDBACK TECHNOLOGY UNDER A NON-SPEECH PARADIGM

A Review of Altered Auditory Feedback Prosthetic Devices

AAF devices reduce stuttering by 40-80% in reading tasks (Lincoln, Packman, & Onslow, 2006; Van Borsel, Reunes, & Van den Bergh, 2003; Ward, 2006). However, there is only evidence of the short-term effect (Armson, Kiefte, Mason, & De Croos, 2006; Pollard, Ellis, Finan, & Ramig, 2009).

Several works have reported a reduction in stuttering, including the enhancement of the speech naturalness by means of AAF, keeping the normal speech rate (R.J. Ingham, et al., 1997; Kalinowski, et al., 2004). It has also been reported that the effect of AAF in reduction of stuttering can decrease (Ward, 2006), even after a few minutes of exposure in some subjects (Armson & Stuart, 1998).

Stutterers report improved fluency and better confidence in speaking, together with less stuttering. Contradictorily, satisfaction reports from subjects of studies are not highly correlated with benefits obtained on measures of fluency (O'Donnell, Armson, & Kiefte, 2008; Pollard, et al., 2009). Other studies reported a difficult in the use of devices in noisy situations and the need of some acclimatization for using them (Pollard, et al., 2009).

In general, the effects of altered feedback can wear off over time and vary from person to person (Armson, et al., 2006; R.J. Ingham, et al., 1997; Lincoln, et al., 2006). Among the most popular AAF approaches, we can highlight the following ones:

- *MAF (masked auditory feedback):* masking provides a synthesized sound, generally a noise of some sort, in user's headphones. This covers up the own auditory feedback. It has demonstrated a reduction in stuttering (Dewar & Dewar, 1979; Kalinowski, Armson, Roland-Mieszkowski, Stuart, & Gracco, 1993; Lincoln, et al., 2006), though that reduction faded with time in many cases (Ward 2006). Furthermore, other AAF approaches, as delayed auditory feedback and frequency altered feedback, seem more effective (Kalinowski, et al., 1993; Lincoln, et al., 2006). The earliest portable MAF device was presented in (Derazne, 1966; Parker & Christopherson, 1963; C. Van Riper, 1965). The Edinburgh Masker was presented afterwards (Dewar & Dewar, 1979).
- *DAF (delayed auditory feedback):* this approach reproduces the user's voice in his headphones delayed a fraction of a second. It has proved its effect in reducing stuttering since 1950s (Molt, 2005; Nessel, 1958). Normally, delays ranges from 50 to 200 milliseconds (Lincoln, et al., 2006). DAF has been used to improve user's fluency at a low speaking rate, reducing subsequently the delay in stages, until the user can speak fluently with normal speaking rate (Bothe, Finn, & Bramlett, 2007; Ward, 2006). It has been found that speakers can maintain fast rates and achieve increased fluency at 50-75 millisecond delays (Kalinowski, et al., 1993; Kalinowski & Stuart, 1996; Lincoln, et al., 2006; Zimmerman, Kalinowski, Stuart, & Rastatter, 1997). DAF has been applied to correct different disorders including apha-

sia, dysarthria, dyspraxia, Parkinson's disease and vocal tremor (Armson & Stuart, 1998; Hargrave, Kalinowski, Stuart, Armson, & Jones, 1994; Saltuklaroglu & Kalinowski, 2006; A. Stuart, Kalinowski, Rastatter, Saltuklaroglu, & Dayalu, 2004). Nowadays there are a number of commercial portable devices that provide DAF.

- *FAF (frequency-shifted auditory feedback):* FAF is the most recent AAF approach. The first work that demonstrates its effect on decreasing the frequency of stuttering was published in 1987 (P. Howell & El-Yaniv, 1987). FAF reproduces user's voice in headphones shifted in frequency. As this approach achieved a reduction of stuttering both at normal and faster-than-normal speaking rates, some authors suggested that altered auditory feedback may correct the neurological abnormality involved (Kalinowski, et al., 1993). However, our model proposes a different causal mechanism. In short reading tasks, variations in pitch ranging from quarter to full octave resulted in 55-74% decrease in stuttering (Armson, Foote, Witt, Kalinowski, & Stuart, 1997; Kalinowski, et al., 1993; Kalinowski, Stuart, Wamsley, & Rastatter, 1999; Zimmerman, et al., 1997). In longer exposures to FAF, only few subjects experience a significative reduction in stuttering (Armson & Stuart, 1998; R.J. Ingham, et al., 1997). FAF has been extensively studied at various speaking rates, shifting frequency in either direction, and combined with other techniques (P. Howell & El-Yaniv, 1987; P. Howell, Wingfield, & Johnson, 1988; Kalinowski, et al., 1993; Kalinowski, et al., 1998).

Among commercial FAF devices, it is worth noting the Fluency Master (R. L. Webster, 1991) developed at HCRI (Hollins communication Research Institute).

- AAF Combination. It has been analyzed the use of DAF and FAF in a combined manner, to improve their effect in reduction of stuttering (Kalinowski, et al., 1998; MacLeod, Kalinowski, Stuart, & Armson, 1995). In fact, the so-called AAF combination category is currently the most used in assistive devices (Molt, 2005).

Casa Futura Technologies, the first company which offered a device which combined AAF approaches, has recently presented the Pocket Speech Lab (PSL), an upgrade of his Pocket Fluency System. PSL provides both DAF and FAF independently or simultaneously, and it can also deliver MAF (www.casafuturatech.com/Catalog/psl.shtml).

It is worth to note here the Digital Speech Aid (DSA), a device which delivers FAF, MAF and a combination of DAF and FAF. Firstly presented in 1992 by Marek Roland-Mieszkowski, Andrzej Czyzewski, and Bozena Kostek, it is now in its 5th generation (www.digital-recordings.com/dsa/dsa.html).

Furthermore, we must cite also the Speech easy device (www.speecheasy.com), developed in 1999 by Michael Rastatter, Joseph Kalinowski and Andrew Stuart among others. There are three versions of Speech easy: BTE (behind-the-ear), ITC (in-the-canal) and CIC (completely-in-the-canal), and all of them provide DAF and FAF in a simultaneous manner. Other devices which belong to this category are shown in Table 1.

There is not a consensus regarding the more effective approach in inhibiting stuttering. Some works have shown that DAF and FAF are more effective than MAF (P. Howell & El-Yaniv, 1987; Kalinowski, et al., 1993). Howell and colleagues reported a better effectiveness of FAF than DAF (P. Howell & El-Yaniv, 1987), whereas other authors showed similar effectiveness in DAF and FAF (P. Howell & El-Yaniv, 1987; Kalinowski, et al., 1993).

Table 1. Commercial AAF devices (adapted from (NHSC, 2007))

Company	product	technology	Features	Cost (estimated)
Janus Development Group	SpeechEasy	DAF	Up to 220 ms, programmed, but not user adjustable	4.100 – 4.900 $
		FAF	500, 1000 or 2000 Hz	
Casa Futura Technolol-gies	Pocket speech lab	DAF	30-200 ms, user adjustable	3.495 $
		FAF	+0.4 to -1.2 octaves in 0.2 octave steps	
		MAF	Manual control button	
	SmallTalk	DAF	30-200 ms, user adjustable	2.495 $
		FAF	+0.4 to -1.2 octaves in 0.2 octave steps	
	Telephone fluency system	DAF	50 ms, fixed	1.495 $
		FAF	+0 to -1.2 octaves in 0.2 octave steps	
	School DAF	DAF	30-200 ms, user adjustable	995 $
VoiceAmp	VoiceAmp 601	DAF	30-200 ms, user adjustable	1.850 $
		FAF	+0.4 to -1.2 octaves in 0.2 octave steps	
A.S. Genstar Limited	Defstut	DAF	-	350 $
		MAF	-	
Digital Recordings Inc	Digital speech aid III & Digital speech aid V	DAF	-	-
		FAF	-	-
		MAF	-	-
Kay Elemetrics	Facilitator model 3500	DAF	-	-
		MAF	-	-

It is worth mentioning here some logopedic-based devices for reduction of stuttering, despite most of them were completely unsuccessful, because these ones complete the perspective of prosthetic and also therapeutic techniques.

- Devices for the alteration of speech motor production patterns

Alteration of speech production patterns can cause a high degree of fluency in stuttering subjects: talking faster or slower than normal, in a softer (louder) voice, with a monotone (mono-loudness) pattern, etc.

The earliest one of these devices was presented by Jean Marc Gaspard Itard in the first years of 19th century. Itard developed different strengthening exercises and utilized a gold or silver "fork" placed under the tongue, holding it in a higher position in the oral cavity (Bobrick, 1996).

The Bates Appliance was patented in 1851, designed to deal with different types of stuttering. It consisted of three parts: a metal plate to keep the lips apart, a hollow tube prevented stuttering on dental phonemes, and a laryngeal compressor (a leather collar) prevented stuttering on guttural phonemes (Molt, 2005). The Idehara "Stutter-Cure" appliance, presented in 1937, was a small whistle placed in the oral cavity and sitting against the hard palate. Whistle provided feedback of the air flux (Charles Van Riper, 1973).

- Feedback of physiological status or production patterns

This class of devices provides visual and (or) auditory feedback of physiological states or speech production patterns. We consider the following categories:

Respiratory kinematics. It has been shown respiratory irregularities in stuttering patients (Bloodstein, 1995). Therefore, some devices were focused on respiratory kinematics to enhance fluency (Molt, 2005). For example, the "Breathing Monitor" (basically, a type of induction plethysmograph) was included in the "Dr. Fluency" computerized stuttering treatment program (A. Friedman, Fetterman, & Jolson, 1999). The CAFET (Computer Aided Fluency Establishment Trainer) is a computer program that tries to improve the control of respiratory and voice production systems. According to authors, the user can coordinate his breathing with the onset of speech and maintain the speech flow (Goebel, 1986). The PFSP (Precision Fluency Shaping Program, http://fluentspeech.com) uses a voice monitor that provides acoustic analysis of sound/speech onset and other parameters, and a "respiration monitor" (abdominal induction plethysmograph) for providing feedback of respiratory kinematics.

Phonatory and articulatory kinematics. Phonation and articulation have received attention as a possible cause of stuttering, as they are altered in many stuttering patients (Molt, 2005). Its modification has been the basis of several therapy approaches:

- *Training of gentle/gradual phonatory onset.* CAFET and Dr. Fluency programs use acoustic monitoring devices for providing real-time feedback of voice onset and characteristics: patterns, duration and amplitude.
- *Training of sustained (continual) phonation.* The "Vocal tactile Feedback Method and Associated Apparatus" (US Patent 4685448, 1987) places a vibrotactile apparatus around the neck for helping to keep a continuous phonation pattern, thanks to the vibration of the device. Recently, transcutaneous electrical nerve stimulation has replaced vibratory signal in the EZ-Speech Sustained Phonation Unit (SPU). We can cite also the Stutter-Free Program (Shames & Florance, 1980).
- *Articulatory tension, timing, and (or) duration.* As stuttering is often accompanied by muscle tension in different structures, EMG measurements provide information which can be used in the training to reduce such tension. Several studies have reported a reduction in frequency of stuttering and tension in different structures, as laryngeal area, lips and jaws.
- *Pacing/Timing devices.* Rhythmic speaking techniques have been focused as an important point of therapy since more than a century (G. A. Lewis, 1897). The *orthophonic lyre* was commercialized in 1830. This is a mechanical metronome which allows the regulation of the speech rhythm. Electronic metronomes became very popular as therapy devices for stuttering in the 60's and 70's. They provide a pacing and rhythmic effect which slows patient's speech to the rhythmic beat, increasing fluency. Several works support the device effectiveness (Beech & Fransella, 1968; Berman & Brady, 1973; Wohl, 1968). Tactual metronomes have been used in stuttering therapy, providing rhythmic vibrotactile pulses instead of auditory signals (Azrin, Jones, & Flye, 1968).

As mentioned in the previous section, there is no evidence that the improvements achieved by these approaches are truly caused by logopedic corrections. In fact, such improvements are probably due to an increase of self-confidence.

An Adaptive Version of AAF: A Bridge to Control Technologies

In the section concerning the implications of our model on treatments was justified the adaptive AAF (A-AAF)) approach because of the accommodative character of sensory system, together with the dependence of stuttering severity on environmental changes. The adaptive version of AAF attempts to improve the effectiveness of the AAF algorithm through the modification of its parameters, according to subject state information (Prado & Roa, 2007). This adaptation pursues an increase in subject's fluency, both external (perceived by the listener) and internal. This new approach takes in consideration the variable character of the stuttering severity for a given subject, in different surroundings, situations, etc., and would led to a substantial advance respect to current devices.

The achievement of a quality real-time quantification of stuttering severity is a key point in the reliability of the A-AAF algorithm. The concept of stuttering severity is not new, and it has been analyzed and discussed in different works (Ludlow, 1990). We can apply different methods to assess stuttering severity. Among these methods, probably the most common is the measurement of stuttering frequency through the quantification of the percentage of stuttered syllables (%SS). However, this measurement just provides information about the number of instances of blocks, and such frequencies are not highly correlated with the internal tension (Charles Van Riper, 1982) and blocking qualia.

Another method to assess stuttering severity is the duration of stuttering, i.e., the percentage of dysfluent speaking-time (C.W. Starkweather, Gottwald, & Halfond, 1990), but this measurement is difficult and time-consuming (Alm, 2005). Several rating scales have been proposed to classify stuttering severity. A scale with a 7-point with four separate concept groups (frequency of stuttering, level of struggle or tension, mean duration of instances of stuttering and level of postponement-avoidance) was proposed in (Charles Van Riper, 1982). A simpler scale with points labelled "mild" and "severe" was proposed in (Martin, Haroldson, & Woessner, 1988). Other method to quantify the stuttering severity is the Stuttering Severity Instrument (SSI) (Riley, 1972). This method evaluates three aspects on a 5-point scale: the percent of stuttered syllables, the estimated length of the three longest blocks and the percent rating of associated behaviours. However, its validity and reliability has been questioned (K. E. Lewis, 1995; Mowrer, 1991).

Probably, the most accurate method is the combination of two or more aspects of stuttering. For example, (Alm, 2005) hypothesized that the severity of stuttering can be described by the proportion of speech time with symptoms of stuttering and the instance of the highest level of superfluous muscular activity of speech, on a rating scale ranging from 0 to 7.

Signal-processing techniques have been successfully applied in screening speech disorders in the last two decades. Voice analysis, EEG analysis and EMG analysis, separately or combined, are appropriate for the assessment of stuttering severity. Furthermore, these techniques can be complemented with kinematic analysis, taking into account the presence of some motor tics suffered by stuttering subjects in severe phases.

- Voice analysis

Acoustic measurement is a non-invasive technique. As a consequence, it is often used for screening and monitoring speech disorders. Furthermore, its effectiveness in speech processing has been demonstrated in a number of works (Baken & Orlikoff, 2000; Eskenazi & Childers, 1990; Klingholz, 1990; Parsa & Jamieson, 2001).

The control of delay and frequency in a A-AAF defined by a combination of DAF and FAF requires the recognition of words and phrases, which can be achieved through a multimodal architecture as presented in (Prado & Roa, 2007). To extract such acoustic characteristics from speech there are two classical approaches: the sustained vowels (Parsa & Jamieson, 2000; Umapathy & Krishnan, 2005) and the continuous speech segments (Hammarberg, Fritzell, Gauffin, Sundberg, & Wedin, 1980; Qi, Hillman, & Milstein, 1999).

Signals involved in the sustained vowel method are controllable and well structured, and their processing is easier. Its main drawback is the loss of the dynamics. In the continuous speech method, on the other hand, it is usually required the segmentation of signals because of its non-stationary nature. However, this difficult has been recently overcome through various computationally efficient time-frequency techniques. Continuous speech approach is expected to achieve an accurate and realistic assessment of pathological speech.

A number of approaches that promise the recognition of voice disorders have been proposed in recent years. Among these, we can cite a neural network based classifier (Godino-Llorente & Gomez-Vilda, 2004), or a classification of pathological speech signals using a local discriminant bases (LDB) algorithm (Umapathy & Krishnan, 2005).

Wavelet transform technique has also been proposed for signal analysis in various speech applications with success. Its multi-resolution capability is appropriate for speech and audio applications. Several works using wavelet approaches for speech coding, enhancement, and classification have been reported (Hsieh, Lai, Chen, & Wan, 2002; Najih, Ramli, Ibrahim, & Syed, 2003; Veselinovic & Graupe, 2003). However, the optimum choice of a wavelet (bases functions) for speech applications remains inconclusive.

- EEG

The electroencephalogram (EEG) technique records the oscillations of brain electric potential recorded from electrodes placed on the human scalp. It provides large-scale measurements of neocortical dynamics function. Robust correlations among EEG signal and different cognitive processes associated with mental calculations, working memory and selective attention, have been observed (Nunez & Srinivasan, 2006).

The EEG activity of people who stutter can provide invaluable information about the severity of subject's stuttering. Effect of stuttering in evoked potentials and EEG was investigated in (Khedr, El-Nasser, Haleem, Bakr, & Trakhan, 2000), finding a reduction of amplitude of visual evoked potentials (P100), as well as a significant prolongation of wave (I, III, V) and interpeak (I-III and I-V) latencies in brainstem auditory evoked potentials compared with the control group. Furthermore, they found the dominant EEG rhythm was slower in stutterers with a significant inter-hemispheric asymmetry. The discoveries of that study correlate EEG recordings with stuttering severity, and point to the possibility of evaluating the stuttering severity of a subject in real-time.

Achim and colleagues placed EEG electrodes at inferior frontal, precentral, and tempo-parietal locations on each hemiscalp of both five right-handed dysfluent speakers and fluent speakers. They found that dysfluent speakers presented overall smaller contingent negative variations (CNVs[1]) that were more marked over the right hemisphere than left (Achim, Braun, & Collin, 2008).

The main drawback of the EEG analysis is the presence of artefacts during stuttered speech that mask the signal of interest. Their sources are mainly due to speech musculature, ocular activity, or face tension. Some recent works have shown the possibility of removing them during stuttering (Tran, Craig, Boord, & Craig, 2004).

- EMG

Electromyography (EMG) is the study of muscle function through its electrical activation. EMG signal can be analyzed to detect neuromuscular functions and diseases or analyze the biomechanics of human movement (including vocal cords), so it can be applied in areas such as computer human interface and in developing intelligent prosthetic devices. Usually their measurements are carried out by surface contact sensors and the electrical signals are transformed into patterns.

Several authors provided the first approaches on the use of EMG to analyze stuttering in the early 70's (Cross, 1977; Guitar, 1975; Hanna, Wilfling, & McNeil, 1975; Lanyon, 1977).

A work of Kumar and colleagues performed the recognition of human speech through an artificial neural network based on EMG recordings acquired from three articulatory facial muscles. The reported results showed an accuracy of 88% (Kumar, Kumar, Alemu, & Burry, 2004). EMG signals have also been applied in subauditory (or unvoiced) speech recognition, interpreting the nervous system signals sent to muscles of vocal tract and providing valuable information complementary to other techniques, such as EEG (C. C. Jorgensen, Lee, & Agabon, 2003). Subauditory speech recognition is targeted for use in acoustically noisy environments (C. Jorgensen & Betts, 2006), and may be helpful for stuttering patients.

These results show the feasibility to extract information about stuttering severity through EMG. For example, EMG signals could assist to detect silent block events, which can be removed then by MAF (Kehoe, 2008).

A Multimodal Wearable Sensor: Actuator Computational Architecture

The A-AAF device is based on the computational architecture depicted in Figure 3. This is an evolution of the technological system presented previously (Prado & Roa, 2007). The system has been designed on the basis of our experience with multimodal intelligent wearable systems for telehealthcare (Prado-Velasco, del Río-Cidoncha, & Ortiz-Marín, 2008). A multimodal intelligent wearable system is composed by a Smartphone that acts as the main node of a wireless personal area network (WPAN) and several intelligent sensors and actuators that act as wireless nodes in WPAN.

Intelligent sensors (IS) acquire biosignals, perform a personalized pre-processing of them, and send results towards the Smartphone. Intelligent actuators (IA) implement personalized and adaptive algorithms on the basis of the inputs from Smartphone, and execute actuations on the target. Any IS or IA device includes sensors or effectors, a microcontroller for operation and signal processing, a wireless transceiver and the associated antenna, and the auxiliary circuitry that depends on their particular functions. The ability of IS and IA to be adapted to the subject and context evolution depends on the processing capacity of the microcontroller.

The operation methodology of this type of multimodal intelligent wearable system is able to reduce the dimensionality of the data to be processed by the Smartphone, making easier to adopt a real time processing approach. It is also

Figure 3. Simplified block diagram of an A-AAF device. IHS and ISs are shown to illustrate the functional devices. In the clockwise, starting above the WPAN label: "In the canal (ITC)" DAF-FAF device from SpeechEasy™, a SmartPhone, a commercial MEMS accelerometer sensor, hybrid EEG sensor adapted from http://www.sensorsmag.com/, and a multiuse EMG electrode

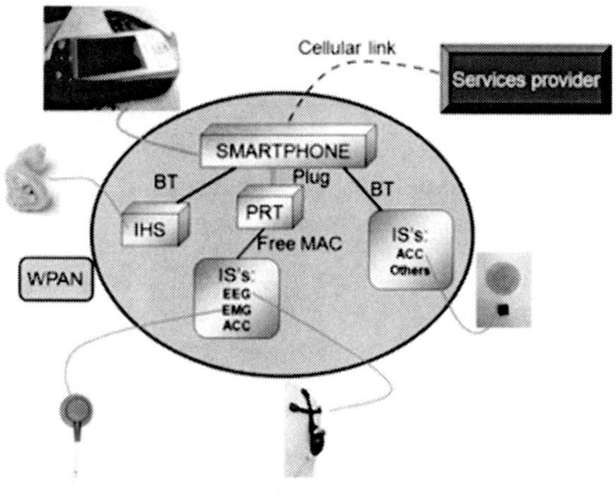

an efficient architecture with the aim of reducing power consumption, circuit sizes, resources allocation, and communication channel capacity requirements (Prado, Reina-Tosina, & Roa, 2002). It allows also the fusion of multimodal data and the design of prosthetic and therapeutic systems that require feedback from multimodal sources.

Our A-AAF is a particular intelligent wearable system composed by the Smartphone, an intelligent headset (IHS) and optionally several ISs to acquire EEG, EMG, and body kinematics through accelerometers based on micro-electromechanical systems (MEMS).

The IHS implements the A-AAF algorithm according to the parameters sent by Smartphone. It comprises an intelligent sensor (microphone) and actuator (speaker) in one autonomous node of WPAN. We have a preliminary design based on a programmable single-chip Bluetooth 2.1 (EDR compliant) solution with on-chip and specialized Digital Signal Processor (DSP), stereo CODEC, and Flash, on-chip lithium battery charger, and DC-DC converter (BlueCore5-Multimedia integrated circuit, http://www.csr.com/ products/bc5range.htm). This is a low cost integrated circuit designed especially for high-end headsets.

The IHS architecture has been defined with the aim of separating the execution of the more basic AAF algorithm from the more advanced features of our device, which are the reactivity to the subject's state through the adaptive parameters of the algorithm, and the possibility to turn off/on some of them (e.g. masking), as a function of the stuttering degree and state. This manner, the IHS is able to perform the basic AAF, whereas the adaptive function is implemented in the Smartphone and supported by data acquired from ISs, included the IHS. Figure 3 shows, as an example, an IHS from SpeechEasy™ (http://www.speecheasy.com/). That is an "In the canal (ITC)" DAF-FAF device cited in the previous Section.

The minimal A-AAF solution is composed by the IHS and the Smartphone, since the technology of these elements allows a discrete design that can be used by the PDS user in any place. However, there is an intense research to achieve wearable and discrete EEG and EMG electrodes, promoted by the last European framework and national programs. As an example, Figure 3 shows an image of a hybrid EEG electrode from Quatum Applied Science & Research (QUASAR). That sensor addresses the problem of triboelectric effect in capacity electrodes by means of a set of "fingers" that reach through hair the scalp. Several relevant international projects are addressing other issues concerning the wearable ability of EEG and EMG electrodes (Casson, Smith, Duncan, & Rodriguez-Villega, 2008).

At the moment, the more complex A-AAF, including EEG and EMG intelligent sensors, is thought to be experimented in a laboratory environment. These ISs will provide relevant information concerning the stuttering severity, associated with neuronal correlates and muscular activity of speech, together with body kinematics in selected segments. That information will optimize the feedback and this way the performance of the adaptive function of the A-AAF.

The adaptive function of the A-AAF device is supported by a multilevel mathematical model that describes the neuronal dynamics of the regions involved in stuttering according to the hypothesis developed in the earlier Section. This model will be developed following an approach similar to that presented by (Izhikevich & Edelman, 2008). However, we will extract a personalized reduced-form of the main model that will be able to run in real-time into the Smartphone, using proper techniques (Bassingthwaighte, Chizeck, & Atlas, 2006).

This methodology was designed with the aim of generating customized knowledge of a chronic patient on a telehealthcare system (Prado, Roa, et al., 2002). It is characterized by the presence of a computational component, called Patient Physiological Image (PPI), which comprises a systemic mathematical model of a patient, and evolves together with him by means of monitored biosignals and other biomedical parameters.

Intelligent sensors and actuators communicate with the Smartphone in the WPAN by two types of wireless technologies: Bluetooth (BT) standard and free Media Access Control (MAC), as a function of the power consumption requirement and autonomy that is required. Current BT technology (v 2.1) allows data transmission up to 3 Mbps, with a typical power consumption of 100 mw, whereas other well-known transmission technology for personal area networks, Zigbee, provides only 0.2 Mbps with 30 mw. Moreover, the specification BT v3.0+HS (based on a UWB modulation technology), is near to be released. This will provide up to 54 Mbps in the same radio frequency band (2.4 GHz), including also a cleaner band (5 GHz) (http://bluetooth.com/). Power consumption in the later will be also low. Interestingly, the Bluetooth Special Interest Group (SIG) is working since 2007 to develop an ultra-low-power version of BT with consumptions like Zigbee, but able to communicate with other BT devices. This technology, previously denoted as Wibree, was considered in (Prado & Roa, 2007). Moreover, BT has been approved by the Continua Health Alliance, an industry coalition of health care and technology companies charged with establishing a system of interoperable personal telehealthcare solutions, as the standard for device interoperability. All these facts compelled us to select Bluetooth for data transmission within the WPAN of A-AAF, for audio or other signals whose frequency sampling overpass clearly 1 - 10 KS/s. This is the case of IHS and some accelerometer sensors (ACC) with specialized functions (see Figure 3).

We have selected a free MAC technology for signals whose sampling frequencies are lower than 10^2 S/s. Zigbee has been rejected, in opposition to our initial proposal in (Prado & Roa, 2007), because the ratio data rate / power consumption is poor (Jin-Shyan, Yu-Wei, & Chung-Chou, 2007). This way EEG, EMG, and the most ACC intelligent sensors use Free MAC in our current architecture (see Figure 3).

Accordingly, ISs with free MAC communication technology are based on the new CC981H Sensium family (previously denoted TZ1030). This is an ultralow power system on chip, including a digital subsystem with the 8051 microprocessor, a very efficient (4 mw) integrated transceiver with 50 kbps data rate (ISM bands), program and data memory, and an 11-bit sigma delta ADC. This IC was designed by Toumaz™ for multimodal monitoring in body area networks applications, and it was also selected by our group (as TZ1030) for a new falling detector based on a triaxial accelerometer sensor (Prado-Velasco, et al., 2008).

The cellular link of Figure 3 is an optional feature of our A-AAF device, which allows sending and even taking feedback from a services provider, where data obtained from the intelligent sensors can feed a more complex multilevel mathematical model. This function extends the A-AAF to be a module of a telehealthcare system, providing richer information and knowledge to professionals and facilitating the development of research studies.

The A-AAF architecture is being developed in two stages. In the first one, a standard headset will be selected and the A-AAF algorithm will be implemented in the Smartphone, together with the adaptive functions. This first prototype pursues the analysis of the current limitations of headsets due to wireless technology, operating systems in the Smartphone (windows mobile, Symbian, Palm, etc.), and processing capacity of the core.

The complete architecture will be developed in a second stage, including the IHS and the others ISs.

SUMMARY AND CONCLUSION

Despite centuries of research the etiology of persistent developmental stuttering is still unknown. Current discoveries based on modern neuroimaging techniques have shown a new and exciting perspective of earlier ideas and hypotheses, but it seems now clear that it is needed a new approach to understand the nature of the disorder (Fox, 2003).

This work presents a new etiological model of persistent developmental stuttering, based on a deep analysis of earlier models and on the stuttering phenomenology, described in basic, clinical, and even ethnographic sources. Our model was developed taking the Occam's razor as criterion for avoiding unnecessary intricacies. One of the more stimulating conclusions has been the suggestion that stuttering is a non-speech based disorder, in opposition to the accepted belief. This is supported by a number of works concerning different expressive communication tasks, including sign language, playing an instrument or handwriting (Snyder, 2006).

The model has guided the design of our new prosthetic and therapeutic device. It is based in the hypothesis of the dynamic core (Edelman & Tononi, 2000; Giulio Tononi & Edelman, 1998), which facilitates the development of the adaptive AAF technology, using neural complexity and other measures over the Patient Physiological Image (PPI) approach (Prado, Roa, et al., 2002). The PPI is a computational component founded on a multilevel systemic mathematical model that it is customized for a user, and executed in an autonomous manner, evolving together with him.

A relevant feature of the PPI approach is the ability to integrate the feedback data into the multilevel mathematical model to generate knowledge, which is used in turn to improve, validate, or reject the hypothesized causal mechanisms. This methodology fills the gap between the therapeutic and prosthetic techniques to treat the stuttering, and the scientific basis on which they must be based, and supposes a new perspective to throw light on the nature of the disorder.

We have presented the preliminary design and computational architecture of the adaptive AAF device. It is being developed within a research project with two technological stages, above described, plus a third line devoted to the research and development of the mathematical model of a neuronal system that embraces the regions involved in stuttering. With that objective, we will take into account the last large-scale neuroanatomic model of (Izhikevich & Edelman, 2008) as reference, together with modern techniques for building reduced-form models (Bassingthwaighte, et al., 2006).

ACKNOWLEDGMENT

We are grateful to Dr. José Ignacio Piruat Palomo, senior researcher of the Institute for Biomedical Research of Seville (IBiS) of the University Hospital Virgen del Rocio, for his valuable comments concerning neuroanatomic details of our stuttering model.

REFERENCES

Achim, A., Braun, C. M. J., & Collin, I. (2008). Event-Related Potentials Distinguish Fluent and Stuttered Speech. *Journal of Neurotherapy, 11*(3), 15–23. doi:10.1080/10874200802126118

Adams, M. R., & Hayden, P. (1976). The Ability of Stutterers and Nonstutterers to Initiate and Terminate Phonation during Production of an Isolated Vowel. *The Journal of Speech and Hearing Disorders, 19*(2), 290–296.

Alm, P. A. (2005). *On the causal mechanisms of stuttering*. Lund, Sweden: Lund University.

Andrews, G., Craig, A., Feyer, A., Hoddinott, S., Howie, P., & Neilson, M. (1983). Stuttering: a review of research findings and theories circa 1982. *The Journal of Speech and Hearing Disorders, 48*(3), 226–246.

Armson, J., Foote, S., Witt, C., Kalinowski, J., & Stuart, A. (1997). Effect of frequency altered feedback and audience size on stuttering. *European Journal of Disorders of communication. The Journal of the College of Speech and Language Therapists*, *32*(3), 359–366.

Armson, J., Kiefte, M., Mason, J., & De Croos, D. (2006). The effect of SpeechEasy on stuttering frequency in laboratory conditions. *Journal of Fluency Disorders*, *31*(2), 137–152. doi:10.1016/j.jfludis.2006.04.004

Armson, J., & Stuart, A. (1998). Effect of extended exposure to frequency-altered feedback on stuttering during reading and monologue. *Journal of Speech, Language, and Hearing Research: JSLHR*, *41*(3), 479–490.

Azrin, N., Jones, R. J., & Flye, B. (1968). A synchronization effect and its application to stuttering by a portable apparatus. *Journal of Applied Behavior Analysis*, *1*(4), 283–295. doi:10.1901/jaba.1968.1-283

Bajaj, A., Hodson, B., & Westby, C. (2005). Communicative ability conceptions among children who stutter and their fluent peers: A qualitative exploration. *Journal of Fluency Disorders*, *30*(1), 41–64. doi:10.1016/j.jfludis.2005.01.002

Baken, R. J., & Orlikoff, R. F. (2000). *Clinical measurements of speech and voice*. San Diego, CA: Singular Thomson Learning.

Barbara, D. (1954). *Stuttering: a psychodynamic approach to its understanding and treatment*. New York: Julian Publishers.

Barker, R. A., & Barasi, S. (1999). *Nuroscience at a Glance*. Blackwell Science.

Bassingthwaighte, J. B., Chizeck, H. J., & Atlas, L. E. (2006). Strategies and Tactics in Multiscale Modeling of Cell-to-Organ Systems. *Proceedings of the IEEE*, *94*(4), 819–831. doi:10.1109/JPROC.2006.871775

Beech, H. R., & Fransella, F. (1968). Explanations of the rhythm effect in stuttering. In B. B. E. Gray, G. (Ed.), *Stuttering and the Conditioning Therapies*. Monterey: The Monterey Institute for Speech and Hearing.

Berman, P. A., & Brady, J. P. (1973). Miniaturized metronomes in the treatment of stuttering: A survey of clinician's experiences. *Journal of Behavior Therapy and Experimental Psychiatry*, *4*(117-119).

Blomgren, M., Roy, N., Callister, T., & Merrill, R. M. (2005). Intensive Stuttering Modification Therapy: A Multidimensional Assessment of Treatment Outcomes. *Journal of Speech, Language, and Hearing Research: JSLHR*, *48*(3), 509. doi:10.1044/1092-4388(2005/035)

Bloodstein, O. (1981). *A handbook of stuttering*. Chicago: National Easter Seal Society.

Bloodstein, O. (1995). *A Handbook on Stuttering*.

Bloodstein, O. (2006). Some empirical observations about early stuttering: a possible link to language development. *Journal of Communication Disorders*, *39*(3), 185–191. doi:10.1016/j.jcomdis.2005.11.007

Bluemel, C. S. (1931). Stammering as an impediment of thought. *Journal of the American Medical Association*, *96*(22), 1846–1848.

Bobrick, B. (1996). *Knotted Tongues: Stuttering in History and the Quest for a Cure*. Kodansha Amer Inc.

Bothe, A. K., Finn, P., & Bramlett, R. E. (2007). Pseudoscience and the SpeechEasy: Reply to Kalinowski, Saltuklaroglu, Stuart, and Guntupalli. *American Journal of Speech-Language Pathology*, *16*, 77–83. doi:10.1044/1058-0360(2007/010)

Brown, S., Ingham, R., Ingham, J., Laird, A., & Fox, P. (2005). Stuttered and fluent speech production: an ALE meta-analysis of functional neuroimaging studies. *Human Brain Mapping*, *25*(1), 105–117. doi:10.1002/hbm.20140

Bryngelson, B., & Clark, T. B. (1933). Left-handedness and stuttering. *The Journal of Heredity*, *24*(10), 387–390.

Büchel, C., & Sommer, M. (2004). What Causes Stuttering? *PLoS Biology*, *2*(2), e46. doi:10.1371/journal.pbio.0020046

Callan, D., Tsytsarev, V., Hanakawa, T., Callan, A., Katsuhara, M., & Fukuyama, H. (2006). Song and speech: brain regions involved with perception and covert production. *NeuroImage*, *31*(3), 1327–1342. doi:10.1016/j.neuroimage.2006.01.036

Casson, A., Smith, S., Duncan, J., & Rodriguez-Villega, E. (2008). *Wearable EEG: what is it, why is it needed and what does it entail?* Paper presented at the Conf Proc IEEE Eng Med Biol Soc.

Chervin, A. (1896). *(Suttering and other pronunciation defects) Tartamudez y otros defectos de pronunciación*. Paris: Société d'Éditions Scientifiques.

Craig, A. (1998). Relapse following treatment for stuttering: a critical review and correlative data. *Journal of Fluency Disorders*, *23*(1), 1–30. doi:10.1016/S0094-730X(97)00027-2

Craig, A. (2000). The Developmental Nature and Effective Treatment of Stuttering in Children and Adolescents. *Journal of Developmental and Physical Disabilities*, *12*(3), 173–186. doi:10.1023/A:1009463703647

Cross, D. E. (1977). Effects of false increasing, decreasing, and true electromyographic biofeedback on the frequency of stuttering. *Journal of Fluency Disorders*, *2*(2), 109–116. doi:10.1016/0094-730X(77)90014-6

Curry, F. K. W., & Gregory, H. H. (1969). The Performance of Stutterers on Dichotic Listening Tasks Thought to Reflect Cerebral Dominance. *Journal of Speech and Hearing Research*, *12*(1), 73–82.

Derazne, J. (1966). *Speech Pathology in the U.S.S.R.* Amsterdam: North Holland.

Dewar, A., & Dewar, A. D. (1979). The long-term use of an automatically triggered auditory feedback-masking device in the treatment of stammering. *The British Journal of Disorders of Communication*, *14*, 219–229. doi:10.3109/13682827909011361

Dodge, D. M. (2009, May 11). *A Reactive Inhibition Model of Stuttering Development & Behavior: A Neuropsychological Theory Based on Recent Research*. Retrieved August 27, 2009 from http://www.veilsofstuttering.com/reactinh.html

Edelman, G. M., & Tononi, G. (2000). *A Universe of Consciousness: How matter becomes imagination*. New York: Basic Books.

Eskenazi, L., & Childers, D. G. (1990). Acoustic correlates of vocal quality. *Journal of Speech and Hearing Research*, *33*, 298–306.

Fenichel, O. (1945). *The psychoanalytic theory of neurosis*. New York: Norton.

Fields, R. (2008). White matter in learning, cognition and psychiatric disorders. *Trends in Neurosciences*, *31*(7), 361–370. doi:10.1016/j.tins.2008.04.001

Foundas, A. L., Bollich, A. M., Corey, D. M., Hurley, M., & Heilman, K. M. (2001). Anomalous anatomy of speech–language areas in adults with persistent developmental stuttering. *Neurology*, *57*, 207–215.

Foundas, A. L., Bollich, A. M., Feldman, J., Corey, D. M., Hurley, M., & Lemen, L. C. (2004). Aberrant auditory processing and atypical planum temporale in developmental stuttering. *Neurology*, *63*(9), 1640–1646.

Fox, P. T. (2003). Brain imaging in stuttering: where next? *Journal of Fluency Disorders*, *28*(4), 265–272. doi:10.1016/j.jfludis.2003.08.001

Fox, P. T., Ingham, R. J., Ingham, J. C., Hirsch, T. B., Downs, J. H., & Martin, C. (1996). A PET study of the neural systems of stuttering. *Nature*, *382*(6587), 158–162. doi:10.1038/382158a0

Friedman, A., Fetterman, E., & Jolson, Y. (1999). *Dr. Fluency Computerized Stuttering Treatment Program User's Guide (Version 2.3)*. Jerusalem, Israel: Speech Therapy Systems, Ltd.

Friedman, S. (1990). *Cartas con un paciente (coautor). Un proceso de terapia para la tartamudez*. Valencia: Promolibro.

García Mila, M. (1987). *Aproximación al síntoma desde una perspectiva de orientación psicoanalítica.* Paper presented at the La tartamudez, IV Simposio.

Gateley, G. (2003). *Johnson's diagnosogenic theory of stuttering: an update*. Retrieved March 22 from http://www.thefreelibrary.com/Johnson's diagnosogenic theory of stuttering: an update

Godino-Llorente, J. I., & Gomez-Vilda, P. (2004). Automatic Detection of Voice Impairments by Means of Short-Term Cepstral Parameters and Neural Network Based Detectors. *IEEE Transactions on Bio-Medical Engineering*, *51*, 380–384. doi:10.1109/TBME.2003.820386

Goebel, M. D. (1986). *A computer-aided fluency establishment trainer*. Annadale Fluency Clinic.

Goldiamond, I., Atkinson, C. J., & Bilger, R. C. (1962). Stabilization of Behavior and Prolonged Exposure to Delayed Auditory Feedback. *Science*, *135*(3502), 437–438. doi:10.1126/science.135.3502.437

Gruart, A., Munoz, M. D., & Delgado-Garcia, J. M. (2006). Involvement of the CA3-CA1 Synapse in the Acquisition of Associative Learning in Behaving Mice. *The Journal of Neuroscience*, *26*(4), 1077–1087. doi:10.1523/JNEUROSCI.2834-05.2006

Guitar, B. (1975). Reduction of stuttering frequency using analog electromyographic feedback. *The Journal of Speech and Hearing Disorders*, *18*(4), 672–685.

Guitar, B. (1998). *Stuttering: An integrated approach to its nature and treatment*. Baltimore, Maryland: Williams y Wilkins.

Hahn, E. F. (1956). *Stuttering: significant theories and therapies* (2nd ed.). Stanford University Press.

Hammarberg, B., Fritzell, B., Gauffin, J., Sundberg, J., & Wedin, L. (1980). Perceptual and acoustic correlates of abnormal voice qualities. *Acta Oto-Laryngologica*, *90*(1), 441–451. doi:10.3109/00016488009131746

Hanna, R., Wilfling, F., & McNeil, B. (1975). A biofeedback treatment for stuttering. *The Journal of Speech and Hearing Disorders*, *18*(2), 270–273.

Hardyck, C., & Petrinovich, L. F. (1977). Left Handedness. *Psychological Bulletin*, *84*(3), 385–404. doi:10.1037/0033-2909.84.3.385

Hargrave, S., Kalinowski, J., Stuart, A., Armson, J., & Jones, K. (1994). Effect of frequency-altered feedback on stuttering frequency at normal and fast speech rates. *Journal of Speech, Language, and Hearing Research: JSLHR*, *37*(6), 1313–1319.

Harrington, J. (1988). Stuttering, delayed auditory feedback, and linguistic rhythm. *Journal of Speech and Hearing Research*, *31*(1), 36–47.

Hashimoto, Y., & Sakai, K. L. (2003). Brain Activations During Conscious Self-Monitoring of Speech Production With Delayed Auditory Feedback: An fMRI Study. *Human Brain Mapping, 20*, 22–28. doi:10.1002/hbm.10119

Hayhow, R., Cray, A., & Enderby, P. (2002). Stammering and therapy views of people who stammer. *Journal of Fluency Disorders, 27*(1), 1–16, quiz 16–17. doi:10.1016/S0094-730X(01)00102-4

Hill, H. E. (1954). An Experimental Study of Disorganization Of Speech And Manual Responses In Normal Subjects. *The Journal of Speech and Hearing Disorders, 19*(3), 295–305.

Howell, P. (2002). The EXPLAN theory of fluency control applied to the treatment of stuttering. In Fava, E. (Ed.), *Clinical Linguistics. Theory and applications in speech pathology and therapy* (pp. 95–115). Amsterdam: John Benjamins.

Howell, P., & El-Yaniv, N. (1987). The effects of presenting a click in syllable-initial position on the speech of stutterers: Comparison with a metronome click. *Journal of Fluency Disorders, 12*, 249–256. doi:10.1016/0094-730X(87)90003-9

Howell, P., Wingfield, T., & Johnson, M. (1988). *Characteristics of the speech of stutterers during normal and altered auditory feedback.* Paper presented at the 7th Federation of Acoustical Societies of Europe Conference, Edinburgh.

Hsieh, C.-T., Lai, E., Chen, W.-C., & Wan, Y.-C. (2002). *Compact speech features based on wavelet transform and PCA with application to speaker identification.* Paper presented at the International Symposium on Chinese Spoken Language Processing

Ingham, R. J., & Bothe, A. K. (2001). Recovery from early stuttering: Additional issues within the Onslow & Packman-Yairi & Ambrose (1999) exchange. *Journal of Speech, Language, and Hearing Research: JSLHR, 44*(4), 862. doi:10.1044/1092-4388(2001/068)

Ingham, R. J., Moglia, R. A., Frank, P., Ingham, J. C., & Cordes, A. K. (1997). Experimental investigation of the effects of frequency-altered auditory feedback on the speech of adults who stutter. *Journal of Speech, Language, and Hearing Research: JSLHR, 40*(2), 361–372.

Ingham, R. J., Warner, A., Byrd, A., & Cotton, J. (2006). Speech Effort Measurement and Stuttering: Investigating the Chorus Reading Effect. *Journal of Speech, Language, and Hearing Research: JSLHR, 49*(3), 660. doi:10.1044/1092-4388(2006/048)

Izhikevich, E. M., & Edelman, G. M. (2008). Large-scale model of mammalian thalamocortical systems. *Proceedings of the National Academy of Sciences of the United States of America, 105*(9), 3593–3598. doi:10.1073/pnas.0712231105

Jhou, T. (2005). Neural mechanisms of freezing and passive aversive behaviors. *The Journal of Comparative Neurology, 493*(1), 111–114. doi:10.1002/cne.20734

Jin-Shyan, L., Yu-Wei, S., & Chung-Chou, S. (2007). *A Comparative Study of Wireless Protocols: Bluetooth, UWB, ZigBee, and Wi-Fi.* Paper presented at the Industrial Electronics Society, 2007. IECON 2007. 33rd Annual Conference of the IEEE.

Johnson, W. (1942). A study of the onset and development of stuttering. *The Journal of Speech Disorders, 7*, 251–257.

Johnson, W. (1959). *The onset of stuttering.* Minneapolis, MN: University of Minneapolis Press.

Jones, M., Onslow, M., Packman, A., Williams, S., Ormond, T., & Schwarz, I. (2005). Randomised controlled trial of the Lidcombe programme of early stuttering intervention. *BMJ (Clinical Research Ed.), 331*(7518), 659. doi:10.1136/bmj.38520.451840.E0

Jones, R. K. (1966). Observations on stammering after localized cerebral injury. *Journal of Neurology, Neurosurgery, and Psychiatry*, *29*(3), 192–195. doi:10.1136/jnnp.29.3.192

Jorgensen, C., & Betts, B. (2006). *Multimodal Platform Control for Robotic Planetary Exploration Missions*. Paper presented at the Second International Conference on Space Mission Challenges for Information Technology.

Jorgensen, C. C., Lee, D., & Agabon, S. (2003). *Subauditory Speech Recognition based on EMG/EPG Signals*.

Kalinowski, J., Armson, J., Roland-Mieszkowski, M., Stuart, A., & Gracco, V. L. (1993). Effects of alterations in auditory feedback and speech rate on stuttering frequency. *Language and Speech*, *36*, 1–16.

Kalinowski, J., Guntupalli, V. K., Stuart, A., & Saltuklaroglu, T. (2004). Self-reported efficacy of an ear-level prosthetic device that delivers altered auditory feedback for the management of stuttering. *International Journal of Rehabilitation Research. Internationale Zeitschrift fur Rehabilitationsforschung. Revue Internationale de Recherches de Readaptation*, *27*(2), 167–170. doi:10.1097/01.mrr.0000128063.76934.df

Kalinowski, J., & Saltuklaroglu, T. (2003). Speaking with a mirror: engagement of mirror neurons via choral speech and its derivatives induces stuttering inhibition. *Medical Hypotheses*, *60*(4), 538–543. doi:10.1016/S0306-9877(03)00004-5

Kalinowski, J., & Stuart, A. (1996). Stuttering amelioration at various auditory feedback delays and speech rates. *European Journal of Disorders of Communication: The Journal of the College of Speech and Language Therapists*, *31*(3), 259–269.

Kalinowski, J., Stuart, A., Rastatter, M., Miller, R., Zimmerman, S., & Shine, R. (1998). *Examination of altered auditory feedback: Therapeutic implications*. Paper presented at the Second World Congress on Fluency Disorders, Nijmegen, The Netherlands.

Kalinowski, J., Stuart, A., Wamsley, L., & Rastatter, M. P. (1999). Effects of monitoring condition and frequency-altered feedback on stuttering frequency. *The Journal of Speech and Hearing Disorders*, *42*(6), 1347–1354.

Kehoe, T. D. (2008). *No Miracle Cures: A Multifactoral Guide to Stuttering Therapy*. University College Press.

Khedr, E., El-Nasser, W. A., Haleem, E. K. A., Bakr, M. S., & Trakhan, M. N. (2000). Evoked potentials and electroencephalography in stuttering. *Folia Phoniatrica et Logopaedica*, *52*(4), 178. doi:10.1159/000021532

Kiefte, M., & Armson, J. (2008). Dissecting choral speech: Properties of the accompanist critical to stuttering reduction. *Journal of Communication Disorders*, *41*(1), 33–48. doi:10.1016/j.jcomdis.2007.03.002

Klingholz, F. (1990). Acoustic representation of speaking-voice quality. *Journal of Voice*, *4*(3), 213–219. doi:10.1016/S0892-1997(05)80016-5

Kumar, S., Kumar, D. K., Alemu, M., & Burry, M. (2004). *EMG based voice recognition*. Paper presented at the Intelligent Sensors, Sensor Networks and Information Processing Conference.

Lanyon, R. I. (1977). Effect of biofeedback-based relaxation on stuttering during reading and spontaneous speech. *Journal of Consulting and Clinical Psychology*, *45*(5), 860–866. doi:10.1037/0022-006X.45.5.860

Le Huche, F. (2000). La tartamudez: Opción Curación: Masson.

Lee, B. S. (1951). Artificial stutter. *The Journal of Speech and Hearing Disorders*, *16*, 53–55.

Lewis, G. A. (1897). *The Origin and Treatment of Stammering*. Philadelphia: The Lewis Phono-Metric Institute.

Lewis, G. A. (1906). *The origin and treatment of stammering*. Detroit, Michigan: Photometer Press.

Lewis, K. E. (1995). Do SSI-3 scores adequately reflect observations of stuttering behaviors? *American Journal of Speech-Language Pathology*, *4*, 46–59.

Limongi, F. P., Subramanian, U., Prabhu, B., Ezrati-Vinacour, R., Amir, O., Kenjo, M., et al. (2005). Stuttering Research and Treatment Around the World. The ASHA Leader, 6-41.

Lincoln, M., Packman, A., & Onslow, M. (2006). Altered auditory feedback and the treatment of stuttering: a review. *Journal of Fluency Disorders*, *31*(2), 71–89. doi:10.1016/j.jfludis.2006.04.001

Loriente Zamora, C. (2006). *La tartamudez como fenómeno sociocultural: una alternativa al modelo biomédico*. UNED.

Ludlow, C. (1990). Research procedures for measuring stuttering severity. *ASHA Reports*, *18*, 26–31.

MacLeod, J., Kalinowski, J., Stuart, A., & Armson, J. (1995). Effect of single and combined altered auditory feedback on stuttering frequency at two speech rates. *Journal of Communication Disorders*, *28*, 217–228. doi:10.1016/0021-9924(94)00010-W

Martin, R. R., Haroldson, S. K., & Woessner, G. L. (1988). Perceptual scaling of stuttering severity. *Journal of Fluency Disorders*, *13*(1), 27–47. doi:10.1016/0094-730X(88)90026-5

Max, L., Guenther, F. H., Gracco, V. L., Ghosh, S. S., & Wallace, M. E. (2004). Unstable or Insufficiently Activated Internal Models and Feedback-Biased Motor Control as Sources of Dysfluency: A Theoretical Model of Stuttering. *Contemporary Issues in Communication Science and Disorders*, *31*, 105–122.

May, A., & Hackwood, A. (1968). Some effects of masking and eliminating low frequency feedback on the speech of stammerers. *Behaviour Research and Therapy*, *6*(2), 219–223. doi:10.1016/0005-7967(68)90010-7

Molt, L. (2005). *A Brief Historical Review of Assistive Devices for Treating Stuttering*. Alabama: Auburn University.

Mowrer, D. (1991). Assessment review. Stuttering severity instrument for children and adults. *Journal of Fluency Disorders*, *16*, 311–314. doi:10.1016/0094-730X(91)90043-C

Najih, A. M. M. A., Ramli, A. R., Ibrahim, A., & Syed, A. R. (2003). *Comparing speech compression using wavelets with other speech compression schemes*.

Nessel, E. (1958). Die verogerts sprachruckklopplung (Lee-effect) bei der stotterern. *Folia Phoniatrica et Logopaedica*, *10*, 199–204. doi:10.1159/000262818

Neumann, K., Preibisch, C., Euler, H. A., Gudenberg, A. W. v., Lanfermann, H., & Gall, V. (2005). Cortical plasticity associated with stuttering therapy. *Journal of Fluency Disorders*, *30*(1), 23–39. doi:10.1016/j.jfludis.2004.12.002

NHSC. (2007). *SpeechEasy Wireless Altered-Auditory Feedback (AAF) device for stammer*. National Horizon Scanning Centre, University of Birmingham.

Nunez, P. L., & Srinivasan, R. (2006). *Electric fields of the brain: the neurophysics of EEG*.

O'Donnell, J. J., Armson, J., & Kiefte, M. (2008). The effectiveness of SpeechEasy during situations of daily living. *Journal of Fluency Disorders*, *33*(2), 99–119. doi:10.1016/j.jfludis.2008.02.001

Ordoñez, J. (1956). *(Stuttering) La tartamudez*. Madrid: Studium.

Ornstein, R. (1991). *The evolution of consciousness: the origins of the way we think*. New York: Touchstone.

Orton, S. T. (1927). Studies in Stuttering: Introduction. *Archives of Neurology and Psychiatry*, *18*(5), 671–672.

Parellada, J. (1978). *Las causas de la tartamudez. Vías hacia su corrección*. Barcelona, Spain: Jims.

Parker, C. S., & Christopherson, F. (1963). Electronic aid in treatment of stammer. *Medical Electronics & Biological Engineering*, *1*(2), 121–125. doi:10.1007/BF02474144

Parsa, V., & Jamieson, D. G. (2000). Identification of Pathological Voices Using Glottal Noise Measures. *Journal of Speech, Language, and Hearing Research: JSLHR*, *43*, 469–485.

Parsa, V., & Jamieson, D. G. (2001). Acoustic Discrimination of Pathological Voice. *Journal of Speech, Language, and Hearing Research: JSLHR*, *44*, 327–339. doi:10.1044/1092-4388(2001/027)

Perkins, W., Rudas, J., Johnson, L., & Bell, J. (1976). Stuttering: Discoordination of Phonation with Articulation and Respiration. *Journal of Speech and Hearing Research*, *19*(3), 509–522.

Perkins, W. H. (1996). *Stuttering and Science*. San Diego: Singular Pub. Group.

Perkins, W. H. (2001). Stuttering: A Matter of Bad Timing. *Science*, *294*(5543), 786a. doi:10.1126/science.294.5543.786a

Phelps, E., & LeDoux, J. (2005). Contributions of the amygdala to emotion processing: from animal models to human behavior. *Neuron*, *48*(2), 175–187. doi:10.1016/j.neuron.2005.09.025

Pichon, E., & Borel-Maisonny, S. (1973). *La tartamudez. Naturaleza y tratamiento*. Barcelona: Toray-Masson.

Pollard, R., Ellis, J. B., Finan, D., & Ramig, P. R. (2009). Effects of the SpeechEasy on objective and perceived aspects of stuttering: a 6-month, phase I clinical trial in naturalistic environments. *Journal of Speech and Hearing Research*, *52*(2), 516–533. doi:10.1044/1092-4388(2008/07-0204)

Prado, M., Reina-Tosina, J., & Roa, L. (2002). *Distributed intelligent architecture for falling detection and physical activity analysis in the elderly*. Paper presented at the 24th Annual International Conference of the IEEE-EMBS and Annual Fall Meeting of the BMES.

Prado, M., Roa, L., Reina-Tosina, J., Palma, A., & Milán, J. A. (2002). Virtual Center for Renal Support: Technological Approach to Patient Physiological Image. *IEEE Transactions on Bio-Medical Engineering*, *49*(12), 1420–1430. doi:10.1109/TBME.2002.805454

Prado, M., & Roa, L. M. (2007). [IOS Pres.]. *Wearable Real-time and Adaptive Feedback Device to Face the Stuttering: a Knowledge-based Telehealthcare Proposal Medical and Care Compunetics*, *4*, 147–156.

Prado-Velasco, M., del Río-Cidoncha, M. G., & Ortiz-Marín, R. (2008). *The Inescapable Smart Impact detection System (ISIS): an ubiquitous and personalized fall detector based on a distributed "divide and conquer strategy"*. Paper presented at the Personalized Healthcare through Technology, 30th Annual International Conference of the IEEE Engineering in Medicine and Biology Society

Preibisch, C., Neumann, K., Raab, P., Euler, H., von Gudenberg, A., & Lanfermann, H. (2003). Evidence for compensation for stuttering by the right frontal operculum. *NeuroImage*, *20*(2), 1356–1364. doi:10.1016/S1053-8119(03)00376-8

Qi, Y., Hillman, R. E., & Milstein, C. (1999). The estimation of signal-to-noise ratio in continuous speech for disordered voices. *The Journal of the Acoustical Society of America*, *105*(4), 2532–2535. doi:10.1121/1.426860

Reed, C. F., Tomkins, S. S., & Alexander, I. E. (Eds.). (1958). *Psychopathology: A Source Book*. Harvard University Press.

Reitzes, P., & Snyder, G. (2006). Response to "Intensive Stuttering Modification Therapy: A Multidimensional Assessment of Treatment Outcomes," by Blomgren, Roy, Callister, and Merrill (2005). *Journal of Speech, Language, and Hearing Research: JSLHR*, *49*, 1420–1422. doi:10.1044/1092-4388(2006/103)

Riley, G. D. (1972). A stuttering severity instrument for children and adults. *The Journal of Speech and Hearing Disorders*, *37*, 314–322.

Rius, A. (1897). *La educación de los niños atrasados (cortos de inteligencia, tartamudos, tartajosos, tardos en el habla, etc)*. Barcelona: F. Sánchez.

Rodríguez Carrillo, P. R. (2002). *La tartamudez desde la perspectiva de los tartamudos*. Caracas: Universidad Central de Venezuela.

Rodríguez Morejón, A. (2003). *La tartamudez: naturaleza y tratamiento*. Barcelona: Herder.

Rosenfield, D. B., & Viswanath, N. S. (2002). Neuroscience of Stuttering. *Science*, *295*(5557), 973b. doi:10.1126/science.295.5557.973b

Ryan, B. (2005). Response to Blomgren, Roy, Callister, andMerrill. *Journal of Speech, Language, and Hearing Research: JSLHR*, *49*, 1412–1414. doi:10.1044/1092-4388(2006/101)

Salgado, A. (2005). *Manual práctico de tartamudez*. Madrid: Editorial Síntesis.

Saltuklaroglu, T., & Kalinowski, J. (2006). *Stuttering*.

Santacreu, J., & Fernandez-Zúñiga, A. (1991). Tratamiento De La Tartamudez: Promolibro.

Schwartz, M. F. (1977). *Stottern ist heilbar: neue und erfolgreiche Behandlungsmethoden* [Stutter is more curable: new and successful working methods]. Düsseldorf: Econ.

Shames, G. H., & Florance, C. L. (1980). *Stutter-Free Speech: A Goal for Therapy*.

Shames, G. H., & Sherrick, C. E. (1963). A discussion of nonfluency and stuttering as operant behavior. *The Journal of Speech and Hearing Disorders*, *28*, 3–18.

Sheehan, J. G., & Voas, R. B. (1957). Stuttering As Conflict: 1. Comparison Of Therapy Techniques Involving Approach And Avoidance. *The Journal of Speech and Hearing Disorders*, *22*(5), 714–723.

Snyder, G. (2006). *The Existence of Stuttering in Sign Language and other Forms of Expressive Communication: Sufficient Cause for the Emergence of a New Stuttering Paradigm?* Paper presented at the International Stuttering Awareness Day Online Conference, Mankato, Minnesota State, USA.

Snyder, G. (2009). The Existence of Stuttering in Sign Language and other Forms of Expressive Communication: Sufficient Cause for the Emergence of a New Stuttering Paradigm? *The Journal of Stuttering Therapy. Advocacy & Research*, *3*, 100–107.

Sommer, M., Koch, M., Paulus, W., Weiller, C., & Buchel, C. (2002). Disconnection of speech-relevant brain areas in persistent developmental stuttering. *Lancet*, *360*(9330), 380–383. doi:10.1016/S0140-6736(02)09610-1

Sporns, O., Almassy, N., & Edelman, G. M. (2000). Plasticity in Value Systems and its Role in Adaptive Behavior. *Adaptive Behavior*, *8*(2), 129–148. doi:10.1177/105971230000800203

Starkweather, C. W. (1987). *Fluency and Stuttering*. Englewood Cliffs, New Jersey: Prentice Hall.

Starkweather, C. W., Gottwald, S. R., & Halfond, M. M. (1990). *Stuttering prevention: A clinical method*.

Stuart, A., Kalinowski, J., Rastatter, M., Saltuklaroglu, T., & Dayalu, V. (2004). Investigations of the impact of altered auditory feedback in-the-ear devices on the speech of people who stutter: initial fitting and 4-month follow-up. *International Journal of language & communication disorders / Royal College of Speech & Language Therapists*, *39*(1), 93-113.

Stuart, A., Kalinowski, J., Saltuklaroglu, T., & Guntupalli, V. (2006). Investigations of the impact of altered auditory feedback in-the-ear devices on the speech of people who stutter: One-year follow-up. *Disability and Rehabilitation*, *28*, 757–765. doi:10.1080/09638280500386635

Suresh, R., Ambrose, N., Roe, C., Pluzhnikov, A., Wittke-Thompson, J., & Ng, M. (2006). New complexities in the genetics of stuttering: significant sex-specific linkage signals. *American Journal of Human Genetics*, *78*(4), 554–563. doi:10.1086/501370

Sussman, E., & Winkler, I. (2001). Dynamic sensory updating in the auditory system. *Brain Research. Cognitive Brain Research*, *12*(3), 431–439. doi:10.1016/S0926-6410(01)00067-2

Takakusaki, K., Saitoh, K., Harada, H., & Kashiwayanagi, M. (2004). Role of basal ganglia-brainstem pathways in the control of motor behaviors. *Neuroscience Research*, *50*(2), 137–151. doi:10.1016/j.neures.2004.06.015

Tononi, G., & Edelman, G. M. (1998). Consciousness and Complexity. *Science*, *282*(5395), 1846–1851. doi:10.1126/science.282.5395.1846

Tononi, G., Sporns, O., & Edelman, G. M. (1992). Reentry and the Problem of Integrating Multiple Cortical Areas: Simulation of Dynamic Integration in the Visual System. *Cerebral Cortex*, *2*(4), 310–335. doi:10.1093/cercor/2.4.310

Tran, Y., Craig, A., Boord, P., & Craig, D. (2004). Using independent component analysis to remove artifact from electroencephalographic measured during stuttered speech. *Medical & Biological Engineering & Computing*, *42*(5), 627–633. doi:10.1007/BF02347544

Travis, L. E. (1978). The cerebral dominance theory of stuttering: 1931--1978. *The Journal of Speech and Hearing Disorders*, *43*(3), 278–281.

Travis, L. E., & Herren, R. Y. (1929). Studies in Stuttering: V. A Study of Simultaneous Antitropic Movements of the hands of stutterers. *Archives of Neurology and Psychiatry*, *22*(3), 487–494.

Umapathy, K., & Krishnan, S. (2005). Feature analysis of pathological speech signals using local discriminant bases technique. *Medical & Biological Engineering & Computing*, *43*, 457–464. doi:10.1007/BF02344726

Van Borsel, J., Reunes, G., & Van den Bergh, N. (2003). Delayed auditory feedback in the treatment of stuttering: clients as consumers. *International Journal of Language & Communication Disorders*, *38*(2), 119–129. doi:10.1080/1368282021000042902

Van Riper, C. (1949). To the Stutterer as he Begins his Speech Therapy. *The Journal of Speech and Hearing Disorders*, *14*(4), 303–306.

Van Riper, C. (1965). Clinical use of intermittent masking noise in stuttering therapy. *ASHA Reports*, *7*, 381.

Van Riper, C. (1973). *The Treatment of the Stuttering*. Englewood Cliffs, New Jersey: Prentice Hall.

Van Riper, C. (1982). *The nature of stuttering*. Englewood Cliffs, New Jersey: Prentice Hall.

Veselinovic, D., & Graupe, D. (2003). A wavelet transform approach to blind adaptive filtering of speech from unknown noises. *IEEE Transactions on Circuits and Systems II: Analog and Digital Signal Processing*, *50*(3), 150–154. doi:10.1109/TCSII.2003.809717

Ward, D. (2006). *Stuttering and Cluttering: Frameworks for understanding treatment*.

Watkins, K. E., Smith, S. M., Davis, S., & Howell, P. (2008). Structural and functional abnormalities of the motor system in developmental stuttering. *Brain*, *131*(1), 50–59. doi:10.1093/brain/awm241

Webster, R. L. (1991). Manipulation of vocal tone: Implications for stuttering. In Peters, H., Hulstijn, W., & Starkweather, C. W. (Eds.), *Speech Motor Control and Stuttering*. Amsterdam: Elsevier-Science.

Webster, R. L., & Lubker, B. B. (1968). Interrelationships Among Fluency Producing Variables in Stuttered Speech. *Journal of Speech and Hearing Research*, *11*(4), 754–766.

Whitebread, G. (2004). *Stuck on the Tip of My Thumb: Stuttering in American Sign Language*. Washington: University of Gallaudet.

Wingate, M. E. (1988). *The Structure of stuttering: a psycholinguistic analysis*. New York: Springer.

Wischner, G. J. (1950). Stuttering Behavior And Learning: A Preliminary Theoretical Formulation. *The Journal of Speech and Hearing Disorders*, *15*(4), 324–335.

Wischner, G. J. (1952). An Experimental Approach To Expectancy And Anxiety In Stuttering Behavior. *The Journal of Speech and Hearing Disorders*, *17*(2), 139–154.

Wohl, M. (1968). The electronic metronome an evaluative study. *The British Journal of Disorders of Communication*, *5*(1), 66–76. doi:10.3109/13682827009011502

Wu, J. C., Maguire, G., Riley, G. D., Fallon, J., LaCasse, L., & Chin, S. (1995). A positron emission tomography [18F] deoxyglucose study of developmental stuttering. *Neuroreport*, *6*(3), 501–505. doi:10.1097/00001756-199502000-00024

Yairi, E., & Ambrose, N. G. (1999). Early childhood stuttering I: Persistency and recovery rates. *Journal of Speech, Language, and Hearing Research: JSLHR*, *42*(5), 1097.

Zimmerman, S., Kalinowski, J., Stuart, A., & Rastatter, M. (1997). Effect of altered auditory feedback on people who stutter during scripted telephone conversations. *Journal of Speech, Language, and Hearing Research: JSLHR*, *40*(5), 1130–1134.

KEY TERMS AND DEFINITIONS

(Stuttering) Etiology: Causal mechanisms underlying the stuttering. This chapter is devoted to the cause of the persistent developmental stuttering.

Expressive Communication: It refers to a supervised sequential motor task like speech, writing, sign language communication, or even playing an instrument.

Mathematical Model: Mathematical description of a physical system. In the framework of this work mathematical models pursue the descriptions of mechanisms underlying stuttering, putting emphasis in the dynamics of neuronal regions involved in the disorder.

Multimodal Intelligent System: Computational system that processes signals from heterogeneous sources and it has the ability to modify its behavior for adapting to the environment or associated subject in an autonomous mode. It is used as a basis for multimodal smart sensors in this work.

Persistent Developmental Stuttering: Disorder that affects between 1 – 2% of world adult population. It impedes that subjects can communicate with others in the manner they wish. From the perspective of the listener, the disturbance is characterized by frequent repetitions or prolongations of sounds and syllables, although it includes also other types of speech dysfluencies, broken words, audible or silent blockings or circumlocutions, among others.

Prosthetic (AAF) Device: Devices designed to improve the fluency of persons who stutter by changing how they hear their voice (speech feedback). There are several well-known distortions to the feedback of speech, like delayed or frequency altered feedback, although the concept is not restricted to them.

Therapeutic (AAF) Device: Devices designed to treat the stuttering disorder and achieve a persistent improvement or even cure. There is not consensus with regard the potential application of AAF as therapy for PDS subjects, but the same occurs with any other current therapy.

ENDNOTE

1 CNV: electrical event associated with an anticipated response to an expected stimulus, and thus indicative of a state of readiness or expectancy

Chapter 7
The Role of Sensory Rhythmic Stimulation on Motor Rehabilitation in Parkinson's Disease (PD)

Pablo Arias
University of A Coruña, Spain

Javier Cudeiro
University of A Coruña, Spain

ABSTRACT

In the last years the role of sensory rhythmic stimulation (SRS) on motor rehabilitation in PD has become a new line of interest for researches and therapists given the promising results reported in scientific literature. This kind of strategies present a whole range of features which make it very appealing for its daily use, namely, they are easy to use, they have not distorting side-effects, and, chiefly, their effectiveness have been reported either in presence as in absence of antiparkinsonian medication.

INTRODUCTION

From a technical point of view SRS can be applied through three different modalities, rhythmic auditory stimulation (RAS), visual stimulation (VS), and somatosensory stimulation (SSS); though the first two modalities have been the most frequently utilized. RAS is a technique by which a series of auditory stimuli are presented at a fixed rhythm, so that patients have to synchronize their movements to the rhythms (i.e. using a metronome). This kind of stimulation has been consistently reported to facilitate gait in PD (Thaut et al. 1996; McIntosh et al. 1997; Thaut 1997; Rochester et al. 2005; Willems et al. 2006; Arias and Cudeiro 2008), though some other motor tasks have also

DOI: 10.4018/978-1-60566-206-0.ch007

been evaluated (Kritikos et al. 1995; Byblow et al. 2002). Recent research efforts are focused on determining rhythm features (mainly frequency (Willems et al. 2006; Arias and Cudeiro 2008)) to better facilitate movement.

VS was firstly depicted as a way to facilitate the movement in PD by Martin in 1967. The author described how colour stripes laid on the floor can induce a better walking pattern in PD when they were asked to walk over them, putting their feet on the stripes. From this work it was clear that stripes should be placed in such a way that their orientation was perpendicular to the walking direction. Subsequently, some other works has reported different results with this kind of stimulation under different conditions and paradigms (Morris and Iansek 1994; Morris et al. 1996; Suteerawattananon et al. 2004; Morris et al. 2005). Several key elements, such as the distance to be set between lines, are still to be determined.

Recently it has been proposed another procedure of VS by means of flashing LEDs (light emitting diodes) integrated into the mount of clear glasses (Rochester et al. 2005; Arias and Cudeiro 2008). This allows administration of VS either in controlled as un-controlled environments, so that it can be use at home or at the clinic, but also in the street. Though VS has been used as a tool to improve gait in PD, some other movements have also been explored, for instance upper limb movements. Some of these studies offer valuable information on the neural mechanism involved in the motor facilitation in presence of sensory stimulation experienced by PD (Cunnington et al. 1999).

SSS has been much less investigated, probably as a consequence of first reports showing poor effects on motor facilitation (Enzensberger and Fischer 1996); however some research groups have re-opened the line recently (Novak and Novak 2006; van Wegen et al. 2006a) as a way of facilitating gait by mean of synchronizing the steps to the rhythm; also new form of SSS - whole body vibration - has been proposed as to ameliorate symptoms in PD (Schmidtbleicher et al. 2004; Haas et al. 2006; Arias et al. 2009)

THE ROLE OF RAS IN FACILITATING MOVEMENTS IN PD

Gait Facilitation in PD by means of RAS

Gait disturbances in PD are a major feature of the disease (Jankovic 2008). Parkinsonian walking is characterized by a series of well documented alterations, which are specific and dependent on the grade of development of the disease (Arias and Cudeiro 2008). Progressing along the disease course, parkinsonian gait develops a whole spectrum of clinical features; step length reduction and slowness in gait (reduction in velocity) are the most recognizable characteristics. However some others, no less important, are also displayed. Prominent among them are: Increase in stride duration variability (i.e. un-ability of maintaining a stable gait cycle from a temporal perspective (Hausdorff et al. 1998; Hausdorff et al. 2002; Hausdorff et al. 2003; Arias and Cudeiro 2008)) which is also related to disease progression (Arias and Cudeiro 2008) and is associated to the risk of falling (Schaafsma et al. 2003b) and to freezing of gait (FOG) (Schaafsma et al. 2003a), a paroxysmal phenomenon commonly seen in advanced Parkinson's disease defined as the inability to start or continue walking.

Different studies have been performed using RAS, either during ON as OFF periods (medicated or un-medicated). Those studies have shown that RAS induces larger steps, higher velocity, and a reduction in the temporal variability of the stride cycle in PD (McIntosh et al. 1997; Suteerawattananon et al. 2004; Rochester et al. 2005; Willems et al. 2006; Arias and Cudeiro 2008). The impact on variability has been described to be relevant, since it seems related to falling, both in PD and in the healthy elderly (Hausdorff et al. 1998;

Schaafsma et al. 2003a; Schaafsma et al. 2003b; Hausdorff 2007). Some works also indicates that RAS can lead to reduce the number and duration of the FOG episodes displayed by some patients (Enzensberger and Fischer 1996). It is progressively clearer that stimulation features, specially the frequency, have a key role in the effectiveness of the technique.

Reports on the effect of RAS in parkinsonian gait have usually been the result of exploring one, or at most two, stimulation frequencies. However, the effect of a whole range of frequencies, in order to clarify the most suitable, has been recently explored (Willems et al. 2006; Arias and Cudeiro 2008). What we know so far is that high stimulation frequencies (well above the frequency of the spontaneous cadence of the patient) produce a change in several of the altered variables in the gait pattern of the patients, for instance step amplitude or velocity. Some other frequencies, around spontaneous cadence, reduce temporal variability and increase step length. Amongst these frequencies, those around 5-10% higher than the spontaneous cadence of the PD beside increasing step length, also raise velocity and reduce variability (Arias and Cudeiro 2008). Interestingly this frequency calculated during ON periods in the PD seems to be useful also when the effect of the medication decreases. Given that variability in stride cycle time is associated, not only to falling, but also to FOG, this frequency slightly above the preferred walking cadence during ON periods might have an effect on FOG (Arias and Cudeiro 2010). It is a remarkable point since a simple device could be used when the patient experience FOG in order to overcome the episode, becoming a valuable tool to improve the quality of life in Parkinson's disease.

RAS in Order to Facilitate Upper Limb Movements in PD

RAS has also been used with movements other than gait. Obviously, the complex nature of upper limb movements, embracing repetitive rhythmic movements, sequential movements, simultaneous movements - which can vary as being in-phase or anti-phase - different movement amplitudes... make this kind of motor behaviour different from a stereotyped pattern like gait. This means systematization of RAS protocols, for instance in the frequency domain, becomes difficult, if feasible. However, it is possible to find in the scientific literature several reports on the positive RAS effects regarding upper limb movements. Patients display faster movements when performing zig-zag in order to press a series of buttons if the movement is done in presence of RAS (Kritikos et al. 1995).

RAS Entrainment in PD

On the basis of previously commented works some researches have approached RAS as a way of entrainment to obtain facilitation of movement lasting beyond the period of stimulation. This therapeutic perspective is based on performing several sessions at which PD have to make different kind of movements, such as unimanual, bimanual, lower limb movements, walking, etc, in presence of RAS. Some report indicates improvement in movements like walking, after a daily period (one hour/day) of entrainment during three weeks at which PD performed different movements in presence of RAS (Thaut et al. 1996; Del Olmo et al. 2006; Nieuwboer et al. 2007). At the end of the programme, PD walked faster and, interestingly, those changes displayed at the end of the programmed lasted for four weeks. Some clinical centres include this kind of therapy within a whole programme of rehabilitation strategies. Stimulation is often provided by means of a metronome, though some other strategies have embedded the metronome sound within a music context.

Later this chapter includes methodological procedures in order to develop a programme which has shown to improve temporal variability in PD, either during upper limb movements as walking; along with changes in brain activity at rest measured by Positron Emission Tomography (PET).

THE ROLE OF VS ON MOTOR PERFORMANCE IN PD

Gait Facilitation by means of VS in PD

As mentioned previously gait facilitation by VS in PD was firstly described by Martin in the sixties. This kind of stimulation has a pure spatial connotation given it is applied by laying colour stripes on the floor, so that PD can walk over them (Morris and Iansek 1994; Morris et al. 1996; Suteerawattananon et al. 2004; Morris et al. 2005; Azulay et al. 2006). This technique is effective in well controlled environments, home for example, where stripes can be lain out on the floor to allow patients to walk from the couch to somewhere else (figure 1).

Based on this technique Lewis (Lewis et al. 2000) has designed a system in order to provide VS anywhere. The system is a light emitting device which projects two lines on the floor, just in front of the subject, so that stimulation "moves" with the patient. Light shafts emerge from the system which is placed on the patient's chest by means of a waistcoat.

Researches have not paid much attention to physical features of the stimuli, i.e. size and colour. However some common characteristics can be drawn from published work. It is obvious than colour must be clearly different from that of the floor, and the size of the stimulus is about 0.55 x 0.05 meters. Another key element in this procedure is inter-stimulus distance. The best results in order to facilitate walking in the PD are found when lines are 0.45 - 0.60 meters apart from each other. This type of stimulation leads to enlarge step amplitude and to walk faster; also it reduces variability of the gait patter in the spatial domain. Interestingly, these effects have been reported either in presence or absence of medication (Morris et al. 2005). This is important given some patients experience fluctuation in the effect of the treatment along the day.

Directly related to this technique another approach has been used to overcome FOG. It simply consists of an extension at the end of one stick (stick with a L shape), so that the extension is directed towards the subject (Kompoliti et al. 2000). This is used as a trigger for PD to pass over one of his legs, re-starting step patterns after the block. Subsequently, the system has been modified so that the stimulation was provided by means of a laser beam (Kompoliti et al. 2000). Despite some report indicates the systems is useful to overcome FOG, same other works reports null effectiveness of the technique.

As mentioned before, some other kind of VS has been recently proposed providing a type of stimulus varying in time. In this case, the rhythmic VS is provided by means of two flashing LED's integrated into an eyeglass frame (on the upper

Figure 1. Colour stripes lain on the floor so that the patient walks perpendicularly to the stripes. Colour stripes are place 40-60 cm apart from each other, and their size is about 5 x 55 cm

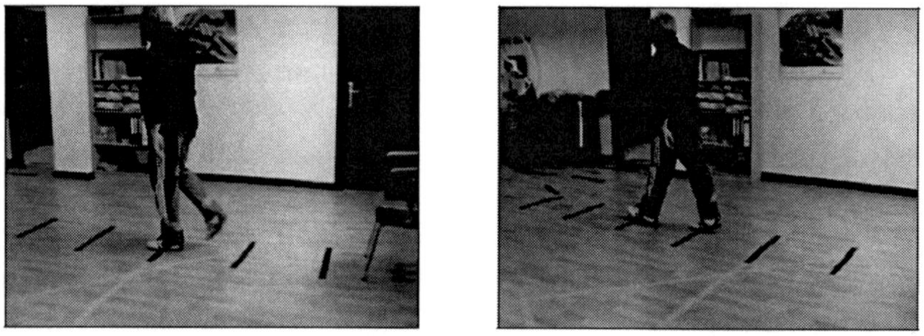

outside corners), so that stimuli can be perceived through peripheral vision (Rochester et al. 2005; Arias and Cudeiro 2008).

Upper Limb Movement Facilitation by means of VS in PD

VS has been widely used in order to evaluate upper limb movements in PD. Tasks including sequential movements are, probably, the most frequently approached. PD are asked to press different arrays of buttons which could be lit or flashing, so that either temporal or spatial cues could be provided. This paradigm has allowed to use neurophysiological techniques like electroencephalogram EEG in order to reveal some features of brain activation in the presence or absence of visual cues (Cunnington et al. 1999).

Therapies Based on VS Entrainment in PD

In contrast to RAS, VS has scarcely been employed with therapeutic purposes, and those works reporting VS entrainment have not been used in isolation (Marchese et al. 2003; Nieuwboer et al. 2007), but in combination with RAS.

SOMATOSENSORY STIMULATION (SSS) IN PD

Rhythmic SSS is, thus far, the less used sensory variety aiming to facilitate movements in PD. This may be due to the fact early reports had not shown any kind of facilitation, in contrast to both auditory and visual varieties. Nevertheless, this approach has recently re-emerged (Novak and Novak 2006; van Wegen et al. 2006b).

SSS has been applied during walking. Tapping at patient's shoulder resulted in impairing gait even when the frequency employed is able to produce good results if applied with RAS (Enzensberger and Fischer 1996). Other authors, using cutaneous stimulation, have achieved better results mainly focused on gait initiation (Burleigh-Jacobs et al. 1997). Some other approaches, with good results, have concentrated their efforts on stimulating the propioceptors through different techniques like walking in treadmills or applying electrical current at the tendons (Frenkel-Toledo et al. 2005; Herman et al. 2009). Another related technique includes vibrating stimulation (at 70Hz) by means of insoles each time that feet are in contact with the ground, which produced an improvement in a number of gait parameters (Novak and Novak 2006).

NEUROPHYSIOLOGICAL BASIS OF MOVEMENT FACILITATION BY MEANS OF SRS IN PD

Earlier in the chapter we have mentioned that, in order to provide further insights about the functional changes which allow better movement performance in PD, some works have used SRS and simultaneously evaluated neurophysiological activity. It has been suggested that SRS permits a switch between different loops related to the control of movement, in such a way that those circuits no damaged in PD can be primarily used.

In this scenario, SRS will involve the cerebellum-premotor cortex loop (implicated in externally triggered movements), avoiding the basal ganglia-supplementary motor area loop related to self-generated movement and severely injured (Jahanshahi et al. 1996; Gerloff et al. 1998; Cunnington et al. 1999; Jenkins et al. 2000).

These assumptions are based, for example, on some studies which analysed the temporal variability of finger-tapping and gait in patients with Parkinson's disease before and after they undertook a physical rehabilitation programme. Positron Emission Tomography (PET) using 2-deoxy-2[18F]fluoro-D-glucose was performed in these subjects to look for changes in metabolic brain activity after completion of the rehabilita-

Figure 2. Location of areas of the brain where increased metabolic activity were displayed in a group of PD after undergoing a therapy based on RAS. A: Right parietal lobe, right temporal lobe, right transverse temporal gyrus, right postcentral gyrus; B: cerebellar lobe, right dentate nucleus (Del Olmo et al. 2006)

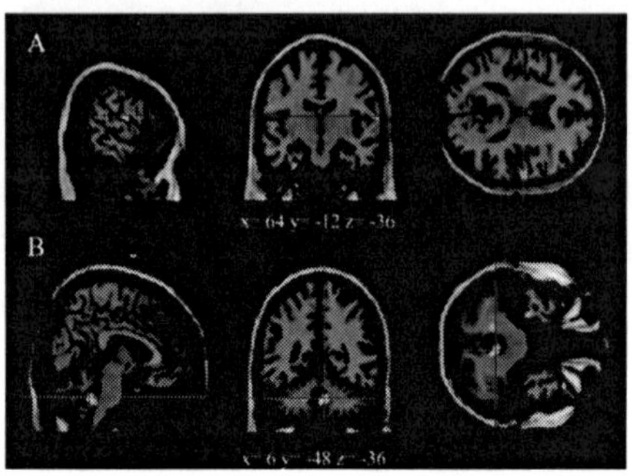

tion program. The results showed improvement in the temporal variability of two types of rhythmic movements after participation in a physical rehabilitation programme, along with changes in glucose uptake in several brain areas involved in sensorimotor processing, including parietal and temporal cortices and cerebellum (Del Olmo et al. 2006) (figure 2).

Other theories have tried to explain the benefits obtained in gait with VS chiefly restricted to the use of visual stimulus with a spatial component (e.g. stripes on the floor). This conception emphasizes the role of the interplay between the stimulus and the dynamic optic flow generated by patient's movement. This is supported by data showing that the improvement induced by colour stripes lain out on the floor during PD gait is cancelled by using a stroboscopic light, which suppress dynamic flow (Azulay et al. 2006). Some other works have indicated that cues help PD by focussing their attention on motor performance (Morris et al. 1996).

Another element that warranties further research is to explain how SRS by means of RAS facilitates movement in PD more efficiently that temporal VS. Figure 3 shows how advance PD modulates their step cadence differently if a range of different stimulation frequencies (above and below their Preferred Walking –PW - cadence) are presented, in contrast to healthy subjects whom adapt their step rhythm to the cue rhythm regardeless the stimulation variety (Arias and Cudeiro 2008)

PROCEDURAL CONSIDERATION FOR USING RAS: THE CASE OF GAIT

As above mentioned there is considerable evidence that RAS has beneficial effects on patient's movement. In this section we will propose a simple procedure in order to utilize RAS in gait. First we

Figure 3. Cadence induced by auditory (dotted line) and visual (solid line) rhythmic stimulation in presence of different stimulation frequencies in advance PD patients (PD III-IV) and in healthy controls (Arias and Cudeiro 2008)

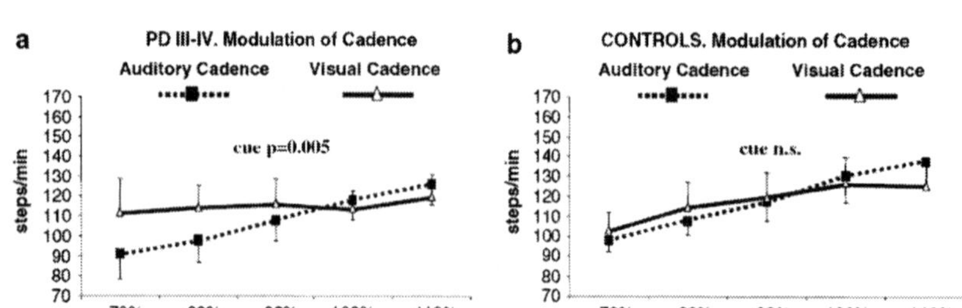

will show a simple way to determine stimulation frequency (for each patient) to be used either to facilitate movements "in situ", (e.g. when the patient freezes) (Arias and Cudeiro 2010) or to develop a training programme. Then we will discuss some methodological principles in order to develop a therapeutic programme based on previous reports.

Best frequencies to facilitate gait are those slightly (5-10%) above the step cadence of each subject measured during preferred walking (in the ON period). This frequency may be used in some other moments, when for instance the effect of medication wears off (Arias and Cudeiro 2008, 2010).

The procedure to calculate the stimulation frequency is simple. Briefly, the subject is asked to walk in a straight path larger enough to achieve stability in their gait pattern, about 7 stride cycles, discounting the first two. A stride is considered from heel strike (or foot contact) to the subsequent contact with the same foot (a stride comprises two steps). Using a stopwatch walking cadence can be easily assessed. So that 5 strides (10 step) in, for instance, 6 seconds, gives a step cadence of 1.66 steps/sec, which multiplied by 60 sec is 100 step/min. This allows matching units usually displayed in metronomes (bpm).

The above mentioned applies when we try to obtain an immediate benefit ("in situ" stimulation). However we might like to include auditory stimulation into a rehabilitation programme of several weeks comprising several sessions in order to practice different movements (gait, upper limb movements and lower limb movements) In this case, a range of different stimulation frequencies have been proposed (from 60 to 150 bpm for gait, frequencies which are above and below PW cadence) (Del Olmo et al. 2006). The programme is structured based on a combination of different elements, like frequencies, presence (synchronization) or absence (reproduction) of stimulation, and performance of single or simultaneous movements, so that task complexity rises along programme progression.

Frequencies of Stimulation

The kind of movement to be done must be taken into account when setting stimulation frequencies. Walking is a repetitive movement which frequency (step cadence) is about 100 step/min; though in some patients, suffering from severe bradykinesia /akinesia may be slower. Thus, the training programme should employ in the beginning a range of frequencies around the "typical" spontaneous cadence and progress from slower to faster frequencies. These variations may be periodically introduced within the task, so that the patient has to modulate step cadence (or finger tapping or any other movement we like to consider) trying to adapt his step pattern to the rhythm.

Presence or Absence of Rhythm

In the beginning of the programme task will be performed in presence of rhythm, and patients have to synchronize their movements to the stimuli (synchronization tasks). Subsequently, along sessions, synchronization-reproduction tasks will be introduced, so that at the beginning of the task patients synchronize their movements to the stimuli, but once the stimuli is suppressed, movement must be kept at the same cadence. Afterwards a third phase may be introduced (reproduction), where subjects have to "catch" the rhythm and once the cue is suppressed they start moving at the rhythm previously proposed.

Simultaneous Movements

Task complexity may be modified by the execution of simultaneous movements along other movements, like for instance gait, or bimanual movements. Sequential simultaneous movement (i.e. opposition of fingers 2-5 against the first) is more complex than simple simultaneous movement, like index-thumb repetition, when performed with just one upper limb. Difficulty will be increased along programme evolution. In the case of performing bimanual movements, complexity will be increased by progressing from in-phase to anti-phase movements, (*in-phase* when the same muscles from homologous limbs are acting at the same time; in prono-supination in-phase execution means both forearms pronate at once, and supinate at once; during anti-phase one forearm pronates while the other supinates). Finally no-repetitive simultaneous movements will be also introduced.

When programming the intervention some other elements should be taken into account in order to optimize it. Most of studies performed sessions of about 45 minutes (Thaut et al. 1996; Del Olmo et al. 2006; Nieuwboer et al. 2007). This point should be carefully address, given an excessive duration might lead to fatigue the patients, or some patients might suffer from medication wearing-off (training is recommended during ON periods). On the other hand, shorter sessions might lead to insufficient stimulation, though most of the works have not specifically assessed this point. Motor facilitation has been reported after programmes of 3 and 5 days per week in experimental settings (Thaut et al. 1996; Del Olmo et al. 2006; Nieuwboer et al. 2007), but it seems advisable to integrate these protocols within daily activity in patient's rehabilitation schedules. This kind of stimulation is useful when performed in an individualized manner, however, if the protocol is going to be carried out in a clinic, attending more than one patient during collective sessions, stimulation may be provided by means of loudspeakers. In this case some other aspects should be considered. Although hardly achievable, it would be needed that patients attending the session have the same level of clinical features. Collective sessions allow therapist to programme tasks to be performed in couples, and to introduce ludic tasks.

PHYSICAL PROPERTIES OF THE STIMULATION

Despite the effect of sensory cueing has been extensively evaluated in PD, the physical properties of the stimuli have been generally left out in the methods sections, and also their putative roles have not been usually evaluated either.

In the case of sensory rhythmic stimulation, frequency has been the only factor that has attracted researcher's attention. In the case of gait, a clear trend has been established in literature towards determining the best frequency to be used. Besides that, and focussing on RAS, the rest of physical properties of the auditory stimulation have not been reported in literature. The waveform frequency has only been reported in few works, for instance Arias and Cudeiro (2008) reported a pulse-wave frequency of 4.625 KHz. Since the same stimulation frequency can be set with different configuration of pulse duration and intra-pulse duration, one might thought a fixed frequency could have different effects by modifying, enlarging and shortening, both parameters at the same extent, but effects due to this modifications on movement facilitation in PD have not been evaluated consistently. Neither stimulus intensity has been systematized in RAS, and available reports sometimes refer to an intensity enough to be clearly perceived avoiding annoying sensation. Pulse wave-form has become another often forgotten parameter as has been usually un-notice by researches, or at least, not reported.

The lack of systematization when reporting physical features is also applicable to visual rhythmic stimulation. In some cases the duration of the stimulus -50ms- has been reported (Arias and Cudeiro 2008), but the possible role of this feature on movement facilitation has not been assessed. Colour is another forgotten characteristic, and this is not a minor point given the loss of colour sensitivity in PD, with impairment for discrimination of blue colours and tonalities.

Somatosensory stimulation provides no further accuracy in terms of depicting the physical properties of the stimuli. For example, some forms of stimulation include cutaneous application (at 1.1 Hz) of a vibrating cylinder (van Wegen et al. 2006a). However the frequency of the vibratory pulse, which often lasted 400ms, is not known. Furthermore, a number of variables, like the spread of the stimulation on the skin, or the hardness of the device providing the stimulation, lacks.

CONCLUSION

In conclusion, the effect of SRS on motor performance, using the auditory and visual varieties, has been deeply evaluated. RAS and VS (in the case of stripes on the floor, spatial VS) have produced good results in order to facilitate movement in Parkinson's disease. In the case of RAS the frequency used seems to be a key element in order to optimize its effect. Spatial VS, apart from being useful, has become available in un-controlled environments by the use of laser devices. SSS need further research in order to prove its effectiveness.

REFERENCES

Arias, P., Chouza, M., Vivas, J., & Cudeiro, J. (2009). Effect of Whole Body Vibration in Parkinson's Disease: A Controlled Study. *Movement Disorders*, *24*, 891–898. doi:10.1002/mds.22468

Arias, P., & Cudeiro, J. (2008). Effects of rhythmic sensory stimulation (auditory, visual) on gait in Parkinson's disease patients. *Experimental Brain Research*, *186*, 589–601. doi:10.1007/s00221-007-1263-y

Arias, P., & Cudeiro, J. (2010). Effect of rhythmic auditory stimulation on gait in Parkinsonian patients with and without freezing of gait. *PLoS ONE*, *5*(3), e9675. doi:10.1371/journal.pone.0009675

Azulay, J. P., Mesure, S., & Blin, O. (2006). Influence of visual cues on gait in Parkinson's disease: Contribution to attention or sensory dependence? *Journal of the Neurological Sciences*, *248*, 192–195. doi:10.1016/j.jns.2006.05.008

Burleigh-Jacobs, A., Horak, F. B., Nutt, J. G., & Obeso, J. A. (1997). Step initiation in Parkinson's disease: Influence of levodopa and external sensory triggers. *Movement Disorders*, *12*, 206–215. doi:10.1002/mds.870120211

Byblow, W. D., Summers, J. J., Lewis, G. N., & Thomas, J. (2002). Bimanual coordination in Parkinson's disease: Deficits in movement frequency, amplitude, and pattern switching. *Movement Disorders*, *17*, 20–29. doi:10.1002/mds.1281

Cunnington, R., Iansek, R., & Bradshaw, J. L. (1999). Movement-related potentials in Parkinson's disease: External cues and attentional strategies. *Movement Disorders*, *14*, 63–68. doi:10.1002/1531-8257(199901)14:1<63::AID-MDS1012>3.0.CO;2-V

Del Olmo, M., Arias, P., Furio, M. C., Pozo, M. A., & Cudeiro, J. (2006). Evaluation of the effect of training using auditory stimulation on rhythmic movement in Parkinsonian patients - a combined motor and F-18 -FDG PET study. *Parkinsonism & Related Disorders*, *12*, 155–164. doi:10.1016/j.parkreldis.2005.11.002

Enzensberger, W., & Fischer, P. A. (1996). Metronome in Parkinson's disease. *Lancet*, *347*, 1337–1337. doi:10.1016/S0140-6736(96)90987-3

Frenkel-Toledo, S., Giladi, N., Peretz, C., Herman, T., Gruendlinger, L., & Hausdorff, J. M. (2005). Treadmill walking as an external pacemaker to improve gait rhythm and stability in Parkinson's disease. *Movement Disorders*, *20*, 1109–1114. doi:10.1002/mds.20507

Gerloff, C., Richard, J., Hadley, J., Schulman, A. E., Honda, M., & Hallett, M. (1998). Functional coupling and regional activation of human cortical motor areas during simple, internally paced and externally paced finger movements. *Brain*, *121*, 1513–1531. doi:10.1093/brain/121.8.1513

Haas, C. T., Turbanski, S., Kessler, K., & Schmidtbleicher, D. (2006). The effects of random whole-body-vibration on motor symptoms in Parkinson's disease. *NeuroRehabilitation*, *21*, 29–36.

Hausdorff, J. M. (2007). Gait dynamics, fractals and falls: Finding meaning in the stride-to-stride fluctuations of human walking. In *3rd European Workshop on Movement Science*, vol 26, Amsterdam, Netherlands (pp. 555-589).

Hausdorff, J.M., Balash, Y., & Giladi, N. (2003). Time series analysis of leg movements during freezing of gait in Parkinson's disease: Akinesia, rhyme or reason? *Physica a-Statistical Mechanics and Its Applications,* 321, 565-570.

Hausdorff, J. M., Cudkowicz, M. E., Firtion, R., Wei, J. Y., & Goldberger, A. L. (1998). Gait variability and basal ganglia disorders: Stride-to-stride variations of gait cycle timing in Parkinson's disease and Huntington's disease. *Movement Disorders*, *13*, 428–437. doi:10.1002/mds.870130310

Hausdorff, J. M., Schaafsma, J. D., Balash, J., Bartels, A., Gurevich, T., & Giladi, N. (2002). Gait dynamics in subjects with freezing of gait and Parkinson's disease: Increased variability during usual walking. In *7th International Congress of Parkinsons Disease and Movement Disorders*, vol 17, Miami, Florida (p. P401)

Herman, T., Giladi, N., & Hausdorff, J. M. (2009). Treadmill training for the treatment of gait disturbances in people with Parkinson's disease: A mini-review. *Journal of Neural Transmission*, *116*, 307–318. doi:10.1007/s00702-008-0139-z

Jahanshahi, M., Jenkins, H., Brown, R. G., Marsden, C. D., Passingham, R. E., & Brooks, D. J. (1996). Self-initiated versus externally triggered movements. 1. An investigation using measurement of regional cerebral blood flow with PET and movement-related potentials in normal and Parkinson's disease subjects - Reply. *Brain*, *119*, 1046–1048.

Jankovic, J. (2008). Parkinson's disease: clinical features and diagnosis. *Journal of Neurology, Neurosurgery, and Psychiatry*, *79*, 368–376. doi:10.1136/jnnp.2007.131045

Jenkins, I. H., Jahanshahi, M., Jueptner, M., Passingham, R. E., & Brooks, D. J. (2000). Self-initiated versus externally triggered movements II. The effect of movement predictability on regional cerebral blood flow. *Brain*, *123*, 1216–1228. doi:10.1093/brain/123.6.1216

Kompoliti, K., Goetz, C. G., Leurgans, S., Morrissey, M., & Siegel, I. M. (2000). "On" freezing in Parkinson's disease: Resistance to visual cue walking devices. *Movement Disorders*, *15*, 309–312. doi:10.1002/1531-8257(200003)15:2<309::AID-MDS1016>3.0.CO;2-P

Kritikos, A., Leahy, C., Bradshaw, J. L., Iansek, R., Phillips, J. G., & Bradshaw, J. A. (1995). Contingent and noncontingent auditory cueing in Parkinsons-disease. *Neuropsychologia*, *33*, 1193–1203. doi:10.1016/0028-3932(95)00036-3

Lewis, G. N., Byblow, W. D., & Walt, S. E. (2000). Stride length regulation in Parkinson's disease: the use of extrinsic, visual cues. *Brain*, *123*, 2077–2090. doi:10.1093/brain/123.10.2077

Marchese, R., Bove, M., & Abbruzzese, G. (2003). Effect of cognitive and motor tasks on postural stability in Parkinson's disease: A posturographic study. *Movement Disorders*, *18*, 652–658. doi:10.1002/mds.10418

McIntosh, G. C., Brown, S. H., Rice, R. R., & Thaut, M. H. (1997). Rhythmic auditory-motor facilitation of gait patterns in patients with Parkinson's disease. *Journal of Neurology, Neurosurgery, and Psychiatry*, *62*, 22–26. doi:10.1136/jnnp.62.1.22

Morris, M., Iansek, R., McGinley, J., Matyas, T., & Huxham, F. (2005). Three-dimensional gait biomechanics in Parkinson's disease: Evidence for a centrally mediated amplitude regulation disorder. *Movement Disorders*, *20*, 40–50. doi:10.1002/mds.20278

Morris, M. E., & Iansek, R. (1994). Characteristics of motor disturbance in Parkinson's disease and strategies for movement rehabilitation. In *Motor Control Symposium, at the Australasian-Winter-Conference-on-Brain-Research Meeting, vol 15*, Queenstown, New Zealand (pp. 649-669).

Morris, M. E., Iansek, R., Matyas, T. A., & Summers, J. J. (1996). Stride length regulation in Parkinson's disease normalization strategies and underlying mechanisms. *Brain*, *119*, 551–568. doi:10.1093/brain/119.2.551

Nieuwboer, A., Kwakkel, G., Rochester, L., Jones, D., van Wegen, E., & Willems, A. M. (2007). Cueing training in the home improves gait-related mobility in Parkinson's disease: the RESCUE trial. *Journal of Neurology, Neurosurgery, and Psychiatry*, *78*, 134–140. doi:10.1136/jnnp.200X.097923

Novak, P., & Novak, V. (2006). Effect of step-synchronized vibration stimulation of soles on gait in Parkinson's disease: a pilot study. *Journal of Neuroengineering and Rehabilitation*, 3.

Rochester, L., Hetherington, V., Jones, D., Nieuwboer, A., Willems, A. M., Kwakkel, G., & Van Wegen, E. (2005). The effect of external rhythmic cues (auditory and visual) on walking during a functional task in homes of people with Parkinson's disease. *Archives of Physical Medicine and Rehabilitation*, *86*, 999–1006. doi:10.1016/j.apmr.2004.10.040

Schaafsma, J. D., Balash, Y., Gurevich, T., Bartels, A. L., Hausdorff, J. M., & Giladi, N. (2003a). Characterization of freezing of gait subtypes and the response of each to levodopa in Parkinson's disease. *European Journal of Neurology*, *10*, 391–398. doi:10.1046/j.1468-1331.2003.00611.x

Schaafsma, J. D., Giladi, N., Balash, Y., Bartels, A. L., Gurevich, T., & Hausdorff, J. M. (2003b). Gait dynamics in Parkinson's disease: relationship to Parkinsonian features, falls and response to levodopa. *Journal of the Neurological Sciences*, *212*, 47–53. doi:10.1016/S0022-510X(03)00104-7

Schmidtbleicher, D., Turbanski, S., & Haas, C. T. (2004). Effects of whole-body vibration on postural control in Parkinson's disease. *Movement Disorders*, *19*, 518.

Suteerawattananon, M., Morris, G. S., Etnyre, B. R., Jankovic, J., & Protas, E. J. (2004). Effects of visual and auditory cues on gait in individuals with Parkinson's disease. *Journal of the Neurological Sciences*, *219*, 63–69. doi:10.1016/j.jns.2003.12.007

Thaut, M. H. (1997). Rehabilitation of gait in Parkinson's disease - Reply. *Journal of Neurology, Neurosurgery, and Psychiatry*, *63*, 556–557. doi:10.1136/jnnp.63.4.556a

Thaut, M. H., McIntosh, G. C., Rice, R. R., Miller, R. A., Rathbun, J., & Brault, J. M. (1996). Rhythmic auditory stimulation in gait training for Parkinson's disease patients. *Movement Disorders*, *11*, 193–200. doi:10.1002/mds.870110213

van Wegen, E., de Goede, C., Lim, I., Rietberg, M., Nieuwboer, A., & Willems, A. (2006a). The effect of rhythmic somatosensory cueing on gait in patients with Parkinson's disease. *Journal of the Neurological Sciences*, *248*, 210–214. doi:10.1016/j.jns.2006.05.034

van Wegen, E., Lim, I., de Goede, C., Nieuwboer, A., Willems, A., & Jones, D. (2006b). The effects of visual rhythms and optic flow on stride patterns of patients with Parkinson's disease. *Parkinsonism & Related Disorders*, *12*, 21–27. doi:10.1016/j.parkreldis.2005.06.009

Willems, A. M., Nieuwboer, A., Chavret, F., Desloovere, K., Dom, R., & Rochester, L. (2006). The use of rhythmic auditory cues to influence gait in patients with Parkinson's disease, the differential effect for freezers and non-freezers, an explorative study. *Disability and Rehabilitation*, *28*, 721–728. doi:10.1080/09638280500386569

KEY TERMS AND DEFINITIONS

Electroencephalogram (EEG): Bioelectrical brain activity recorded non-invasively from electrodes placed on the scalp.

Freezing of Gait (FOG): Paroxysmal phenomenon commonly seen in advanced Parkinson's disease defined as the inability to start or continue walking.

LEDs: Light emitting diodes.

PD: Parkinson's disease.

Positron Emission Tomography (PET): Scanning technique used in conjunction with small amounts of radiolabeled compounds (tracers) to visualize brain (or other body parts) anatomy and function.

Preferred Walking (PW): Walking pattern preferred by each patient.

Rhythmic Auditory Stimulation (RAS): Technique by which a series of auditory stimuli are presented at a fixed rhythm, so that patients have to synchronize their movements to the rhythms.

Sensory rhythmic stimulation (SRS): Strategy used for motor rehabilitation that can be provided to the patients using different inputs: visual, auditory or somatosensory.

Somatosensory Stimulation (SSS): Technique by which a series of tactile stimuli are presented at a fixed rhythm, so that patients have to synchronize their movements to the rhythms.

Visual Stimulation (VS): Technique by which a series of visual stimuli are presented mainly to improve gait.

Chapter 8
Transcranial Magnetic Stimulation (TMS) as a Tool for Neurorehabilitation in Parkinson's Disease

Pablo Arias
University of A Coruña, Spain

Nelson Espinosa
University of A Coruña, Spain

Javier Cudeiro
University of A Coruña, Spain

ABSTRACT

Transcranial Magnetic Stimulation (TMS) is a stimulation technique introduced to clinical practise by Anthony Baker in 1985. TMS has become very valuable either for neurophysiological examination as for research. When use in a repetitive way it has shown to have a therapeutic role for treatment of neurological and psychiatric disorders. This chapter summarizes the basic principles of the technique focusing on its interaction with the neural tissue along with the analysis of different stimulation protocols, potential risks, and its effectiveness on Parkinson's disease.

INTRODUCTION

TMS is based on the generation of magnetic fields to induce currents in the cortical tissue (or any excitable tissue) interfering, therefore, with the electrical activity of neurons. TMS was introduced by Anthony Barker in 1985 as a painless and non-invasive technique that, based on the principles of electromagnetic induction, is able to generate currents in the brain and modulate the function of the cortex. The prototype presented by Barker was capable of generating current pulses of 110μsec at a frequency of 0.3Hz and an intensity of 4kA.

DOI: 10.4018/978-1-60566-206-0.ch008

This device (developed by Magstim and under an exclusive license to the University of Sheffield) was the first magnetic stimulator built for commercial purposes. Today there are new versions of magnetic stimulators manufactured by different companies specially designed for clinical and research applications and able to work with higher current and frequency ranges. The following is a review of the technique that includes the general aspects of the device, the physics behind TMS and its main applications in both, clinical and experimental protocols, focused on Parkinson's disease.

Basic Setup of TMS

A TMS apparatus is composed by (see Figure 1):

A: A capacitive systems of charge-discharge current designed to store an electric charge at high potential (in the kV range) and to supply a high current (in the kA range).

B: A control system which allows to determine the current level, according to the user needs, and generates a magnetic stimulus either manually or by an external trigger circuit. In addition, it governs all electric and thermal protections for a safe operation.

C: A stimulating coil whose design is crucial because it determines the profile of the induced magnetic field and because it is the only component in direct contact with the subject to study.

Figure 1. Transcranial magnetic stimulator Magstim model Rapid. A: two capacitive systems to accumulate electric charge above 2.8 kV. B: control system to adjust stimulation parameters and safeguards. C: circular coil and two figure-eight coils with different diameters, each of them induces a magnetic field with different characteristics

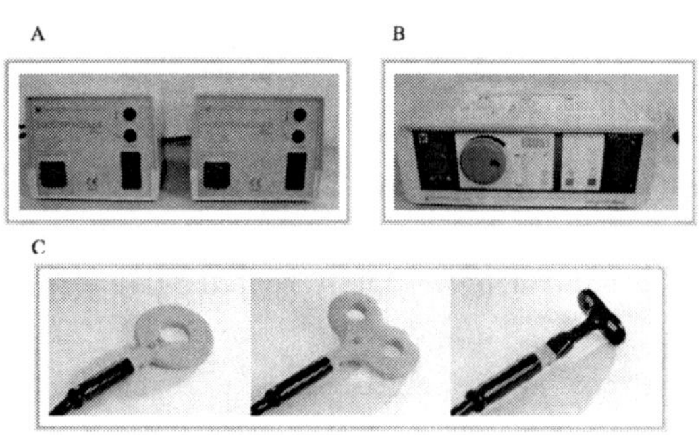

Operating Principles

Whenever the capacitor bank is discharged by the action of the control system, a pulse of current I flows through the stimulating coil and, according to Ampère's Law (eq. [1]), induces a magnetic field $\vec{H}$ surrounding the coil. Figure 2A shows a simplified circuit equivalent to a *figure of eight* (or *butterfly*) coil (Figure 1C, center & right). Note that the induced magnetic field is greater (*2H*) where the more current flows.

Because I varies with time (pulse) so does $\vec{H}$ and, by virtue of the Faraday's law (eq. [2] in Figure 3), an electric field is induced in the air (see Figure 3) and all tissues located on the coil vicinity. Then, if the coil is placed on the scalp, the magnetic field crosses the scalp, skull, cerebrospinal fluid and brain. As a result, the induced electric field gives rise to eddy currents whose

Figure 2 A. a circulating current I induces a magnetic field H. The magnetic field is greater (2H) at points with greater current flow and is zero where the net current is zero. B: The right-hand rule is a mnemonic rule to determine the spatial relationship between current and magnetic field. The Ampère's law (eq. [1]) expresses the relation between the current and the magnetic field

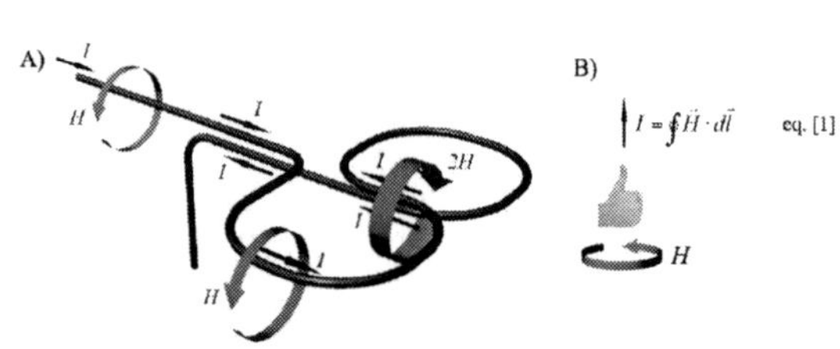

magnitude depends on the conductivity of each medium (Wagner et al., 2004).

TMS stimulus intensity can be inferred from the equation [2] in such a way that the bigger the slope of the current pulse, the higher the electric field intensity. Therefore, both the capacitive charge-discharge system design and the electrical parameters of the stimulation coil determinate the stimulus strength. The characteristics of the spatial distribution of the induced electric field (i.e. the precision and penetration depth of the stimulus) depend on the region where the eddy currents are induced (Starzynski et al., 2002, Miranda, Hallett and Basser, 2003, Roth et al., 1991, Nadeem et al., 2003) as well as on the geometric characteristics of the stimulation coil.

Coil Configurations and Companies

Different coil shapes (see Figure 1C) are available from different companies and the choice depends on the objective of the study. "Figure of eight" or "round" coils are those more often used in clinical practise, though some other shapes are also being developed.

Circular coil: Circular coils (Figure 1C, left) are developed in different sizes and produce a wide electric field, allowing bihemispheric stimulation.

Figure 3. Electric field A: 3D and B: 2D induced by a figure of eight coil (Fig 1C, right) at 100% of the capacity of the Magstim Rapid. The maximum value is located at the center of the coil (Jalinous, 1996). Equation [2] shows the relation between the electric field E and the magnetic field H. ∇× is the curl operator and μ is the permeability of the medium

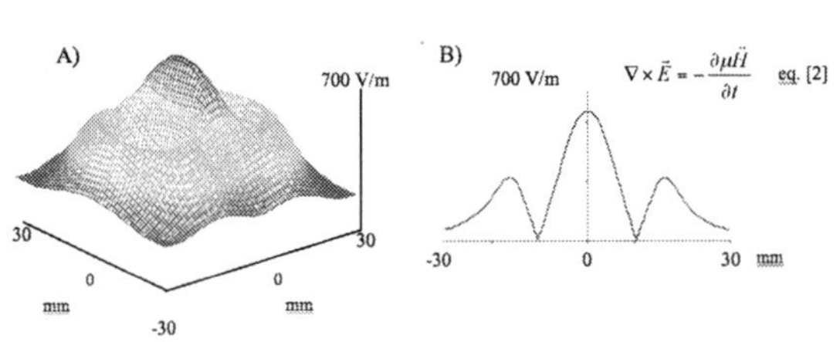

Large 90mm mean diameter coil is most effective in stimulating the motor cortex and the spinal nerve roots. Using this kind of coil the stimulation is maximum under the winding of the coil, but tends to zero at the center. It is important to point out the role of current direction in the case of applying stimulation with a circular coil; given both sides of the coils have stimulating properties the appropriate direction must be chosen in order to preferentially activate each hemisphere. When the coil powered from a monophasic stimulator is placed centrally over the vertex of the skull and the current induced in the tissue flows clockwise, the stimulated hemisphere is chiefly the left one, and viceversa; given the motor cortex is more sensitive when current flows from posterior to anterior (Hovey and Janilous, 2008).

Figure of eight coil: eight-shaped coils (see Figure 1C, center & right) are built from two windings place side by side, so that the induced tissue current reaches its maximum under the centre with a lower electric field in the remaining area, allowing a very good definition of the stimulated area. At this point, coil orientation critically influences the way stimulation interferes with the stimulated area, if a monophasic pulse is applied with this coil with latero-medial orientation corticospinal activity emerges from activation of either activation of the cortico-spinal tract directly, as well as from trans-synaptic activation of the piramidal cells, whereas stimulation with a posterior-anterior orientation elicits only the latter (Patton and Amassian, 1954; Kaneko et al., 1996; Nakamura et al., 1996; Di Lazzaro et al. 2004)

Some other coil shapes: Apart from these classic coil shapes some other special configurations have been devised, allowing a more focused stimulation on the lower limb areas; some dedicated to sham stimulation or a recently developed coil to deeper stimulation.

Double Cone Coil: it has two large cup shaped windings side by side that allows a very good coupling to the skull, so that the induced current at the central fissure is very high, and the areas controlling lower limbs and torso are better stimulated (Hovey and Janilous, 2008).

Sham Coil: it looks like a standard coil but just a very small portion of the energy is delivered to the head of the coil, since the coil is routed via a special box. Inside the box most of the energy is discharged but the characteristic 'click' is heard when the stimulator is fired (Hovey and Janilous, 2008).

Sham coils have been a matter of debate, given a perfect sham coil should match a number of features to perfectly mimic real stimulation (i.e. identical coil positions on the scalp, acoustic artefacts, and identical sensations evoked on the scalp). Traditionally sham stimulation has been performed by tilting the coil 90º, however this technique is known not to fulfil the conditions mentioned beforehand. In addition some degree of real stimulation might also be present. To overcome the problems some works have proposed to use two superimposed coils (Okabe et al., 2003), and new sham coils are being developed such as the one composed by joining two coils, one real coil, and one sham coil, place upside-down so that the real coil provides some key elements to achieve realistic sham stimulation, like noise artefacts, and the sham coil some others, like coil's position on the skull.

Despite these steps forward the development of sham stimulators keeps on being a target given the devices developed so far do no match side-effect scalp stimulation provided by real coils. Some researches (Okabe et al. 2003) have dealt with this issue by applying cutaneous electrical stimulation of the scalp. For instance, Rossi et al., (2007) have recently presented an adaptation of the traditional figure of eight coil which is built in compact wood. This is attached to the real coil by Velcro strips, so that the first one acts as a physical spacer between the real coil and the scalp; also the latter houses a bipolar electrical stimulator within the surface which is in contact with the scalp to reproduce cutaneous sensations felt by the subject when is really stimulated.

H-coil: recently a way to obtain deeper TMS stimulation of the brain has been proposed, it is based on a new configuration of the coil. This coil allows to generate a summation of the evoked electric fields in a given brain region by means of placing several coil elements around this area; all this elements induce a electric field in the same direction (Roth, et al., 2002; Zangen et al. 2005)

Coil companies: From a theoretical point of view one coil-shape will generate a given magnetic field, and will induce a characteristic electric field. However based on everyday practice things are not so easy and a new source of variability appears given several companies have developed differently the same kind of coil. For instance, figure of eight coils have been developed with both windings in the same plane, side by side, or in different plane and overlapping.

The difference in configuration has been proved to have different neurophysiological effects when generating a pulse to interact with the cortex. Figure 4 illustrates how the output intensity from the stimulator at which motor threshold is determine varies depending on the coil manufacturer, regardless pulse waveform or the current direction (Kammer et al., 2001). This is a critical point to take into account when interpreting data, given motor thresholds are usually the key point in order to determine stimulation intensity in experimental or clinical procedures.

STIMULATION PARAMETERS

Pulse Waveform

Pulse waveform: this feature is also a basic element to take into account during TMS. According to the technical specifications of the equipments, single pulse may be monophasic, biphasic and polyphasic. Each type leads to different neurophysiological interactions with the tissue, and leads to different applications (Di Lazzaro et al., 2001). Monophasic pulse is more accurate, and produces

Figure 4. Variation in motor threshold in 8 subjects expressed as percentage of the stimulator as a function of the manufacturer, the pulse waveform and the current direction (anterior-posterior or postero-anterior) (modified from Kammer et al., 2001)

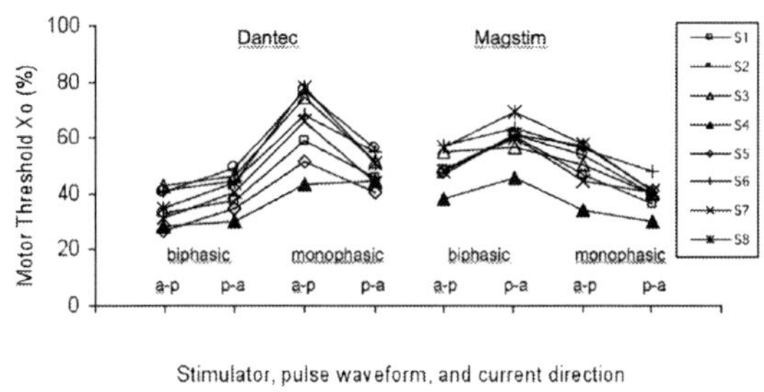

lower noise and heat, but bilateral responses are not easy achievable (Hovey and Janilous, 2008). Neurophysilogical studies demonstrated that monophasic and biphasic pulses require different output intensities in order to determinate the motor threshold (MT), either active (AMT), or at rest (RMT) (Sommer et al., 2006).

Stimulation Frequency

Depending on the frequency of the pulses there are three possible stimulation protocols:

Simple stimulation: TMS is applied with a frequency below 1Hz (Barker, 2002). This is suitable for studies of peripheral nerves, being able to depolarize neurons in the motor cortex and to induce a motor evoked potential (MEP) that can be measured in a given muscle of the contralateral hemibody (usually in the hand). This type of stimulation is applied, for example, to evaluate the motor conduction time, which is altered in cases of multiple sclerosis or amyotrophic lateral sclerosis (de Noordhout et al., 1998).

Paired pulse stimulation: It consist of two TMS pulses applied in the same or different brain areas. Pulses are usually of different intensities and presented within an interval of milliseconds (Kujirai et al., 1993). When applied to motor cortex and varying the interval or intensity of the first pulse, the response to the second pulse can be inhibited or facilitated (Ziemann et al., 1998, Di Lazzaro et al., 1999, Ilic et al., 2002). These two phenomena are known respectively as intracortical inhibition and facilitation since, supposedly, it would be mediated by intracortical connections in pyramidal neurons, being inhibitory or excitatory depending on the interval between stimuli (Kujirai et al., 1993, Ziemann, Rothwell and Ridding, 1996). For other applications, further studies have proposed a range of protocols, varying the number of pulses, intensity and the interval between stimuli (Ziemann et al., 1998, Bestmann et al., 2004, Tokimura et al., 1996).

Repetitive stimulation: Repetitive TMS (rTMS) consists of pulse trains delivered with a maximum frequency of 50 Hz during tens, hundreds or thousands of milliseconds. It is useful to modify the excitability of brain areas at the site of stimulation or in other cortical areas due to cortico-cortical connections (Jalinous, 1991), lasting even several minutes after the end of the rTMS protocol (Robertson, Theoret and Pascual-Leone, 2003), "off-line effect" or "after effect" (Siebner and Rothwell, 2003)). Depending on the frequency of stimulation, rTMS have been classified as of low and high frequency, being the separation between types around 5 Hz. This division is not random and is due mainly to results obtained in experiments devoted to analyze this frequency range. They concluded that frequencies above 5 Hz tended to increase corticospinal excitability (Berardelli et al., 1998, Maeda et al., 2000a, Pascual-Leone et al., 1994, Pascual-Leone et al., 1998). In contrast, frequencies below 5 Hz tended to depress the excitability (Pascual-Leone et al., 1998, Chen et al., 1997, Muellbacher et al., 2000). One special type of repetitive stimulation is called "theta burst" and consists of trains of pulses of short duration applied with a repetition rate of 5 Hz (it has also been tested in humans with 10 and 20 Hz, see De Ridder et al., 2007). Each train consists normally

Table 1. Maximal rTMS train duration (secs) as a function of stimulation frequency to be bound to safety guidelines. Values have been calculated from data obtained from motor cortex stimulation; therefore it is worth remarking cortical excitability varies from area to area (Wassermann, 1998)

Frequency (Hz)	Stimulation Intensity (% RMT)												
1	>1800	>1800	360	>50	>50	>50	>50	27	11	11	8	7	6
5	>10	>10	>10	>10	7.6	5.2	3.6	2.6	2.4	1.6	1.4	1.6	1.2
10	>5	>5	4.2	2.9	1.3	0.8	0.9	0.8	0.5	0.6	0.4	0.3	0.3
20	2.05	1.6	1.0	0.55	0.35	0.25	0.25	0.15	0.2	0.25	0.2	0.1	0.1
25	1.28	0.84	0.4	0.24	0.2	0.24	0.2	0.12	0.08	0.12	0.12	0.08	0.08

of 3 to 5 pulses with an intra-train frequency of 100 Hz; although human safety restrictions (Wassermann, 1998, Rossi et al. 2009, Table 1) limits the stimulation trains to 3 pulses with an intra-train frequency of 50 Hz (Huang and Rothwell, 2004). Its effect can be controlled, being facilitator in the "intermittent mode" (using groups of trains of 2 sec duration every 10 sec) or inhibitor in the "continuous mode" (Huang et al., 2005, Di Lazzaro et al., 2005). Its main advantage is that to achieve a specific period of delayed effect it requires a comparatively smaller period of stimulation than conventional rTMS (Huang and Rothwell, 2004).

Other Parameters

Other parameters to be determined are the current that flows through the stimulation coil (i.e. the magnitude of the magnetic field, see eq. [1]) and the period of stimulation. Several studies have shown that frequency, intensity and duration are closely dependent variables. For example, a facilitatory effect similar to that obtained using 10 TMS pulses at 20 Hz and 150% of motor threshold (Pascual-Leone et al., 1994) is obtained by applying a train of 240 pulses at the same frequency but with an intensity of 90% (Maeda et al., 2000a, Maeda et al., 2000b). On the other hand, interdependence between frequency and duration of the stimulus is revealed in a second study devoted to analyze visual evoked potentials after rTMS applied on occipital cortex of the cat at low and high frequencies during periods ranging from 1 to 20 minutes (Aydin-Abidin et al., 2006). Trains of low frequency (1 to 3 Hz) require a long period of application (20 min) to significantly decrease the amplitude of the evoked potential; in contrast, high frequency trains (10 Hz) require less time (1 to 5 min) to increase the amplitude of evoked potentials and appear to be more effective than longer trains (20 min).

CLINICAL APPLICATIONS OF TMS

The use of TMS as a tool for clinical diagnosis is widely recognized. It has become a regular technique in neurology and neurophysiology, with application in the study of central conduction in multiple sclerosis, diagnosis of psychogenic disorders, study of facial paralysis, diagnosis and monitoring of spine injury, or as an operating room monitoring system. Likewise its application for basic research has grown exponentially in the last decade, given it is a suitable tool for exploring visual system physiology, language, learning, memory, and of course, motor system, for which it was originally developed.

However, the effectiveness of TMS as a therapeutic tool is an issue of debate. Some researchers have stated that no treatment based on rTMS has consistently improved any disorder in the last decade. Despite, it is clear the technique is very attractive, given the possibility of stimulating cerebral circuitry through a non-invasive way with proved effect on functional re-organization, which can become of clinical utility. The technique has been used in several neurological and psychiatric diseases, like depression, stroke, migraine, or tinnitus. Results have been variable.

Part of scepticism around the therapeutic effectiveness of TMS might be due to a wrong choice of the disorders to be treated; probably these are still to be determined. Wassermann and Lisanby (2001) reviewed the therapeutic use of rTMS, Pascual-Leone et al. (2002) and Hallet and Chokroverty (2005) have edited excellent monographs also.

Some disorders have been the subject of research applying rTMS at low frequency with the aim of depressing neuronal activity of abnormally hyperexcitable cerebral circuits. This is the case, for instance, of focal dystonia, epilepsy, or auditory hallucinations present in schizophrenia, which might be good targets to be treated with rTMS (Lefaucheur et al., 2004, Poulet et al., 2005; Allam et al., 2007; Joo et al., 2007). On the other hand, in some other disorders which affect (diffusely) larger areas of the brain, the hope of succeeding should be more modest.

An intermediate example is Parkinson's disease, where histological and neurochemical deficits are subcortical (beyond the direct TMS pulses influence), but with concomitant cortical dysfunctions well documented. Some of the affected cortical areas are the dorsolateral prefrontal cortex, the supplementary motor area, the lateral premotor cortex, the parietal cortex, the sensorimotor cortex, and also the motor cortex. Therefore, it seems conceivable that some of these areas can represent a target for rTMS application with the aim to relieve parkinsonian symptoms.

TMS over the Motor Cortex (Area 4)

This area was the first target for TMS application in PD and some other movement disorders. Several of the parameters that can be evaluated with this technique are impaired in PD:

- Motor threshold: The minimum stimulation intensity that can produce a motor output of a given amplitude from a muscle at rest (RMT) or during a muscle contraction (AMT). It reflects excitability within the corticospinal system (Rossini et al. 1994). It is usually registered by electromyography recordings of the Motor Evoked Potential (MEP). Some works report normal threshold in PD; though some other reports RMT to be reduced in PD (Cantello et al. 2002).
- MEP amplitude: size (peak-to-peak) of MEP which increases in direct proportion to stimulus intensity. Most of the published works have reported that MEP is enlarged at rest; this may reflect an excitation-inhibition unbalance in the corticospinal system and desinhibition would be increased (Cantello et al. 2002).
- Cortical silent period: this parameter has become a key element of the use of TMS in PD. If a TMS pulse is delivered over the motor cortex whilst a muscle is voluntary contracted, a period of silent EMG activity is displayed following the muscular evoked potential (Figure 5) (Cantello et al. 2002). Its duration reflects the functionality of the cortical inhibitory mechanisms; it is shortened in PD, and increased by antiparkinsonian drugs.
- Neurophysiological evaluation of cortical physiology by mean of paired pulse stimulation: Stimulation with two distinct stimuli through the same coil over the cerebral cortex at a range of different intervals; the intensities can be varied independently. In

Figure 5. Cortical silent period obtained after stimulation of M1. After the MEP, a period without electrical activity is observed

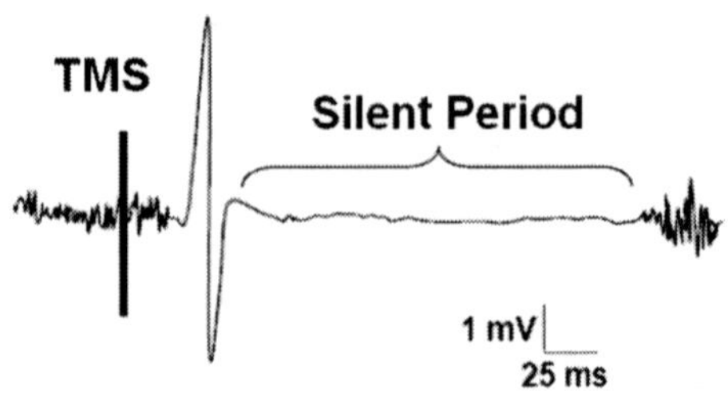

this technique, a subthreshold conditioning stimulus (CS) is applied prior to a suprathreshold test stimulus (TS). The effect of the conditioning stimulus depends critically on the interstimulus interval (ISI) between CS and TS but also on CS strength. The motor-evoked response (MEP) elicited by the test stimulus is reduced if CS precedes TS by approximately 1–4 ms, while facilitation of the MEP results in ISIs of 7–20 ms (Ziemann et al., 1996). This phenomenon is commonly referred to as intracortical inhibition (and facilitation, since it is thought that either inhibitory or excitatory intracortical connections to the pyramidal tract neurones are activated in an ISI-dependent way. More recently, this kind of inhibition has been termed short-interval intracortical inhibition to distinguish it from another kind of cortically mediated inhibition observed with longer (50–200 ms) interstimulus intervals (Valls-Solé et al., 1992) both altered in PD (Cantello et al. 2002).

- Repetitive TMS (rTMS) in PD: Alvaro Pascual Leone and collaborators in 1994 were the first to describe the effects of rTMS on PD signs. They showed how stimulation the motor cortex at 5 Hz, with an intensity of 90% of the RMT sped up movements in a hand dexterity test (Grooved Pegboard). However, other authors using similar protocols have not been able to reproduce those results (Ghabra et al. 1999).

Some other stimulation paradigms, more complex from a methodological point of view, have yielded promising results. In a placebo controlled trial by Siebner et al., (1999), rTMS with an intensity of 90% RMT resulted in significant improvement of hand movements. Stimulation was applied by means of 15 trains of 30 seconds each at 5 Hz, for a total of 2250 pulses over the motor cortex contralateral to the evaluated hand. In the task, patients had to perform balistic movements to a target in front of them. Movement time, accuracy, and velocity variability improved after real stimulation, but not in the case of those patients receiving sham stimulation. Though the experiment was carefully designed, it has been criticised given real stimulation facilitates ongoing movement, a fact that has not been achieved in the case of sham stimulation.

Based on studies showing long lasting effects on parkinsonian sings obtained with just one session of rTMS, it seems conceivable to look for cumulative effects after different sessions. Recently, data obtained in a well controlled study have shown an improvement in clinical signs in PD after several sessions of rTMS at high frequency applied bilaterally over the motor cortex. The effects lasted for several days (Kherd et al., 2006).

Stimulation over Some Other Areas Involved in Motor Control

Some other areas than the motor cortex have been also stimulated in order to ameliorate motor and non-motor sings in PD.

- Supplementary motor area (SMA): This area is involved in sequencing complex movements along with motor planning. When SMA was stimulated at 5 Hz (intensity 110% AMT) delivered by a figure of eight coil with a slight improvement in clinical signs was found (Hamada et al., 2008).

- Dorsolateral prefrontal cortex (DLPFC): This region mediates cognitive processes, like decision making or working memory. It is also related to movement given it connection to the basal ganglia-SMA loop. DLPFC has become a target for stimulation in PD given that stimulation of this area induces dopamine release in the caudate nucleus. Also some reports have shown improvement in symptoms of depression, which are common in PD. Although early reports indicate that motor sings might be improved after stimulation of DLPFC, a later placebo controlled study has pointed out that placebo effect could be responsible for the observed improvement in several motor task (arm movements, grip strength, and gait) after DLPFC stimulation of the contralateral hemisphere for several days (del Olmo et al. 2007).

DLPFC and Motor Cortex

rTMS stimulation delivered over these areas may be beneficial and with long-lasting effects. Stimulation (25 Hz at 100% RMT) was applied twice per week, for 4 weeks, resulting in a significant improvement in gait, and bradykinesia in the PD receiving real stimulation, but not in the sham group. This was a double-blind study with a positive outcome which reinforces the view that TMS might be a promising tool to treat PD (Lomarev et al. 2006).

Cerebellum

Recently the use of rTMS has been explored with promising results in order to control some side effects of antiparkinsonian medication. Kock et al., 2009 have shown how rTMS applied over the cerebellum under continuous theta-burst protocol reduced levodopa induced diskynesias in the patients, as well as modified some altered cortical excitability parameters in the PD.

CONCLUSION

Any kind of therapeutic approach must fulfil at least three main requirements in order to be consider useful from a clinical perspective: (i) the effect must last, hours or days, (ii) the improvement must be measurable and, finally (iii) benefit/risk ratio must be clearly positive. rTMS (even with the existing discrepancies) seems to match all requirements to be taken into account as a therapeutic tool in order to treat PD, the topic keeps on being matter of research. Some reports indicate improvements in clinical sings lasting several days after the last rTMS session with minor side effects, which are chiefly restricted to headache just after stimulation, which lasts a few minutes and appears seldom.

In spite of the promising results, some questions remain open. What is it mechanism of action? What is the best protocol of stimulation? Is it suitable for all PD or is it phenotype dependent? Is the effect observed really different to that obtained by placebo? So far, the main conclusions to be drawn are: the technique allows a better knowledge of the disease from a neurophysiological point of view and it gives hope to find a new way to ameliorate parkinsonian symptoms.

REFERENCES

Barker, A. T. (1999). The history and basic principles of magnetic nerve stimulation. *Electroencephalography and Clinical Neurophysiology. Supplement*, *51*, 3–21.

Bartres-Faz, D., Junque, C., Tormos, J. M., & Pascual-Leone, A. (2000). Aplicación de la estimulación magnética transcraneal a la investigación neuropsicológica. *Revista de Neurologia, 30*(12), 1169–1174.

Boylan, L. S., Pullman, S. L., Lisanby, S. H., Spicknall, K. E., & Sackeim, H. A. (2001). Repetitive transcranial magnetic stimulation to SMA worsens complex movements in Parkinson's disease. *Clinical Neurophysiology, 112*(2), 259–264. doi:10.1016/S1388-2457(00)00519-8

Calvo-Merino, B., & Haggard, P. (2004). Estimulación magnética transcraneal. Aplicaciones en neurociencia cognitiva. *Revista de Neurologia, 38*(4), 374–380.

Cantello, R., Tarletti, R., & Civardi, C. (2002). Transcranial magnetic stimulation and Parkinson's disease. *Brain Research. Brain Research Reviews, 38*(3), 309–327. doi:10.1016/S0165-0173(01)00158-8

Del Olmo, M. F., Bello, O., & Cudeiro, J. (2007). Transcranial magnetic stimulation over dorsolateral prefrontal cortex in Parkinson's disease. *Clinical Neurophysiology, 118*(1), 131–139. doi:10.1016/j.clinph.2006.09.002

Di Lazzaro, V., Oliviero, A., Mazzone, P., Insola, A., Pilato, F., & Saturno, E. (2001). Comparison of descending volleys evoked by monophasic and biphasic magnetic stimulation of the motor cortex in conscious humans. *Experimental Brain Research, 141*(1), 121–127. doi:10.1007/s002210100863

Di Lazzaro, V., Oliviero, A., Pilato, F., Saturno, E., Dileone, M., & Mazzone, P. (2004). The physiological basis of transcranial motor cortex stimulation in conscious humans. *Clinical Neurophysiology, 115*, 255–266. doi:10.1016/j.clinph.2003.10.009

Espinosa, N., de Labra, C., Rivadulla, C., Mariño, J., Grieve, K. L., & Cudeiro, J. (2007). Effects on EEG of Low (1Hz) and High (15Hz) Frequency Repetitive Transcranial Magnetic Stimulation of the Visual Cortex: A Study in the Anesthetized Cat. *The Open Neurosci Journal, 1*, 20–25.

Fitzgerald, P. B., Fountain, S., & Daskalakis, Z. J. (2006). A comprehensive review of the effects of rTMS on motor cortical excitability and inhibition. *Clinical Neurophysiology, 117*(12), 2584–2596. doi:10.1016/j.clinph.2006.06.712

Fregni, F., Simon, D. K., Wu, A., & Pascual-Leone, A. (2005). Non-invasive brain stimulation for Parkinson's disease: a systematic review and meta-analysis of the literature. *Journal of Neurology, Neurosurgery, and Psychiatry, 76*(12), 1614–1623. doi:10.1136/jnnp.2005.069849

Ghabra, M. B., Hallett, M., & Wassermann, E. M. (1999). Simultaneous repetitive transcranial magnetic stimulation does not speed fine movement in PD. *Neurology, 52*(4), 768–770.

Hamada, M., Ugawa, Y., & Tsuji, S. (2008). Effectiveness of rTMS on Parkinson's Disease Study Group, Japan. High-frequency rTMS over the supplementary motor area for treatment of Parkinson's disease. *Movement Disorders, 23*(11), 1524–1531. doi:10.1002/mds.22168

Hovey, C., & Janilous, R. (2008). *The guide to magnetic stimulation*. The Magstims Company UK.

Jalinous, R. (1991). Technical and practical aspects of magnetic nerve stimulation. *Journal of Clinical Neurophysiology, 8*(1), 10–25. doi:10.1097/00004691-199101000-00004

Joo, E. Y., Han, S. J., Chung, S. H., Cho, J. W., Seo, D. W., & Hong, S. B. (2007). Antiepileptic effects of low-frequency repetitive transcranial magnetic stimulation by different stimulation durations and locations. *Clinical Neurophysiology, 118*(3), 702–708. doi:10.1016/j.clinph.2006.11.008

Kammer, T., Beck, S., Thielscher, A., Laubis-Herrmann, U., & Topka, H. (2001). Motor thresholds in humans: a transcranial magnetic stimulation study comparing different pulse waveforms, current directions and stimulator types. *Clinical Neurophysiology*, *112*(2), 250–258. doi:10.1016/S1388-2457(00)00513-7

Kaneko, K., Kawai, S., Fuchigami, Y., Morita, H., & Ofuji, A. (1996). The effect of current direction induced by transcranial magnetic stimulation on the corticospinal excitability in human brain. *Electroencephalography and Clinical Neurophysiology*, *101*, 478–482. doi:10.1016/S0013-4694(96)96021-X

Khedr, E. M., Rothwell, J. C., Shawky, O. A., Ahmed, M. A., & Hamdy, A. (2006). Effect of daily repetitive transcranial magnetic stimulation on motor performance in Parkinson's disease. *Movement Disorders*, *21*(12), 2201–2205. doi:10.1002/mds.21089

Kobayashi, M., & Pascual-Leone, A. (2003). Transcranial magnetic stimulation in neurology. *The Lancet Neurology*, *2*(3), 145–156. doi:10.1016/S1474-4422(03)00321-1

Koch, G., Brusa, L., Carrillo, F., Lo Gerfo, E., Torriero, S., & Oliveri, M. (2009). Cerebellar magnetic stimulation decreases levodopa-induced dyskinesias in Parkinson disease. *Neurology*, *73*(2), 113–119. doi:10.1212/WNL.0b013e3181ad5387

Lefaucheur, J. P., Fénelon, G., Ménard-Lefaucheur, I., Wendling, S., & Nguyen, J. P. (2004). Low-frequency repetitive TMS of premotor cortex can reduce painful axial spasms in generalized secondary dystonia: a pilot study of three patients. *Neurophysiologie Clinique*, *34*(3-4), 141–145. doi:10.1016/j.neucli.2004.07.003

Lomarev, M. P., Kanchana, S., Bara-Jimenez, W., Iyer, M., Wassermann, E. M., & Hallett, M. (2006). Placebo controlled study of rTMS for the treatment of Parkinson's disease. *Movement Disorders*, *21*(3), 325–331. doi:10.1002/mds.20713

Machii, K., Cohen, D., Ramos-Estebanez, C., & Pascual-Leone, A. (2006). Safety of rTMS to non-motor cortical areas in healthy participants and patients. *Clinical Neurophysiology*, *117*(2), 455–471. doi:10.1016/j.clinph.2005.10.014

Mally, J., & Stone, T. W. (1999). Improvement in Parkinsonian symptoms after repetitive transcranial magnetic stimulation. *Journal of the Neurological Sciences*, *162*(2), 179–184. doi:10.1016/S0022-510X(98)00318-9

Nakamura, H., Kitagawa, H., Kawaguchi, Y., & Tsuji, H. (1996). Direct and indirect activation of human corticospinal neurons by transcranial magnetic and electrical stimulation. *Neuroscience Letters*, *210*, 45–48. doi:10.1016/0304-3940(96)12659-8

Pascual-Leone, A., Valls-Sole, J., Brasil-Neto, J. P., Cammarota, A., Grafman, J., & Hallett, M. (1994). Akinesia in Parkinson's disease. II. Effects of subthreshold repetitive transcranial motor cortex stimulation. *Neurology*, *44*(2), 892–898.

Patton, H. D., & Amassian, V. E. (1954). Single and multiple-unit analysis of cortical stage of pyramidal tract activation. *Journal of Neurophysiology*, *17*, 345–363.

Poulet, E., Brunelin, J., Bediou, B., Bation, R., Forgeard, L., & Dalery, J. (2005). Slow transcranial magnetic stimulation can rapidly reduce resistant auditory hallucinations in schizophrenia. *Biological Psychiatry*, *57*(2), 188–191. doi:10.1016/j.biopsych.2004.10.007

Ridding, M. C., & Rothwell, J. C. (2007). Is there a future for therapeutic use of transcranial magnetic stimulation? *Nature Reviews. Neuroscience*, *8*(7), 559–567. doi:10.1038/nrn2169

Rossi, S., Ferro, M., Cincotta, M., Ulivelli, M., Bartalini, S., & Miniussi, C. (2007). A real electro-magnetic placebo (REMP) device for sham transcranial magnetic stimulation (TMS). *Clinical Neurophysiology*, *118*(3), 709–716. doi:10.1016/j.clinph.2006.11.005

Rossi, S., Hallett, M., Rossini, P. M., & Pascual-Leone, A. (2009). The Safety of TMS Consensus Group. Safety, ethical considerations, and application guidelines for the use of transcranial magnetic stimulation in clinical practice and research. *Clinical Neurophysiology, 120*(12), 2008–2039. doi:10.1016/j.clinph.2009.08.016

Rossini, P. M., Barker, A. T., Berardelli, A., Caramia, M. D., Caruso, G., & Cracco, R. Q. (1994). Non-invasive electrical and magnetic stimulation of the brain, spinal cord and roots: basic principles and procedures for routine clinical application. Report of an IFCN committee. *Electroencephalography and Clinical Neurophysiology, 91*(2), 79–92. doi:10.1016/0013-4694(94)90029-9

Roth, Y., Amir, A., Levkovitz, Y., & Zangen, A. (2007). Three-dimensional distribution of the electric field induced in the brain by transcranial magnetic stimulation using figure-8 and deep H-coils. *Journal of Clinical Neurophysiology, 24*(1), 31–38. doi:10.1097/WNP.0b013e31802fa393

Rothwell, J. C. (1997). Techniques and mechanism of action of transcranial stimulation of the human motor cortex. *Journal of Neuroscience Methods, 74*(2), 113–122. doi:10.1016/S0165-0270(97)02242-5

Rothwell, J. C., Thompsom, P. D., Day, B. L., Boyd, S., & Marsden, C. D. (1991). Stimulation of the human motor cortex through the scalp. *Experimental Physiology, 76*(2), 159–200.

Shimamoto, H., Morimitsu, H., Sugita, S., Nakahara, K., & Shigemori, M. (1999). Therapeutic effect of repetitive transcranial magnetic stimulation in Parkinson's disease. *Rinsho Shinkeigaku. Clinical Neurology, 39*(12), 1264–1267.

Siebner, H. R., Mentschel, C., Auer, C., & Conrad, B. (1999). Repetitive transcranial magnetic stimulation has a beneficial effect on bradykinesia in Parkinson's disease. *Neuroreport, 10*(3), 589–594. doi:10.1097/00001756-199902250-00027

Siebner, H. R., Rossmeier, C., Mentschel, C., Peinemann, A., & Conrad, B. (2000). Short-term motor improvement after sub-threshold 5-Hz repetitive transcranial magnetic stimulation of the primary motor hand area in Parkinson's disease. *Journal of the Neurological Sciences, 178*(2), 91–94. doi:10.1016/S0022-510X(00)00370-1

Sommer, M., Alfaro, A., Rummel, M., Speck, S., Lang, N., Tings, T., & Paulus, W. (2006). Half sine, monophasic and biphasic transcranial magnetic stimulation of the human motor cortex. *Clinical Neurophysiology, 117*(4), 838–844. doi:10.1016/j.clinph.2005.10.029

Tormos, J. M., Catalá, M. D., & Pascual-Leone, A. (1999). Estimulación magnética transcraneal. *Revista de Neurologia, 29*(2), 165–171.

Valls-Solé, J., Pascual-Leone, A., Wassermann, E. M., & Hallett, M. (1992). Human motor evoked responses to paired transcranial magnetic stimuli. *Electroencephalography and Clinical Neurophysiology, 85*(6), 355–364. doi:10.1016/0168-5597(92)90048-G

Wassermann, E. M. (1998). Risk and safety of repetitive transcranial magnetic stimulation: report and suggested guidelines from the international Workshop on the Safety of Repetitive Transcranial Magnetic Stimulation. *Electroencephalogr Clin Neurophysiol, 108*(1), 1-16.

Wassermann, E. M., & Lisanby, S. H. (2001). Therapeutic application of repetitive transcranial magnetic stimulation: A review. *Clinical Neurophysiology, 112*(8), 1367–1377. doi:10.1016/S1388-2457(01)00585-5

Zangen, A., Roth, Y., Voller, B., & Hallett, M. (2005). Transcranial magnetic stimulation of deep brain regions: evidence for efficacy of the H-coil. *Clinical Neurophysiology, 116*(4), 775–779. doi:10.1016/j.clinph.2004.11.008

Ziemann, U., Rothwell, J. C., & Ridding, M. C. (1996). Interaction between intracortical inhibition and facilitation in human motor cortex. *The Journal of Physiology*, *496*, 873–881.

Zimmermann, K. P., & Simpson, R. K. (1996). 'Slinky' coils for neuromagnetic stimulation. *Electroencephalography and Clinical Neurophysiology*, *101*(2), 145–152. doi:10.1016/0924-980X(95)00227-C

KEY TERMS AND DEFINITIONS

AMT: Motor threshold (MT) during a muscle contraction.

Dorsolateral Prefrontal Cortex (DLPFC): Part of the cerebral cortex involved in cognitive processes, like decision making or working memory. It is also related to movement given it connection to the basal ganglia-SMA loop.

Interstimulus Interval (ISI): Time between consecutive stimulus.

Motor Cortex (Area 4): Part of the cerebral cortex involved in controlling muscle contraction.

Motor Evoked Potential (MEP): Electrical activity recorded from muscles following direct stimulation of motor cortex.

Motor Threshold (MT): The minimum stimulation intensity that can produce a motor output of a given amplitude from a muscle at rest (RMT) or during a muscle contraction (AMT).

PD: Parkinson's disease.

Repetitive TMS (rTMS): Modality of TMS in which pulse trains are delivered with a maximum frequency of 50 Hz during tens, hundreds or thousands of milliseconds.

RMT: Motor threshold at rest.

Subthreshold Conditioning Stimulus (CS): Stimulus with an intensity below the motor threshold.

Supplementary Motor Area (SMA): In sequencing complex movements along with motor planning.

Supra-Threshold Test Stimulus (TS): Stimulus with an intensity above the motor threshold.

Transcranial Magnetic Stimulation (TMS): Stimulation technique based on the generation of magnetic fields to induce currents in the cortical tissue (or any excitable tissue) interfering, therefore, with the electrical activity of neurons.

Chapter 9
A Feedback Controlled FES in Rehabilitation

Yu-Luen Chen
National Taipei University of Education, Taiwan

Te-Son Kuo
National Taiwan University, Taiwan

ABSTRACT

A feedback control functional electrical stimulation (FES) system was proposed to prevent quadriceps weakness and drop-foot of the hemiplegia during gait training. The FES system is triggered by a foot-switch on the heel of the affected foot to stimulate the tibialis anterior muscle for dorsi-flexion and to turn-off the knee locker in the swing phase through the main controller. The footswitch on the heel of the affected-side can be used to stimulate the quadriceps and turn-on the knee locker for quadriceps weakness in the stance phase. It was revealed that the mean velocity, cadence, stride length, active ankle motion range and functional ambulation category (FAC) were significantly improved. A paired t-test indicated that the differences in the electromyography (EMG) of the tibialis anterior and the quadriceps muscles between patient's affected foot and unaffected foot were not significant (p>0.05) after 16 weeks of training. The proposed knee locker device with closed-loop FES system is capable of providing a hemiplegic patient with regular walking restoration after appropriate gait training.

INTRODUCTION

In this chapter, targeted commonly seen problems in stroke patients, carrying out a discussion on knee joint weakness and drop-foot. The goal was to design a more convenient knee lock device combined with closed loop control FES. On one hand, it was hoped to improve the weak knee joint support problem in stroke victims using a knee locker. On the other hand, it was hoped to rectify the drop-foot problem in stroke victims using sensors(footswitch, position sensor)closed loop control. After system construction was completed, before and after gait analysis documentation of stoke victims using this system in walking train-

DOI: 10.4018/978-1-60566-206-0.ch009

ing, the system's actual benefit to stroke victims in walking was evaluated.

BACKGROUND

The development of functional electrical stimulation (FES) has a history of more than 40 years. Along with improvements in hardware technology and software control, FES now occupies an important role in rehabilitation medicine. In 1961, to rectify the drop-foot problem in hemiplegics, Liberson and Holmquest used FES to stimulate the peromeal nerve of the hemiplegics paralyzed side and discovered that this method was able to effectively correct drop-foot on the patient's paralyzed side. In those days, the method was simply called functional electrotherapy. It was not until 1962 that Liberson and Holmquest named this kind of therapy functional electrical stimulation (Liberson et al. 1961). From this time on, FES provided another favorable option for rehabilitation medicine and numerous correlated FES studies were subsequently undertaken.

In 1988, Andrews used sensory feedback combined with closed loop control. A standing state control study was carried out in which FES was administered to the lower limbs of two spinal cord injured (SCI) patients. The results of the study were then compared to results from conventional rehabilitative aids. Aids combined with FES were able to allow spinal cord injured patients to stand for relatively long periods of time (Andrews et al. 1988). In 1996, Rongching Dai (Rongching et al. 1996) used tilt sensors to replace conventional footswitches to detect angular variations in the movement of the lower limbs of stroke and SCI patients. These angular variations were used to control the current of the electric stimulus, thereby enabling the patient's walking movements to approach a more normal state. The gait analysis experiment results also proved that this method was superior to conventional ankle support orthosis combined with a footswitch control.

Apart from using tilt sensors and sensory feedback control as a means of control, other methods such as machine learning, fuzzy control, EMG myoelectrical signal control and neural network control were combined with FES to stimulate patient functional movement generation, all producing favorable results (Vodovnilc et al. 1984; Peckham et al. 1992; Chen et al. 2001).

Of the various aids commonly seen on the market, more than half rely on movement from the patient's own residual motor function, which is then corrected using aids. The rectifying ability of these kinds of passive correctional aids is limited. However, in the majority of studies, FES has already been acknowledged in rehabilitation medicine as having reasonably good effects in dealing with increased muscle force shrinkage, promoting muscle activation and the reestablishment of auxiliary motor function. FES is therefore often used in rehabilitation treatment (Kostov et al. 1995; Chen et al. 2004; Miyamoto et al. 1999; Abbas et al. 1995). In the rehabilitation of stroke, the most commonly seen problem during standing and walking movement training is inadequate knee joint support strength (knee back) and drop-foot. When the knee joint support strength is inadequate in walking, patients are prone to fall due to unstable support when standing on the hemiplegic side. The patient's fear of falling results in different step lengths for the left and right feet when walking. Drop-foot can affect patient abilities when walking. Apart from the toes coming into contact with the ground first and resulting in patient tripping, it also has affects the step length when walking and influences the esthetic appearance of the patient's walk.

FEEDBACK CONTROL FES

Instrumentation

The configuration of the proposed a feedback control FES system is shown in Figure 1. This

Figure 1. The configuration of the feedback control FES system for hemiplegia in gait training

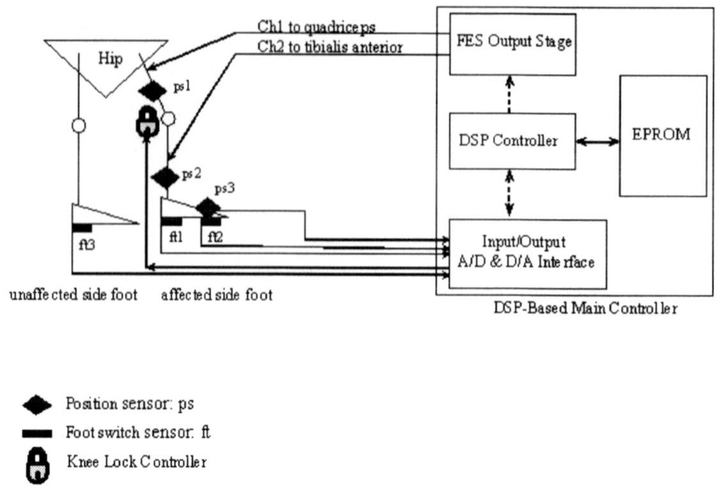

four-channel high performance FES system was developed in the laboratory. The system includes a waveform generator, a current amplifier, a voltage amplifier and a power isolation circuit. A DSP-Based main controller was installed to control and record the output current intensity, delay time, pulse duration and the FES frequency.FES can produce pulses at an amplitude's range from 0 to 100 mA using a 9V battery with frequency f = 0-100 Hz, and pulse duration t = 70-1000 μs. In addition, the FES can execute feedback-controlled functions using the main controller, DSP-TMS320C32.

The mechanical structure of the self-produced knee lock device includes a major support aid that enables the hemiplegic patient to stand. The major design consideration was whether patients could support their own body weight with the assistance of this structure. At the initial design phase, steel was used as the primary material for the structure. However, during testing on able-bodied persons after design completion, we discovered that the device weight was excessive, causing the muscles on which it was worn to fatigue. We therefore redesigned the device, changing the material to an aluminum alloy. This design is shown in Figure 2. This device having has a weight of approximately 600g to 700g. After design was completed, we again invited several able-bodied persons to wear the device and test it while walking. The aluminum alloy design posed no problems as concerning structural strength (Chen et al. 2003).

Figure 2. The mechanical structure of the knee locker

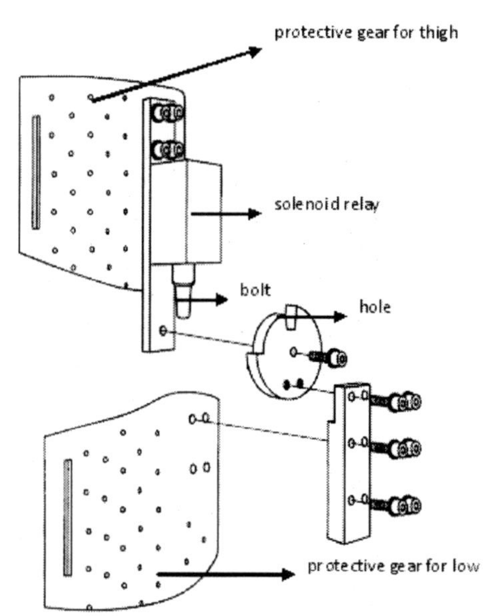

Figure 3. (a)The knee locker in stance phase, (b) the knee locker in swing phase

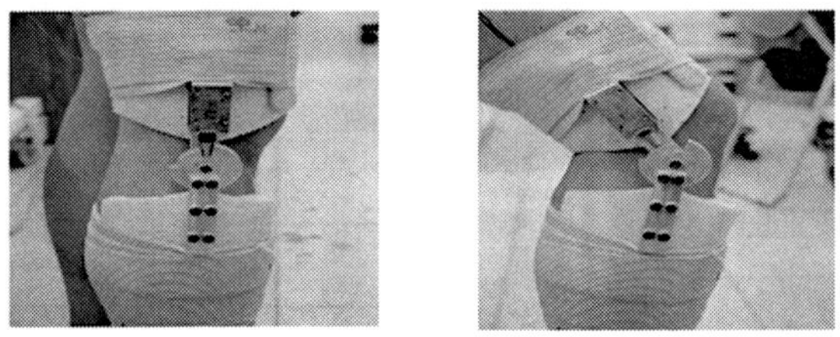

(a) (b)

The solenoid relay used in this experiment was produced by the Summit Company with a weight of 205g. It uses a voltage of DC12V to conduct electricity for movement. When the hemiplegic patient is standing, as shown in Figure 3(a), the solenoid relay installed in the mechanical structure does not conduct magnetism. The bolt in the solenoid relay falls into the hole (turn-on) of the mechanical structure by gravity and, in doing so, locks the hemiplegic knee joint, assisting the stroke victim in standing. When the patient's lower limb in the swing phase, the bolt in the solenoid relay is turned-off due to magnetism conduction, allowing the hemiplegic's knee joint to move freely, as shown in Figure 3(b).

The footswitches placed on the heels of the unaffected and affected-sides and on the first metatarsal of the affected-side, can turn on when a pressure of approximately 150 grams is applied. The FES system is triggered by a footswitch on the heel of the affected foot to stimulate the tibialis anterior muscle for dorsi-flexion and to turn-off the knee locker device in the swing phase through the main controller. The footswitch on the heel of the affected-side can be used to stimulate the quadriceps and turn-on the knee lock device for quadriceps weakness in the stance phase.

This system uses three position sensors. The position sensors that have been used as angular sensors for applications such as detection of angular position of the steering wheel in automobiles are Magneto-Resistive (M.R.) elements. In this study, UV-1W position sensor (from Midori Precision Co., Ltd., Japan) was integrated into this system. In model UV-1W the magnet pieces are attached to a pendulum, which forms a total mass of 10 g. When the sensor tilts away from the vertical direction, the mass moves toward the direction of gravity and rotates the pendulum that displaces the magnets over the MR element. The displacement of the magnets changes the magnetic flux density across the MR elements. As a result, a tilted angle is formed to reflect the resistance change of the MR elements. Three position sensors are needed for the system, and their associated locations are placed on the lateral sides of thigh, low leg, and fifth metatarsal of affected-side foot to detect the angular displacement of both knee and ankle, respectively. As shown in Figure 4(a) and Figure 4(b), the angles of knee and ankle can be calculated from ($\theta h - \theta' k$) and ($\theta a - \theta k$). In the Figure 5(a) and Figure 5(b), the side-view of the position sensors placement and the front-view of the position sensors and electrodes placement are demonstrated, respectively.

The closed-loop FES system can monitor in real time the angular movements of knee and ankle in stance phase and swing phase of the disabled foot, respectively. Moreover, the FES system constantly takes the output parameters to adjust properly the angular movements of knee and ankle after a set of angles' parameters being programmed by clinician beforehand.

The D/A and A/D interface is integrated into the main controller. The interface that integrates the knee lock controller, the footswitches, the position sensors and main controller. The FES system is a multi-functional DAS card. This card provides features such as a 8ms 12 bits A/D converter, a DC to DC converter, a 12 bits double-buffered D/A converter and 16 digital inputs and outputs. The control system sampling rate is approximately 15Hz. The therapist can set up the upper boundary for the output current intensity for the FES. The upper output current intensity boundary can be

Figure 4. The angles of the lower limb during gait training: (a) the affected-side foot in loading response (stance phase), and (b) the affected-side foot in terminal swing (swing phase)

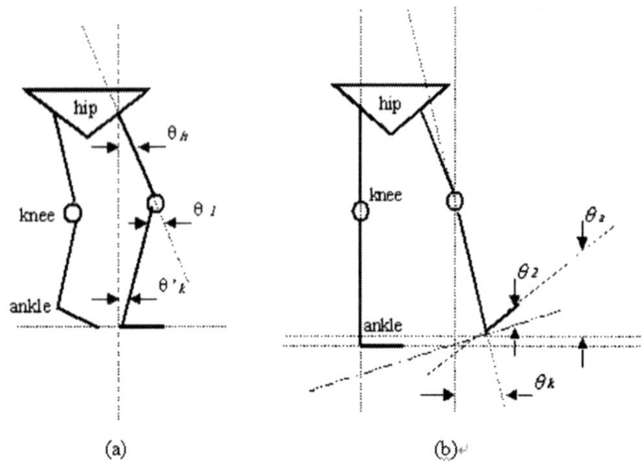

obtained by testing the patient's current tolerance before gait training. By comparing data obtained from the footswitch and position sensor, a set of optimal stimulation parameters are generated by the FES using control rules after considering the predetermined parameters previously set up. Analytically, the control rules that use the on-line signals from monitoring sensors (footswitches and position sensors) as a "current intensity of controlled constraint" for inputs has presented a deterministic and logic expression. The control rule output is the safely adjusted current. Because the EPROM can record both patient data and each parameter generated at the end of the training program using the FES automatically, the clinician must set up the FES parameters only at the beginning of the patient's first training session. In future training, the patient will automatically receive a set of optimal stimulation parameters based on the data collected by FES from the previous training.

Figure 5. (a) The side-view of the position sensors placement, and (b) the front-view of the position sensors and electrodes placement are demonstrated

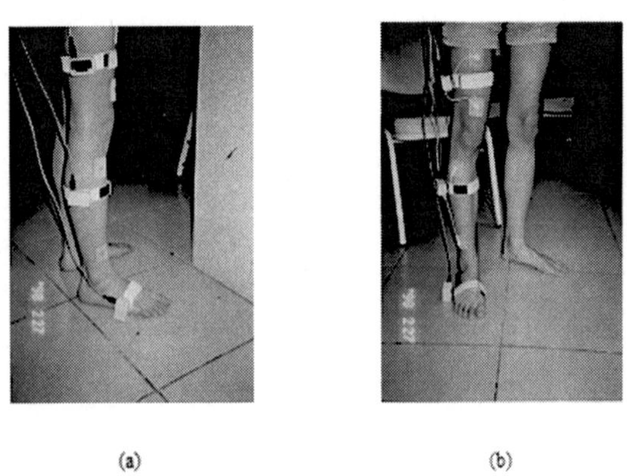

Once the function of each individual component and the control software module are completed, the system and the sensors can be further tested for performance. The testing items include

Figure 6. The timing sequence of the affected-side and unaffected-side of the hemiplegic patient

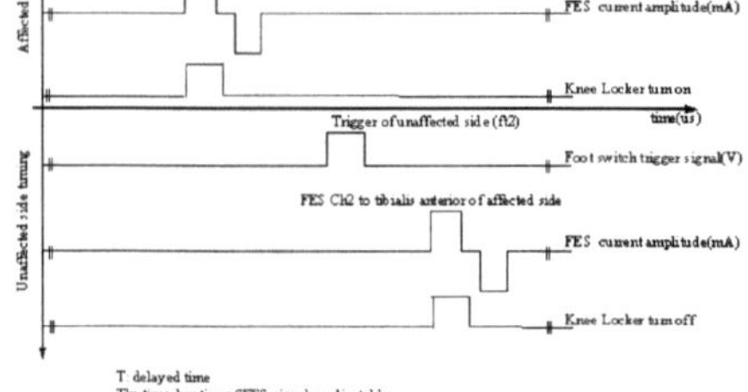

Table 1. Functional Ambulation Category (FAC)

Level0	-Patient cannot walk, or requires help of two or more people
Level1	-Patient requires firm continuous support from one person who helps with carrying weight and with balance
Level2	-Patient needs continuous of intermittent support of one person to help with balance and coordination
Level3	-Patient requires verbal supervision of stand-by help from one person without physical contact
Level4	-Patient can walk independently on level ground, but requires help on stairs, slopes, or uneven surface
Level5	-Patient can walk independent anywhere

FES outputs to the quadriceps and tibialis anterior muscles, real-time closed-loop control and FES signals' monitor and display. A delay time that controls the timing sequence between footswitch trigger signals and FES outputs is controlled by a time counter, as shown in Figure 6. The purpose of designing the delay time is to help the patient acquire enough time to transfer his body's center of gravity and change his gait from the swing phase into stance phase.

A Case Report

One patient (male, 58 years old, right-sided hemiplegia for three months) was recruited and gave his formal consent in this study. This patient was level 2 of Functional Ambulation Category (FAC) (Chen et al. 2001). He requires intermittent support from one person to help him with balance or coordination all of the time. All levels of FAC are shown in Table 1. The patient was treated with this new system for 15 minutes per day, every other day, for a period of 16 weeks. The dynamic EMG and FAC of the patient were recorded at the end of each training every 4 weeks. After the gait training program (16 weeks training), the patient received gait motion analysis via a VICON system (Oxford Metrics Limited Company). The VICON system contains six-cameras for recording the translational and angular kinematics of the lower segments of the affected limb in the sagittal, frontal and horizontal planes. Generally, the training is initiated with the normal foot first. The knee angle (flexion at the knee) and ankle angle (plantar flexion) were both set at 15 degrees during the gait training. For data analysis, the average integrated EMG of the quadriceps and the tibialis anterior muscles for the affected or unaffected feet were taken from six gait cycles, respectively.

The integrated system performance and its individual functions were tested before clinical assessment. Ten normal individuals were tested using the position sensor and footswitch to prove that these sensors were functional and reliable. Each normal subject was attached to position sensors and footswitches and walked ten strides. The timing sequences of the position sensors and footswitches were monitoring in real time. After identifying, the timing sequences by experienced clinician examined the system.

During the clinical test, the patient wearing the apparatus and the FES outputs on the quadriceps and tibialis anterior muscles are recorded whenever the affected foot or the unaffected foot triggered the footswitches. If the footswitches were not re-triggered for 5 sec, audio alarms would be activated.

Table 2, Figure 7 and Figure 8 show that the average integrated EMGs for both the quadriceps and the tibialis anterior of affected foot or unaffected foot show no significant difference ($p>0.05$) after the 16th week of treatment using the paired t-test. This indicates that each factor measurement such as mean velocity, cadence, stride length, and active ankle motion span changed from 0.15±0.04m/sec, 43.3±15.4steps/

Table 2. The results of muscle activities (tibialis anterior and quadriceps),and FAC of experimental subject during 16-weeks of gait training

	Experimental group (Tibialis)				Experimental Group (Quadriceps)			FAC
Week	affected-sided	unaffected-sided	P		affected-sided	unaffected-sided	P	
Pre-training	7.90±2.07	11.43±2.07	*		7.18±2.33	12.03±2.93	*	2
Post-training								
4	8.64±1.89	11.43±2.18	*		8.55±1.93	12.21±2.10	*	2
8	9.57±2.59	11.58±2.44	*		9.17±1.01	11.98±2.03	*	3
12	10.69±2.00	11.78±3.00			11.23±2.66	12.01±1.78		3
16	11.16±2.78	11.38±1.97			12.38±2.08	12.48±2.03		4

Figure 7. The average integrated EMG of tibialis anterior muscle is demonstrated during four weeks ambulation training for patient under experiment

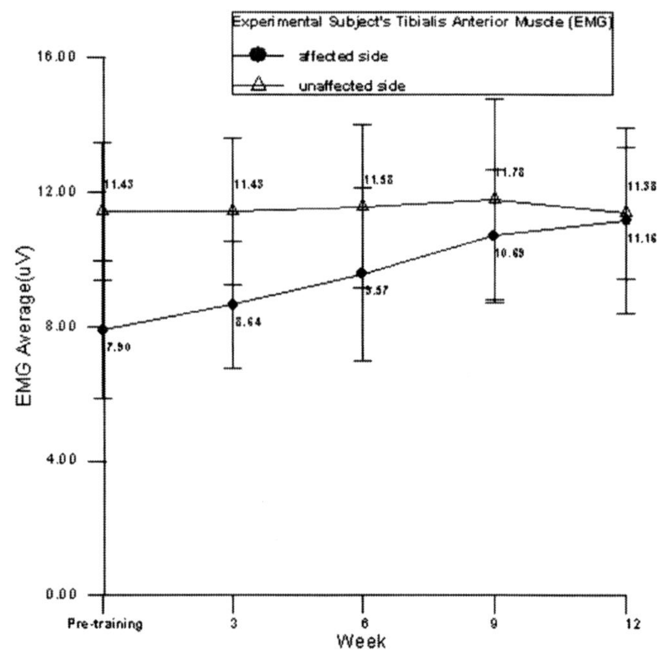

min, 0.36±0.11m, 15°to 0.43±0.21m/sec, 69.4±19.1steps/min, 0.73±0.17m, 40° improved significantly for the patient. The FAC data for patient of level 2 to level 4 during 16-weeks of gait training using the proposed knee lock device with closed-loop FES system are shown in Table 2 and Figure 9.

FUTURE TRENDS

According to the results of this study, using the knee lock device combined with the electrical stimulator provides positive benefits to improving the gait of stroke victims. In the future, a greater number of patients must be recruited for testing. The time for each patient's testing should also be prolonged. An evaluation of the physi-

Figure 8. The average integrated EMG of quadriceps muscle is demonstrated during four weeks ambulation training for patient under experiment

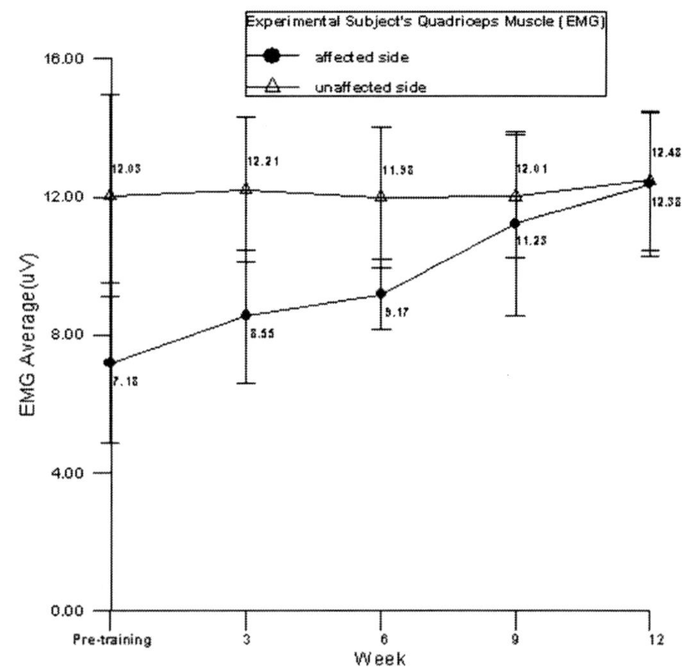

Figure 9. The FAC during four weeks ambulation training for patient under experiment

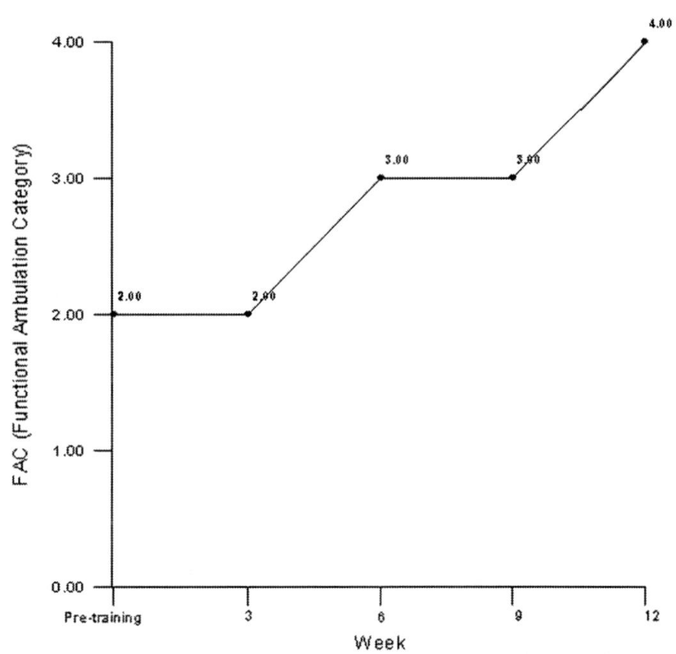

ological aspect could be incorporated, including VO_2, blood oxygen concentration analysis, blood pressure change etc. and muscle supporting force measurements, to more subjectively examine how the knee lock device and electrical stimulation effectively assists with hemiplegic patient standing and walking.

CONCLUSION

When hemiplegics joined this experiment, in the beginning, he encountered problems with unsteady steps, not being accustomed to the device. However, after several training sessions, the hemiplegic patients gradually became accustomed to the knee lock device and the FES control mechanism and gradually recovered stepping stability and balance. It was only at this time that the difference in the pace for the hemiplegic side and non-hemiplegic side could be accurately measured during patient walking. From the documentation recorded from hemiplegic patients, after using the device continually for 16 weeks, the proposed knee locker device could increase the supporting force of the knee joint for hemiplegic patients that suffered strokes approximately three months previously. The quadriceps weakness and drop-foot improvement in hemiplegic patients was also greatly improved.

REFERENCES

Abbas, J. J., & Chizeck, H. J. (1995). Neural network control of functional neuromuscular stimulation systems: computer stimulation studies. *IEEE Transactions on Bio-Medical Engineering, 11*, 1117–1127. doi:10.1109/10.469379

Andrews, B. J., Baxendale, R. H., Barnett, R., Phillips, G. F., Yamazaki, T., & Freeman, P. A. (1988). Hybrid FES orthosis incoporating closed loop control and sensory feedback. *Journal of Biomedical Engineering, 10*, 253–259. doi:10.1016/0141-5425(88)90099-4

Chen, Y. L., Chang, W. H., Chen, S. C., Sheu, P. F., & Chen, W. L. (2003). The development of a knee locker with closed-loop functional electrical stimulation (FES) for hemiplegia in gait training. *Disability and Rehabilitation, 25*(16), 916–921. doi:10.1080/0963828031000122230

Chen, Y.L., Chen, S.C., & Chen, W.L., Hsiao Chin-Chih, Kuo, T.S., & Lai, J.S. (2004). Neural network and fuzzy control in FES-assisted locomotion for the hemiplegic. *Journal of Medical Engineering & Technology, 28*(1), 32–38. doi:10.1080/03091900310001211523

Chen, Y. L., Li, Y. C., Lai, J. S., & Kuo, T. S. (2001). The development of a closed-loop controlled functional electrical stimulation (FES) in gait training. *Journal of Medical Engineering & Technology, 25*(2), 41–48. doi:10.1080/03091900110043612

Kostov, A., Andrews, B. J., Popovic, D. B., & William, W. (1995). Machine learning in control of functional electrical stimulation systems for locomotion. *IEEE Transactions on Bio-Medical Engineering, 42*, 541–551. doi:10.1109/10.387193

Liberson, W. T., Holmquest, H. J., Scot, D., & Dow, M. (1961). Functional electrotherapy: stimulation of the personal nerve synchronized with the swing phase of the gait of hemiplegic patients. *Archives of Physical Medicine and Rehabilitation, 42*, 101–105.

Miyamoto, S., Shimada, Y., Sato, K., & Kagaya, H. (1999). Hibrid functional electrical stimulation for energy-efficient restoration of standing-up motion. *Archives of Physical Medicine and Rehabilitation, 2*, 536–541.

Peckham, P. H., & Creasey, G. H. (1992). Neural prostheses: clinical applications of functional electrical stimulation spinal cord injury. *Paraplegia, 30*, 996–1001.

Rongching, D., Richard, B., Stein, B., Andrews, B. J., James, K. B., & Wieler, M. (1996). Application of tilt sensors in functional electrical stimulation. *IEEE Transactions on Rehabilitation Engineering*, *4*, 63–71. doi:10.1109/86.506403

Vodovnilc, L., Bowman, B. R., & Hufford, P. (1984). Effects of electrical stimulation on spinal spasticity. *Scandinavian Journal of Rehabilitation Medicine*, *16*, 29–34.

KEY TERMS AND DEFINITIONS

Drop-Foot: Drop foot, sometimes called foot drop, is a general term used to describe difficulty lifting the front part of the foot, may be caused by spinal of neurological disorders.

Feedback Control: A control method which can monitor the system effect (outputs) and real-time feedback controlling and modifies its output accordingly.

Functional Electrical Stimulation: A clinical technique that uses external electrical currents to activate nerves innervating extremities affected by paralysis resulting from spinal cord injury (SCI) or other neurological disorders, restoring function in people with disabilities.

Hemiplegia: Person who is a condition in which half of a body is paralyzed, that is more severe than hemiparesis, wherein one half of the body is weakened but not paralysed.

Position Sensor: An electronic element that permits position or movement measurement, it can either be an absolute position sensor or a relative one (displacement sensor), position sensor can be either linear or angular.

Stance Phase: Stance phase represents about 60% of the gait cycle, stance phase has five parts: contact, loading, midstance, terminal stance, and preswing.

Swing Phase: Swing phase represents about 40% of the gait cycle, the beginning of the swing phase of gait is signaled by toe off, and the end of the swing phase is just prior to the heel making contact with the ground.

Chapter 10
Human-Centered Metal Hydride Actuator Systems for Rehabilitation and Assistive Technology

Shuichi Ino
National Institute of Advanced Industrial Science and Technology (AIST), Japan

Mitsuru Sato
Showa University, Japan

ABSTRACT

Metal hydride materials can store a huge amount of hydrogen and can convert energy due to enthalpy change through a hydride reaction. Artificial actuation systems that employ this special physicochemical property are named metal hydride actuators. The actuators utilize the mechanical energy formed from hydrogen equilibrium pressure through thermal energy given to the metal hydride alloys as output. Metal hydride actuators have a simple structure and a number of features that make them attractive for use in rehabilitation engineering and assistive technology. They provide a high power-to-weight ratio, high strain actuation, human-compatible softness and noiselessness, and they are environmentally benign. The behavior of metal hydride actuators is also useful for overall human-machine interface applications. This article reviews the motivation for the development of some of the leading artificial muscle-like actuators, outlines the metal hydride actuators and describes its applications in quality-of-life technology.

INTRODUCTION

In an aging society with a falling birthrate, there is an increased need for home-based rehabilitation systems and human-centered robots for healthcare services (Gardner-Bonneau & Gosbee, 1997). In particular, elderly patients who are required to lie in a reclined position due to stroke or bone fracture may suffer from disuse syndromes, such as bedsores, joint contracture and muscular

DOI: 10.4018/978-1-60566-206-0.ch010

atrophy (Bortz, 1984). It is difficult for these elderly patients to actively exercise for preventive rehabilitation. Thus, to manage these disuse syndromes, rehabilitation equipment and assistive devices, such as bedside apparatuses for continuous exercise of joints, power assistance devices for standing and transfer hoists must be developed. These equipment demands powerful and soft actuators, as well as human muscles.

Currently, however, no commercially available actuators with the desired characteristics, which are human-compatible, softness for safety, noiseless and having a high power-to-weight ratio exist (Burdea, 1996). These technical requirements present a challenge to the development of rehabilitation and personal autonomy systems. To solve this challenge, various types of artificial muscle-like actuators, such as pneumatic muscle actuators (Caldwell et al., 2000), shape memory alloy actuators (Huang, 2002) and polymer actuators (Shankar, 2007) have been actively studied by material scientists and biomedical engineers. However, a satisfactory result for artificial muscle technologies for rehabilitation or healthcare devices has not been achieved yet.

In order to fulfill the above demands for the design of a human-centered actuator, we originally developed some actuator systems using metal hydride materials as a flexible mechanical power source (Wakisaka et al., 1997). Metal hydride actuators (MH actuators) can produce a powerful and soft force, even if it is a small and light package, because the metal hydride materials can store a large amount of hydrogen gas by controlling heat energy; this energy is about a thousand times larger than the volume of the metal hydride alloy itself. Moreover, MH actuators have human-compatible softness and noiseless motion, which derived from a reversible thermochemical reaction of metal hydrides. An additional potential merit is that hydrogen is a clean energy carrier candidate because it does not have adverse effects on the environment (Sakintuna et al., 2007).

The purpose of this chapter is threefold: first, to overview soft artificial muscle-like actuators to support personal physical activity; second, to describe the properties of metal hydride materials, the structure and motion control technique of the MH actuator and the performance upgrade with installed soft bellows made of a multilayer laminate film; third, to show some applications of the MH actuators in rehabilitation and assistive technologies, which require a continuous passive motion machine for joint rehabilitation and a power assistance system for people with restricted mobility.

Finally, we present future works related to further improvements of the MH actuators for more suitable devices in rehabilitation engineering and assistive technology.

BACKGROUND

Current Actuator Technologies of Artificial Muscles

For many industrial machines and robots, actuators are very important elements (Alciatore & Histand, 2003). The actuators convert energy from an electrical, hydraulic or pneumatic power source to mechanical energy for rotational or linear motion. The main types of actuators are hydraulic, pneumatic and electrical motors. Muscles are actuators in the body. Electric motors have good controllability and high-energy efficiency, so they are in widespread use for practical applications, such as various industrial machinery and household electrical appliances. However, in the ratio of torque to mass in motors is low compared to that of muscle, making them bulky for medical and biomimetic robot applications (Smela, 2003).

Moreover, no commercial actuators fit together well for human motion assistance and rehabilitation in daily life. Rehabilitation equipment and assistive devices that patients directly wear on their body strongly require softness, quiet functioning, reduced size and weight and hygienic treatment. These ergonomic requirements differ vastly from those of industrial application design. First, we describe some unique actuators that take for the need to assist human into account, which can also perform quietly and powerfully enough. Although there are still no established definitions in terms of artificial muscles, the term refers to "actuators with similar properties to biological muscle" or "actuators modeled after the mechanism of animal muscle" in biomedical engineering and robotics.

Artificial muscle-like actuators can be classified into different types, such as pneumatic muscle actuators using a rubber tube and an air compressor, a shape memory alloy (SMA) actuators that deform to apply heat to the installed SMA strings, polymer actuators using electroactive polymers (EAPs) and metal hydride (MH) actuators that apply the hydrogen storage effect of metal hydride materials.

In this chapter, the operating principles and basic configurations of these artificial muscle-like actuators, which are the pneumatic muscle actuators, the SMA actuators and the EAP actuators, are outlined to validate commercial actuator devices. In particular, the MH actuators and its applications in rehabilitation and personal autonomy technology are described in the following section.

Pneumatic Muscle Actuators

A pneumatic muscle actuator mainly consists of a cylindrical rubber tube covered with a braided plastic sheath with helical winding swaged by metal stoppers at both ends and an air compressor. When compressed air is sent into the spindly tube inside, the rubber tube expands asymmetrically because the motion of the rubber tube resists the special knitted sleeve and thus experiences directionally dependent stretching. The expansion power of the rubber tube is transferred into a longitudinal flexion force, not an expansion force. Thus, to increase the pressure inside the tube with the air compressor, the pneumatic muscle actuator generates a contraction force like that of a human muscle. This type of pneumatic actuator is named the McKibben artificial muscle (Daerden & Lefeber, 2002).

The other type of pneumatic rubber actuator is shown in Figure 1. The silicone rubber tube of the actuator has three separate pressure chambers inside (Kure et al., 2008). This rubber tube can bend any direction by controlling the pressure in each chamber because of its isotropic elasticity because of radial fiber reinforcement. Therefore, this pneumatic rubber actuator can be used as a soft manipulator to perform as a human finger and is suitable for handling fragile or irregular objects.

Figure 1. Conformation and deformation image of a flexible micro actuator (FMA) with three separated pressure chambers in a fiber-reinforced silicone rubber tube. (© 2009, Koichi Suzumori. Used with permission.)

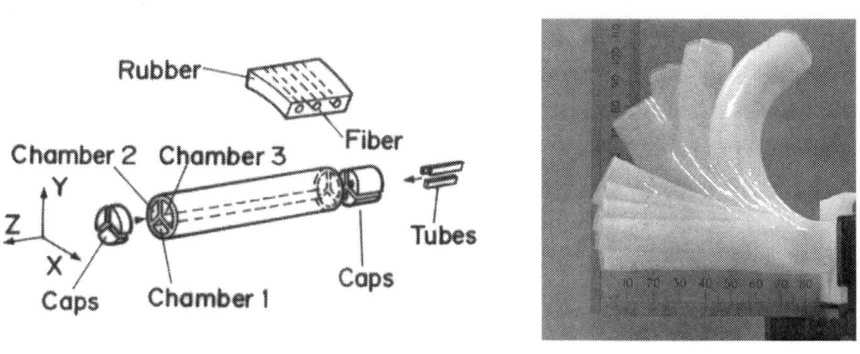

Using limber rubber materials as the main structure and air pressure as the driving power, the pneumatic muscle actuator can produce flexible deformation and soft motion, as described above. Therefore, it may be applied in humanoid robots, rehabilitation equipment and assistive devices. However, the pneumatic rubber actuator requires an air compressor or a high-pressure gas cylinder to obtain compressed gas. High-pressure apparatuses usually generate noise caused by gas emission. To develop a practical pneumatic muscle actuator for rehabilitation and assistive technologies, the problems of noisy exhaust and excessive size and weight of the air compressor or gas cylinder will have to be solved.

Shape Memory Alloy Actuators

Shape memory alloy (SMA) is a smart material that can remember its original shape. The SMA can return to a previously defined shape when heated above a certain critical temperature after having been deformed. In 1932, A. Olander discovered an alloy of gold and cadmium could be plastically deformed when cool and then be heated to return to the original configuration (Olander, 1932). This interesting phenomenon is known as the Shape Memory Effect (SME) and the alloys that exhibit this behavior are called Shape Memory Alloys. In 1961, W. Beuhler et al. stumbled across a significant discovery in the field of SME and SMA. While testing an alloy of Nickel and Titanium for heat and corrosion resistance, they found that it too exhibited the SME. The Ni-Ti alloy proved to be significantly less expensive, easier to work with and less dangerous from a health standpoint than previously discovered SMAs (Otsuka & Xiaobing, 1999).

The SME occurs due to a temperature and stress dependent shift in the material's crystalline structure between two different phases: martensite and austenite. In the martensite phase, the low temperature phase, the alloy is relatively soft, whereas during the austenite phase, the high temperature phase, the alloy is relatively hard. For a simple example of the SME in action, consider the following. If a straight bar made of a SMA in its austenitic phase is allowed to cool below the phase transition temperature, the crystalline structure will change to martensite. If this bar is subsequently plastically deformed and then reheated above the phase transition temperature, it will return to its original straight configuration.

Recently, some ceramic or polymer materials with a similar function of the SME have been studied in material science (Gall et al., 2002). However, currently, the most beneficial and flexible inter-metallic compounds for a practical actuator system are Ni-Ti based alloys, which have suitable mechanical properties for force output and cyclic motion behavior. Figure 2 shows a typical configuration of a SMA actuator with a bias spring. A SMA wire of this actuator was shaped like a spring coil. When the SMA spring is cooled or heated, a rod connected the SMA spring is moved from side to side, and its force output can be transmitted externally.

With all of these features, the SMA actuator has been recently applied as a prosthetic limb, an orthodontic wire and an intravascular surgery device in the medical field (Kuribayashi et al., 2006).

Polymer Actuators

The various types of polymer actuators can be divided into two major groups (Mirfakhrai, 2007). In the first group, actuation dimensional change

Figure 2. A typical configuration of a shape memory alloy (SMA) actuator with a bias spring

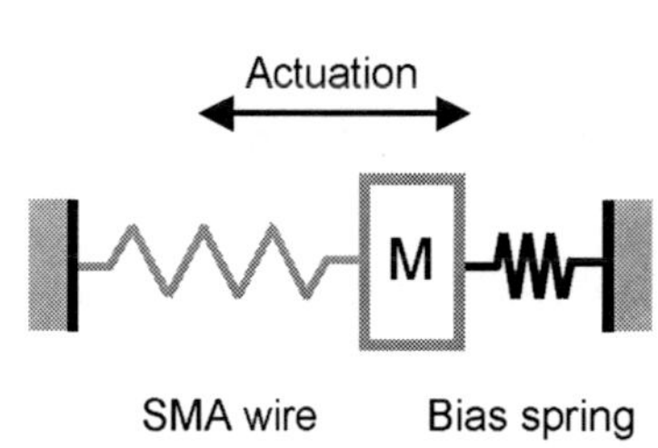

occurs in response to an electric field. These materials are commonly known as electronic electroactive polymers (EAPs) or dry EAPs. Some of the technology in this category includes dielectric elastomer actuators (DEAs), relaxor ferroelectric polymers and liquid crystal elastomers. The second group of polymer actuators is a class of materials in which the presence and movement of ions is necessary to make actuation possible. This group is referred to as ionic EAPs. For the ions to be able to move, an electrolyte phase is necessary, which is often liquid. These types of actuators are also known as wet EAPs. In this section, the described DEAs are a practical example of polymer actuators (Pelrine, 2002).

The DEAs are capable of generating large strains and strain rates. They are one of the most studied polymer actuators, and numerous applications are being developed, including fluid pumps, Braille screens and biomimetic robots. This actuator is a capacitor with compliant dielectrics and electrodes. When a voltage is applied across the DEA materials, the attraction between opposite charges and the repulsion of like charges generates stress in the dielectric, known as Maxwell stress, which compresses and elongates the dielectric, as shown in Figure 3. This stress is proportional to the square of the applied field and the dielectric constant. A low elastic modulus and high dielectric strength can lead to strains of up to 380% at high applied fields (Prahlad et al., 2005).

The high electric field drives the DEAs. Thus, some safety issues may arise in large devices where high voltages and currents are applied by a power source. It is important to develop a low voltage device, which is a materials challenge in itself.

Figure 3. Actuation mechanism of a dielectric elastomer actuator (DEA)

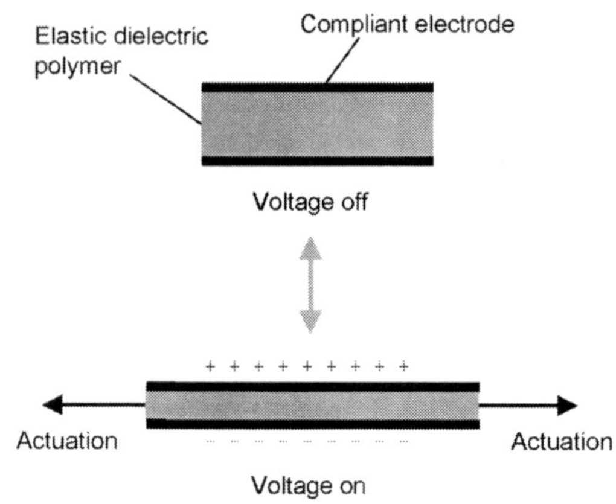

METAL HYDRIDE ACTUATORS

Metal Hydride Alloys

Metal hydride (MH) alloys have the ability to store a large amount of hydrogen, which is about 1000 times as large as the volume of the alloy itself. The compressibility of hydrogen in the MH alloy is higher than that of a high-pressure gas cylinder and liquid hydrogen. The first practical MH alloy, which is an inter-metallic compound, magnesium-nickel (Mg_2Ni), was discovered in 1968 at Brookhaven National Laboratory, USA (Reilily & Wiswall, 1968). Shortly thereafter, a rare-earth based MH alloy, which is an inter-metallic compound, lanthanum-nickel ($LaNi_5$), was coincidentally discovered in 1969 at Philips Research Laboratories, the Netherlands (Zijlstra & Westendrop, 1969). These successive big discoveries triggered research on many MH alloys and opened new possibilities for industrial developments, such as a fuel battery, a chemical heat pump and an actuation device.

We describe the general hydrogen absorbing/desorbing properties in the MH alloy. First, a reversible chemical reaction between metal (M) and hydrogen gas (H_2) generates metal hydrides (MH_x) according to the following reaction formula:

$$M + \frac{x}{2}H_2 \leftrightarrow MH_x + Q \tag{1}$$

where Q is the heat of reaction, and thus, $Q > 0$ J/mol for H_2. As shown in Figure 4, if this reaction succeeds at a constant temperature, then it will advance up to an equilibrium pressure, which is called the plateau pressure. This graph, the PCT diagram (*P*: hydrogen pressure, *C*: hydrogen content, *T*: temperature), shows the basic characteristics of the MH alloy. As demonstrated in the PCT diagram, the plateau pressure is controlled by changing the MH alloy temperature.

Next, the hydrogen equilibrium pressure (*P*) is related to the changes ΔH and ΔS in enthalpy and entropy, respectively, as a function of temperature (*T*) by the Van't Hoff equation:

$$\log_e P = \frac{\Delta H}{\mathrm{R}} \cdot \frac{1}{T} - \frac{\Delta S}{\mathrm{R}} \quad (2)$$

where R is the gas constant. Then, the relationship between the hydrogen equilibrium pressure and the temperature of the MH alloy can be coordinated by adding mishmetal (Mm) and aluminum (Al) to the alloy. Mishmetal is a common name for a mixture of unrefined rare earth elements.

Furthermore, the MH alloy is not combustible and is inflammable, so it is safe as a hydrogen storage material for a fuel battery in road vehicles and other mobile applications (Schlapbach & Züttel, 2001).

Actuator Configurations

The MH alloy can store and release a large amount of hydrogen by changing its temperature. If this reversible reaction between absorbing and desorbing hydrogen gas is carried out in a hermetically sealed system, heat energy applied to the MH alloy is converted into mechanical energy via a pressure change in the system. Thus, the MH actuator acts by directly using the hydrogen pressure derived from the MH alloy through the heat energy.

The MH actuator is composed of a solidified MH alloy powder, Peltier elements to electrically control the temperature of the MH alloy, a hermetically sealed MH module container and flexible bellows to transfer the hydrogen pressure into a force output (Ino et al., 1992). Figure 5 shows an MH actuator using a metal bellows for

Figure 4. Pressure-content-temperature (PCT) diagram of metal hydride materials

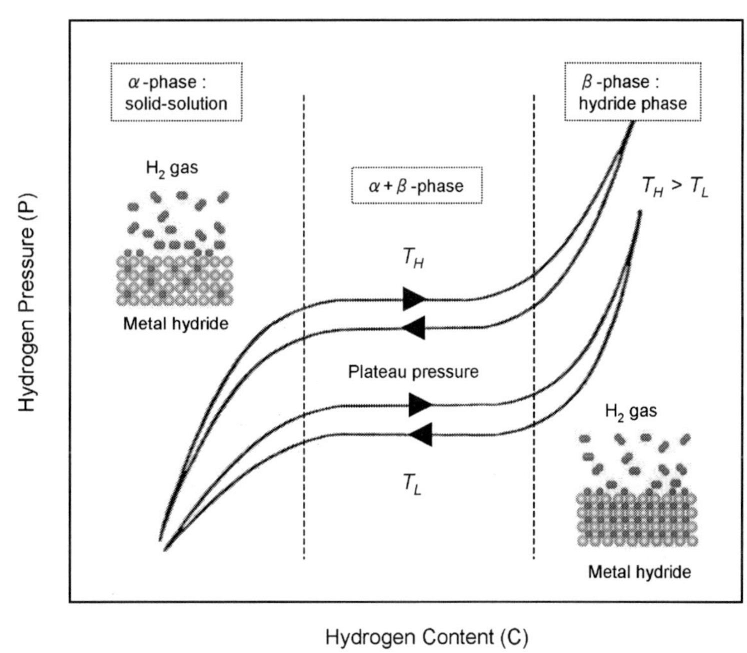

a flexible end-effector and the MH module with Peltier elements.

Operation Properties

For example, for an MH actuator attached to a metal bellows, which contains a 6-g MH alloy, the maximum force output is about 600 N. This force output is 10,000 times the weight of the MH alloy. Generally, the power-to-weight ratio of the MH actuator is very large compared to those of conventional actuators, such as electric motors and hydraulic actuators.

The motion speed of the MH actuator depends on the heat conductivity of the solidified MH alloy powder (MH powder compact). The heat conductivity of the MH alloy is typically low because of pulverization during the cyclic hydrogen storage process. To improve this low heat conductivity, the powdered MH alloy was coated with a thin copper layer with chemical plating and formed by a 3-ton press for solid construction. Moreover, the MH powder compact and the Pletier module were unified to accelerate the heat transfer. The surface of the MH compact was coated with alumina, which is an electric insulator, using plasma spray, and an electric circuit pattern for the Peltier module was drawn on the alumina-coated layer.

From experimental results, it was found that the hydrogen pressure of the MH actuator rose smoothly from 0.3 to 1.0 MPa, and the time delay from the onset pressure change was about 0.1 s (Wakisaka et al., 1997). Therefore, the MH actuator is sufficient for applications that require slow, safe motion, such as joint rehabilitation or transfer assistance.

Control Techniques

In human joints, muscles or muscle groups are arranged to be mutually antagonistic to each other at the axis of rotation and contract to generate the torque in both directions (extension and flexion) of the joint (Kapandji, 2007). Likewise, in the MH actuator system, the rotational movement of a single axis has the same effect. An antagonistic MH actuator system is composed of two metal bellows arranged in opposition with each other.

The translational motion produced by the deformation of two bellows is converted into rotational motion by a rack-and-pinion mechanism (Sato et al., 1996). By modeling the MH actuator as a spring with a variable elastic coefficient, the force outputs F_1 and F_2 of each MH actuator are expressed as follows:

$$F_1 = (aP_1 + K_b)\Delta L + cP_1 + d \quad (3)$$

Figure 5. Block diagram of an MH actuator system with a metal bellows and a photograph of its actuator and MH alloy powders

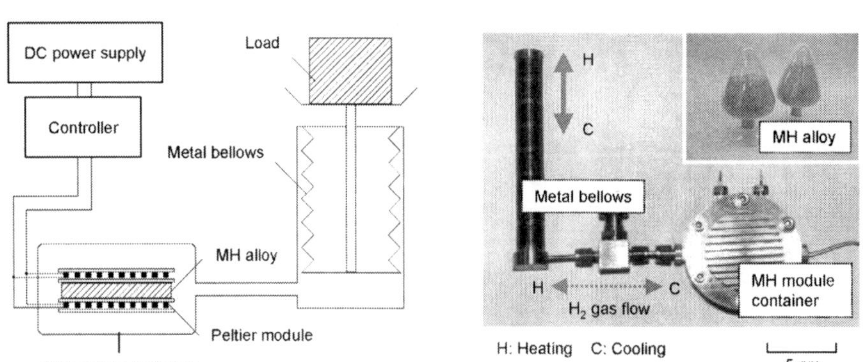

$$F_2 = (aP_2 + K_b)(-\Delta L) + cP_2 + d \quad (4)$$

where P_1 and P_2 are the hydrogen pressure of the two MH actuators, $L(=r\theta)$ is the displacement of the bellows from the middle point of expansion and contraction, r is the radius of the pinion, θ is the angle of the pinion, and a, *kb* c and d are constants. The values of a, *kb* c and d were determined from experimental data. From equations (3) and (4), the torque τ is shown as follows:

$$\tau = (F_1 - F_2)r = \{a(P_1 + P_2) + 2K_b\}r^2\theta + c(P_1 - P_2)r \quad (5)$$

In equation (5), if there is no external torque, the angle in equilibrium is shown as follows:

$$\theta = \frac{c(P_2 - P_1)}{a(P_1 + P_2)r + 2K_b r} \quad (6)$$

Because $a(P_1+P_2)$ is small enough compared to $c(P_2 - P_1)$ and $2K_b$, equation (6) is approximated as follows:

$$\theta = \frac{c(P_2 - P_1)}{2K_b r} \quad (7)$$

Therefore, the rotation angle (position) of the antagonistic MH actuator system is almost proportional to the relative difference of the two hydrogen pressures $(P_2 - P_1)$.

On the other hand, from equation (5), the angular stiffness K_r is shown as follows:

$$K_r = \frac{\partial \tau}{\partial \theta} = \{a(P_1 + P_2) + 2K_b\}r^2 \quad (8)$$

In equation (8), K_r changes in proportion to (P_1+P_2) because *a*, K_b and *r* are constants. The angular stiffness of the antagonistic MH actuator system varies in proportion to the sum of the internal pressure of both MH actuators.

Thus, the position and stiffness of a pair of MH actuators arranged antagonistically are independently controlled by altering the difference and sum values, respectively, of the pressures in the bellows, P_1 and P_2. This means that the antagonistic MH actuator system can operate the joint torque and stiffness with a similar structure to that of the musculoskeletal system around human joints.

Wearable Design

The MH actuators are required to be constructed with metallic components to ensure impermeability against hydrogen gas, which is the pressure transfer medium in the MH actuator. However, using metallic components restricts the weight, elongation rate and usability of the MH actuator. In particular, rehabilitation equipment and power assistance devices for daily life support must be light and soft to a human body. Therefore, we have attempted to design a wearable bellows made of primarily non-metal materials.

The wearable bellows for the MH actuators must be flexible, lightweight and impermeable to hydrogen. However, fulfilling these requirements using only non-metal materials is very difficult because of the diminutive size of hydrogen molecules. Alternatively, a polymer-metal laminate composite was selected to improve the usability of the MH actuator (Ino et al., 2009). The laminate composite is a multilayer structure film of polyethylene, aluminum and polyester. The hydrogen impermeability of the laminate film should be proportional to the thickness of the metal layer, but the compliance of the film decreases as the thickness increases. These properties of the laminate film are in a trade-off relationship with the metal layer thickness. The metal layer thickness was heuristically adopted to be about 10 μm for a wearable bellows.

The weight and the elongation range of the laminate film bellows were 20 times lighter and

30 times larger than that of the metal bellows, respectively. These mechanical properties of the laminate film bellows are useful in designing a human-centered MH actuator. Here, the MH actuator with the laminate film bellows is called the soft MH actuator to distinguish it from the conventional MH actuator using the metal bellows.

The hydrogen impermeability is very important for the bellows of the soft MH actuator. Therefore, we continuously monitored the inner pressure and displacement of the bellows filled with high purity hydrogen gas for a long time. The decompression rate of the laminate film bellows after 10 days was less than 1% of the initial pressure. Thus, the laminate film bellows is a capable barrier against hydrogen gas. At the same time, a flex durability test was performed to determine how long the laminate film bellows could continuously contract and expand in length and volume. The laminate film did not break down due to repeated motion for ten days. The laminate film bellows had good hydrogen impermeability and flex durability for actuation derived from the MH alloys.

The passive elasticity of the soft MH actuator built in the laminate film bellows was measured by a universal tester. The stiffness increased with increasing strain on the laminate film bellows, and the rate of the stiffness change decreased as the initial inner pressure of the MH actuator increased. Moreover, the range of the variable stiffness of human muscle at full activation (Cook, C. S. & McDonagh, M. J. N., 1996) was included in that of the MH actuator using the laminate film bellows, as shown in Figure 6 (right bottom). Thus, the soft MH actuator may be suitable for a human power assistance and rehabilitation device from the viewpoint of mechanical impedance matching and passive elasticity safety to reduce any potential danger.

The other merit of the laminate film bellows is the production cost. The laminate film bellows can be produced at a very low cost compared to a metal bellows because a mass-produced polymer-metal laminate film is not typically expensive in the packaging industry. Therefore, it is possible to create a disposable version of the laminate film

Figure 6. Image of an elbow CPM machine using the laminate film bellows (left) and its motion pattern (center top), and stiffness comparison between human muscle and the soft MH actuator with laminate film bellows (right bottom)

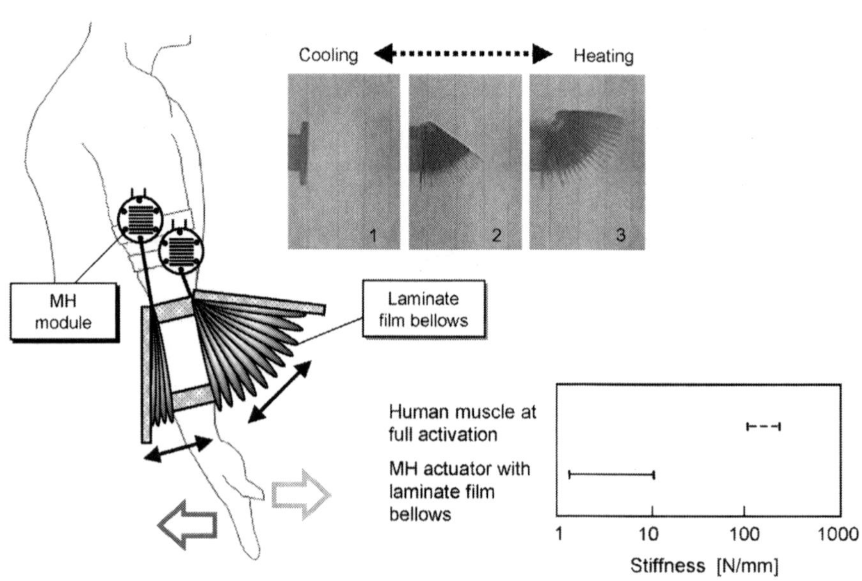

bellows, which would also satisfy the hygienic requirements of medical and rehabilitation devices.

APPLICATIONS FOR REHABILITATION ENGINEERING AND ASSISTIVE TECHNOLOGY

Joint Rehabilitation

In an aging society, there is a significant need for home healthcare equipment for rehabilitation of a stroke or joint injury. Joint rehabilitation techniques include manual therapy by physical and occupational therapists and range of motion (ROM) exercises using a continuous passive motion (CPM) machine. Some therapeutic effects of the CPM machine were clinically suggested in previous studies (Salter et al., 1984). However, current CPM machines have some problems, such as a lack of mechanical flexibility that mimics the human body, bulky size for home medical care and noise from the electric motors. These problems disturb the safe, easy usage of the CPM machine at home. Thus, we have designed a compact MH actuator and prototyped a CPM machine that uses it.

The prototyped CPM machine for elbow joints and hands is shown in Figure 7. This CPM machine utilizes a compact MH actuator with a small metal bellows cylinder. The output torque around an elbow was maximally about 7 Nm, which was adopted based on the clinical data obtained by the manual therapy motion provided by a physical therapist. The weight was about 1.7 kg lighter than that of a conventional CPM machine with electric motors. Although the prototyped CPM machine has the potential to care for joint disease, it is still not durable enough for a clinical or home setting.

In order to solve this problem, we have proposed a different type of CPM machine, which uses a laminate film bellows integrated into a soft MH actuator (Ino et al., 2008), as shown in Figure 6 (left). The antagonistic mechanism is composed of two soft MH actuators, which allows for flexible actuation of the elbow joints, and its stiffness can easily be controlled based on the sum of the inner pressure of both bellows. Moreover, the range of the variable stiffness of human muscle at full activation was included in that of the soft MH actuator, as mentioned above. Thus, the soft MH actuator is also suitable for a physical rehabilitation apparatus with mechanical impedance matching.

Furthermore, by using the MH actuator, an extremely slow motion that is not available manually can be applied to a patient's joint, so it could provide effective exercise for early ROM

Figure 7. A prototyped elbow (left) and hand (right) CPM machine using a double-acting compact MH actuator

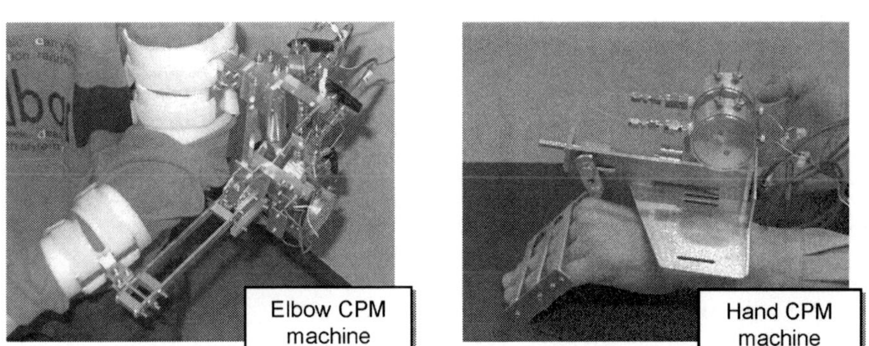

rehabilitation after joint surgery, the cure of clubfoot and other joint diseases.

Prevention of Disuse Syndrome

Elderly patients who must rest in bed because of a stroke or bone fracture may suffer from disuse syndrome, which includes bedsores, joint contracture and muscular atrophy (Bortz, 1984). However, it is difficult for these elderly patients to actively exercise for preventive rehabilitation. Thus, an apparatus for continuous joint exercise to facilitate blood flow in subcutaneous tissues and joints at bedside is devised to prevent disuse syndrome.

A prototype of a bedside power assist system for toe exercise is composed of a couple the soft MH actuators. The laminate film bellows of the soft MH actuator weighed 40 g. The extension and flexion motion of toe joints is derived from a pair of yielding laminate film bellows spread out in a fan-like cage. The motion of the toes in the power assist system was properly gentle and slow for multiple-joint exercise. During the operation of the system, the subject's toes were constantly held and moved between the two soft bellows.

Thus, some toe joint exercises could be easily actualized by a simple pressure control of the soft MH actuators with antagonistic allocation. In addition, we have measured the cutaneous blood flow before and during exercise to examine the preventive effect on bedsore formation by passive motion exercise (Ino et al., 2009). These results show that the simple toe exercise can elicit a significant blood flow increase at the frequent sites of decubitus ulcers. The passive motion at toe joints using such soft MH actuators may be useful for preventing disuse syndrome.

Transfer Assistance

When it is difficult for people to stand up by themselves due to some illness or injury, they need help transferring from a bed to a wheelchair, toilet seat, or bath. Transfer assistance systems must be both strong and safe. In the transfer motion, a physical and mental load exists between a patient and a helper at any time. However, securing mobility by transfer assistance tools facilitates the patient's personal autonomy in daily life. Thus, we developed a transfer hoist based on ergonomic motion analysis of transfer behavior. A high-powered MH actuator was implemented into a mobile floor hoist.

The mobile floor hoist using the high-powered MH actuator is shown in Figure 8 (left). A kneepad, an arm pad and a chest pad with cushioning material were built into the transfer hoist to prevent a fall because of a knee-flexed motion and to move the user's body stably and safely.

Figure 8. A mobile floor hoist using a high-powered MH actuator (left), and a toilet seat lifter using an MH actuator system with a cooling jacket that utilizes flowing tap water (right)

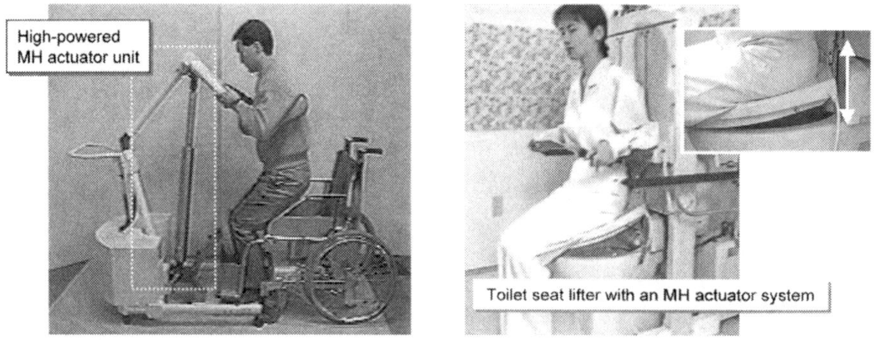

The support pads were designed based on the motion analysis measurements of elderly people (Tsuruga et al., 2001). The kneepad had a variable position mechanism using springs to take into account changes in the ankle joint angle through the transfer motion. The transfer hoist consists of some module parts to customize the fit to the user's body. The high-powered MH actuator adopted double-acting (antagonistic) MH modules for the flexible lifting mechanism of the transfer hoist. Thus, this MH actuator can easily control its own stiffness and position by changing the balance between the inner and outer hydrogen pressures of a metal bellows in a cylindrical housing. This high-powered MH actuator provides a maximum lifting weight of 200 kg and a stroke of 350 mm.

Seat Lift for Wheelchair and Toilet

A wheelchair is a popular assistive device for persons with a lower limb disability or the elderly. Recently, the wheelchair has been significantly improved, and many types have been developed to conform to the life style of wheelchair users. When using a wheelchair, however, some fundamental tasks that require a standing position, such as reaching a tall shelf and cooking in the kitchen are difficult in daily life. Thus, a wheelchair with a seat lift system using the MH actuator was developed to improve the quality of life for wheelchair users (Wakisaka et al., 1997).

These assistive systems for lifting must secure long stroke motion for users. Therefore, a hybrid MH actuator system that uses a tandem piston cylinder with a hydraulic converter was developed. When hydrogen gas flows into a lower piston, silicone oil in the lower piston moves to the upper piston, depending on the inflow of the hydrogen gas. By using such a hybrid driving mechanism with a hydrogen-hydraulic system, the stroke displacement is doubled in comparison with a MH actuator-driven system using only hydrogen gas.

This hybrid MH actuator, which uses a 40-g MH alloy, can produce approximately an 800-N force output and a 40-cm stroke. The lift speed was about 20 mm/s and the total weight of the seat lifting unit, including the MH actuator with the tandem piston cylinder, was about 5 kg.

Our collaborative company has also developed a toilet seat lifter using an MH actuator, as shown in Figure 8 (right) (Wakisaka et al., 1997). This toilet with a seat lifting function has a similar hybrid MH actuator system to that described above. This toilet seat lifter was installed in a smart house, the Welfare Techno House, in Japan (Tamura, 2006), which was built to investigate the well being of elderly people.

FUTURE TRENDS

Globally, society is aging or aged because of a reduction in infections and improved healthcare; many countries face difficult problems in medical and social welfare policy. Here, a sustainable social security service and healthcare program must be further improved and expanded, and supportive life environments for elderly people and the physically challenged with user-selectable rehabilitation and assistive technologies are required. In particular, it is important to take integrated measures against (a) healthcare costs for health maintenance and preventive care with progressive aging of our populations, (b) a shortage of human resources such as caregivers and nurses and (c) social support for empowerment of autonomy.

Some actuators producing soft and powerful motions are necessary for most rehabilitation equipment and assistive technologies that serve an aging society. The actuators for better and safer living demand the following features and functions:

- Human compatible size, high power to weight ratio and lithe body.

- Low impact for a living environment (e.g., noiseless, non-exhaust gas and high-voltage free).
- Safe enough for users.

Traditional actuators largely consist of electrical, hydraulic and pneumatic systems. Construction machinery, processing machinery and precision instruments are built into hydraulic, pneumatic actuators and electric motors, respectively. These actuators are mainly used in factories or inside the machines, but are seldom used in a tangible space or daily living environment.

To overcome the drawbacks of a living environment, various types of artificial muscles such as a polymer actuator, a shape memory alloy actuator and a polymer actuator have been studied. These new actuators must have the following features: minimal noise, output, size and life cycle; moreover, they must be optimized for actual assistive devices for elderly people and physically handicapped persons.

Because of the above background, we have developed a novel soft actuator using metal hydride alloys, which has a nonconventional operating principle for actuation. The MH actuators utilize the tremendous hydrogen storing ability, structure simplicity, high force to weight ratio, low stiffness, noiselessness, good durability, slow actuation and advantage of environmental sustainability by hydrogen energy of MH alloys. Moreover, by using laminate film for external contact at the movable operating parts, the MH actuators can be assembled in wearable structures and fit the human body. They also experience reversible contraction and expansion in length and volume by the antagonistic arrangement of two actuators (bellows), which functions similarly to natural muscles. From these various unique aspects, the MH actuator is one of the new human-centered actuators with a high potential for practical applications in rehabilitation and assistive technologies.

The current MH actuators, however, have some technical issues: low energy conversion efficiency and a slow contraction phase (Ino et al., 2009). Both causes are derived from the performance of a thermoelectric Peltier device for the temperature control of the MH alloy. Actuation performance improvement demands the development of new Peltier devices that are highly efficient in thermoelectric energy conversion, alternative devices for thermal control and cooling circuits with good waste heat processing. The new materials for elastic piping and easy connection with high hydrogen permeability are strongly desired for flexible fabrication.

Rehabilitation equipment and personal autonomy techniques that are expected to be applied in artificial muscle technology do not only contain the CPM machine, the prevention system of disuse syndromes and the transfer hoist as previously described, but also a functional prosthetic limb, a power assistance system, a nursing robot and a home elevator. In different fields, it is also considered for use in haptic interface devices in virtual reality (Bicchi et al., 2008) and a submarine robot that requires a low speed and high torque operation.

In the future, human-centered actuator technology for active health promotion and the personal autonomy of elderly people and physically handicapped people, which can accommodate human physical characteristics and daily living environments, is expected to improve social welfare and address the declining birthrate and the aging population.

CONCLUSION

In this chapter, we explained some emerging artificial muscle-like actuators for rehabilitation and assistive technology. Pneumatic muscle actuators, shape memory alloy actuators and polymer actuators have been developed for human-friendly biomimetic actuations over the years but none of them had fully yielded practical applications. To include all the functions of a high force-to-mass ratio, large strain actuation, an adjustable and wide ranging stiffness for mechanical impedance matching at the human body and noiselessness, like natural muscles, is difficult for these types of artificial muscle actuators. It is also difficult for conventional actuators, such as hydraulic, pneumatic and electrical motors, to satisfy these specific performance criteria.

Because there are no optimal actuators for rehabilitation and assistive technology devices, we have developed a new actuator that exploits metal hydride materials as a mechanical energy source. This metal hydride actuator can fulfill all requirements for softness, compactness, quietness and cleanness. Moreover, the combination use of laminate film bellows adds the advantage of lightness, wearability and low cost. Technical challenges also remain regarding the working speed and energy efficiency of the MH actuators, most of which can be overcome through improvement in Peltier devices and radiative cooling materials to achieve effective waste heat management.

We have applied metal hydride actuators to various types of rehabilitation and assistive technology equipment, such as a CPM machine, a bedsore prevention device, a wheel seat lifter and a transfer hoist. Initial applications of the metal hydride actuators are being developed, but further work with an interdisciplinary approach among rehabilitation engineering, material science, medicine and robotics should help the metal hydride actuators become applicable in a wide range of devices in which human-like motion is desirable for quality-of-life technologies.

REFERENCES

Alciatore, D. G., & Histand, M. B. (2003). *Introduction to mechatoronics and measurement systems*. New York: McGraw-Hill, Inc.

Bicchi, A., Buss, M., Ernst, M. O., & Peer, A. (2008). *The Sense of Touch and Its Rendering: Progress in Haptics Research*. Berlin: Springer. doi:10.1007/978-3-540-79035-8

Bortz, W. M. (1984). The disuse syndrome. *The Western Journal of Medicine*, *141*(5), 691–694.

Burdea, G. C. (1996). *Force and touch feedback for virtual reality*. New York: John Wiley & Sons, Inc.

Caldwell, D. G., Tsagarakis, N., & Medrano-Cerda, G. A. (2000). Bio-mimetic actuators: polymeric pseudo muscular actuators and pneumatic muscle actuators for biological emulation. *Mechatronics*, *10*(4-5), 499–530. doi:10.1016/S0957-4158(99)00071-9

Cook, C. S., & McDonagh, M. J. N. (1996). Measurement of muscle and tendon stiffness in man. *European Journal of Applied Physiology*, *72*(42), 380–382. doi:10.1007/BF00599700

Daerden, F., & Lefeber, D. (2002). Pneumatic artificial muscles: actuators for robotics and automation. *Journal of the American Chemical Society*, *54*(1), 11–21.

Gall, K., Dunna, M. L., Liua, Y., Fincha, D., Lakeb, M., & Munshib, N. A. (2002). Shape memory polymer nanocomposites. *Acta Materialia*, *50*(20), 5115–5126. doi:10.1016/S1359-6454(02)00368-3

Gardner-Bonneau, D., & Gosbee, J. (1997). Health care and rehabilitation. In Fisk, A. D., & Rogers, W. A. (Eds.), *Handbook of human factors and the older adult* (pp. 231–255). San Diego: Academic Press.

Huang, W. (2002). On the selection of shape memory alloys for actuators. *Materials & Design*, *23*(1), 11–19. doi:10.1016/S0261-3069(01)00039-5

Ino, S. Hosono. M., Sato, M., Nalajima, S., Yamashita, & Izumi, T. A Preliminary Study of a Power Assist System for Toe Exercise using a Metal Hydride Actuator, In Schlegel, W. & Dössel, O. (Eds.), *Proceedings of the World Congress on Medical Physics and Biomedical Engineering2009* (vol. 25/IX, pp. 287-290), Munich, Germany: Springer.

Ino, S., Hosono, M., Sato, M., & Nalajima, S. Yamashita, & Izumi, T. (2009). A Soft Metal Hydride Actuator Using $LaNi_5$ Alloy and a Laminate Film Bellows. In Ibrahim, Y. (Ed.), *Proceedings of the 2009 IEEE International Conference on Industrial Technology* (pp. 1215-1220), Gippsland, Australia: IEEE.

Ino, S., Izumi, T., Takahashi, M., & Ifukube, T. (1992). Design of an actuator for tele-existence display of position and force to human hand and elbow. *Journal of Robotics and Mechatronics*, *4*(1), 43–48.

Ino, S., Sato, M., Hosono, M., & Izumi, T. (2009). Development of a Soft Metal Hydride Actuator Using a Laminate Bellows for Rehabilitation Systems. *Sensors and Actuators. B, Chemical*, *B-136*(1), 86–91. doi:10.1016/j.snb.2008.10.054

Ino, S., Sato, M., Hosono, M., Nalajima, S., Yamashita, K., Tanaka, T., & Izumi, T. (2008). Prototype Design of a Wearable Metal Hydride Actuator Using a Soft Bellows for Motor Rehabilitation, In Dumont, G. & Galiana, H. (Eds.), *Proceedings of the 30th Annual International Conference of the IEEE Engineering in Medicine and Biology Society* (pp. 3451-3454), Vancouver, Canada: IEEE.

Kapandji, I. A. (2007). *The Physiology of the Joints*. New York: Churchill Livingstone.

Kure, K., Kanda, T., Suzumori, K., & Wakimoto, S. (2008). Flexible displacement sensor using injected conductive paste. *Sensors and Actuators. A, Physical*, *143*(2), 272–278. doi:10.1016/j.sna.2007.11.031

Kuribayashi, K., Tsuchiya, K., You, Z., Tomus, D., Umemoto, M., & Ito, T. (2006). Self-deployable origami stent grafts as a biomedical application of Ni-rich TiNi shape memory alloy foil. *Materials Science and Engineering A*, *419*(1-2), 131–137. doi:10.1016/j.msea.2005.12.016

Mirfakhrai, T., Madden, J. D. W., & Baughman, R. H. (2007). Polymer artificial muscles. *Materials Today*, *10*(4), 30–38. doi:10.1016/S1369-7021(07)70048-2

Olander, A. (1932). An electrochemical investigation of solid cadmium-gold alloys. *European Journal of Mechanical and Environmental Engineering*, *47*(10), 3819–3833.

Otsuka, K., & Ren, X. (1999). Recent developments in the research of shape memory alloys. *Intermetallics*, *7*(5), 511–528. doi:10.1016/S0966-9795(98)00070-3

Pelrine, R., Kornbluh, R., Pei, Q., Stanford, S., Oh, S., & Eckerle, J. (2002). Dielectric Elastomer Artificial Muscle Actuators: Toward Biomimetic Motion. In Bar-Cohen, Y. (Ed.), *Proceedings of SPIE: Vol. 4695* (pp. 126-137). San Diego: SPIE.

Prahlad, H., Pelrine, R., Kornbluh, R., Guggenberg, P. V., Chhokar, S., & Eckerle, J. (2005). Programmable surface deformation: thickness-mode electroactive polymer actuators and their applications. In Bar-Cohen, Y. (Ed.), *Proceedings ofSPIE: Vol. 5759* (pp. 102-113). San Diego: SPIE.

Reilly, J. J. Jr, & Wiswall, R. H. Jr. (1968). Reaction of hydrogen with alloys of magnesium and nickel and the formation of Mg_2NiH_4. *Inorganic Chemistry*, *7*(11), 2254–2256. doi:10.1021/ic50069a016

Sakintuna, B., Lamari-Darkrimb, F., & Hirscherc, M. (2007). Metal hydride materials for solid hydrogen storage: A review. *International Journal of Hydrogen Energy*, *32*, 1121–1140. doi:10.1016/j.ijhydene.2006.11.022

Salter, R. B., Hamilton, H. W., Wedge, J. H., Tile, M., Torode, I. P., & O' Driscoll, S. W. (1984). Clinical application of basic research on continuous passive motion for disorders and injuries of synovial joints: A preliminary report of a feasibility study. *Journal of Orthopaedic Research*, *1*(3), 325–342. doi:10.1002/jor.1100010313

Sato, M., Ino, S., Shimizu, S., Ifukube, T., & Izumi, T. (1996). Development of a compliance variable metal hydride (MH) actuator system for robotic mobility aid for disabled persons. *Transactions of the Japan Society of Mechanical Engineers: Part C*, *62*(597), 1912–1919.

Schlapbach, L., & Züttel, A. (2001). Hydrogen-storage materials for mobile applications. *Nature*, *414*, 353–358. doi:10.1038/35104634

Shankar, R., Ghosh, T. K., & Sponta, R. J. (2007). Dielectric elastomers as next-generation polymeric actuators. *Soft Matter*, *3*, 1116–1129. doi:10.1039/b705737g

Smela, E. (2003). Conjugated polymer actuators for biomedical applications. *Advanced Materials (Deerfield Beach, Fla.)*, *15*(6), 481–494. doi:10.1002/adma.200390113

Tamura, T. (2006). A Smart House for Emergencies in the Elderly. In Nugent, C., & Augusto, J. C. (Eds.), *Smart homes and beyond* (pp. 7–12). Amsterdam: IOS Press.

Tsuruga, T., Ino, S., Ifukube, T., Sato, M., Tanaka, T., Izumi, T., & Muro, M. (2001). A basic study for a robotic transfer aid system based on human motion analysis. *Advanced Robotics*, *14*(7), 579–595. doi:10.1163/156855301742021

Wakisaka, Y., Muro, M., Kabutomori, T., Takeda, H., Shimiz, S., Ino, S., & Ifukube, T. (1997). Application of hydrogen absorbing alloys to medical and rehabilitation equipment. *IEEE Transactions on Rehabilitation Engineering*, *5*(2), 148–157. doi:10.1109/86.593282

Zijlstra, H., & Westendrop, F. F. (1969). Influence of hydrogen on magnetic properties of $SmCo_5$. *Solid State Communications*, *7*(12), 857–859. doi:10.1016/0038-1098(69)90427-X

KEY TERMS AND DEFINITIONS

Actuator: A device used to produce a motion or action. The major actuators in industrial applications are electric motors, hydraulic and pneumatic cylinders.

Artificial Muscle: An actuation device with similar (biomimetic) properties to animal muscle or modeled after the mechanism of biological muscle.

Assistive Technology: Devices and services used in the daily lives of people with a disability to enhance their ability to function independently, such as wheelchairs, transfer hoists, environmental control devices, or communication aids.

Bedsore: A chronic ulcer of the skin caused by prolonged pressure of the weight of one's own body because of lack of movement; occurs primarily in bedridden people and wheelchair users.

Continuous Passive Motion: A medical treatment in orthopedics, which moves a joint continuously and slowly after injury or a surgical operation and promotes recovery of the range of motion.

Disuse Syndrome: A pattern of symptoms as a result of long-term disuse, which is characterized by both physical and psychosocial effects of inactivity. Typical symptoms of disuse syndrome include muscle weaknesses, restricted range of motion (ROM) of joints, declined respiratory function, altered blood flow in the peripheral tissue, reduction of bone density and mental function disorder.

Metal Hydride Alloy: Inter-metallic compounds having the reversible ability to store and release large amounts of hydrogen when cooled and heated, respectively. They are inherently safer than compressed gas or liquid hydrogen and have a higher volumetric hydrogen storage capacity.

PCT Diagram: A diagram that summarizes the property of hydrogen concentration (C) in an equilibrium state when an HM alloy is exposed to various hydrogen pressures (P) while maintaining a certain alloy temperature (T). This shows the fundamental character of the hydrogen absorption ability of the MH alloy.

Peltier Device: A device that uses a thermo-electrical effect for cooling or heating. When the current flows through the junction between two metals, heat is absorbed or liberated at the junction.

Rehabilitation Engineering: A discipline of biomedical engineering concerned with the application of science and technology to improve the quality of life of individuals with disabilities because of sickness or aging.

Section 3
Internet Accessibility

Chapter 11
Web Accessibility:
Current Trends

Simon Harper
University of Manchester, UK

Yeliz Yesilada
University of Manchester, UK

ABSTRACT

Web accessibility conjures the vision of designers, technologists, and researchers valiantly making the World–Wide–Web (Web) open to disabled users. While this maybe true in part, the reality is a little different. Indeed, Web accessibility is actually about correcting our past mistakes by making the current Web fulfill the original Web vision of access for all. It just so happens that in the process of trying to re-engineer these corrections, that have for the most part ignored, we may solve a number of 'larger–scale' usability issues faced by every Web user. Indeed, by understanding disabled–user's interaction we enhance our understanding of all users operating in constrained modalities where the user is disabled by both environment and technology. It is for this reason that Web accessibility is a natural preface to wider Web usability and universal accessibility, it is also why 'main–stream' technologist take it so seriously and understand its cross-over benefits.

INTRODUCTION

We may imagine that there are many reasons for the Web to be accessible ranging from moral necessity, through ethical requirement, to legal obligation. However, the two most compelling are solid main–stream considerations; the business–case and the 'über–use–case'.

The business–case for Web accessibility is strong on three fronts. Firstly, one in five people over the age of 65 are disabled. Population demographics indicate that our populations are ageing across the board. As the population ages the financial requirement to work longer is increased, but the ability to work longer is reduced because

DOI: 10.4018/978-1-60566-206-0.ch011

disability becomes a bar to employment (European Union Policy Survey, 2005). Secondly, an ageing and disabled, but Web literate, population indicates a large market for online shopping and services especially when mobility is a problem for the shopper (Disability Rights Commission, 2004). A final benefit for business, keeping in mind that disability does not equal unskilled, is a highly motivated and skill rich workforce (Westwell et al. 2006). With the growth of the knowledge economy through many developed countries, and a move from manual work to more thought and communication based activities, there is the very real possibility of disabled Web users being able to find productive, fulfilling, and social empowering employment; if only technology, and specifically the Web, where available to them (European Union Policy Survey, 2005). Web accessibility means commercial success.

Web accessibility is really just an 'über–use–case' because in the end we will all be disabled by the technology or the environment (Novick et al. 2002; Ivory et al., 2002); we become 'situationally impaired'. Work on Web accessibility is helping us address many other domains including those centered around user mobility and digital inclusion. For instance, work on physical disability and the Web is helping solve problems of the usability of mobile technology (Trewin, 2006; Harper, 2007). By applying the same technology, used to counter a physically disabled users tremors and jerky movements, to the mobile Web, the operational problems of mobile interaction in moving environments are being solved (Trewin, 2006). Similarly, mobile Web access suffers from the interoperability and usability problems that make the Web as difficult to interact with for main–stream users as it is for visually impaired users. Again, solutions proposed 3–4 years ago in the Web accessibility community are now being applied to main–stream mobile devices. A more concrete example is the Firefox browser extension for 'mouseless browsing' which adds "small boxes with unique ids behind every link and/or form element. You just have to type in the id to trigger the corresponding action i.e. following a link, pressing a button or selecting a text-field" [1]; this work, has roots in accessibility 'access-keys' (Robinson, 2003) and 'auto access-keys' (Yesilada, 2008).

A fact often forgotten is that we are all unique. The disabled user serves as a reminder that Web accessibility is a truly individual experience and that by understanding the flexible and personalization required by disabled users we can understand that at some-point this same flexibility and personalization will be required by all (Panayiotou, 2004).

To understand the needs of disabled users is to understand the needs of everyone (Raskin, 1997; Raskin, 2000). With this in mind we will split this chapter into three main parts. First we will examine the intersection between accessibility, disability, and technology in an effort to understand the differing needs of users, and the technology provided to fulfill those needs (see § 'Web Accessibility Primer'). Next, we will investigate Web accessibility from a more practical orientation. We will set out the current trends in the tools, techniques and technologies in use to help build, check, and transform Web pages into accessible forms; and from this investigation understand the extent and use of each of these activities (see § 'Current Trends in Practical Web Accessibility'). Finally, we present an overview of possible future directions in Web accessibility (see § 'Future Trends'). We suggest that to understand accessibility the developer must take account a number of truths: (1) there is never just one solution; (2) solutions are not simple; (3) a single solution will never work, instead, combinations of solutions are required; and finally, (4) you do not know the user or their requirements at the granularity required to make assumptions. We remember that work in the Web accessibility field is not only for disabled people; organizations and people without disabilities can also benefit.

We conclude with the understanding that to build applications and content that allows for heterogeneity, flexibility, and device independence is incredibly difficult, incredibly challenging, but incredibly necessary.

WEB ACCESSIBILITY PRIMER

Pre-eminent when discussing Web accessibility is visual impairment and profound blindness, however it should be remembered that visual disability is just one aspect of accessibility and the Web. Other disabilities also exist which require changes to the Web to enable a greater degree of accessibility. Before considering these thought, it is important to consider just what accessibility really means and why it is necessary to think about 'access' when building Web sites.

Many disabled users consider the Web to be a primary source for information, employment and entertainment (European Union Policy Survey, 2005). Indeed, from questioning and contact with many disabled users we have discovered that the importance of the Web cannot be under-estimated.

"For me being online is everything. Its my hi-fi, my source of income, my supermarket, my telephone. Its my way in."

This quote, taken from a blind user, sums up the sentiments we experience when talking with many disabled users, and drives home the importance of Web accessibility in the context of independent living. Indeed, by making sites accessible we help people live more productive lives (Jacobs et al., 2005). So how does this work in practice? Disabled Web 'surfers' user intermediate technologies to provide access to Web and computer functionality. In general this technology exists to provide access to any generic software on the computer, however this is not always the case for Web interaction. These 'Assistive Technologies' form a bridge from the user to the computer, much like a keyboard and monitor, the keyboard provides input, the monitor, output. In the case of say physical disability the input device, the keyboard, is not accessible to the user and so a software keyboard is substituted. This keyboard can then be tailored depending on the physical characteristics of the user. A mouse or joystick may be used to place the cursor, or a simple switch is used to interact with a software keyboard exhibiting a 'scanning' behavior (Cook et al., 2001). However, the Web tends to be seen as special case because programmatic elements are build directly into the document and dynamic functionality, such as hyper-links, are included in the document design. This means that in some cases assistive technology exists as a solution just to the unique problems found when interacting with the Web as opposed to more general system accessibility (Cook et al., 2001). Most assistive technology focuses on output and input-interaction driven by output (the monitor) and so assistive technology for users with input problems, such as profound physical disability, tends to be focused on the computer and software in general and does not normally impact on Web accessibility specifically (Laux et al., 1996).

This output accessibility is developed independently along two fronts, both as part of the Web page design along with assistive technology on the users computer. However, due to the design effort needed to build Web pages, along with their shear number, the focus is primarily on the accessibility of the content or the tailoring of the content to a specific audience. Indeed, this later case tends to be the focus of accessibility for cognitive disability and hearing impairment (Lewis, 2005).

In these cases, very little work is focused specifically on Web accessibility mainly because a perception exists that both user groups can interact with Web content visually as per a 'conventional' user. This is however an incorrect assumption, hearing impaired users primary language is 'sign-language' be that British, American, International, or any one of the many others that exist. In this case the textual rendering is not accessible to a hearing impaired user because it is not their language (Huenerfauth, 2005). Therefore, written language is not appropriate and so a translation is required however this translation is to a linear form (similar to the spoken word) and so the problems inherent in visual to audio translations are also applicable. Along with the difficulty of forming signed animation based on text and natural language processing, 'native tongue' accessibility for hearing impaired users is very low. Cognitive impairments (termed learning disability in the United Kingdom and intellectual disability in Australia, Europe, Canada) are also based on an inability of comprehend certain types of information. In this case simpler content or audio-visual renderings may be more appropriate to ease the cognitive load. Again, very little work has been targeted at users with cognitive impairments and so for both hearing and cognitively impaired users most solutions to enhance Web accessibility are based on thoughtful but generic design.

Visual impairment is perhaps the most addressed disability in the Web accessibility spectrum. It is a challenging area because it requires the visual interaction model, and XHTML structure created to support this model, to be moved into an audio interaction paradigm (World Health Organisation, 2004). To bridge this gap, assistive technologies called 'screen–readers' address text to speech translations by audibly reading documents, top–left to bottom–right, through a text-to-speech synthesizer. This is acceptable in most instances as the screen reader also translates the focused user event handler (such as a toolbar or menu system), and so the applications normal user event mechanisms can be used for interaction by the visually impaired user. Initial attempts at screen reading technology only read the screen as presented to a visual use, and was called 'screen scraping' as it only produced superficial information regarding the text being translated. As the visual complexity of Web pages increased these screen–readers become inadequate because of the reliance of Web documents on context, linking, and the deeper document structure to convey information in a useful way. In this case Web browsers and Web page readers for visually impaired users have been created to access this deeper document structure, by directly examining the XHTML or the Document Object Model (DOM). By examining the precise linguistic meaning of the text it was hoped that more complex meanings (associated with style, colour etc.) could be derived. However, when interacting with complex Web documents these readers, although better than screen-scrapers, still do not enable an understanding of the meaning of the underlying structure which is vital for the cognition of information.

Finally, we come to a group who are often included in Web accessibility research because they often exhibit unique combinations of all of the disabilities covered so far; 'seniors' (Czaja, 2006). The ageing population presents a huge challenge for Web accessibility as older people often have multiple disabilities that are usually not particularly sever but can cause decreased Web accessibility in combination (Hawthorn, 2000). In these cases some assistive technology is available especially Web browser additions that assist with interaction and cognitive load. A major problem is the perceived stigma in using assistive technologies; this follows from the tendency for an older person to no admit to a limitation or disability, and to associate access technology with implied weakness. In these cases the assistive technology developer must achieve Web accessibility along with a level of camouflaging of the access technology itself.

In summary, there is no 'catch–all' solution to providing accessibility to Web based resources for disabled users. Each disability requires a different set of base access technologies and the flexibility for those technologies to be personalized by the end–user. To date, the main focus has been on visual impairment, however there are moves to investigate accessibility and hearing and cognitive impairments.

CURRENT TRENDS IN PRACTICAL WEB ACCESSIBILITY

Designing and building Web documents are perhaps the most important parts of the Web accessibility cycle. Only by expecting a clean technical design can the access technology developer create approaches which fully interact with the content of the document. The World-Wide-Web Consortium (W3C) has recognized the importance of correctly engineering the document by recommending a separation between content as well as structure, encapsulated within the extensible hypertext language (XHTML) mark–up (Pemberton et al. 2002), and its presentation, using cascading style-sheets (CSS) (Lie et al. 1999). While this separation does provide the building blocks for increasing access to Web based documents, additional guidelines, techniques, and best practice are sometimes required to facilitate a documents increased accessibility.

Design and Build

The design and build of a Web document is the starting point of Web accessibility, and as such much effort and attention was focused on guidelines, techniques, and best practice in an effort to facilitate greater accessibility. This initial effort has resulted in the accelerated development of these tools and techniques to support document creation, along with guidelines to design against. Indeed, the literature suggests that work theorizing new guidelines, techniques, and practice has now moved to the practice arena in which the application of these design and build elements to different motivational problems such as Web portals (Gappa et al. 2004) and mobile device design is emerging.

Importance / User Perspective

Design and build is of extreme importance from the perspective of the user. If the design and build process conforms to the set guidelines and takes account of user testing and evaluation (Colwell et al. 2001, Petrie et al. 2004) then the user experience and site usability are both enhanced. By undertaking visual design with an eye toward accessibility designers can still create appealing sites but that also facilitate and respect the user (Meyer, 2005). All too often, designers rely on their experience of 'print' to inform their design, and whilst this immutable view of design–creation has served well in the past, it does not translate to the electronic domain (Regan, 2004). Design and build best practice therefore encourages designers to think differently about their work, and provides a checklist, in the work of guidelines, to enable the inexperienced designer to understand the particular requirements of disabled users.

Overview

From its first beginnings Web accessibility focused on good design, and this good design split initially into guidelines and techniques with best practice becoming more important as the field moved from research into development. Initially, Web accessibility was conflated with good design (Ohnemus, 1997) and more generalized HCI usability (Nielsen, 1993). However, Web access for disabled, mainly visually impaired, users began to develop with the formation of the W3C's Web Accessibility Initiative (WAI) based in work toward Web accessibility being undertaken mainly in University research groups pre–1996.

This accessibility research grew from the more specific hypertext / hypermedia field and first started to be though about more separately around 1995 / 1996 (Laux et al. 1996, Morkes et al. 1997) when the challenge was seen as adapting browsers to make the Web more accessible to 'special' user groups and to ensure that Web pages conform to the Standardized General Markup Language (SGML); a common hypertext technology[2]. This work (Laux et al. 1996) proposed lessening the development load for accessible Web documents and deciding on appropriate interaction techniques and guidelines. It proposed user adaptability and interface specification tools, standards and an accessible infrastructure along with presentation independent information. In hindsight this work set the general tone for the coming ten years of research, and latterly practice, in Web accessibility (Robertson et al. 2005).

Through the late 1990's and into the turn of the new millennium researchers and research groups started to work on novel ideas for guidelines, techniques, and practice. While these resulted in some notable projects such as HARMONY (Engelen et al. 1999) and NOVA (Craven et al. 2003) much research effort proceeded on an ad-hoc basis with the WAI serving as a focal point. However, being a 'Standards Body' the WAI mainly dealt with the formulation of guidelines and their dissemination to industry as best practice.

With the formulation of the Web Content Accessibility Guidelines (WCAG) version 1.0 (Chisholm, 2001) in 1999 the WAI's initial mission was fulfilled and these guidelines have become pre-eminent in the Web Accessibility community. These guidelines and techniques included those initially developed by national special interest groups concerned with communities who found Web document interaction to be difficult or impossible. These guidelines, supplied by agencies such as the Royal National Institute for the Blind (RNIB) in the UK (RNIB, 2004) and the American Foundation for the Blind in the USA, meant that the WCAG became, some would say necessarily, skewed toward visually disabled users.

While there are some reservations (Colwell et al. 2001) these guidelines are generally seen as assisting the Web accessibility of disabled users and as such parts of them have been adopted by various national governments. For instance, the Americans with Disabilities Act (ADA–508) legislation (Justice, U. D. of. 1998) picks a subset of WCAG guidelines which is acknowledged to be an enhanced set of WCAG 'A' conformance tests[3], likewise the UK's Disability Discrimination Act looks at WCAG guidelines but is less prescriptive in stating conformance rules, while the Publicly Available Specification (PAS) 78 (DRC, 2006) uses them to guide best practice in commissioning Website designs that are accessible to and usable by disabled people.

The current state of the art in design practice encompasses a separation of presentation and content along with usability (Meyer, 2002) and Web accessibility good practice (Nielsen, 1999; Coyne et al. 2001). Indeed so successful has this move into the mainstream of design practice been that the focus is moving onto the accessibility of more general Web based electronic information (Gonzalez et al. 2005; Chisholm et al. 2005).

While alternate[4] Web formats start to become accessible the WAI accessibility effort is moving into a more mature phase with the development of WCAG version 2.0 guidelines, techniques, and best practice. These are set to become far less prescriptive and cover a wide range of issues and recommendations for making Web content more accessible. While WCAG 2.0 contains similar information to WCAG 1.0 they differ in that they contain principles, guidelines, success criteria, benefits, and examples written as testable statements that are not technology-specific. Key to WCAG 2.0 are the four principles of accessibility: Content must be perceivable; User interface components in the content must be operable; Content and controls must be understandable; and Content must be robust enough to work with current and future technologies. While these principles are high-minded it has yet to be seen if they can indeed be followed in real-world deployments.

As a consequence of recent developments and the 'ease' with which Web documents can be made to conform to accessibility standards, design has moved into a socio–political phase firmly routed in practice. Legal issues of non-conformance are now beginning to emerge along with debate as to the effectiveness in a legal situation of Web standards. This socio-political phase does come with some problems, because there is a proliferation of standards both from special interest groups, governments, and non-governmental organizations that there is a very real prospect of standards becoming unenforceable. Indeed so real is this threat that the WAI has started to look at how standards legislation can be harmonized across international boarders (Brewer, 2004).

One final aspect does effect build, more than design, and this is tooling and tool quality in particular. More particularly, the quality of the generated output from design–and–build tools especially 'What You See Is What You Get' (WYSIWYG) developer tools. These have been notoriously bad at generating clean, succinct, and standards compliant Web code with developers often required to manually modify the output or in some extreme cases re–code by hand. Thankfully, these tools have evolved through the 'nought-ies' with small-shop developed Web authoring tools pushing large corporate tools to be increasingly compliant. However, problems do still exist in that while Web design tools do generate 'good' content, those which generate content from more complicated standard documents (such as Microsoft Word, and Adobe Acrobat) still do not output Web code which is succinct and compliant enough for Web assistive technologies to parse and produce intelligible results. Finally, author tools do not have the concept of either linguist or structural semantics, and so information is generated that may seem accessible but is not semantically correct[5].

In summary, design and build has moved on substantially since the publication of WCAG version 1.0. With the dissemination of these materials to mainstream Web design effort, Web accessibility has become a 'cause célèbre' in some corners. While WAI Web best practice are set to become de-facto standards, advances in guidelines, design techniques, and best practice continue to come from the Web design and practice community (Shneiderman et al. 2004; Paciello, 2000; Pilgrim, 2002; Thatcher et al. 2003). While small changes in practice do occur from time to time we are currently in a state of consolidation and homogenization. In this case practitioners should follow the technical specifications (of XHTML, CSS, and other Web technologies) and the human focused guidelines thereby using the best practice encapsulated in design guidelines for their deployed Web sites. In effect, guideline driven design and build has become firmly rooted within generic Web development best practice to such an extent that we are now waiting for all Web practitioners to catch–up with accessibility leaders.

Evaluation, Validation and Repair

Evaluation and document validation are key to building standardized documents. Once standards have been established there needs to be someway to decide if a document has been designed and created so as to meet them. Without document validation and evaluation tools, and the techniques encoded within them, true accessibility can never be reached. Therefore, validation to standards was seen as being the next job for the Web accessibility research community (Levi et al. 1996) as standards evolved into practice.

Importance / User Perspective

The importance of testing cannot be underestimated with regard to the user. By enabling the automated evaluation, validation and repair of Web pages best practice and guidelines, introduced earlier, can be checked and documents automatically re-engineered to conform. This conformance is important if a holistic user experience across the Web landscape is to be accomplished. By capturing the guidelines and best practice as part of a software tool the expert knowledge used to create and implement them can be transferred to an automated process. This process then removes the burden on the designer and encourages design conformance. Indeed, without automated evaluation, validation and repair the user often experiences a reduced ability to interact with the page, although research suggest that this automated approach still does not work sufficiently well for it to be the only testing carried out (Disability Rights Commission, 2004).

Overview

Initial techniques for Web document validation (suggested by many) tried to provide Web developers and maintainers with a practical basis for considering Web accessibility (Boldyreff, 2002). Techniques have ranged from the Cognitive Walkthrough for the Web (CWW) using Latent Semantic Analysis (Blackmon et al. 2002), through The Barrier Walkthrough Method (BW) (Brajnik, 2008), to the application of Web accessibility heuristics used to help understand which areas of a document have accessibility issues and provide useful insights into how to create a solution (Paddison et al. 2003).

Some techniques evolved to address the technical problems of often changing guidelines. These techniques (Abascal, 2004) proposed well-defined XML structures which could be easily replaced or updated. In this way differing standards sets along with changing mainstream guidelines could all be applied from a single tool both individually or as a battery of techniques.

Other novel approaches rely on separating guidelines evaluation logic from the evaluation engine. Due to this separation, the whole evaluation process can be divided into two main phases: (1) Specifying formal guidelines in terms of Unified Guideline Languages (UGL); and (2) Web page evaluation analyses of content and structure to define which guidelines are to be evaluated on the page parsed (Vanderdonckt et al. 2004). To assist these processes, the Evaluation And Report Language (EARL) (McCathieNevile et al. 2005) was created using the Resource Description Framework (RDF) for recording, transferring and processing data regarding automatic and manual evaluations of resources. The purpose of this is to provide a framework for generic evaluation description formats that can be used in generic evaluation and report tools. EARL is aimed as a practical solution for tools and developers and as such faces industry more than science, however, uptake in EARL compatibility has been patchy at best.

To be of any use, techniques for Web accessibility validation must be encapsulated in tools. These validation engines evolved from state of the art tools made to automatically evaluate user interfaces for usability (Ivory, 2001). While most tools do acknowledge the primacy of the WCAG guidelines some evaluation techniques include additional sets of user test often evolved from mainstream HCI principles (Leporini et al, 2003). Indeed, numerous, automated, evaluation and transformation tools have been created to assist Web developers build better sites for users with diverse needs (Ivory et al. 2003).

The Center for Applied Special Technology's (CAST) 'Bobby'[6] online validation tool was one of the first fully-functional validation service and greatly served in exposing badly built Web documents (Cooper et al. 2001). Bobby, analyzed Web pages against the WCAG 1.0 and ADA 508 guidelines and suggested ways to fix documents that did not conform along with lists of things which could not be checked automatically. Paradoxically, this kind of checking has remained both standard and static across most validators, which check straight standards compliance. Other validation engines, such as 'WAVE' (Kasday, 2000) and 'Cynthia Says' quickly followed (Chisholm et al. 2005). Both differ slightly from Bobby, for instance WAVE helps people perform those tasks that require human judgment (e.g. 'Does this ALT text a functional equivalent for this image?' 'Does this reading order make sense?'). Documents are displayed graphically to show the linearized reading order while WAVE shows the ALT text of images and AREAS on the page for comparison. While 'Cynthia Says' main purpose is to educate Web site developers about accessible Web design.

It validates one page at a time and identifies errors related to ADA 508 and WCAG standards.

Finally, increased information density within Web documents has lead to increased visual complexity and, in turn, an increase in the complexity of the underlying structure of the documents. New techniques have therefore been formulated to take into account this increased complexity and encoded into newly developed tools (Fukuda et al. 2005). Indeed a number of validation tools are available all looking at standards conformance from slightly differing perspectives however some novel approaches, such as OCAWA, do exist on the boundaries. OCAWA runs accessibility tests based on the WCAG 1.0 with audits cross-referenced to other rule-sets (e.g. ADA 508, AccessiWeb, FT OCAWA, etc) by virtue of a built-in expert system (Chene, 2002). This cross referencing to an expert system is intended to provide enhanced checking and feedback and recognizes that other non-WAI standards do still exist. Different techniques and tools claim different performances and so side by side tool evaluations (Brajnik, 2004) have also been established to measure correctness, completeness and specificity in supporting the task of assessing the conformance of a Web site with respect to established guidelines. These have shown differing results but, as we shall see, in most cases the problems have centered around the inability to wholly encode the standards in a machine understandable format.

Even though standards conformance is the focus of much validation tool research and, latterly, development, tools directed a specific document evaluation tasks have been released; most notably 'aDesigner' from IBM Japan (Takagi, 2004). aDesigner is a disability simulator that helps Web designers ensure that their pages are accessible and usable by the visually impaired. Because screen-reader in effect linearise complex or multicolumn documents the time to read a document can be substantial. aDesigner enables the Web designer to indicates the length of time it will take to get a specific parts of the document thereby enable designers to reformat their work.

Many of these tools also include repair capabilities which try to guide the developer through the often complicated process of reengineering documents to conform with standards or to encourage good Web accessibility. While succeeding to a greater or lesser extent the repair process is never fully automated, except for small tasks, because the complexity of a Web document combined with an inability to wholly encode the standards in a machine understandable format makes the analysis and correct process to difficult. Herein lays the problem for all Web accessibility evaluation and validation tools. While these tools are useful for demonstrating errors in simple Web accessibility or, more correctly, deviations from some standards, a deep analysis of the document compared to the standards is not yet available. This means that seemingly simple issues such as the presence of appropriate text within an ALT element is not machine decidable because an intelligent analysis of the image and the wording is not available. While the WCAG standards declare that appropriate text must be present to gain, say, WCAG 1.0 'A' conformance, tools can only assert that text is present, its appropriateness cannot be analyzed.

In summary, evaluation, validation & repair of Web documents is commonplace, semi–automated, and industry facing. While research is on going it is lessening and in reality, apart from the seemingly intractable problems of 'semantics', has moved mainly into practice. While these semi–automated approaches have focused on technical solutions, increasing emphasis is being placed on qualitative analysis. Indeed, to support the vision of Web accessibility, designers and instructors of assistive technology often need to go beyond the limited constructs of engineering standards and integrate actual users of assistive technology as participants into both the design and delivery processes (Marsico et al. 2004, Wattenberg, 2005).

Client–Side Approaches

The main way to render content on the client is to use a standard Web Browser and join the visual rendering specified in the CSS with the DOM specified in the XHTML document. However, conventional renderings are often not appropriate for disabled users.

Importance / User Perspective

Client–side approaches are seen to be the most important, with regard to user interaction, because the client side agent is the application the user knows intimately and uses whenever interacting with the Web. Indeed, this is the tool that allows the user to interact with Web content in exactly the way that suits them. This personalization of interaction is the great 'leveler' of users, brought by the Web and the 'e'–revolution. By understanding that the user decides what and how to 'see' content the designer must understand that their work cannot carry the immutable characteristics of print. However, this understanding mostly does not happen. Content is badly created without: user participation; reference to guidelines; or user evaluation. In this case users need a way of accessing content and bye–passing the designer (and their bad design), ergo Client–Side approaches.

Overview

Browsers such as IBM's Home page Reader and Oxford Brookes University's BrookesTalk (Hanson et al. 2008) were created to get around these problems. While these have met with some success, and indeed work still continues on browser such as HearSay and Emacspeaks, bespoke browsing solutions have dropped away and work is now refocusing to use bespoke browsers along with document annotation and transformation[7] technologies.

Simply, transcoding (Asakawa et al. 2008) is a technology used to adapt Web content so that it can be viewed on any of the increasingly diverse devices found on today's market. It has been used for a number of years in the context of making incomplete or badly written hypertext accessible to visually impaired users and their accessibility technologies. Transcoding in this context normally involves: (1) Syntactic changes like shrinking or removing images, (2) Semantic rearrangements and fragmentation of pages based on the mean of a section (Lunn et al. 2008), (3) Annotation of the page created by a reader or algorithm (Yesilada et al. 2007), (4) and Generated annotations created by the content management system (Buyukkokten et al. 2000).

There are a number of different ways that transcoding can take place. In one example, the original material (an HTML document, for example) is analyzed by a program that creates a separate version containing annotations. The annotations include information that will instruct the reformatting process, and inaccessible elements will be removed or altered. Systems are often based along similar lines and address set problems, some are annotation based, others generate text only versions, some filter the content (Various, 2004), and others are specifically used for small scale device interaction (Buyukkokten et al. 2000). Whatever system is used it invariably does not transform all inaccessible elements but just a subset leaving holes in the accessibility of their transcode.

The goal of annotations for Web content transcoding is to provide better support either for audio rendering, and thus for visually impaired users, or for visual rendering in small screen devices. However, there are major differences and requirements. Although the amount of information that could be accessed at once in a small-screen device is also limited, the interaction is still visual. The provided visual rendering is still persistent, screen acts as an external memory, as opposed to audio rendering which is transient. Additionally, compared to visual rendering, audio is less focused and more serial in nature, the user cannot easily and quickly shift the focus.

Various proxy-based systems to transcode Web pages based on the external annotations for visually impaired users have also been proposed (Takagi et al. 2000, Asakawa et al. 2000). The main focus is on extracting visually fragmented groupings, their roles and importance. Eight different roles such as proper content, header and footer are proposed for annotation. These roles are mainly at abstract level and are not rich enough to fully annotate the page to enhance the mobility support. They do not support deep understanding and analysis of pages, in consequence the supported transcoding is constrained by these proposed roles.

Other work centers on small-screen devices and proposes a system to transcode an HTML document by fragmenting it into several documents (Hori et al. 2000). The transcoding is based on an external annotation framework. Since the focus is the small-screen devices, physical and performance constraints of the devices need to be considered, such as screen size, memory size, and connection bandwidth. However, these are not the main requirements of the users accessing Web pages in audio and there are differences as explained above.

In summary, most current client–side rendering occurs in the form of a proxy or mainstream browser extension that alters and manipulates the DOM and then applies a new tailored rendering to it. Most current transformation uses annotation or makes a best–guess and breaks documents into fragments and then re-assembles them into a new tailored format.

FUTURE TRENDS

We can see that Web accessibility is, at present, mainly based around the design and build stage: tools to build pages, guidelines to relate best practice to designers and authors, checkers and validators to warn of errors, and finally repair tools to help change and correct the errors found. At this point technology is centered on helping the designers and authors of Web sites, but this places an unfair burden on page creators because they cannot possibly design for the combination of every device and every user. In good faith, all a creator can build is a device and user agnostic site and leave the rest to technologists who can encapsulate specific knowledge of devices and users into assistive device and technologies. Currently this can be accomplished for large sections of the community and developers are only just learning how to accurately transform visually centric resources into presentation neutral resources that scale.

Web accessibility has previously been characterized by the correction of our past mistakes to make the current Web fulfill the original Web vision of access for all. Indeed, we can see that Web accessibility is currently characterized by 'catch–up'. This catch–up is necessary because when new aspects of the Web were emerging, enough consideration was not given to their accessibility from the outset. This explains why the current focus of Web accessibility work is mainly based around the design and build stage: tools to build pages, guidelines to relate best practice to designers and authors, checkers and validators to warn of errors, and finally repair tools to help change and correct the errors found. At this point technology is centered on helping the designers and authors of Web sites.

Designers often design for the most popular browser, which common knowledge suggests is Microsoft's Internet Explorer (IE), however, according to the W3CShools statistics IE and its derivatives accounted for 91% of browser usage in January 2005; this figure had reduced to 62% by October 2006. These statistics blow away conventional wisdom which suggests we only need to consider one browser maker, indeed as the Web moves mobile these statistics will change even further with percentage browser market being reduced as a function of the number of devices and embedded browsers in use. Designing for one browser, for one user group, and expecting to know all technologies and formats will soon become outdated. In the future the luxury of expecting creators to know multiple guidelines and best practice will evaporate as the technologies, applications, and user devices they are used to create will be expanding exponentially (Power et al.2007).

All this catch-up because, new technologies where not designed with accessibility in mind, and technologies that could be useful for addressing accessibility issues were not identified or adopted by the accessibility community. In this case consider what we will need to address in the future if the Web is to maintain and increase it's accessibility; look at what new technologies are on the horizon, and ask the question 'how will Web accessibility research and development cope with them?' To help answer these questions we provide a short overview of each emerging technology or area which we think will be important in the future.

Semantics & Linkdata: The key idea is to have data on the Web defined and linked in such a way that its meaning is explicitly interpretable by software processes rather than just being implicitly interpretable by humans. This may be useful from an accessibility perspective in that understanding the explicit semantics of layout or interactions may make complex interfaces more accessible;

Animation & Rich Media: Describe a whole range of interactive digital media that exhibit dynamic motion and dynamic interaction. These proprietary behaviors are notoriously hard to expose in an accessible format to correct the content authors mistakes. This area is one of the more difficult areas to address from an accessibility standpoint;

Digital Television & the Mobile Web: Constrained operating hardware combines suffers from interoperability and usability problems that make the Web difficult to interact with for disabled users. However, the possible inclusion benefits of using no general computation resources for enhanced access is appealing. The question is how to achieve inclusion without excluding disabled users;

ARIA, AJAX, & Mash-ups: Documents, once created from a single source and delivering static client-side content, are now evolving into composite documents created from multiple third party sources delivering dynamically changing content. Asynchronous JavaScript and XML (AJAX) has facilitated this change, however Document Object Model (DOM) updates on the client means assistive technology does not 'see' the change. Accessible Rich Internet Applications (ARIA) tries to make updates visible in 'live regions' and suggests how updates are handled;

HTML5 and XHTML 2.0: HTML5 was created from the 'WHATWG' splinter group formed by the user agent manufacturers; Apple, Opera, and Mozilla. It is very interactive and it's 'roles' feature hints at a move to a declarative application platform. While ARIA may be integrated the specification allows bad code by encouraging bad practice. Incubated in the W3C, XHTML 2.0 on the other hand, is more document focused and standards based with an emphasis on encouraging good coding practice. The tussle between these standards should be closely observed by the accessibility researcher;

Microformats: Microformats are built using existing standards compliant technology and are intended to solve simple problems without the need for full language and technology redesigns. This suggests that they could be useful for capturing information in the context of accessibility and the provision of annotated page information;

UML and EARL: The UGL was proposed at the 2009 W4A conference and proposes an abstract guidelines language so that sets of guidelines can be created easily and de-coupled from the testing software. Coupled with the imminent version two EARL, which facilitates the production and embedding of page testing and conformance reports, suggest a certain maturity and completeness in the testing cycle; and

Guidelines v2: While WCAG was the first set of accessibility guidelines to reach version 2.0 status, both the Authoring Tool Accessibility Guidelines (ATAG) and the User Agent Accessibility Guidelines (UAAG) are currently in version 2.0 development with lead times of a little over 2 years. These guidelines and in some case the harmonization of conformance and principles across them, is set to push conformance checking, validation and repair to the next stage with holistic checks of the software user agent, content, and generated content.

The areas listed above are those that we expect will influence Web accessibility in the future. In some cases they will provide the tools to enable accessibility; for instance the semantic Web. In some case they will provide the business case to address accessibility problems due to shared problems; for instance the mobile Web. In other case they will be the focus of our efforts to build accessibility and address the problems which are created by their inception; for instance HTML5. In all cases, the solutions will be challenging, and we will learn more about development for the wider community in the far future by addressing the problems of disabled users in the close future.

CONCLUSION

Web accessibility aims to help people with disabilities to perceive, understand, navigate, and interact with, as well as contribute to, the Web. There are millions of people who have disabilities that affect their use of the Web. Although Web guidelines direct designers and authors to best practice, currently, most Web sites have accessibility barriers that make it either difficult or near impossible for many people with disabilities to use these sites.

Evaluation, validation, and repair tools exist to check and actual pages against best practice. Validation tools analyze pages against accessibility guidelines and return a report or a rating. Repair tools, in addition to validation, try to repair the identified problems. While it is likely that there are certain accessibility issues that cannot be fully automated (e.g., checking the quality of alternative text provided for images), these tools still provide incomplete automation and complex outputs. So, although there has been extensive work in the degree and development of evaluation, validation, and repair tools, automation is still limited.

Finally, client–side rendering and transformation tools try to remold Web pages into user centric presentations. This may either be in the form of a custom browser built to enhance the interaction of people with specific disabilities or as, extensions to mainstream browsers, or as proxies which modify Web documents as they are delivered to the user. While overcoming some of the problems of the targeted disability most solutions fall down for three main reasons: (1) building for individuals is difficult; (2) understanding heterogeneous content without explicit semantics is difficult; and (3) because they use bespoke technology which cannot be maintained in a commercial setting. Addressing these reasons for failure, gives us a better chance at an accessible future.

ACKNOWLEDGMENT

This work was undertaken as part of the RIAM project funded by EPSRC (EP/E002218/1) and conducted in the Human Centred Web Lab part of the School of Computer Science at the University of Manchester (UK).

About: http://hcw.cs.manchester.ac.uk/research/riam/

Reports: http://hcw-eprints.cs.man.ac.uk/view/subjects/riam.html

REFERENCES

Abascal, J., Arrue, M., Fajardo, I., Garay, N., & Tomes, J. (2004). The use of guidelines to automatically verify web accessibility. *Univers. Access Inf. Soc.*, *3*(1), 71–79..doi:10.1007/s10209-003-0069-3

Asakawa, C., & Takagi, H. (2000). Annotation-based transcoding for nonvisual web access. In *Proceedings of the fourth international acm conference on assistive technologies* (pp. 172-179). ACM Press.

Asakawa, C., & Takagi, H. (2008, September). Transcoding. In S. Harper & Y. Yesilada (Eds.), Web accessibility: A foundation for research (1st ed., pp. 231–260). London: Springer. doi:10.1007/978-1-84800-050-6_14

Blackmon, M. H., Polson, P. G., Kitajima, M., & Lewis, C. (2002). Cognitive walkthrough for the web. In *Chi '02: Proceedings of the sigchi conference on human factors in computing systems* (pp. 463-470). New York: ACM Press. doi:10.1145/503376.503459

Boldyreff, C. (2002). Determination and evaluation of web accessibility. In *Wetice '02: Proceedings of the 11th IEEE international workshops on enabling technologies* (pp. 35-42). Washington, DC, USA: IEEE Computer Society.

Brajnik, G. (2004). Comparing accessibility evaluation tools: a method for tool effectiveness. In *Universal access in the information society* (Vol. 3, pp. 252–263). London: Springer-Verlag. doi:10.1007/s10209-004-0105-y

Brajnik, G. (2008). A comparative test of web accessibility evaluation methods. In *Assets '08: Proceedings of the 10th international ACM Sigaccess conference on computers and accessibility* (pp. 113-120). New York: ACM.

Brewer, J. (2004). Web accessibility highlights and trends. In *W4a '04: Proceedings of the 2004 international cross-disciplinary workshop on Web accessibility* (W4A) (pp. 51-55). New York: ACM Press.

Buyukkokten, O., Molina, H. G., Paepcke, A., & Winograd, T. (2000). Power browser: Efficient web browsing for PDAs. In *Proceedings of the SIGCHI conference on human factors in computing systems* (pp. 430-437). ACM Press.

Chene, D., & Hoel, M. (2002). Web site accessibility auditing tool for visually deficient persons OCAWA. In *ICCHP '02: Proceedings of the 8th international conference on computers helping people with special needs* (pp. 27–32). London: Springer-Verlag.

Chisholm, W., & Kasday, L. (2005). Evaluation, Repair, and Transformation Tools for Web Content Accessibility. Retrieved 2005 from http://www.w3.org/ WAI/ER/existingtools.html

Chisholm, W., Vanderheiden, G., & Jacobs, I. (1999). Web Content Accessibility Guidelines 1.0. Retrieved 2005 from http://www.w3.org/TR/WCAG10/

Chisholm, W., Vanderheiden, G., & Jacobs, I. (2001). Web content accessibility guidelines 1.0. *Interaction*, *8*(4), 35–54. doi:10.1145/379537.379550

Chisholm, W. A., & Henry, S. L. (2005). Interdependent components of web accessibility. In *W4a '05: Proceedings of the 2005 international cross-disciplinary workshop on web accessibility* (w4a) (pp. 31-37). New York: ACM Press.

Colwell, C., & Petrie, H. (2001). Evaluation of guidelines for designing accessible web content. *SIGCAPH Comput. Phys. Handicap.*, *70*, 11–13.. doi:10.1145/501078.501082

Cook, A. M., & Hussey, S. (2001). *Assistive technologies: Principles and practice* (2nd ed.). St. Louis: Mosby.

Cooper, M., & Rejmer, P. (2001). Case study: localization of an accessibility evaluation. In *Chi '01: Chi '01 extended abstracts on human factors in computing systems* (pp. 141–142). New York: ACM Press. doi:10.1145/634067.634154

Coyne, K. P., & Nielsen, J. (2001). *Beyond ALT text: Making the web easy to use for users with disabilities*. Nielson Norman Group.

Craven, J., & Bophy, P. (2003). *Non-visual access to the digital library: the use of digital library interfaces by blind and visually impaired people. Library and Information Commission Research Report 145*. Manchester Centre for Research in Library and Information Management.

Czaja, S. J. (2006). Technology and older adults: Designing for accessibility and usability. In *Assets '06: Proceedings of the 8th international ACM Sigaccess conference on computers and accessibility*. New York: ACM.

Department of Justice. (1998). Workforce Investment Act SEC. 508. Electronic and Information Technology. Retrieved 2005 from http://www.usdoj.gov/crt/508/508home.html

Disability Rights Commission. (2004). *The Web: Access and inclusion for disabled people* (Tech. Rep.). UK: Disability Rights Commission (DRC).

DRC. (2006). PAS 78: A guide to good practice in commissioning accessible websites.

Engelen, J., Evenepoel, F., & al, G. B. et. (1999). Producing Web Pages that Everyone can Access. TIDE-Harmony project (DE1226). Retrieved 2005 from http://www.stakes.fi/cost219/webdesign.htm Pemberton, S., et al. (2002). Xhtml 1.0 the extensible hypertext markup language (2nd ed.). Retrieved 2005 from http://www.w3.org/TR/2002/REC-xhtml1-20020801

European Union Policy Survey. (2005, November). eaccessibility of public sector services in the European union (European Union Policy Survey). UK Government Cabinet Office (RNIB and AbilityNet and DCU and RNID and Socitm). Retrieved from http://www.cabinetoffice.gov.uk/e-government/resources/eaccessibility/index.asp

Fukuda, K., Saito, S., Takagi, H., & Asakawa, C. (2005). Proposing new metrics to evaluate web usability for the blind. In *Chi '05: Chi '05 extended abstracts on human factors in computing systems* (pp. 1387–1390). New York: ACM Press. doi:10.1145/1056808.1056923

Gappa, H., & Nordbrock, G. (2004). Applying web accessibility to internet portals. *Univers. Access Inf. Soc.*, *3*(1), 80–87. doi:10.1007/s10209-003-0070-x

Gonzalez, A., & Reid, L. G. (2005). Platform-independent accessibility api: accessible document object model. In *W4a '05: Proceedings of the 2005 international cross-disciplinary workshop on Web accessibility* (w4a) (pp. 63-71). New York: ACM Press. doi: 10.1145/1061811.1061824

Hanson, V. L., Richards, J. T., & Swart, C. (2008, September). Browser augmentation. In S. Harper & Y. Yesilada (Eds.), Web accessibility: A foundation for research (1st ed., pp. 215–229). London: Springer. doi:10.1007/978-1-84800-050-6_13

Harper, S. (2007). Is There Design-For-All? *Universal Access in the Information Society, 6*(1), 111–113. Retrieved from http://www.simonharper.info/publications/Harper2007vn.pdf

Hawthorn, D. (2000). Possible implications of aging for interface designers. *Interacting with Computers*, *12*(5), 507–528. Retrieved from http://www.sciencedirect.com/science/article/B6V0D-3YKKDNJ-5/2/9e0ae58d2d9be3ed8302fa25fc4a482f. doi:10.1016/S0953-5438(99)00021-1

Hori, M., Kondoh, G., Ono, K., & Hirose, S. ichi, & Singhal, S. (2000). Annotation-based web content transcoding. In *Proceedings of the 9th International World Wide Web Conference on Computer Networks: The International Journal of Computer and Telecommunications Networking* (pp. 197-211). Amsterdam, The Netherlands, The Netherlands: North-Holland Publishing Co.

Huenerfauth, M. (2005). Representing coordination and non-coordination in an American Sign Language animation. In *Assets '05: Proceedings of the 7th international ACM sigaccess conference on computers and accessibility* (pp. 44–51). New York: ACM.

Ivory, M. Y., & Hearst, M. A. (2001). The state of the art in automating usability evaluation of user interfaces. *ACM Computing Surveys, 33*(4), 470–516. doi:10.1145/503112.503114

Ivory, M. Y., Mankoff, J., & Le, A. (2003). Using Automated Tools to Improve Web Site Usage by Users with Diverse Abilities. In *IT & Society* (p. 195236). USA: Stanford University.

Jacobs, J., Hammerman-Rozenberg, R., Maaravi, Y., Cohen, A., & Stessman, J. (2005, Aug). The impact of visual impairment on health, function and mortality. *Aging Clinical and Experimental Research, 17*(4), 281–286.

Kasday, L. R. (2000). A tool to evaluate universal web accessibility. In *Cuu '00: Proceedings on the 2000 conference on universal usability* (pp. 161-162). New York: ACM Press. doi:10.1145/355460.355559

Laux, L. F., McNally, P. R., Paciello, M. G., & Vanderheiden, G. C. (1996). Designing the World Wide Web for people with disabilities: A user centered design approach. In *Assets '96: Proceedings of the second annual ACM conference on assistive technologies* (pp. 94–101). New York: ACM Press. doi:10.1145/228347.228363

Leporini, B., & Paterno, F. (2003). Criteria for usability of accessible web sites (LNCS 2615, pp. 43-55). London: Springer-Verlag.

Levi, M. D., & Conrad, F. G. (1996). A heuristic evaluation of a World Wide Web prototype. *Interactions, 3*(4), 50–61. doi: 10.1145/234813.234819

Lewis, C. (2005). Bridges for the mind: opportunities for research on cognitive disabilities. In *Assets '05: Proceedings of the 7th international ACM Sigaccess conference on computers and accessibility*. New York: ACM.

Lie, H. W., & Bos, B. (1999). Cascading Style Sheets, level 1. Retrieved 2005 from http://www.w3.org/TR/CSS1

Lunn, D., Bechhofer, S., & Harper, S. (2008, September). Experiences of exposing semantics to drive transcoding. In M.-M. Bouamrane, S. Luz, & M. Masoodian (Eds.), *Proceedings of first international workshop on ontologies in interactive systems* (p. 9-17). IEEE Computer Society. Retrieved from http://www.simonharper.info/publications/Harper2008gs.pdf

Marsico, M. D., & Levialdi, S. (2004). Evaluating web sites: exploiting user's expectations. *International Journal of Human-Computer Studies, 60*(3), 381–416..doi:10.1016/j.ijhcs.2003.10.008

McCathieNevile. C., & Abou-Zahra, S. (2005). Evaluation and Report Language (EARL) 1.0. Retrieved 2005 from http://www.w3.org/TR/EARL10/

Meyer, E. (2002). *Eric Meyer on CSS: Mastering the Language of Web Design*. New Riders Press.

Meyer, E. A. (2005). Is accessible design a myth? In *W4a '05: Proceedings of the 2005 international cross-disciplinary workshop on Web accessibility* (W4a) (pp. 60-62). New York: ACM Press.

Morkes, J., & Nielsen, J. (1997). Concise, Scannable, and Objective: How to Write for the Web. Retrieved from http://www.useit.com/papers/webwriting/writing.html

Nielsen, J. (1993). *Usability engineering*. San Diego, USA: AP Professional.

Nielsen, J. (1999). *Designing Web Usability: The Practice of Simplicity*. New Riders Press.

Novick, D. G., & Scholtz, J. C. (2002). Editorial - universal usability. *Interacting with Computers*, *14*(4), 269–270. doi:10.1016/S0953-5438(01)00057-1

Ohnemus, K. R. (1997). Web style guides: who, what, where. In *Sigdoc '97: Proceedings of the 15th annual international conference on computer documentation* (pp. 189–197). New York: ACM Press. doi: 10.1145/263367.263392

Paciello, M. G. (2000). *Web Accessibility for People With Disabilities*. CMP Books.

Paddison, C., & Englefield, P. (2003). Applying heuristics to perform a rigorous accessibility inspection in a commercial context. In *Cuu '03: Proceedings of the 2003 conference on universal usability* (pp. 126–133). New York: ACM Press. doi:10.1145/957205.957228

Panayiotou, C., & Samaras, G. (2004). mpersona: personalized portals for the wireless user: An agent approach. *Mobile Networks and Applications*, *9*(6), 663–677. doi:10.1023/B:MONE.0000042505.07003.e6

Petrie, H., Hamilton, F., & King, N. (2004). Tension, what tension? Website accessibility and visual design. In *Proceedings of the international cross-disciplinary workshop on Web accessibility* (pp. 13-18).

Pilgrim, M. (2002). Dive Into Accessibility. Retrieved 2005 from http://diveintoaccessibility.org/

Power, C., & Petrie, H. (2007). *Accessibility in non-professional Web authoring tools: A missed Web 2.0 opportunity?* In *W4a '07: Proceedings of the 2007 international cross-disciplinary conference on Web accessibility* (W4a) (pp. 116-119). New York: ACM Press.

Raskin, J. (1997). Looking for a humane interface: will computers ever become easy to use? *Communications of the ACM, 40*(2), 98–101. doi:10.1145/253671.253737

Raskin, J. (2000). The humane interface (book excerpt). *Ubiquity, 1*(14), 3. doi:10.1145/341836.342022

Regan, B. (2004). Accessibility and design: a failure of the imagination. In *Proceedings of the international cross-disciplinary workshop on Web accessibility* (pp. 29–37).

RNIB. (2004). See It Right Guidelines. Retrieved 2005 from http://www.rnib.org.uk/xpedio/groups/public/documents/code/public rnib008789.hcsp

Robertson, S., Beesley, S., Byrne, J., Richards, J., Koechley, N., & Sloan, M. (2005). Accessible Design in the Digital World Conference, Dundee, UK. (Panel Session – Legislation? Standards? How do we tell people to design technology that supports inclusion?)

Robinson, S. (2003, June). Accesskeys: Unlocking hidden navigation. *A List Apart, 1*(158). Retrieved from http://www.alistapart.com/articles/accesskeys/

Shneiderman, B., & Plaisant, C. (2004). *Designing the User Interface: Strategies for Effective Human-Computer Interaction* (4th ed.). Addison Wesley.

Takagi, H., & Asakawa, C. (2000). Transcoding proxy for nonvisual web access. In *Proceedings of the fourth international ACM conference on assistive technologies* (p. 164-171). ACM Press.

Takagi, H., Asakawa, C., Fukuda, K., & Maeda, J. (2004). Accessibility designer: visualizing usability for the blind. In *Assets '04: Proceedings of the 6th international ACM Sigaccess conference on computers and accessibility* (pp. 177–184). New York: ACM Press.

Thatcher, J., Waddell, C., & Burks, M. (2003). *Constructing Accessible Websites*. Rebound by Sagebrush.

Trewin, S. (2006). Physical usability and the mobile web. In *W4a: Proceedings of the 2006 international cross-disciplinary workshop on web accessibility (W4a)* (pp. 109–112). New York: ACM Press.

Trewin, S., Keates, S., & Moffatt, K. (2006). Developing steady clicks: a method of cursor assistance for people with motor impairments. In *Assets '06: Proceedings of the 8th international acm sigaccess conference on computers and accessibility* (pp. 26–33). New York: ACM.

Vanderdonckt, J., Beirekdar, A., & Noirhomme-Fraiture, M. (2004). Automated evaluation of web usability and accessibility by guideline review (LNCS 3140, pp. 17–30). London: Springer-Verlag.

Various. (2004). WebCleaner. Retrieved from http://webcleaner.sourceforge.net

Wattenberg, T. (2004). Beyond standards: reaching usability goals through user participation. *SIGACCESS Access. Comput.*, 79, 10-20. doi: 10.1145/1040053.1040055

Westwell, J., Andrews, M., McLean, J., & Mitchell, K. (2006). Baker & Mckenzie's annual review of developments in EU law relating to IP, IT and telecommunications. *Computer Law & Security Report*, *22*(1), 20–25. Retrieved from http://www.sciencedirect.com/science/article/B6VB3-4J335VH-3/2/b77693178b70913e89a31a-c951afd359. doi:10.1016/j.clsr.2005.11.008

World Health Organisation. (2004, 11). Magnitude and causes of visual impairment (No. 282). Retrieved from http://www.who.int/mediacentre/factsheets/fs282/en/

Yesilada, Y., Jay, C., Stevens, R., & Harper, S. (2008). Validating the use and role of visual elements of web pages in navigation with an eye-tracking study. In *WWW '08: Proceeding of the 17th international conference on World Wide Web* (pp. 11–20). New York: ACM. Retrieved from http://www.simonharper.info/publications/Harper2008yu.pdf

Yesilada, Y., Stevens, R., Harper, S., & Goble, C. (2007). Evaluating DANTE: Semantic transcoding for visually disabled users. *ACM Transactions on Computer-Human Interaction*, *14*(3), 14. Retrieved from http://www.simonharper.info/publications/Harper2007fk.pdf. doi:10.1145/1279700.1279704

KEY TERMS AND DEFINITIONS

AJAX / ARIA: Asynchronous JavaScript and XML (AJAX) has facilitated the creation of multi-source dynamic documents. However, the Document Object Model (DOM) updates on the client means assistive technology does not 'see' the change. Accessible Rich Internet Applications (ARIA) tries to make updates visible in 'live regions' and suggests how updates are handled

Conformance: Conformance testing is application of guideline checkpoints to an instance of a webpage to decide if the website conforms to the guidelines.

Design Guidelines: Guideline specifications in support of good practice when trying to create accessible web pages and sites.

HTML5: HTML5 is the next version of HTML, created from the 'WHATWG' splinter group formed by the user agent manufacturers;

Apple, Opera, and Mozilla, it is now housed under the w3c umbrella.

Transcoding: A technology used to adapt Web content so that it can be viewed on any of the increasingly diverse devices found on today's market. It has been used for a number of years in the context of making incomplete or badly written hypertext accessible to visually impaired users and their accessibility technologies.

User Agent: A user agent is the client application used to access the World Wide Web. Web user agents range from web browsers to search engine crawlers,, as well as mobile phones, screen readers and Braille browsers used by people with disabilities.

Validation: The determination of a valid or invalid web page or site and repair tools, techniques, or advice which attempts to enable the correction of parts of a site which are not valid.

Web Accessibility: Making the World Wide Web accessible to people with disabilities.

ENDNOTES

1 https://addons.mozilla.org/en- US/firefox/addon/879 viewed 06 July 2009.

2 Notably, the Extensible Mark-up Language (XML) is a less rigorous implementation of SGML.

3 WCAG version 1.0 has fourteen guidelines that are general principles of accessible design. Each guideline has one or more checkpoints that explain how the guideline applies in a specific area. Each checkpoint is assigned a priority, enabling it to be ranked into (3) conformance levels 'A'–'AAA' with a site being ranked 'AAA' if it reaches all WCAG 1.0 guidelines (Chisholm et al. 1999).

4 By alternate we mean none XHTML / CSS formats.

5 For instance and XHTML ALT attribute maybe present in an image element but the alternative text may not semantically represent the image it relates to, or indeed anything intelligible to a human.

6 Now called WebXACT.

7 called Transcoding.

Chapter 12
Catering for Personal Autonomy with E-Mentoring Supported by Recommendations

Olga C. Santos
UNED, Spain

Carmen Barrera
UNED, Spain

Emanuela Mazzone
UNED, Spain

Jesus G. Boticario
UNED, Spain

ABSTRACT

This chapter presents a technology solution based on a recommender system supporting people with intellectual disabilities in their work integration and independent life, in the scope of the CISVI and AMI4Inclusicion research projects. Information and Communication Technologies are essential for supporting personal autonomy and improving the quality of life of disabled people. The technology can contribute in a twofold way: (1) facilitating the work of the human mentor when training people with intellectual disabilities and (2) automatically offering them advice and recommendations in response to certain cues/actions detected in the environment.

INTRODUCTION

Education and work are inextricably linked to people's lives in our society, and they are the key agents towards successful social integration. However, people with disabilities still find barriers to inclusion in employment and education which weigh against independent living. One approach to help them overcome these barriers is through mentoring. A mentor is someone who

DOI: 10.4018/978-1-60566-206-0.ch012

supervises the career and development of another person through teaching, advising and providing psychological support. Nevertheless, this definition is limited because it does not take into account certain relationships and obstacles such as organizational structure, geographic location, interpersonal skills and the challenging nature of work. The use of Information and Communication Technologies (ICT) to provide electronic mentoring, or e-mentoring, may help overcome these problems (Hamilton et al., 2003). Moreover, this mentoring behaviour can not only be supported, but also reproduced by the technology. In this way, the systems perceive what the users are doing in the environment and can support personal autonomy. Technology can be used to support this twofold approach: (1) facilitating the mentoring work for human mentors, and (2) reproducing some of this support and offering it dynamically when certain user actions are detected in the environment. In particular, this chapter presents how this can be achieved with the use of a recommender system developed for educational purposes.

The objective of this chapter is to present a technology solution based on a recommender system to support the needs of people with intellectual disabilities towards their integration into work and independent life. First, we comment the background that supports the need for researching in ICT to support personal autonomy and improve the quality of life of disabled people. Next, we comment on the research work carried out in the scope of the CISVI and AMI4Inclusicion projects, where the aDeNu research group is engaged in fostering independent living through ICT. Next, we comment how personal autonomy can be supported through recommendations offered within the mentoring approach from both perspectives: the mentor and the mentored. Finally, future trends are commented, and conclusions are provided at the end of the chapter.

BACKGROUND

According to article 26 of the Universal Declaration of Human Rights, "everyone has the right to education" (UN, 1948). More recently, the "Convention on the Rights of Persons with Disabilities", approved by the General Assembly of the United Nations (UN, 2006a), in its article 4 takes account of all major legal and political instruments for the safeguarding of the rights of disabled people including those relevant for their participation in education. In Europe, the Ministerial Conference "ICT for an inclusive society" in Riga resulted in a common Ministerial Declaration in 2006 (EU, 2006a), where the prominent role of ICT in education is mentioned in the preamble, as well as the need for accessibility to services available through a range of devices. Many barriers to access education are mentioned along with service design and personal capacity. The needs of older workers and elderly people and the need to enhance e-accessibility and usability are also addressed here.

These initiatives have great relevance and impact in contemporary society since about six hundred million people in the world live with a functional diversity, or so called disability. They are supposed to have the same rights and obligations as any other member of the society, but unfortunately, due to the lack of support to specific needs, they usually face obstacles that prevent them from enjoying their rights. In Europe, the estimated percentage of the population with intellectual disabilities is about 3% (Inclusion@eu, 2004).

The European Ministerial e-Inclusion Conference of Vienna, in 2008 recognises the progress and success already achieved in the field of e-Inclusion in Europe and, at the same time, the challenges that still remain. The conclusion is that, in these difficult economic times, it is more than ever essential to support vulnerable people in our society, and ICT constitute an essential tool to achieve this objective. Better digital inclusion will contribute to strengthen Europe's main asset, its human capital. Through adopting the communication 'Towards and accessible information Society' (EU, 2009), the European Commission has set out a clear, common European direction for e-Accessibility.

When referring to disability, we do not only consider physical impairments, for the most part we will focus on intellectual and developmental dysfunctions that affect an individual's social, conceptual and practical skills. Most people with an intellectual disability, if diagnosed on time, can have the opportunity to achieve a sufficient level of independence in everyday life activities if they are supported with appropriate programmes (i.e. BIT Project, Promentor Project). Many studies have been developed in this direction, mainly promoted by research centres or independent communities of specific disabilities (i.e. Down Syndrome Online, Fundación Syndrome de Down de Madrid, ILSMH, FEAPS). Lately, the question has achieved a public dimension and governmental regulations encourage companies to recruit workers with disabilities. This increase in social awareness has boosted the interest of research institutions and private companies to exploit the potential of information technologies towards supporting disabled people in their work, personal and leisure daily activities (Loyd 2006, Valverde, 2005).

Independence for people with intellectual disabilities will be most effectively enhanced by a supportive environment with sound economic, social and environmental conditions, including adequate income, social security provisions and public policies that affect the level of independence in individual lives for all (EU-IST 034707 – http://www.mpower-project.eu).

Although the interrelationship between education and work is one of the main agents for a successful social integration, this may also bring up barriers to the inclusion of people with disabilities. Traditionally, time and space were the main barriers for attending a classroom. Nowadays, with the application of ICT to the learning process, time and space barriers can be removed. Nevertheless, according to European reports, "only 3% of European public web sites surveyed comply with the minimum web accessibility standards and guidelines, hindering access to web content and services for people with disabilities who comprise some 15% of the EU population" (EU, 2006a). Currently, e-Inclusion has become a widely used term to refer to accessibility features provided by ICT based products and services. These services are to be used by people with disabilities as well as older people with age-related changes in functional capacities, they cover a wide range of disabilities, such as cognitive sensorial (sight, hearing), cultural and mobility. It is crucial to ensure that ICT products and services are not a further obstruction to access and can be used by those disabled. The concept of ALL (accessible lifelong learning) focuses on access to education and lifelong learning which are both more and more mediated through ICT.

However, even though the technology is applied so that everyone can use it by taking into consideration the existing functional diversity of students (research efforts in this line are addressed, such as the EU4ALL project (Santos et al., 2008)), specific support is required to cater for the needs of people with intellectual disabilities. Support will be provided through appropriate mentoring processes, encouraging the individual's progress towards independent living (EU, 2006b).Efforts have been carried out to offer solutions concerning ICT and ageing services (ICT & Ageing, 2009). However, research towards supporting independent living for people with intellectual disabilities is not so extensive. Within this target group, user needs vary widely, and there is potentially a very broad range of e-Accessibility challenges that need to be addressed.

CURRENT RESEARCH DIRECTIONS AT ADENU FOR CATERING PERSONAL AUTONOMY

Research in advanced learning technologies have an impact on the improvement of the quality of life of disabled people since it can provide them with the means to increase their personal autonomy. In this way, the quality of life represents the degree to which an individual can establish and sustain a viable self in the social world (Brown and Brown, 2003). Unfortunately, technology is very often not ready to support the final user in this way.

In this context, at the aDeNu group we are doing advanced research on ICT to foster the inclusion of people with cognitive and physical disabilities in society. At present, we are involved in the CISVI (TSI-020301-2009-20) and AMI4Inclusion (TSI-020100-2009-172) projects, which face different issues related to the inclusion of disabled people using ICT.

In the ICT research area, a consensus has emerged that user involvement is very important during the design and the development phases of novel applications and services. When users are drawn in, the solutions developed will be practical and address concrete user needs. Despite this, developers and users are very often disconnected from each other. However, there is a persistent need for research on how to integrate all users (each person involved in the real scenario, from carers to public agents, including also family and fellowships). CISVI and AMI4Inclusion projects are in this path, and are within the Social Spaces for Innovation (EsdI – Espacios Sociales de Innovación - http://www.espaciossociales.es/) Spanish Initiative.

In both projects, aDeNu's research is focused on the accessibility, usability, e-learning, e-mentoring and user modelling through diverse implementations, developments and evaluations. Although we are faced with different scenarios, (1) employment of people with cognitive disabilities (Santos et al., 2009a) and (2) addressing independent life (Barrera et al., 2009); all of them share a common challenge: to help people with intellectual disabilities to easily learn the activities of daily living. The first solution consists on a set of didactic units for the reinforcement of these activities.

To assist learning in this digital context we decided to introduce a recommender system. Recommender systems are largely used in commercial contexts to suggest suitable options amongst all the possibilities available in an information-rich environment. The recommender system's potential can also be applied in learning and training contexts to help the users deal with the content and services.

In this paper, we focus on the support offered by the recommender system, one of the key research lines of the aDeNu work (Santos and Boticario, 2008). The recommender system support is mainly offered taking into account both the learner's interactions with the lessons and the events that occur in the environment.

Before going into details on the application of the recommender system in the CISVI and AMI4Inclusion projects, we introduce briefly the objectives of both projects.

CISVI Project

CISVI stands for Communities for Health and Independent Living Research (in Spanish, "Comunidades de Investigación para la Salud y la Vida Independiente"). The project is funded by the Spanish Ministry of Industry, Tourism and Commerce (Secretaría de Estado de Telecomunicaciones y para la Sociedad de la Información. Proyectos Singulares y de Carácter Estratégico del Plan Avanza 2008). The main objective of CISVI is to identify, test and validate a new methodological research framework named Social Spaces for Innovation (ESdI) in three scenarios: (1) labour integration of people with cognitive disabilities, (3) home healthcare for elderly people s, (3) living independently and (4) rural e-inclusion. At aDeNu, we have started by contributing mainly to (1) and (2), but obtained outcomes are planned to be extended to (2) and (4) at the next stages. The primary objective of ESdIs research framework is to encourage the involvement -from the very beginning of the research activities- of the end user as co-creator of the services (Tansey and Stembridge, 2005).

The research activity carried out within the scope of these ESdIs pose important contributions in the following areas of technology and its adaptation for the elderly or for people with intellectual disabilities:

- Intelligence Environmental Technologies: RFID, mobile sensors, etc.
- Mobile devices for accessing ICT suitable for meeting the needs of people with disabilities and dependence
- Accessibility, usability and user modelling technologies
- e-learning and e-mentoring ubiquitous technologies, adapted to people with disabilities and dependence
- Tracking and geographic information technologies
- IT security and identity

AMI4Inclusion Project

AMI4Inclusion is the acronym of Environments of Ambient Intelligence for the Labour Integration of Youth with Intellectual Disabilities, a research project funded by the Spanish Ministry of Industry, Tourism and Commerce (Programa Nacional de Tecnologías de Servicios de la Sociedad de la Información, Acción Estratégica e-inclusión y e-asistencia). The goal of this project is to foster the integration in the workplace for all young people and especially for those with intellectual disabilities, since this provides a better social integration and a complete development of the individual. Currently, training and learning is merely offered at university level, but there is a need for specific training for young people with intellectual disabilities about 18-20 years old that allows them to gain access to decent jobs and become more skilled. The project aims at the following main objectives to uphold independent living and train young disabled and potential professionals:

- Full integration of people with intellectual disabilities into working life, family and independent living.
- Coaching and mentoring support through virtual management of everyday life (including employment support) for people with intellectual disabilities.
- Profit from Intelligence Environmental Technologies (such as RFID) to monitor the people activities in the physical environment.

FOSTERING INDEPENDENT LIVING THROUGH ICT

In this section we introduce the scenarios approached in both projects and a description of the e-learning system used for the mentoring process.

Current Scenarios

Three differentiated scenarios are defined:

- Scenario 1: Young people with minor intellectual disabilities who are starting to work in a new workplace. The labour integration involves a mentoring process with a social assistant, to adapt the work-site to her needs. The physical scenario is the workplace where RFID technology is available, one of the activities to be done is filing paper documents, and.
- Scenario 2: Adults (sometimes, nearly elderly) with major intellectual disabilities who live in an occupational centre, receive training on how to perform basic daily life

activities (ADL). They receive this training in different places: within the class-room, in simulated rooms at the centre (simulating a real home), and within their real home or residence. RFID technology and other sensors are available.

- Scenario 3: Young people with low level intellectual disabilities at a school are to be prepared as future workers (they learn practical, social and emotional skills) to handle their first jobs. Several psycho-educational experts give them the needed support. There is also RFID technology available.

Within the mentoring process a deep knowledge of the user is required; the mentor supervises the user's actions (and thus directly plays a role); the aim is to perceive how the user, understands the context, to be aware of the user's abilities, skills and troubles in daily life activities. Next, the mentor offers the user emotional feedback, advices and also some tools and facilities to overcome any difficulties.

The E-Learning System

The initial technology implemented as a baseline consists on a set of learning units jointly designed with the participation of technology experts (graphical designers, web developers), psycho-pedagogical experts, but also the direct users are involved in the scenario. The didactic units are designed taking into account the specific needs of the learner when she/he is faced with a particular task. The units are designed as reinforcement units when the user needs to remember the different actions. These units are available everywhere and the learner can access them when needed. This is not a traditional educational system, where the learner acquires concepts and knowledge, but it serves as a continuous reinforcement in time to acquire skills and behaviours.

The procedural learning units are complemented with training activities, which use a very attractive and interactive interface, these interactive units seek to train the learner in the relevant skills.

The diversity of learners' behaviours and needs requires the system to incorporate a learner profile that is continuously enriched with the use of the system.

On the other hand, the e-learning system monitors the interactions that take place between the learner and the system and generates a report for the mentor regarding the actions of each learner. Also, the system receives events coming from the physical environment (from the RFID technology) that provide additional information about the result of those tasks performed manually by the learner.

SUPPORTING PERSONAL AUTONOMY WITH RECOMMENDATIONS DURING THE MENTORING PROCESS

This section introduces how personal autonomy can be supported with recommendations offered within the mentoring process, at two levels: (1) facilitating the mentoring work for human mentors (Santos et al., 2009a), and (2) reproducing some of this support and offering it dynamically when certain actions produced by people with disabilities are detected in the environment, these require a direct support (via recommendations which are offered to them) that complement the human component of the traditional mentoring process. Both levels are applied in the three scenarios presented above, the first one (filing documents in the labour integration context) is mainly focused on level 2. The independent life context is focused on "hand washing" as a basic daily life activity ADL (see Roldan et al., 2009), and due to the high degree of cognitive needs of the target group, recommendations are only intended for mentors (level 1) Finally, level 1 and 2 are both applied in the third scenario, where alphabetic, numeric and chronological classification are the skills meant to be acquired and trained in the educational context.

The Recommender System

The technological support to provided for the mentoring process is a recommender system for educational purposes, which has been developed to offer personalized support for users in an inclusive and interoperable way (Santos and Boticario, 2008). This system is based on a recommendations model originally defined for general use, so it can be applied in a diverse set of circumstances. The recommendations model describes:

- what should be recommended (different recommendation types have been identified and can be offered, they relate to the actions produced by the users),
- when a recommendation is deemed appropriate (considering the user and course context, the conditions for the application and the timeout restrictions),
- how a recommendation should be displayed (considering accessibility and usability criteria) and
- why a recommendation has been produced (in terms of what category the recommendation applies to, what technique has been used to generate it, and the source that originated the recommendation).

In the past, it has been applied to e-learning scenarios to plug adaptive navigation capabilities to existing learning management systems. As commented in this chapter, it can also be used to support the mentoring process aiming to provide personal autonomy for people with disabilities.

In any case, the idea behind the recommender system is to offer suggestions to the people (both the mentor and the people with disabilities) on what to do next taking into account the current context of use and the individual characteristics of the user. The former (i.e. the current context) requires tracking the users' interactions. The interactions carried out within the traditional learning management systems, are complemented with external interactions, that is, in the physical environment where the user is placed. The later (i.e. the individual characteristics of the user) requires the modelling of the user features in a standard way. For this, existing specifications can be used, such as IMS Learner Information Packaging, IMS Accessibility for Learner Information Packaging and ISO/IEC 24751 Individualized adaptability and accessibility in e-learning, education and training (part 2 on Personal Needs and Preferences). With this information available, the recommender system can work.

The process for designing the recommendations followed a user centred methodology (Santos et al., 2009b) where users are involved in the process of identifying the appropriate recommendations. This approach differs from the one used in non-educational recommenders where the recommendation generation process takes into account the users preferences and their past interactions (Draschler et al., 2007). In an educational scenario like the one required for the mentoring process, psycho-educational considerations are to be taken into account, and not solely the user preferences (Bloch et al., 2003). The methodology proposed is to be used at the recommendations' design time, that is, when the recommendations are created.

The methodology applies scenario-based methods (Rosson and Carroll, 2001) to involve psycho-educational experts in writing stories (i.e. scenarios) about the problems taking place in relevant situations that may occur during the users' interaction with the environment. The information obtained from the psycho-educational experts is used to transform the predefined recommendation types (i.e. any action that can be potentially recommended to the person) into recommendations that have associated the applicability conditions and restrictions. Moreover, in order to increase the confidence in the well-behaving of the system, the justifications of the recommendations (by means of metadata information) are also provided to the user. This information is also relevant to facilitate a future automation process of the generation of the recommendations using artificial intelligence techniques.

At runtime, that is, when the person is in the environment, the recommender is called in at certain moments to look for appropriate recommendations for the current user in the current context. Then, the recommender checks if the current context for this user matches the conditions defined for each of the recommendations that were produced during the design phase. The recommendations that match the conditions are instantiated and offered to the person in the appropriate graphical user interface and modality.

To facilitate the management of the recommendations generation process, a template has been proposed to describe the recommendations obtained with the methodology. Three sets of information have to be provided:

- Description of the recommendation type, by showing the action to be done on the selected object
- Translation of the text associated to the recommendation type in the appropriate spoken language(s) so the system can be used by users with different language skills and knowledge
- Description of the recommendation according to the model, assigning the specific element to be recommended and filling in the metadata for the recommendation: type, category, origin, explanation and conditions (positive and negative).

A usable interface is being developed to facilitate the manual generation process of the recommendations by the mentors.

At aDeNu, we are mainly working with people with intellectual disabilities in a working environment providing them with an interactive support for daily living and working activities. In this context, the recommender system has to be developed together with the mentor inline with whatever traditional tools they have worked with so far. In this way, the new tool can help the workers to complete their tasks. At the same time, it will provide useful information for the mentor on how the worker has interacted with the device, for what and in what specific moment. This type of automated information is essential for improving the personalization and the efficiency of the worker's life long training and support. The recommender system detects problems after analysing the interaction of a specific user with the system in his/her context and suggests possible actions for the mentor to provide support for any problems arising or for improving a specific situation.

Hereafter, we comment how the recommendations can support the mentoring process in both complementary levels: (1) facilitating the mentoring work for human mentors, and (2) reproducing some of this support, and offering it dynamically when certain user actions are detected in the environment.

Facilitating the Mentoring Work for Human Mentors (Recommendations for Mentors)

In this scenario, the mentor is considered as the person in charge of training and providing workplace guidance for people with disabilities and is supported by the mentoring process to provide the most efficient support for those mentored (Santos et al., 2009a). In order to design these recommendations within this scenario, a group of key players from the social community were identified, and a focus group session with three mentors was set up, here the methodology described earlier was applied. A SCORM course on how to use the platform for the mentor's collaborative work was published in a learning management system and shown to the focus group. As part of this course, a training space with workers was simulated as a virtual community to show the mentors the main interactions that the users may have in this scenario. The feedback obtained in the focus group session served to identify a set of relevant recommendations. The recommendations identified were expressed as natural language statements to allow the verification by the users involved in the experience. After the recommendations were expressed as natural language statements, they were translated to the recommender system model (Santos et al., 2009a). The recommendations identified were:

- Recommendations for 'New mentor introduction'
- Recommendations for 'Inter-mentor coordination'
- Recommendations for 'Mentor course design'
- Recommendations for 'Mentor teaching'
- Recommendations for 'Mentor guidance'
- Recommendations to follow-up the mentored progress, which should take into account the particularities of the mentored

In this scenario, recommendations are very much related to those proposed for learning management systems (since mentors can be seen as members of virtual learning communities), where potentially any action can be recommended to be done on any object in the learning management system.

Dynamic Mentoring to Support People with Cognitive Disabilities in Their Tasks (Recommendations for People in Their Daily Activities, at Home, at School or at Work)

In turn, dynamic monitoring can be also used to reproduce some of this support by offering it dynamically to users during their daily activities when certain actions are detected in the environment. Three activities are considered: (i) filing documents (labour integration context), (ii) hand washing (independent life context) and (iii) document classification (educational context). This approach can be used to support disabled people for independent life.

In implementing recommender systems in these specific contexts of use, it is necessary to pay special attention when designing the interface for end-users with an intellectual disability, given that cognitive and visual overload is the main concern for an optimal use of the product.

The e-learning system offers structured reinforced learning by providing learning objects for users. The learning objects deal with specific concepts and may contain interactive exercises considering the level of difficulty. The goal of the recommender system is to propose that the learner re-views a didactic unit for reinforcement or suggest further training with interactive exercises.

The recommendation is fired when certain events occur in the environment (external conditions outside the learning system, which are captured using RFID techniques) and also during the interaction between the learner and the e-learning system.

Sometimes, depending on the learner profile, the same recommendation is addressed to the mentor, advising her/him when the learner comes across any trouble or strain.

The recommender system includes a general repository of initial recommendations, some of them of general-purpose, others were obtained from the focus groups (see last section) conducted with experts mentors. But also, the study has identified the convenience of providing a tool for the mentor in order to configure recommendations on-the-fly, these are commonly addressed to a particular user.

The recommender system behaviour is based on:

- conditions regarding the learner's profile
- conditions regarding past interactions between the learner and didactic units

- conditions regarding the results of exercises
- conditions regarding events within the physical environment

The recommender system provides the user recommendations such as:

- motivational messages for the learner (positive reinforcement, a congratulation message for encouragement)
- proposing to work on a concept (to revise a learning object and to interact with a set of exercises).
- advising the learner to contact the mentor (by phone, chat).

In this case, recommendations are not so diverse, and focus on recommending specific contents and actions in the course design. The effort here has to be put on the recommender system's interface (a young person with cognitive disabilities) should be offered a very simple interface that the user can easily understand and use.

In the third scenario, the focus is on the training environment, where future workers learn the practical, social and emotional skills needed to handle their jobs. In this domain we are working on two scenarios for the final user. One is completely screen based, where the students practise the exercise the unit taught in the lessons. The system is °tailored to the profile and the needs of the specific students. A set of suggestions is offered, bearing in mind the type of exercise and the user errors detected, in order to improve his/her performance. Recommendations in this context can direct the user to go over the syllabus of a specific lesson or increase/decrease the level of difficulty of the exercise. The information of the interaction stored by the system will also inform the mentor on any suitable actions concerning the needs of the specific student.

In a similar scenario, the student interacts within the physical environment while training for the work task. One of the exercises includes filing documents in the correct order and storing them in the corresponding tray. In the training environment, the students work with documents tagged with RFID and intelligent trays with an RFID reader and writer. When the trainee completes the filing task and put the documents in the tray, the system detects the accuracy of the activity. The feedback provided to the user (and/or the mentor) is integrated with the recommender system which suggests what actions should be taken according to the specific user profile and needs.

FUTURE TRENDS

The support of personal autonomy though mentoring processes is bound to undergo dramatic changes in the coming years. In this key working area the purpose is to introduce the possibility of managing the mentoring processes themselves in an accessible and standard-based way, supporting both the mentor and the mentored. In particular, the following issues are to be solved:

- Responsiveness of the environment: being able to react quickly to the requirements of learners (motivate, engage, inspire). In this sense, the current recommender system presented in this chapter should be extended to consider further areas of motivation, engagement and inspiration.
- Covering different approaches: from individual to collaborative support and from desktop management to ubiquitous activities.
- Adaptive and intuitive response: adapting to behaviours that reflect relevant people's features such as learning styles, learners' competences and skills, preferences and specific needs, diverse functional issues, etc. The objective of the system is to guide the students from their initial intuitions to the final learning

- Intelligent monitoring process of users with the aim of providing sensible reports to mentors, who can then improve the support provided. Auditing facilities will include support for identifying, defining, and evaluating any type of situation that needs to be audited.
- Evidence on effective support for personal autonomy, with special emphasis on the management of the effectiveness and its evolving features.

Mentoring process for people with intellectual disabilities could be applied to people with other disabilities and also to the general population.

CONCLUSION

This chapter has presented a solution based on a recommender system to address the technological challenges to support the needs of people with intellectual disabilities towards their work integration and independent life, in the scope of the CISVI and AMI4Inclusicion research projects.

Personal autonomy can be supported with recommendations offered within the mentoring process, in two complementary scenarios: (1) facilitating the mentoring work for human mentors, and (2) reproducing some of this support and offering it dynamically when certain actions of the users are detected in the environment. The first scenario (facilitating the mentoring work for human mentors) is applied in the research route that promotes the labour integration of people with cognitive disabilities. The second one (reproducing some of this support and offering it dynamically when certain actions of the users are detected in the environment) is applied to support independent life.

The recommender system offers (1) a general system for the mentor to "configure" adaptations or help adjusted to the needs of one particular user, in the form of recommendations, (2) direct recommendations to the mentor and the user in their own activities, and (3) help to the mentor to detect troubles and possible next actions for the user.

ACKNOWLEDGMENT

Authors would like to thank her colleague Cecile Finat from the aDeNu Research Group for her suggestions to clarify the readability of the contents of the chapter. Moreover, they would also like to thank the Spanish Government for funding the research projects that support this research: AMI4Inclusion (TSI-020100-2009-172), CISVI (TSI-020301-2009-20) and A2UN@ (TIN2008-06862-C04-01/TSI). Details of the projects are at aDeNu website.

REFERENCES

Barrera, C., Santos, O. C., Gutierrez y Restrepo, E., Boticario, J. G., Moranchel, J., Roldán, J. R., & Casas, R. (2009). Empowering disabled people: e-learning challenges for independent life. In *Proceedings of the 3rd Workshop Towards User Modeling and Adaptive Systems for All: Modeling and Evaluation of Accessible Intelligent Learning Systems (TUMAS-A 2009) held in conjunction with AIED 2009* (pp. 38-44).

Blochl, D., Rumershofer, H., & Wob, W. (2003). Individualized e-learning systems enabled by a semantically determined adaptation of learning fragments. In *Proceeding of the 14th International workshop on Database and Expert Systems Applications* (pp. 640-645).

Brown, I., & Brown, R. (2003). *Quality of Life and Disability. An Approach for Community Practitioners*. Jessica Kingsley Publishers.

Down syndrome online (n.d.). Retrieved from http://www.down-syndrome.org/about/

Drachsler, H., Hummel, H. G. K., & Koper, R. (2007). Personal RS for learners in lifelong learning: requirements, techniques and model. *International Journal of Learning Technology*. eInclusion@EU project (2004). D1.1 Analytic Framework - eInclusion and eAccessibility priority issues, October 2004. Available from http://www.einclusion-eu.org/Document.asp?View=TRUE&MenuID=77#_ftnref62

European Union. Declaration on eInclusion 11-13 June (2006a). Ministers of the European Union Member States and accession and candidate countries, European Free Trade Area (EFTA) countries and other countries. Retrieved April 20, 2008, from http://europa.eu.int/information_society/events/ict_riga_2006/doc/declaration_riga.pdf

European Union. (2006b) *User Needs in ICT Research for Independent Living, with a Focus on Health Aspects*. Retrieved from http://ec.europa.eu/information_society/activities/health/docs/events/indep-living-nov2005/24-25nov-report-final-draft-june2006.pdf

European Union. (2009). e-Inclusion Ministerial Conference (Dec 2008, Vienna, Austria.) DG Information Society and Media – Unit H.3 ICT for Inclusion, Report (June 2009). Retrieved from http://ec.europa.eu/information_society/events/e-inclusion/2008/doc/final_report.pdf

FEAPS. (Confederación Española de Organizaciones en favor de las Personas con Discapacidad Intelectual). (n.d.). Retrieved from http://www.feaps.org/

Hamilton, B. A., & Scandura, T. A. (2003). E-Mentoring: Implications for Organizational Learning and Development in a Wired World. *Organizational Dynamics*, *31*(4), 388–402. doi:10.1016/S0090-2616(02)00128-6

ICT & Ageing. (2008) European Study on Users, Markets and Technologies. Empirica & WRC. Retrieved from http://www.ict-ageing.eu/ict-ageing-website/wp-content/uploads/2008/11/ictageing_vienna_handout_final2.pdf

ILSMH (Formerly International League of Societies for Persons with Mental Handicap). (n.d.). Retrieved from http://www.siwadam.com/hmm/euie.htm

IMS Global Consortium. (n.d.). Retrieved from http://www.imsglobal.org/

ISO/IEC 24751. (2008). Individualized adaptability and accessibility in e-learning, education and training. ISO/IEC 24751-1:2008 Part 1: Framework and reference model. Part 2: "Access for all" ISO PNP (Personal Needs and Preferences). Part 3: "Access for all" digital resource description. Lloyd, J., Moni, K.B., & Jobling, A. Breaking the hype cycle: Using the computer effectively with learners with intellectual disabilities. Retrieved from http://www.down-syndrome.org/practice/296/practice-296.pdf.

Roldán, J. R., Moranchel, J., Barrera, C., & Casas, R. (2009) Aprendizaje de las actividades de la vida diaria mediante el uso de tecnología adaptada, ESSAAC'2009 2nd National Congress on Augmentative Communication and Technology for life, September, 2009, Zaragoza, Spain.

Rosson, M. B., & Carroll, J. M. (2001). *Usability engineering: scenario-based development of human computer interaction*. Morgan Kaufmann.

Santos, O. C., & Boticario, J. G. (2008). Users' experience with a recommender system in an open source standard-based learning management system. In *Proceedings of the 4th Symposium of the WG HCI&UE of the Austrian Computer Society on Usability & HCI for Education and Work (USAB 2008)* (LNCS 5298).

Santos, O. C., Boticario, J. G., del Campo, E., & Saneiro, M. (2008). Personalised support for students with disabilities based on psycho-educational guidelines. *In Proceedings of the IEEE international conference on advance learning technology (ICALT 2008): workshop on advanced learning technologies for disabled and non-disabled people (WALTD)*. Santander, Spain, IEEE Computer Society Press

Santos, O.C., Couchet, J., & Boticario, J.G. (2009a). Personalized e-learning and e-mentoring through user modelling and dynamic recommendations for the inclusion of disabled at work and education. *ICALT 2009*.

Santos, O. C., Martin, L., del Campo, E., Saneiro, M., Mazzone, E., Boticario, J. G., & Petrie, H. (2009b). User-Centered Design Methods for Validating a Recommendations Model to Enrich Learning Management Systems with Adaptive Navigation Support. In S. Weibelzahl, J. Masthoff, A. Paramythis, & L. van Velsen (Eds.), *Proceedings of the Sixth Workshop on User-Centred Design and Evaluation of Adaptive Systems*, held in conjunction with the International Conference on User Modeling, Adaptation, and Personalization (UMAP2009) (pp. 64-67).

Tansey, M., & Stembridge, B. (2005). The challenge of sustaining the research and innovation process. *World Patent Information*, *27*(3), 212–226. doi:10.1016/j.wpi.2004.12.006

United Nations. (1948). Universal Declaration of Human Rights. Adopted and proclaimed by General Assembly resolution 217 A (III) of 10 December 1948. Retrieved April 28, 2008, from http://www.un.org/Overview/rights.html

United Nations. (2006). Convention on the Rights of Persons with Disabilities. General Assembly. Retrieved September 20, 2009, from http://www.un.org/esa/socdev/enable/rights/convtexte.htm

Valverde, S. (2005). El aprendizaje de las tecnologias de la información y la comunicación en personas con síndrome de down. Tesis doctoral. Universidad Complutense de Madrid. Retrieved from http://eprints.ucm.es/tesis/edu/ucm-t28915.pdf.

KEY TERMS AND DEFINITIONS

Accessible Lifelong Learning (ALL): focuses on access to education and lifelong learning which are both more and more mediated through ICT.

e-Inclusion: Approach to preventing digital exclusion, i.e prevent that disadvantaged people and disadvantaged groups could be left behind in the development of the information society.

Independent Living: ability to perform the activities of daily life with no or little help from others.

Information and Communication Technologies (ICT): use of electronic computers and computer software to convert, store, protect, process, transmit, and securely retrieve information.

Mentor: someone who oversees the career and development of another person through teaching, advising and providing psychological support.

Radio Frequency Identification (RFID): an portable storage system that uses an object (tag) applied to a product for the purpose of identification and tracking using radio waves.

Recommender Systems: systems that guide people to interesting materials or services based on information from other people, providing recommendations based on opinions/behaviours of others.

Section 4
Computer Access

Chapter 13
Blind User Interfacing:
Requirements, Models and a Framework

Fernando Alonso
Technical University of Madrid, Spain

José L. Fuertes
Technical University of Madrid, Spain

Ángel L. González
Technical University of Madrid, Spain

Loïc Martínez
Technical University of Madrid, Spain

ABSTRACT

There are specific usability requirements for developing dual interfaces, that is, graphical user interfaces that are also adapted for blind users. These include task adequacy, dimensional trade-off, behavior equivalence, semantic loss avoidance and device-independence. Consequently, the development of human-computer interfaces based on task, domain, dialog, presentation, platform and user models has to be modified to take into account these requirements. This paper presents the requirements for blind user interfacing, the changes to be made to the human-computer interface models and a framework that improves the development of dual user interfaces. The framework includes a set of guidelines for interface design, a toolkit for the low effort implementation of dual user interfaces, and a programming library for the inclusion of speech and Braille in applications. A case study of the development of one such dual interface application is also presented.

DOI: 10.4018/978-1-60566-206-0.ch013

INTRODUCTION

Graphical user interfaces were designed to increase the usability and improve the functionality of applications (Cox and Walker, 1993). These interfaces are generally user friendly and easy to use. However, blind and visually-impaired people may find them hard to manage. Not only does this group of people find the items on screen difficult to access, but also many items whose meaning is important for users to be able to understand the application are represented as images only and are, therefore, not directly accessible for blind users. On top of this, this group of users cannot operate a mouse. A graphical interface is, therefore, obviously a barrier for blind people, although screen readers solve many of the problems they come up against. Making an application accessible for blind users involves, firstly, putting each item into a proper text-based format and, secondly and more importantly, reproducing the visual interface in a structure that can be understood by users.

To do this, designers must be familiar with the needs and capabilities of blind users and with the assistive technologies they use. Synthesized speech, Braille displays, Braille and QWERTY keyboards and speech recognition are the major, albeit not the only, assistive technologies used by blind people. One feature that all these elements have in common is linearity (these devices can only interchange information sequentially). Nevertheless, they all have their own peculiarities and behaviors (think about the volatility of the information that the user receives through speech messages as opposed to the persistence of Braille displays). Therefore, these behaviors need to be analyzed when trying to develop effective interfaces.

Hence an adequate graphical user interface for blind people sets some specific usability requirements for these users. This means that the designer has to present the interface information in an appropriate structure that blind users can understand, none of the meaning of the interface content should be lost during the adaptation and the information supplied should be adapted for the assistive technologies used by blind people. These requirements have an impact on HCI modeling, involving the creation of the task, domain, dialog, presentation, platform and user interface models (Szekely et al., 1993). Model design is therefore affected by this adaptation.

Based on the above, this chapter describes some usability requirements for blind users and sets out what actions have to be taken in each of the above-mentioned HCI models to incorporate these requirements to develop applications with a graphical interface that is also adapted for blind people. The paper also describes a framework for developing graphical user interfaces for blind people based on the actions described for each of the HCI models. The experience in developing this kind of applications (Alonso et al., 1997a; Alonso et al., 1997b; Alonso et al., 1998) gathered over the years has served as input for defining this framework.

The chapter is organized as follows. Section 2 shows the background about applications for blind people. Section 3 describes the requirements, models and framework for blind user interfacing. Section 4 describes the future trends. The chapter ends with some general conclusions.

BACKGROUND

The development of user interfaces for blind people has taken two complementary research and development paths: (1) adapting existing visual interfaces for blind users and (2) building dual interfaces or interfaces especially adapted for blind or visually impaired users.

The adaptation of visual interfaces for blind people emerged in response to the need to adapt the directly manipulated graphical environments that were proliferating to enable people with impaired vision to use common development software. The pioneering projects on this subject include OutSpoken (Edwards, 1991) and Mercator (Mynatt and Edwards, 1992a), which aimed to adapt MacOS and X-Windows, the most commonly used graphical environments in the early 90s. These projects encouraged the development of the Off Screen Model (Mynatt and Edwards, 1992b), the adaptation model on which most of the tools available for adapting interfaces for blind users are based. Tools like Orca help provide access to applications and toolkits that support the AT-SPI (e.g., the GNOME desktop) (GNOME, 2009), VoiceOver gives blind people access to MacOS X systems (Apple, 2009), and using Hal Screen Reader (Dolphin Computer Access, 2009), JAWS (Freedom Scientific BLV Group, 2008) and Window-Eyes (GW Micro, 2009) non-sighted users can access Windows environments.

The installation or use of such tools does not in itself guarantee that blind users will be able to access all the environment or applications. Both the environment (operating system) and the applications need to be built following special design rules (ISO, 2008).

The drawback of this approach is that the original dialog design addresses the specific needs and abilities of sighted users, and syntax has to be restructured during adaptation to a non-visual form to meet the needs and abilities of blind users. The problem is that "no knowledge can be extracted on the application domain and, consequently, the idiosyncrasy of the application, for instance, additional error prevention methods, is not taken into account in this adaptation" (Savidis and Stephanidis, 1995a). A clear example of an application that cannot be adapted according to this approach would be a musical score editing application. For it to be usable, the blind user-adapted tasks and dialog process need to be defined.

A second approach is focused on creating applications with special-purpose interfaces for blind users or with dual interfaces, one visual and another adapted for blind people enabling them to use assistive technology directly. Toolkits like HAWK (Stephanidis et al., 2009), which provides a set of standard non-visual interaction objects and interaction techniques that have been especially designed to support high quality non-visual interaction, have been created to facilitate this process. HAWK is suitable for developing not only interfaces targeting blind users, but also interfaces for a variety of situations in which dialogs not relying on visual communication and standard input devices are required (e.g., driving, telephone-based applications, home control auditory interaction). Another tool aiding the development of dual interfaces suitable for both sighted people and blind users is the User Interface Management System (UIMS) (Savidis and Stephanidis, 1995a). HOMER (Savidis and Stephanidis, 1998), for example, is a UIMS that eases the development of dual user interfaces for sighted and visually impaired users.

In any case, we have found, as pointed out by (Moreley, 1999), that it is essential to examine the fundamental accessibility issues for blind people at length and define appropriate usability guidelines in order to design an interface suited for use by blind people. These guidelines, which should be based on experimental evidence (Casali, 1995), should not only be formulated as general design principles or low-level and platform-specific recommendations, but also added to the actual HCI models that define a user interface. Additionally, the use during the analysis, design and implementation phases of development tools (toolkits, UIMS…) to build applications with non-visual interfaces is essential for efficiently and systematically developing these applications.

REQUIREMENTS, MODELS AND FRAMEWORK FOR BLIND USER INTERFACING

Requirements for Blind User Interfaces

As a primary premise in usability requirements specification for blind people, note that these requirements have to coexist with those of other user types in accordance with Design for All principles (equitable use, flexibility in use, simple and intuitive use, perceptible information, error tolerance, low physical effort, size and space for approach and use) (Connell et al., 1997) and HCI dialog principles (suitability for the task, self-descriptiveness, conformity with user expectations, suitability for learning, controllability, error tolerance, suitability for individualization) (ISO, 2006).

The usability requirements for blind and non-blind people differ a lot. One characteristic that makes such a difference is the fact that, at the current state of the art, blind people cannot perform all tasks. Outside a computing setting, a blind person cannot as yet drive a car, for example, which means that this task would not have to be adapted for this group of people. This question is referred to as *task adequacy*.

Additionally, blind people and non-blind people access information in a computer differently. This is a consequence of a blind person not being able to see the 2D screen.

The dimensional access scheme of sighted people is 2+1: they access graphical interfaces where the information items are distributed in two-dimensional regions (the screen, a page, a window…) and their position on the plane normally provides additional semantics about each item. The transition (navigation) from one 2D region to another is performed by selecting and opening elements (the +1 component). In this respect, any application will be formed by a set of linked 2D regions, making up a navigation graph.

The dimensional access scheme of blind people is 1+1: unfortunately, devices for blind people (synthesized speech and Braille displays) are one-dimensional, which means that an item is selected following a list structure and an item is opened as a link, usually to another list. Hence, for a blind person, an application is more like a set of structured linked lists of items (forming a tree). This is what we have called the *dimensional trade-off*.

There is another requirement closely related to the dimensional trade-off: *behavior equivalence*. A sighted person interacts by directly manipulating a graphical interface following a procedure that is nothing like how a blind person interacts using the linear interface resulting from interface adaptation for the respective assistive technologies. Apart from linearization, the process should also deal with how to make each interactive object accessible for blind users. Extra actions need to be added for all objects in the tree, including the messages that must be sent to assistive technologies, the mechanism for accessing each part of the item, and any review functions that are performed.

It will not be enough either just to adapt each interactive object to the blind person's procedure of interaction. The information provided to blind users as they perform the different tasks allowed by the system also has to be adapted. This should assure that there will be no semantic loss, because a lot of the information may be conveyed by means of images or the spatial distribution of objects located in a window. This is what we have termed the *semantic loss avoidance* requirement.

Finally, the assistive technologies used by blind people are not standardized. Speech devices and Braille displays differ not only as regards what functionality they offer to users but, most importantly, as to the protocols they use to communicate with applications. We call this the *device independency* requirement.

In sum, it can be said that to improve the usability of applications for blind users, they have to be given access to all contents and the additional semantic information they require to guarantee that the application will be consistent with how visually impaired users needs to interact.

USER INTERFACE MODELING FOR BLIND USERS

The HCI model most widely accepted by researchers and designers is the modeling-based definition by Szekely (Szekely, 1993) that includes six models: task, domain, dialog, presentation, platform and user model (Myers, 2000). The *task model* gives a structured representation of what activities the software user may want to perform. The *domain model* describes the syntactic sequence of the interaction and is implemented as a sequence of windows. The *dialog model* describes the interaction between the different objects making up the interface. The *presentation model* describes the user interface's visual appearance. The *platform model* describes the various computer systems that may run a user interface. The *user model* describes the characteristics of the user or group of users.

There are several issues for which each model has to account when developing interfaces for blind users. These issues are derived from the usability requirements for blind people described above (Figure 1).

Task model. The task model is a formal description of the services the user accesses. It is organized hierarchically and contains information regarding task activation, preconditions, postconditions, and the actual task action (Menkhaus and Fischmeister, 2003).

During problem analysis the tasks described should be checked for incompatibility with what blind people can do (task adequacy requirement). Blind people cannot do activities that require hand-eye coordination, or activities that require simultaneously controlling the state of more than one visual item, because they communicate with the computer serially.

Figure 1. Influence of blind-user interfacing on HCI models

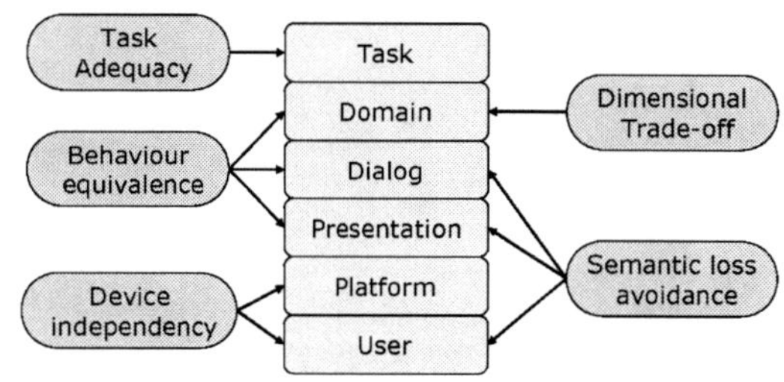

Domain model. The domain model describes the syntactic sequence of human-computer interaction through user interface objects and determines how the set of tasks and actions are ordered (Menkhaus and Fischmeister, 2003). This model is usually implemented as a sequence of windows consisting of a set of user interface objects and a set of transitions for navigating from one window to the next.

The domain model should define a sequence of windows and window content and structure that is compatible with 1 + 1 navigation (dimensional trade-off requirement). Also, the domain model should include the information to be output as speech and Braille in the transition from one window to another (behavior equivalence requirement).

In the first place, the domain model should be represented hierarchically as a series of trees linked by transitions between windows. Each window is described as a tree and the window components (title bar, main menu, button bar, etc.) will be its children. Each of these nodes will be decomposed into other objects (each of the buttons in the bar, for example) until the objects can be decomposed no further. Any leaf objects whose activation leads to the appearance of a new window will have a link to the tree of this new display unit. Figure 2 shows an example of part of this graph for an application.

One important question is the tree's depth level for each software window. Because blind users must necessarily navigate by levels within

Figure 2. Example of a tree-based domain model

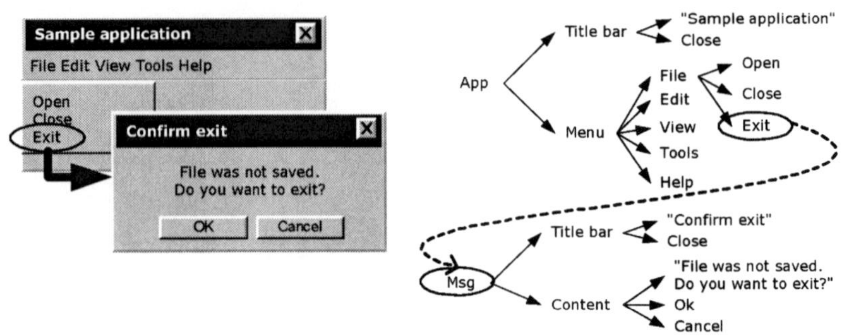

the above tree and cannot "take a look" to find out where to go, the windows should be designed to assure that their navigation tree is not overly complicated.

To cater for the behavior equivalence requirement, blind users should also be given information about what happens when transitions between tree levels or trees take place. This includes messages about the features of an open item, the type of process that is taking place, the type of objects in the new level or, generally, any information that helps blind users to manage or understand the interface. For example, when a message window is opened, the following information could be speech synthesized: window title, message text and active user interface object.

Dialog model. The dialog model defines the commands as well as the purpose of each one. Commands are executed via interaction techniques and may produce one or more system responses (Puerta, 1996).

The dialog model should enable keyboard-only access, define each user interface object's interaction process, define the access mechanisms to the object's properties (behavior equivalence requirement), and should incorporate additional interaction techniques to give access to important semantic information (semantic loss avoidance).

First, the dialog model should be developed taking into account the fact that blind users cannot use pointing devices (they require hand-eye coordination) and have to use the keyboard or keyboard equivalents (such as speech recognition, Braille keyboards, etc.).Therefore, the type of interaction techniques that this model can use is limited.

It is especially important in this respect that the dialog model retains the target platform keyboard usage conventions. For example, if a key combination is assigned a given function by convention (for example, CTRL+P for printing), then the applications should not attempt to use these combinations for other purposes.

Second, each user interface object's interaction procedure must be defined in line with blind people's capabilities. There should be two chief rules in this interaction procedure: keyboard-based interaction and speech or Braille access to the most important attributes of each user interface object.

Therefore, it is necessary to define which of each user interface object's attributes should be accessed through speech or Braille. In the case of a menu option, for example, access should be given to the text, the mnemonic (underlined letter), the associated keyboard accelerator, its state (active or inactive) and, finally, its type: direct command, open dialog or open a submenu. Figure 3 shows an example of menu options and their attributes.

Thirdly, and as regards the semantic loss avoidance requirement, a number of additional interaction commands should be incorporated to enable non-sighted users to access extremely useful semantic information:

Figure 3. Examples of menu item attributes

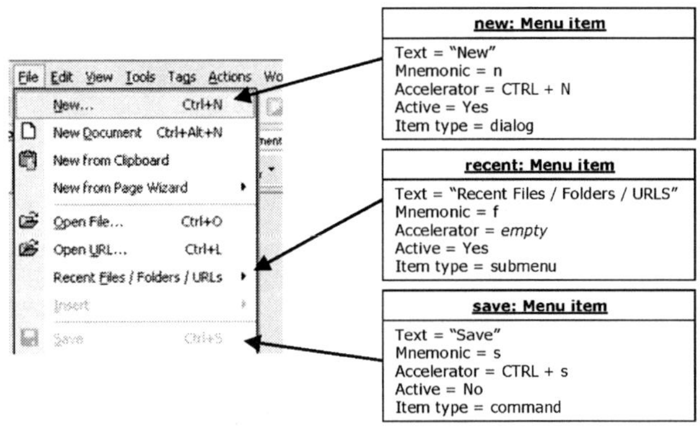

- Inform users about current location (speech and Braille)
- Repeat the last message (speech only)
- Spell the last message (speech only)
- Provide context-sensitive help including what actions users can take in the current window (speech and Braille)
- Progress report for tasks being performed by the system (speech and Braille).

Finally, and under certain circumstances, alternative interaction techniques need to be provided to perform a given command. This type of actions affects both the dialog and the presentation model (for example, a musical composition program for blind people should offer special-purpose non-visual mechanisms for editing the score).

Presentation model. This model is usually defined as the model that describes the visual appearance of the user interface (Eisenstein et al., 2000). This way of looking at the presentation model is good for graphical interfaces, but blind users perceive the interface using other senses, like hearing or touch.

Therefore, we propose another definition for this model, which is compatible with the diversity of presentations that an interface may have: the presentation model describes the perceptual appearance of the user interface.

Taking into account this definition, the presentation model should define the speech and Braille output for each user interface object (behavior equivalence requirement) and several detail levels for different user experience levels. It should also guarantee that non-standard objects containing graphical content provide enough semantic information (semantic loss avoidance).

As part of this philosophy it is essential to take into account what differences there are between the speech and Braille outputs, differences that lead to different messages.

Some examples of these differences follow: information persists in Braille displays until the user takes an action, which is not the case with speech; access to spoken information is sequential (the user has to wait for the voice to reach the fragment of the target information), whereas it is direct in Braille displays (users can move through the displayed information however they like); character attributes (bold, italic, underlined, etc.) can be represented in Braille displays using points 7 and 8 of the 8-point Braille code. These attributes cannot be represented in speech without interrupting the dialog.

The presentation should make provision for several detail levels, from novice to expert users. Novice blind users will want to receive as much information as possible on each interface element as they learn to use the application. Expert users

Table 1. Presentation of menu item attributes in speech and Braille

	Speech output	Braille output
Menu item	"item"	"MI"
Text	The text	The text
Mnemonic	A separate character	Underlined letter in the text
Accelerator	Accelerator with full wording for the modifier keys ("control")	Accelerator with abbreviated wording for modifiers ("ctrl")
State	"" or "inactive"	"" or "inactive"
Item type	"dialog", "submenu" or "command"	"...", ">" or ""

will only want to receive the information that they need to do the job. Our experience has led us to define three detail (or help) levels: beginner, intermediate and advanced.

The designer has to take all this into account to define the speech and Braille representation of every user interface object. This is a two-step process:

1. Define the presentation of each user interface object attribute for speech and Braille. For example, the object type is represented by full text in speech ("Button") and in abbreviated form in Braille ("BT"). Table 1 shows the presentation of menu item attributes.

2. Define the *object attributes combination* to generate the output message for each detail level. The designer has to use different sorting techniques for speech and Braille. For instance, the object's name has to appear first in speech to enhance navigation speed. Table 2 shows the presentation messages for menu items.

Figure 4 shows the presentation of some menu items using the rules defined in Tables 1 and 2.

The designer has to take special care to assure that the information sent to the user via speech or Braille is semantically equivalent to what is given visually in the graphical user interface. This way, blind users will have all the information they need to use the application to do their job.

Platform Model. The platform model contains information about the target platform capabilities, constraints and limitations (Menkhaus and Fischmeister, 2003). When developing user interfaces for blind people, the platform model is affected by the device independency requirement.

For this purpose, the platform model should include speech and Braille output capabilities through standardized APIs, such as but not limited to:

Table 2. Speech and Braille presentation of menu items

Speech output	
Beginner	<text> <mnemonic> <accelerator> <state> <item type> <menu item>
Intermediate	<text> <mnemonic> <accelerator> <state> <item type>
Advanced	<text> <mnemonic> <accelerator> <state>
Braille output	
Beginner	<menu item> <text + mnemonic> <accelerator> <state> <item type>
Intermediate	<text + mnemonic> <accelerator> <state> <item type>
Advanced	<text + mnemonic> <accelerator> <state>

Figure 4. Examples of menu item presentation

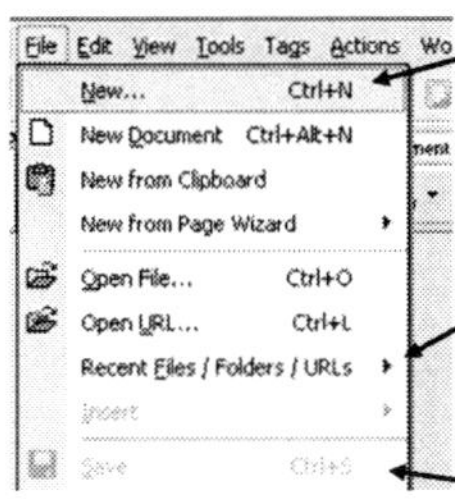

	Speech	Braille
1	New n control n dialog menu item	MI New CTRL n ...
2	New n control n dialog	New CTRL n ...
3	New n control n	New CTRL n

	Speech	Braille
1	Recent Files / Folders /URLs f submenu menu item	MI Recent Files / Folders /URLs >
2	Recent Files / Folders /URLs f submenu	Recent Files / Folders /URLs >
3	Recent Files / Folders /URLs f	Recent Files / Folders /URLs

	Speech	Braille
1	Save s control s inactive command menu item	MI Save CTRL s inactive
2	Save s control s inactive command	Save CTRL s inactive
3	Save s control s inactive	Save CTRL s inactive

- For speech: text to speech output, stop speech, spelling management of queued speech messages, management of speech progress, changing speech parameters
- For Braille: text to Braille output, information about display characteristics (such as the display size), automatic management of text that is bigger than the Braille display size, management of keys pressed in the Braille display, changing Braille parameters.

Examples of such APIs for speech are SAPI in Microsoft Windows (Microsoft, 2009) and Java Speech for the Java platform (Sun Microsystems, 2009).

User model. The user model is a description of the characteristics of an individual user or of a stereotype user group (Puerta, 1996). The user model is not intended to be a description of the mental state of a user.

The user model has to include configuration parameters related to the semantic loss avoidance and device-independency requirements, such as speech parameters (the device used, speed, tone, volume, etc.) and Braille parameters (the device used, Braille code type, cursor type, presentation of character attributes, etc.) or the detail level of the output messages (for beginner, intermediate and advanced).

A FRAMEWORK FOR BLIND USER INTERFACING

Based on this model, we have developed a Framework for BLind user INterface Development (FBLIND). This framework has three components (Alonso et al., 2006):

1. A set of user interface design guidelines, based on software accessibility standards.
2. A programming library providing support for Speech and Braille Input and Output (SBIO).
3. An interface development toolkit with automatically adapted user interface objects (BVCL).

Figure 5 shows the relationship between the blind user requirements, the HCI models and our framework.

Blind user interfacing guidelines. These guidelines are based on the International Standard on Software Accessibility (ISO, 2008). This standard, in whose development we participated as experts, along with other tips picked up over the years are incorporated into the framework.

The guidelines affect all the HCI models to a different extent and contain useful information for all the stages of interface development. One important aspect of these guidelines is that the application should be compatible with screen

Figure 5. FBLIND and HCI models

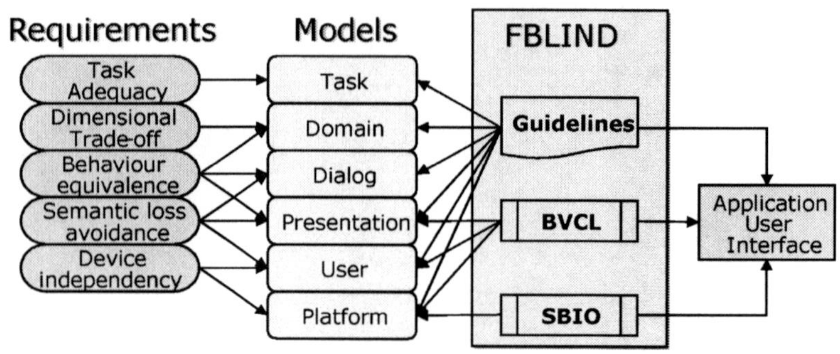

readers and other assistive technologies that blind people use.

SBIO. There was a need for synthesized speech and Braille output capability, and standardized APIs should be provided for this functionality. Another requirement is for programming libraries that make this functionality as easy as possible to use. This is the goal of SBIO.

SBIO contains several programming components that improve speech and Braille input and output. This package was developed for the Microsoft Windows platform, as this is the platform most commonly used by blind people in Spain. It was developed jointly by the Spanish National Organization for the Blind, Microsoft and the Technical University of Madrid.

SBIO contains the following components (Figure 6):

- SAPI (Speech API): Microsoft SAPI enables the use of both device-independent synthesized speech and speech recognition. The device is accessed by its respective driver. A series of drivers were developed for the most common external voice synthesizers.
- BAPI (Braille API): the API for using Braille displays enables the use of any Braille display provided its respective driver is available.
- SBIO-Core: set of ActiveX components offering a unified speech and Braille interface that is simpler than the interfaces provided by SAPI and BAPI. This interface offers less functionality, including only really useful objects for developing applications for blind people. Additionally, SBIO-Core offers new services for coordinating applications and screen readers and improving their compatibility.
- SBIO-Lib: dynamic link library that facilitates the use of SBIO for those programming languages in which it is complicated to use ActiveX objects. SBIO-Lib contains a series of C functions that can be used to easily control all the SBIO objects.

BVCL. The usability requirements for blind people applicable to the presentation, platform and user models have been built into a blind user adapted VCL (BVCL) toolkit (Varela, 1998; Guede 2002; García, 2005), which improves the development of these user interfaces:

- *Presentation model*: BVCL incorporates user interface objects including automated behavior for presentation in speech and Braille.
- *Platform model*: BVCL improves the programming of additional speech and Braille

Figure 6. SBIO components

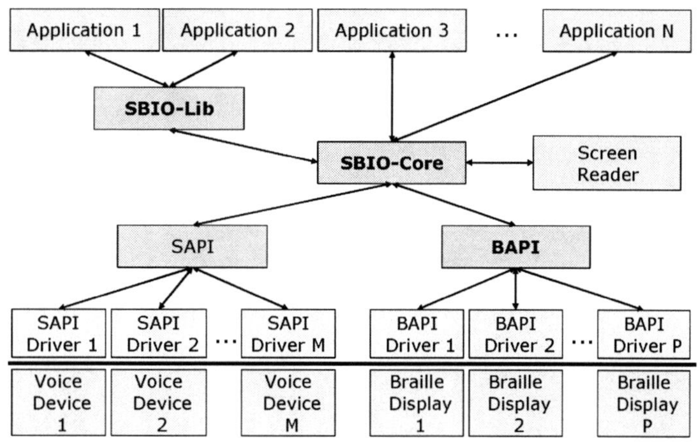

outputs that go beyond what is offered by the user interface objects.

- *User model*: BVCL improves the configuration of the user interface parameters and especially the specific messages in speech and Braille generated for each user interface object.

BVCL is an extension of the Borland C++ Builder development environment VCL (Visual Component Library), to which a series of components adapted to the needs of blind users have been added.

As VCL is an object-oriented library, an inheritance mechanism has been used to build specialized versions of the most used VCL components (buttons, edit-boxes, lists, etc.) which are capable of automatically using speech and Braille, and reacting properly to the events in the user interface. Figure 7 shows some BVCL components and their relation to the VCL components.

The TAdaptation class, based on SBIO-Lib, enables programmers to make use of speech and Braille in those cases where the information provided automatically by BVCL components is insufficient.

The output messages are configured by means of format files for improving the flexibility of the applications developed using BVCL. The output of each interface object attribute and whole objects can be changed without having to recompile the application.

Finally, BVCL also offers services for automatically managing the layout and size of the user interface objects when there are changes to the font size. This is highly important for visually impaired people, who usually use large fonts. In this case, it is often difficult to reorganize and size the interface objects. Therefore, BVCL incorporates a number of layout manager classes integrated into the C++ Builder design interface so the programmer does not have to write code for this functionality.

Note also that BVCL allows big savings on development effort for applications adapted for blind users. In most cases, all programmers have to do is use BVCL (instead of VCL) components at design time, and the application built will have a graphical interface that will also be automatically adapted for use by blind people with very little specific effort.

CASE STUDY: DABIN

DABIN is an environment that accommodates a range of bilingual dictionaries, allowing users to choose the translation source and target languages,

Figure 7. BVCL components

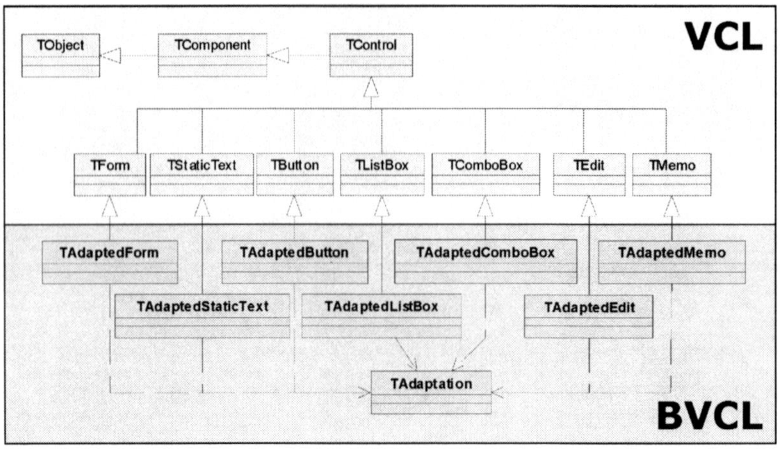

as well as the user interface language. It has a dual user interface, and can run word searches, returning all the information about their translation in another language, including grammatical categories, examples, etc. It now includes a Spanish-English and English-Spanish dictionary, and a Spanish-French and French-Spanish dictionary, and has user interfaces in Spanish, English and French (Alonso et al., 2008).

The application follows the Design for All principles and the special-purpose usability requirements for blind people. DABIN uses speech synthesis and Braille to provide users with all the information they need.

DABIN has a generic interface, combining visual and blind interfaces to assure that the user interface is fully accessible for blind users, without detracting from its graphical quality. Figure 9 shows the graphical user interface.

The different HCI models adapted for blind people were built to model the user interface. The actions taken for each model to build DABIN are discussed in the following.

Task model. During software requirements specification, we checked that all the tasks were adequate for blind users and accessible by means of the keyboard, synthesized speech and Braille display.

In no case do these tasks require hand-eye coordination or the simultaneous control of different visual objects. All the operations performed by users are confined to text input (using a keyboard), the activation of functions using buttons or menus (using the keyboard or mouse) and navigation through different interface objects, such as edit boxes, windows, buttons, etc. (using the keyboard or mouse).

Domain model. The information in each window has been represented in the domain model, taking special care not to go into too much depth and breadth at each level.

Figure 8 shows an example of two windows: a search term has been entered in the first (a), and the result of this search is shown in the second (b).

Figure 8 (i) illustrates the navigation tree for the window in Figure 8 (a) and Figure 8 (ii) shows the navigation tree for the window in Figure 8(b), displayed after finding the translation. New information appears in the "Content" node.

Looking at Figure 8, we find that the trees are not very deep (4 levels) and not very wide (5 nodes) in line with the guidelines. The button bar has been omitted from the tree description, as, not being able to operate a mouse, blind people cannot use these buttons directly. This does not detract from the functionality offered to blind people, as all

Figure 8. Search windows and navigation trees

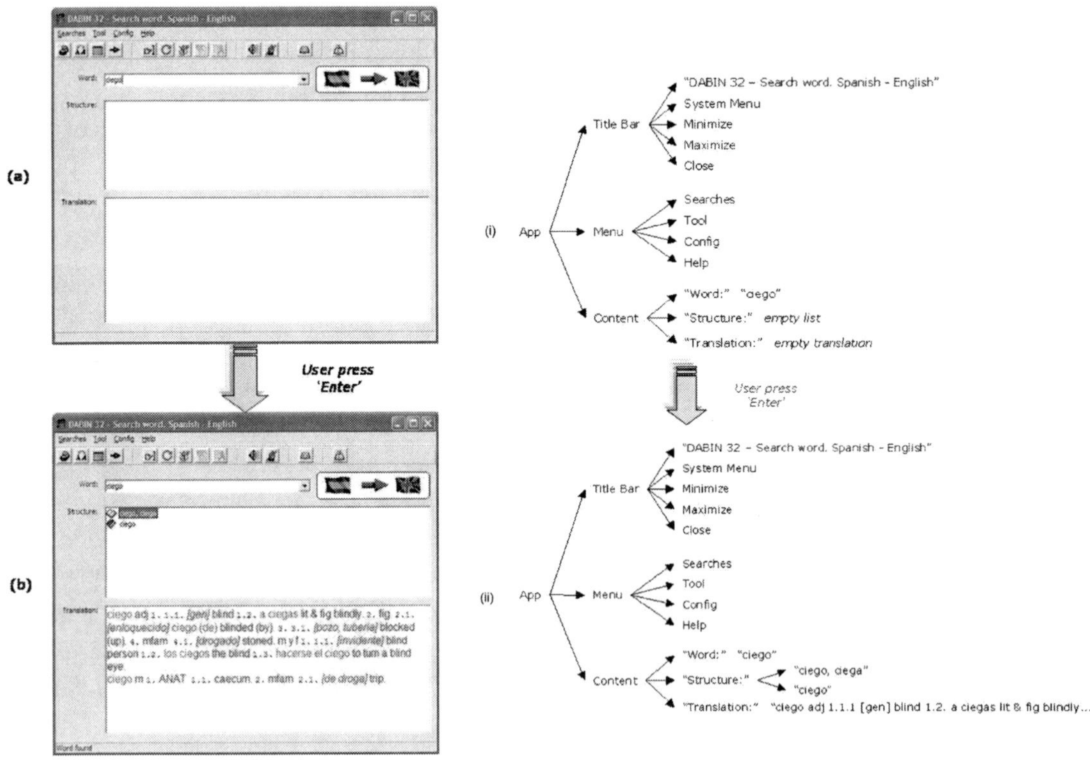

the button-activated operations can be performed using menus or by means of key combinations.

Additionally, as it may take a few seconds to search the database for the term (depending on computer speed), the user is informed by voice or Braille that the operation is in progress.

This model follows the 1+1 dimensional access scheme, but without omitting the 2+1 dimensional scheme for users who can make use of their sight to operate the system.

Dialog model. Based on the list of operations for the task model, each operation has been associated with its respective command. Taking into account that blind users cannot interact with the objects displayed on screen like a sighted user can, mechanisms have been enabled to allow them to do the same tasks efficiently. The commands for the operations are composed of system menus or key combinations (e.g. Ctrl+1 to configure synthesized speech), function keys (e.g. F1 for help).

The interaction procedure for each user interface object also had to be defined for adaptation to blind people. First, we identified the interface objects like: menus, menu items, push buttons, edit boxes, static texts, etc. They were standard components and had already been used in earlier projects, which meant that they could all be classed as accessible objects, with the advantage that they were all available in the BVCL toolkit. The only exception was a new complex component needed to display all the information from a translation ("translation browser") (Figure 9b – Translation Region).

The usual way of navigating components like these is to move around using the mouse. This meant that they were originally classed as inaccessible. Additionally, there could be semantic information loss (some information is conveyed by color and text style). Therefore, jointly with experts on vision-related issues, we defined an interaction procedure to make it a natural and simple activity for blind users to read a translation. This procedure is based on enabling several ways of getting the information using the keyboard only, allowing users to move forwards and backwards over the translation, to select the target text and even to start a search for the word on which the cursor is positioned.

The next step was to define the access attributes. No additional effort was needed for the standard interaction objects, as they had already been defined in BVCL, including all the information needed for a blind user.

The access attributes of the non-standard component give access to the full text of the translation, including the expansions of abbreviations and acronyms, together with all the semantic information.

To define the behavior of the components, we used the standard behavior of the standard components. For the "translation browser", the defined behavior is compatible with a standard edit box, save that the texts are presented in different styles depending on their meaning. In both cases, all the access attributes are sent to the assistive technologies, together with the additional context-sensitive information for the non-standard component.

Commands that can be used to access additional semantic information, such as user location in the application, repetition of the last message issued by speech, spelling or context-sensitive help, have been added to the system interaction techniques for all interaction objects. Consequently, blind users will receive all the system information without semantic information loss.

Presentation model. The design of the presentation model has been divided into two parts. The first part is related to the visual appearance of the system, for which purpose it was decided to follow the Windows systems standards. The second part is related to the non-visual appearance of the system, where we have focused on the speech and Braille display presentation.

In DABIN we decided to include only one detail level in the presentation, this being the one that provides the least amount of information. This decision was taken when we found that the potential users of this tool were blind people used to operating Windows applications. In any case, there is no loss of information because full and satisfactory information for use of the application is provided in any case.

We have defined the speech and Braille interface for each interface item using BVCL functionality. By not modifying its operation, we are improving the learning of other applications also built using BVCL. Additionally, the outputs defined by BVCL are similar to the ones that other environments or assistive technologies offer.

With respect to the non-standard component, the "translation browser", the output in response to the different actions taken by the user has been defined in detail in each case. This definition is a

Table 3. Effect of line down

Description	The user decides to move (down) a line.
Keys	↓ (Cursor down)
Screen	The cursor will appear on the next line down, more or less underneath the original cursor position. If the original position is further to the right than the end of the next line, the cursor will appear at the end of the next line. If the cursor is already on the last line, it will not move.
Speech	If the cursor has moved, the line to which it has moved will be synthesized. If the cursor has not moved, the "Last line" message will be synthesized (followed by a beep).
Braille	It will show the content of the next line (on screen), updating the cursor to the respective position.

product of the authors' earlier experience in developing similar components as part of products for blind people. Additionally, this same component has been reused to create an encyclopedia for blind people.

The "translation browser" can automatically transmit all its content to the assistive technologies or the user can run through it manually. By way of an example, Table 3 and Table 4 show the visual, speech and Braille effects in response to different user actions.

The interface was tested by blind users, as a result of which the model was refined.

User Model. Within the user-specific model, we identified three user types:

- Sighted users: no special-purpose adaptation is required.
- Visually impaired users: the colors of the whole system and the sizes of the texts follow the operating system configuration. Additionally, it provides the option of modifying the text and background colors of each of the displayed text types, as well as the size of this text, for the special case of the "translation browser". Also a number of default color combinations and text sizes, which are useful for most potential users, have been provided.
- Blind users: the voice parameters (speed, tone and volume) can be configured for each of the languages used allowing full personalization of system interface (for example, Spanish users learning French would set the speed of the French language pronunciation slower than they would for the Spanish language). Additionally, they are allowed to configure the general appearance of the Braille output.

FUTURE TRENDS

The issue of *accessibility* as the right of *all* citizens to obtain and maintain access to a society-wide pool of information resources and interpersonal communication facilities given the varieties of context (Stephanidis et al., 1998) is the basis of the future development of blind user interfacing. Accessibility for blind people has been addressed through three collaborative efforts. The first, which is also known as the reactive approach, aims to adapt products for blind people. The second aims to develop *dual user interfaces* as an appropriate basis for "integrating" blind and sighted users in the same working environment by taking the proper actions during the early phases of a product's life cycle. The third, more recent and future approach has proposed the concept of *User Interfaces for All* (Stephanidis, 2001), following the concept of *Design for All*, as the vehicle for efficiently and effectively addressing the numerous and diverse accessibility problems. Design for All is an inclusive and proactive approach seeking to

Table 4. Effect of abbreviation expansion

Description	The user wants to know the expansion of an abbreviation in the translation when the cursor is positioned over one of the letters of the abbreviation.
Keys	F8
Screen	It will have no effect (if a sighted user needs to know the expansion of an abbreviation, a tooltip with its meaning will appear when the mouse cursor is placed over the abbreviation).
Speech	The expansion of the abbreviation, if any, will be synthesized. Otherwise, the "It is not an abbreviation" message will be spoken.
Braille	The expansion of the abbreviation, if any, will be displayed. Otherwise, the "It is not an abbreviation" message will be displayed. These messages will disappear and the original text will be displayed again when the user presses any key.

accommodate diversity in the users and usage contexts of interactive products, applications and services, starting from the design phase of the development life cycle. The underlying principle of *User Interfaces for All* is to ensure accessibility at design time and to meet the individual needs, abilities and preferences of the user population at large, including blind people and other disabled and elderly users.

CONCLUSION

The development of graphical user interfaces that can be used by blind people involves taking into account a set of specific requirements: task adequacy, dimensional trade-off, behavior equivalence, semantic loss avoidance and device-independent interface. In the case of dual interfaces, those requirements must, of course, coexist with the standard dialog principles and Design for All guidelines.

In this chapter we have defined the specific requirements and described their influence when using HCI models based on our experience in the development of software for blind people. As has been discussed, all six models have to deal with specific issues in order to build user interfaces that provide effectiveness, efficiency and satisfaction for both sighted and blind users.

We have also presented FBLIND, a framework to improve the development of dual user interfaces. This framework includes a set of guidelines, a development toolkit for self-adaptive user interface objects and an API for the use of assistive technologies (speech and Braille). The use of this framework has been explained through a case study, a software environment enabling blind users to access bilingual dictionaries. Experience in others projects has demonstrated that FBLIND is very useful for developing dual user interfaces.

REFERENCES

Alonso, F., & Barreiro, J. M. (2008). Investigación y Desarrollo en el campo de la Accesibilidad-CETTICO. In J. Pereira, L. A. Martínez, J. L. Fuertes & J. M. Vázquez (Eds.), *Tecnologías de la Información y las Comunicaciones en la Autonomía Personal, Dependencia y Accesibilidad* (pp. 497-538). Colección Informática 16. Santiago de Compostela, Spain: Fundación Alfredo Brañas.

Alonso, F., Barreiro, J. M., Caraça-Valente, J. P., López, G., Montes, C., & Navajo, R. J. (1998). An Electronic Newspaper for the Blind. In A. D. N. Edwards, W. Zagler & A. Arato (Eds.), *Computers and Assistive Technology: ICCHP '98 Proceedings of the XV IFIP World Computer Congress,* Vienna (Austria) and Budapest (Hungary), Vienna, Austria: Osterreichische Computer Gesellschaft.

Alonso, F., Frutos, S., Fuertes, J. L., Martínez, L. A., Montes, C., & Sánchez, A. (1997b). Un Diccionario Automático Bilingüe para Invidentes (DABIN). *Integración, 25,* 14–31.

Alonso, F., Frutos, S., & Montes, C. (1997a). Interfacing for the Blind. The DILE Model. In *Proceedings 12th Annual CSUN Conference: Technology and Persons with Disabilities*, Los Angeles, CA: California State University-Northridge.

Alonso, F., Fuertes, J. L., González, A. L., & Martínez, L. (2006). A Framework for Blind User Interfacing. In *Computers Helping People with Special Needs* (LNCS 4061, pp. 1031-1038). doi: 10.1007/11788713_151

Apple (2009). Apple - Accessibility - VoiceOver - In-Depth. Retrieved September 25, 2009 from http://www.apple.com/accessibility/voiceover/

Casali, S. P. (1995). A physical skills-based strategy for choosing an appropriate interface method. In Edwards, A. D. N. (Ed.), *Extra-ordinary Human Computer Interaction: Interfaces for People with Disabilities* (pp. 315–342). New York, NY: Cambridge University Press.

Connell, B. R., Jones, M., Mace, R., Mueller, J., Mullick, A., & Ostroff, E. (1997). *The Principles of Universal Design*. Raleigh, NC: NC State University, The Center for Universal Design.

Cox, K., & Walker, D. (1993). *User interface design*. Singapore: Prentice Hall.

de Investigación, C. Desarrollo y Aplicación Tiflotécnica [CIDAT] (1998). *Diccionario para Invidentes de la Real Academia Española*, ONCE-CETTICO, product no. 0209020033912. Retrieved February 19, 1999 from http://cidat.once.es/home.cfm?excepcion=52&idproducto=241&idseccion=10).

Dolphin Computer Access. (2009). Hal Screen Reader, Version 11.0, April 2009. Retrieved September 25 2009 from http://www.yourdolphin.com/manuals/v11hal00044.pdf

Edwards, A. D. N. (1991). *Evaluation of Outspoken software for blind users*. (Tech. Rep. YCS150). York, England: University of York, Department of Computer Science.

Eisenstein, J. Vanderdonckt, J. & Puerta, A. (2000). Adapting to Mobile Contexts with User-Interface Modeling. In *Proceedings of the 3rd IEEE Workshop on Mobile Computing Systems and Applications* (pp. 83-92). Los Alamitos, CA: IEEE Press.

Freedom Scientific BLV Group. (2008). JAWS(r) for Windows(r) Quick Start Guide, 11800 31st Court North, St. Petersburg, Florida 33716-1805 USA.

García, M. (2005). *Adaptación de Entornos Visuales para Invidentes. Unpublished final-year project*. Madrid, Spain: Facultad de Informática, Universidad Politécnica de Madrid.

Geary, D. M. (1999). *Graphic Java. Mastering the JFC* (3rd ed.). Upper Saddle River, NJ: Prentice Hall.

GNOME. (2009). Orca GNOME Live. Retrieved August 5, 2009 from http://www.baum.ro/gnopernicus.html.

Grammenos, D., Savidis, A., & Georgalis, Y. (2007). Dual educational electronic textbooks: the starlight platform. In *9th International ACM SIGACCESS Conference on Computers and Accessibility* (pp. 107-114). New York: ACM. doi: 10.1145/1296843.1296863.

Guede, Á. (2002). *Proyecto PEIN: Lector de Periódicos de 32 bits para Ciegos. Unpublished final-year project*. Madrid, Spain: Facultad de Informática, Universidad Politécnica de Madrid.

International Standards Organization [ISO] (2003). *Ergonomics of human-system interaction – Guidance on accessibility for human-computer interfaces*, Technical Specification ISO TS 16071.

International Standards Organization [ISO] (2006). ISO 9241-110:2006 Ergonomics of human-system interaction -- Part 110: Dialogue principles. Retrieved September 25, 2009 from http://www.iso.org/iso/iso_catalogue/catalogue_tc/catalogue_detail.htm?csnumber=38009

International Standards Organization [ISO] (2008). ISO 9241-171:2008 Ergonomics of human-system interaction -- Part 171: Guidance on software accessibility. Retrieved September 25, 2009 from http://www.iso.org/iso/catalogue_detail.htm?csnumber=39080

Menkhaus, G., & Fischmeister, S. (2003). *Dialog Model Clustering for User Interface Adaptation.* Paper presented at the 3rd International Conference on Web Engineering, Oviedo, Spain.

Micro, G. W. (2009). GW Micro - Window-Eyes, Version 7.1. Retrieved September 25, 2009 from http://www.gwmicro.com/Window-Eyes/

Microsoft. (2009). Speech API Overview (SAPI 5.4). Retrieved September 25, 2009 from http://msdn.microsoft.com/en-us/library/ee125077(VS.85).aspx

Microsystems, S. (2009). Java Speech API. Retrieved September 25, 2009 from http://java.sun.com/products/java-media/speech/

Morley, S. (1999). *Design and Evaluation of Non-Visual Information Systems for Blind Users*. Unpublished doctoral dissertation, University of Hertfordshire, UK.

Myers, B., Hudson, S. E., & Pausch, R. (2001). Past present and future of user interface software tools. *ACM Transactions on Computer-Human Interaction*, *7*(1), 3–28. doi:10.1145/344949.344959

Mynatt, E. D., & Edwards, W. K. (1992a). *The Mercator Environment: A Nonvisual Interface to X Windows and Unix Workstations*. (Tech. Rep. GIT-GVU-92-05). Atlanta, GA: Georgia Institute of Technology, Graphics Visualization & Usability Center.

Mynatt, E. D., & Edwards, W. K. (1992b). Mapping GUIs to Auditory Interfaces. In *Proceedings of the 5th annual ACM Symposium on User Interface Software and Technology*. (pp. 61-70). Monterey, CA: ACM.

Puerta, A. (1996). The MECANO Project: Comprehensive and Integrated Support for Model-Based Interface Development. In Vanderdonckt, J. (Ed.), *Computer-Aided Design of User Interfaces* (pp. 19–36). Namur, Belgium: Namur University Press.

Savidis, A., & Stephanidis, C. (1995a) Developing dual user interfaces for integrating blind and sighted users: the HOMER UIMS.I. In *Proceedings of the SIGCHI Conference on Human Factors in Computing Systems* (pp. 106-113). New York: ACM Press/Addison Wesley Publishing Co. doi:acm.org/10.1145/223904.223918

Savidis, A., & Stephanidis, C. (1995b) Building non-visual interaction through the development of the Rooms metaphor. In *Conference Companion on Human factors in Computing Systems* (pp. 244-245). New York: ACM.

Savidis, A., & Stephanidis, C. (1998). The HOMER UIMS for dual user interface development: Fusing visual and non-visual interactions. *Interacting with Computers*, *11*, 173–209. doi:10.1016/S0953-5438(98)00025-3

Stephanidis, C. (2001). User Interfaces for All: New perspectives into HCI. In Stephanidis, C. (Ed.), *User Interfaces for All – Concepts, Methods and Tools*. Mahwah, NJ: Lawrence Erlbaum Associates.

Stephanidis, C., Salvendy, G., Akoumianakis, D., Bevan, N., Brewer, J., & Emiliani, P. L. (1998). Toward an Information Society for All: An International R&D Agenda. *International Journal of Human-Computer Interaction*, *10*(2), 107–134. doi:10.1207/s15327590ijhc1002_2

Stephanidis, C., & Savidis, A. (2009). Interface Development Toolkits for Non-visual and Switch-based Interaction, *ERCIM News 46*. Retrieved August 18, 2009 from http://www.ercim.org/publication/Ercim_News/enw46/stephanidis2.html.

Szekely, P., Luo, P., & Neches, R. (1993). Beyond Interface Builders: Model-Based Interface Tools. In *Proceedings of the INTERCHI '93 Conference on Human factors in Computing Systems* (pp. 383-390). Amsterdam, The Netherlands: IOS Press.

Varela, J. I. (1998). *Modelo de Interfaz para Aplicaciones Adaptadas para Invidentes Basado en Componentes. Unpublished final-year project*. Madrid, Spain: Facultad de Informática, Universidad Politécnica de Madrid.

KEY TERMS AND DEFINITIONS

Dialog Model: Model that defines the commands as well as the purpose of each one. Commands are executed via interaction techniques and may produce one or more system responses.

Domain Model: Model that describes the syntactic sequence of human-computer interaction through user interface objects and determines how the set of tasks and actions are ordered.

Dual User Interface: A graphical user interface that can also accommodate blind users.

HCI Modeling: A method for developing user interfaces. One key HCI modeling method is based on six models: task, domain, dialog, presentation, platform and user.

Platform Model: Model that contains information about the capabilities, constraints and limitations of the target platform.

Presentation Model: Model that describes the perceptual appearance of the user interface.

Task Model: A formal description of the services the user accesses. It is organized hierarchically and contains information regarding task activation, preconditions, postconditions, and the actual task action.

Usability: The extent to which a product can be used by specified users to achieve specified goals with effectiveness, efficiency and satisfaction in a specified context of use.

User Interfaces for All: The principle of ensuring accessibility at design time and to meet the individual needs, abilities and preferences of the user population at large, including blind people and other disabled and elderly users.

User Model: Description of the characteristics of an individual user or of a stereotype user group. The user model is not intended to be a description of the mental state of a user.F

Chapter 14
Sensors in Assistive Technology

Yu-Luen Chen
National Taipei University of Education, Taiwan

Walter H. Chang
Chung Yuan Christian University, Taiwan

Te-Son Kuo
National Taiwan University, Taiwan

ABSTRACT

This chapter reports on the development of an eyeglass-type infrared-controlled computer interface for the disabled. This system may serve to assist those who suffer from spinal cord injuries or other handicaps to operate a computer. This system is comprised of three major components: (A) an infrared transmitting module; (B) an infrared receiving / signal-processing module; and (C) a main controller, the Intel-8951 microprocessor. The infrared transmitting module utilizes tongue-touch circuitry which is converted to an infrared beam and a low power laser (<0.1mW) beam. The infrared receiving / signal-processing module, receives the infrared beam and fine tunes the unstable infrared beam into standard pulses which are used as control signals. The main controller is responsible for detecting the input signals from the infrared receiving / signal-processing module and verifying these signals with the mapping table in its memory. After the signal is verified, it is released to control the keys of the computer keyboard and mouse interface. This design concept was mainly based on the idea that the use of an infrared remote module fastened to the eyeglasses could allow the convenient control of the input motion on the keys of a computer keyboard and mouse which are all modified with infrared receiving / signal-processing modules. The system is designed for individuals with spinal cord injuries and disabled in which the subjects' movement are severely restricted. The infrared transmitting module can be easily mounted on eyeglasses or artificial limbs.

DOI: 10.4018/978-1-60566-206-0.ch014

INTRODUCTION

The infrared-controlled human-computer interface utilizes a small infrared- transmitting module mounted on the user`s eyeglasses, and a tongue-touch panel on the input headset was developed and designed for this system. The user utilizes the tip of the tongue to gently touch the panel which is attached to one side of the mouth in order to turn the power switch of the infrared transmitting module on or off. The infrared transmitting module generates an infrared beam and a low power laser beam. The infrared beam is used for selecting the keys from a keyboard, while the laser beam allows the user to see which keys are selected. All the keys of the computer keyboard have been replaced with infrared receiving / signal-processing modules. By aiming the laser beam at the desired number, letter, or function key, the user can select the key. After verification for error, a main controller, the Intel-8951 microprocessor, carries out the signal reception processing and input functions. The microprocessor is also responsible for controlling the computer keyboard interface and providing feedback to the user that the input motion has been completed.

BACKGROUND

Patients with spinal cord injuries (SCI) and persons with disabilities involving paralysis increasingly utilize electronic assistance devices to improve their ability to perform certain essential functions. The functional areas in which the disabled most commonly utilize electronic equipment are: communications, environmental control and powered wheelchairs. A wide range of interfaces between the user and the device are available. The interface may be an enlarged keyboard or a complex system that allows the user to operate or control a function with the aid of a mouthstick, eye movements, an eye imaged input system and electroencephalogram (EEG) signals (Peizer et al. 1982; Vasa, 1982; Perkins et al. 1986; Ranu, 1986; Andrews et al. 1980; Kilgallon et al. 1987; Lacourse et al. 1990; Keirn et al. 1990) etc.. In many disabilities such as quadriplegia, the mouthstick method has poor accuracy and is uncomfortable. The eye movement and EEG methods provide few available controlled movements, can have slow response time for signal processing and requires substantial motor coordination. However, these instruments all tend to be highly specialized and are generally cost prohibitive. Thus, alternative systems which utilize commercially available electronics to assist in the performance of special tasks such as computer operation and environmental control are sorely needed.

The ability to operate a computer is becoming increasingly more important to the disabled persons and to those with SCI as advances in technology allow more and more functions to be computer controlled. There are many reasons for operating a computer. These include acquiring new knowledge and communicating with the outside world. However, they also include doing work at home, leisure activities, and many other things. This paper reports on the design of an infrared-controlled (Chen et al. 1999; Chen et al. 1999) human-computer interface for patients who are paralyzed from a cervical cord injury with quadriplegia but retain the ability to rotate the neck and perform shrugging movements.

INFRARED IN COMPUTER ACCESS

The configuration of the infrared-controlled computer interface is shown in Figure 1. This system replaces the keys of the original computer keyboard with infrared receivers and mounts an infrared transmitting module onto the eyeglasses of the disabled user. The user employs neck rotation movement to aim the infrared beam at the key of the computer keyboard in order to input data and perform all computer functions. The computer keyboard was divided into three parts: two

Figure 1. The configuration of the infrared-controlled human-computer interface

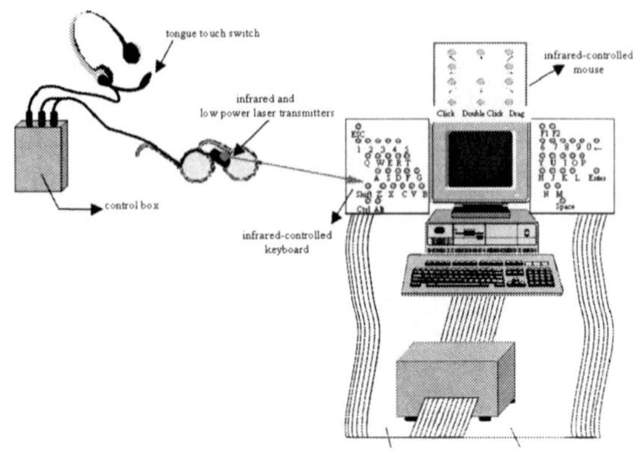

Figure 2. The schematics of (a) an infrared transmitting module mounted on a eyeglasses is used to generate a infrared beam and a low power laser beam; (b) a tongue-touch switch is played as a power switch; and (c) a control box

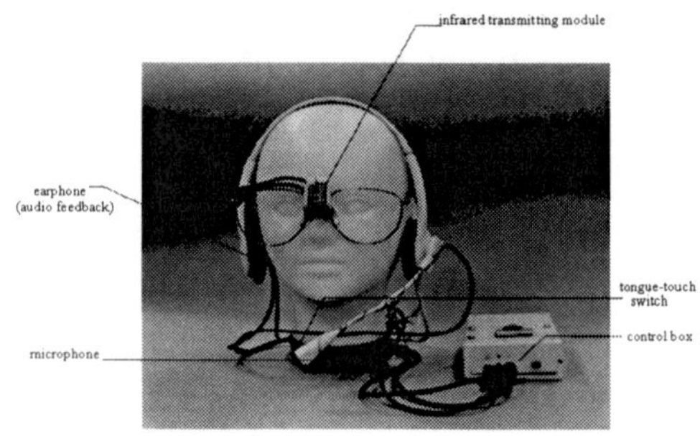

parts are placed beside the monitor, for numbers, letters and function key input, and the third part is situated upon the monitor for mouse control, which utilized the assistant tool in the control console of Windows98, using keyboard instead of mouse controlling. The mouse-controlled functions include: up, low, left, right, upper-left, upper-right, lower-left, lower-right, single click, and double clicks.

This circuit for the infrared-controlled human-computer interface is composed of three major elements: (A) an infrared transmitting module; (B) an infrared receiving / signal-processing module; and (C) a main controller, the Intel-8951 microprocessor. The infrared transmitting module utilizes tongue-touch circuitry to activate an infrared beam and a low-power laser beam. The infrared receiving / signal-processing module, apart from receiving the infrared beam, also processes any unstable component of the infrared beam into standard pulses that are then used as control signals. The main controller is responsible for detecting the input signals, verifying the mapping table in its memory, and releasing correct signals to control the computer keyboard or other electronic interfaces.

The Infrared Transmitting Module

The infrared transmitting module links the computer keyboard and mouse interface with the disabled user. The infrared transmitting module includes three main elements: an infrared transmitter and circuitry, a low-power laser transmitter, and tongue-touch circuitry. Its dimensions are 3.0 * 2.0 * 1.5 cm^3. It weighs about 8 grams and can be easily mounted onto a pair of eyeglasses, as shown in Figure 2(a).

The system adapts to an infrared receiver with a HC-377M model, therefore, the receiving frequency is 37.9 KHz or higher. The oscillating frequency of the infrared transmitter through the unstable multivibrator circuitry must be designated at 37.9 KHz or higher. The infrared beam, an invisible beam, has a wavelength which ranges from 0.75μm to 1000μm. The projected angles of the infrared beam are in a positive relation ship to the distance of the projection. Because the beam is invisible, it is difficult to determine whether it is accurately aimed at the infrared receiver's window. In order to solve this problem, a low-power laser is incorporated below the infrared transmitter to aid in positioning the infrared beam. In addition, a tongue-touch switch was included to facilitate coordinated use. This makes it convenient for the disabled user to turn on or turn off the power of the infrared-transmitting module, as shown in Figure 2(b).

To alleviate refraction of the infrared beam, the viewing angle of the LTE-209 infrared transmitting diode is positioned at ±8°. After appropriate filtration, the radius area of its projection within a distance of 50 ~ 100 cm, is approximately 0.5 cm. An optic filter is used to regulate the characteristics of the infrared beam closer to a paralleled beam. The transmitting focus of the infrared transmitting diode is about 0.2 cm from that of the low-power laser transmitter. Thus, the target of the low-power laser beam projection is 0.2 cm from the target of the infrared beam projection.

One 9V and two 1.5V batteries are used to supply the power needed for all of the devices contained in the control box apart from the infrared transmitter oscillating circuitry, the low-power laser transmitting circuitry, and the tongue-touch circuitry of the circuitry control box. The control box measures 12.5 * 8 * 3 cm^3, and weighs roughly 150 grams, as shown in Figure 2(c). This allows the operator to conveniently attach it to the waist or over other body areas.

Infrared Receiving / Signal-Processing Module

The infrared receiving / signal-processing module consists primarily of two parts: an infrared receiver, and the infrared signal processing circuitry. In order to replace all manual input motion, all keys of the computer keyboard were replaced by infrared receivers. A total of 60 infrared receivers are used in this system. A common infrared receiver, HC-377M optic receiver module, Vcc=5.8V, Icc = Max. 3mA with a receiving range: 10 M, θ=45°, resolution frequency = 37.9KHz, and λp = 9,400 mm are employed.

In order to utilize the infrared beam to perform control and calculating functions, an infrared receiving / signal-processing interface is designed into this system, as shown in Figure 3. The unstable signals are received via the infrared receiver and converted into fixed timing, cyclical pulsation (with a cycle of 1 per second) through use of the non-retriggered circuitry. The relationship between the input and output of the HC-377M and the use of non-retriggerable circuit is shown in Figure 4. As shown in Figure 4(a), the output of the HC-377M is at a high level (+5V) when there is no infrared input. After the infrared beam is received by the HC-377M, the output of HC-377M

Figure 3. Circuit diagram of the infrared receiving / signal processing module

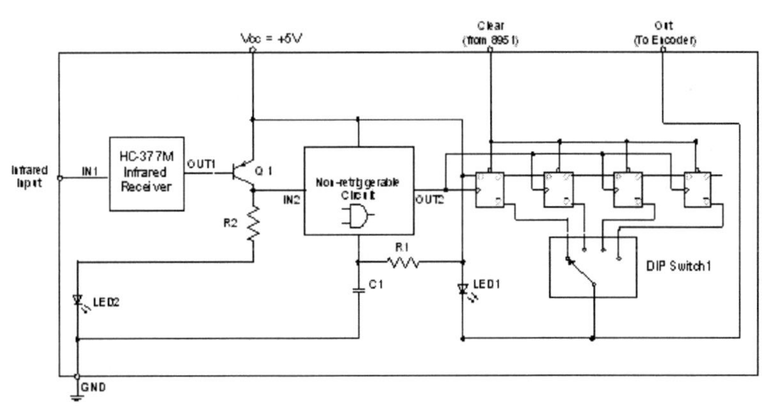

Figure 4. Input and output signals at the infrared receiving/signal-processing module

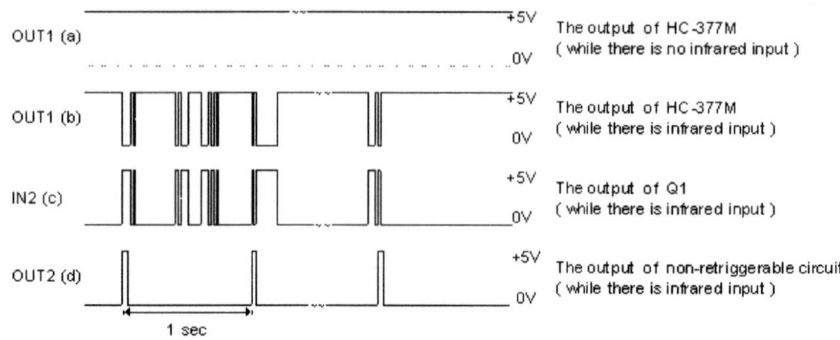

becomes unstable, as shown in Figure 4(b). The non-retriggerable circuit converts this unstable signal, shown in Figure 4(c), into a standard pulse train, as shown in Figure 4(d). The duration and duty cycle of the standard pulse depends on the values for R1 and C1, as shown in Figure 3. The standard pulse is set like a clock and sent to the shift registers (D-type flip-flops), which act as a delayed time counter while the user focuses on the infrared receiver. The LED1 (Light Emitting Diode) remains lit while the input processing is completed, and at the same time all the infrared receiving / signal-processing modules receive a control signal to clear their shift registers from Port2 of the Intel-8951. This can be set according to the user's preference for aiming the infrared receiver key for 1, 2, 3 or 4 seconds of uninterrupted or continuous aiming before it is recognized and input. Otherwise, no input will be processed. This design in response to the infrared receivers of the infrared-controlled computer keyboard, is configured using a two-matrix alignment method. The margins between any two keys are all set at 1 cm. Thus, when the user operates the system, the infrared transmitting module will not inadvertently select a non-targeted key. Therefore, to incorporate this function into the design, the user must aim at the target key by maintaining the beam continuously on the target for one second or more as per the designated activation time. The timing of the focus can be designated through the user's control of the infrared transmitting module sensitivity by adjusting the dual-in-line package (DIP) switch on the infrared receiving / signal-processing module.

In the design of the main structure of the computer keyboard, due to the restricted or stiff neck movement of the users, we added certain special function to the main structure with a design and production concept in order avoid the need to alter the keyboard's own schematics, and for ease of installation. An ordinary computer keyboard can be plugged into the system for immediate use. The infrared-receiving keyboard includes the basic 60 keys on a common modern computer keyboards.

The Main Controller, Intel 8951, Micro-Processor

The Intel-8951 microprocessor is the main controller of the system. The Intel-8951's Port1 and Port3 utilize decoders to intersect the remote input signals transmitted via the infrared receiving / signal-processing module. A table-verifying method is deployed via Port0 to dispatch signals commensurate to control input motion of the computer keyboard. At the same time, Port2 dispatches all control signals which are required by the surrounding circuits, including LED1 and buzzer control as a visual and audio feedback, respectively, to the operator for confirming that his input motion has been completed. The infrared-controlled, computer keyboard software and hardware installation have been completed, and this equipment is shown in Figure 5, including an infrared transmitting module, and an infrared receiving / signal-processing module, and a main controller, the Intel-8951 micro-processor. The infrared transmitting module and the tongue-touch switch are shown in Figure 2(a) and Figure 2(b), respectively. The disabled user needs only to put on the new developed eyeglass-type infrared transmitting module in order to accomplish the objective of operating the computer and communicating a message through the World Wide Web (WWW).

For system evaluation, six subjects (all men, 26~39 years old, 3 are normal subjects and 3 are SCI with quadriplegia) who had operated computer were selected and gave their informed consent in this study. The 3 normal subjects whose neck movements are constrained below a fixed and stationary position were assigned as the control group. The other 3 SCI subjects with quadriplegia were assigned as the experimental group.

Figure 5. The schematic of the infrared-controlled computer interface used by a SCI subject with quadriplegia

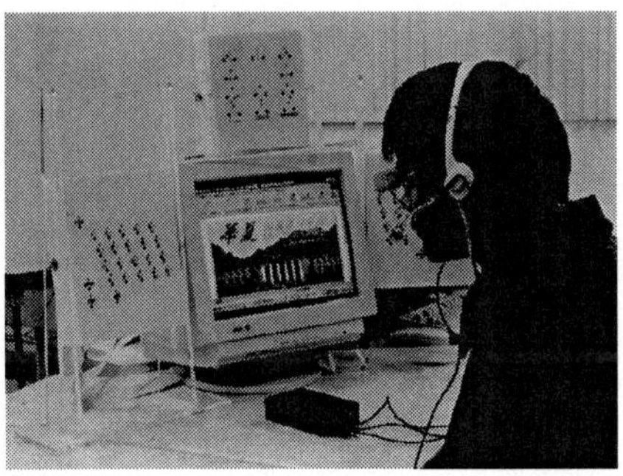

All of the subjects were given 10 minutes instruction and training for operation prior to using this new developed infrared-controlled human-computer system. Then, give them a short article with 97 letters (The short article is following: this is a test, for evaluation of the new developed infrared-controlled human-computer interface). The test results were shown in Table 1 and Figure 6. The average accuracy of the control group and the experimental group are 97.4±5.3% and 94.6±7.6%, respectively. The average time cost of the control group and the experimental group are 3.6±1.5 min and 4.9±2.0 min, respectively. An independent t-test revealed that the differences in the average accuracy and the average time cost of the control group and the experimental group are no significant ($p>0.05$).

FUTURE TRENDS

This infrared-controlled human-computer interface utilizes current circuit technology to effectively accomplish the control of a computer keyboard system. In the future, this interface could potentially be introduced into many control systems at home including home appliances, telephones, and electronics, as shown in Figure 7, the design of an infrared-based communication board interface for patients who are nonspeaking with paralyzed from a cervical cord injury with quadriplegia but retain the ability to rotate the neck and perform shrugging movements (Chen et al. 2007; Chen et al. 2004).

The cost of all parts of the infrared-controlled human-computer interface is approximately U.S.

Table 1. The test results of the infrared-controlled human-computer interface

	Control group (3 normal subjects)	**Experimental group (3 SCI subjects and quadriplegia)**	**p**
average accuracy (%)	97.4±5.3	94.6±7.6	p>0.05
average time cost (min)	3.6±1.5	4.9±2.0	p>0.05

Figure 6. The test results of the control group and the experimental group of the newly developed infrared-controlled human-computer interface

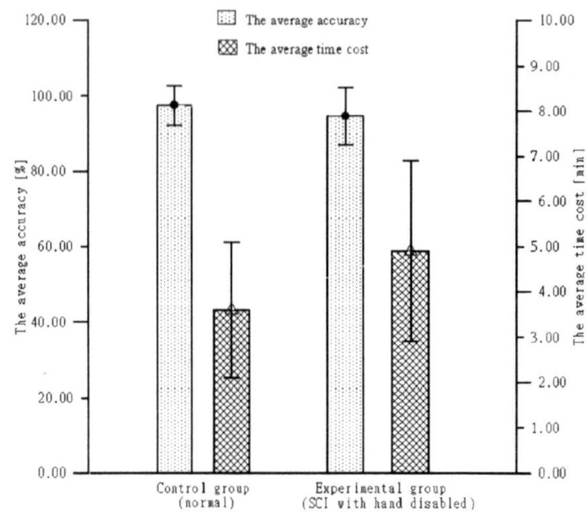

$450.00. This cost could be used to estimate the production costs of this device. In comparison, an IR modular eye movement monitor produced by Universal Initram Corporation costs about U.S. $12,175.00. Also, the response time of the new infrared-controlled human-computer interface is shorter than other systems, and the response time could be set from 1 sec. to 4 sec. adjustable.

CONCLUSION

The increasing number of various accidental injuries over the years has resulted in a dramatic increase in the disabled population. Although there are many devices which can supplement the loss of function in patients suffering from spinal cord injuries, there are substantial differences in their

Figure 7. The configuration of the infrared-based communication system

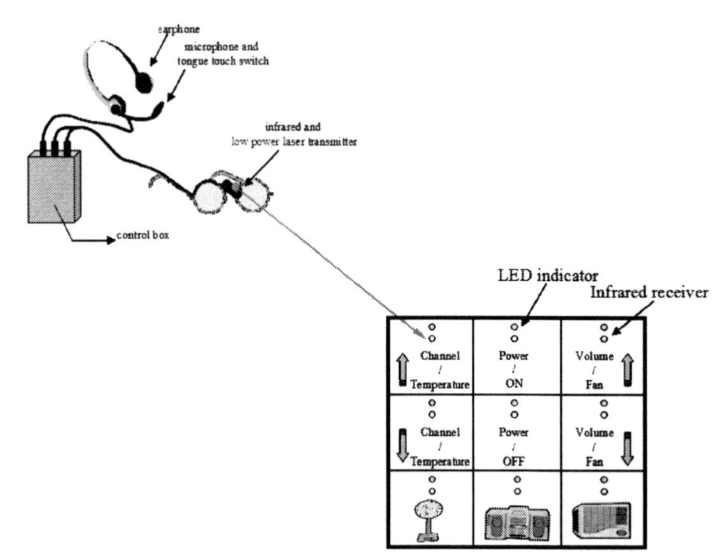

convenience and accuracy. Most devices intended to serve as computer keyboard supplements for the disabled utilize mouthstick, eyeball movements, or eyeball-imaging methods to complete the input motion (Peizer et al. 1982; Vasa, 1982; Perkins et al. 1986; Ranu, 1986; Andrews et al. 1980). Although many of these systems provide reasonable function and allow successful input through the computer keyboard, they frequently lack good sanitation or convenience because they are orally activated. Eyeball movement and eyeball-imaging based systems rely on high-level imaging analysis, provide questionable accuracy, and need a longer operating time to input a number or a letter. In addition, these systems have the disadvantage of expensive instrument costs and may require extended operational training.

In today's era of leaps in electronics and computer technologies, we hope the disabled will not become technological orphans in this era. We hope to utilize the least amount of circuitry design with highly accurate control systems to provide devices for the disabled to overcome the inconveniences in their daily lives. The system presented in this paper allows the disabled person to avoid the need to use uncomfortable input methods such as clutching a mouthstick. The system utilizes the remaining neck rotating function, directly applying an infrared transmitting module to control the computer keyboard and mouse. It has several user-friendly features, such as allowing the user to check if his input motion is correct and providing a LED indication and buzzer as visual and audio feedback to the user when input motion is completed. Thus, this system has the definite advantages of convenience, accuracy, and sanitation over the mouthstick-based system. In addition, an eyeglass-type control method is especially suitable for those who suffer from quadriplegia due to spinal cord injuries. Disabled users can also mount the infrared transmitting module on a prosthesis, on protective gear, or on a power wheelchair to achieve the objective of administering control.

REFERENCES

Andrews, B., Miller, S., Horrocks, D., & Chawla, J. C. (1980). Electronic communications and environmental control systems for the severely disabled. *Paraplegia*, *17*, 153–156.

Chen, S. C., Tang, F. T., Chen, Y. L., Chen, W. L., Li, Y. C., & Shih, Y. Y. (2004). Infrared-based communication augmentation system for the people with multiple disabilities. *Disability and Rehabilitation*, 1105–1109. doi:10.1080/09638280410001713025

Chen, W. L., Andy Liou, A. H., Chen, S. C., Chung, C. M., Chen, Y. L., & Shih, Y. Y. (2007). A novel home appliance control system for people with multiple disabilities. *Disability and Rehabilitation*, 201–206.

Chen, Y. L., Chang, W. H., Tang, F. T., Wong, M. K., & Kuo, T. S. (1999). The new design of an infrared-controlled human-computer interface for the disabled. *IEEE Transactions on Rehabilitation Engineering*, *7*(4), 474–481. doi:10.1109/86.808951

Chen, Y. L., Shih, Y. Y., Chang, W. H., Tang, F. T., Wong, M. K., & Kuo, T. S. (1999). A novel infrared-controlled telephone communication interface for the disabled. *IEICE Transactions on Information and Systems*, *82*(10), 1417–1424.

Keirn, Z. A., & Aunon, J. I. (1990). Man-machine communications through brain-wave processing. *IEEE Engineering in Medicine and Biology*, *3*, 55–57. doi:10.1109/51.62907

Kilgallon, M. J., Roberts, D. P., & Miller, S. (1987). Adapting personal computers for use by high-level quadripegics. *Medical Instrumentation*, *21*(2), 97–102.

Lacourse, J. R., & Hladik, F. C. Jr. (1990). An eye movement communication -control system for the disabled. *IEEE Transactions on Bio-Medical Engineering*, *37*(12), 1215–1220. doi:10.1109/10.64465

Peizer, E., Lorenze, E. J., & Dixon, M. (1982). Environmental controls to promote independence in severely disabled elderly persons. *Medical Instrumentation*, *16*(3), 171–173.

Perkins, W. J., & Stenning, B. F. (1986). Control units for operation of computers by severely physical handicapped persons. *Journal of Medical Engineering & Technology*, *10*(1), 21–23. doi:10.3109/03091908609044332

Ranu, H. S. (1986). Engineering aspects of rehabilitation for the handicapped. *Journal of Medical Engineering & Technology*, *10*(1), 16–20. doi:10.3109/03091908609044331

Vasa, J. J. (1982). Electronic aids for the disabled and the elderly. *Medical Instrumentation*, *16*(5), 263–264.

KEY TERMS AND DEFINITIONS

Disabilities: The term is defined by the Americans with Disabilities Act of 1990 as a physical or mental impairment that substantially limits one or more major life activities.

Human-Computer Interface: The interaction methods between people (users) and computers.

Infrared Receiving Module: There are Photo detector and preamplifier in one package, which can sense infrared light.

Infrared Transmitting Module: There are Photo generator and transmitter in one package, which can infrared light.

Infrared: Infrared light is a form of electromagnetic waves. Infrared can be visible light or can be in the form of microwaves. In its visible form, infrared can be seen as red or violet. Visible infrared waves are very short, measuring about 750 nm in length.

Spinal Cord Injuries (SCI): People who are damage to the spinal cord that results in a loss of function such as mobility or feeling.

Tongue-Touch Switch: A switch can for the people with severely impairments to control any device by his tongue.

Chapter 15
Non-Manual Control Devices:
Direct Brain-Computer Interaction

Reinhold Scherer
University of Washington, USA & Graz University of Technology, Austria & Judendorf-Strassengel Clinic, Austria

Rajesh P. N. Rao
University of Washington, USA

ABSTRACT

Brain-computer interface (BCI) technology augments the human capability to interact with the environment by directly linking the brain to artificial devices. The first generation of BCIs provided simple 1D control in order to select targets on a screen or trigger pre-defined motion sequences of paralyzed limbs by means of functional electrical stimulation. BCIs today can provide users on-demand access to assistive robotic devices, Virtual Reality environments, and standard software applications such as Internet browsers. Here, we introduce readers to BCIs and review basic principles and methodologies underlying their operation. We illustrate the capabilities and limitations of modern BCI systems by discussing two practical examples: BCI-based control of a humanoid robot for physical manipulation and transport of objects in an indoor environment, and BCI-based interaction with the popular global navigation program Google Earth.

INTRODUCTION

Communicating and interacting with the environment are fundamental human capabilities. However, damage to the central nervous system due to neuromuscular disease, stroke, or traumatic brain injury can result in loss of these motor capabilities to varying degrees. In a majority of cases, individuals have largely unaltered cognitive functions, but are left with physical impairment and disability ranging from paralysis of specific parts of the body to being completely "locked-in." Exemplars of this situation include individuals suffering from degenerative neurological diseases such as amyotrophic lateral sclerosis (ALS), individuals with spinal cord injury, or survivors of a stroke.

DOI: 10.4018/978-1-60566-206-0.ch015

To manage activities of their daily lives, these individuals usually have to rely on the assistance of others. In some cases, individuals may even be unable to use conventional interfaces such as a keyboard or a computer mouse. Depending on the remaining motor function, some alternative communication aids are available, such as systems that track eye-gaze in order to select options on a computer screen, or switches that can be activated by respiration (e.g., by sucking on a straw) to give "yes" or "no" answers.

Brain-Computer Interface (BCI) technologies provide a novel way for humans to interact with machines. BCIs are not dependent on actual movements; instead, BCIs process the user's intent directly and translate the corresponding brain activity into control commands for devices (Wolpaw, 2002; Dornhege, 2007). The information transfer rate (ITR) of BCIs is low compared to muscle operated devices, usually less than 30 bit min^{-1}. Disabled and able-bodied individuals, however, have learned to successfully operate BCI-based devices to compose messages on a computer (Birbaumer, 1999; Neuper, 2003; Scherer, 2004; Piccione, 2006; Sellers, 2006; Williamson, 2009), browse the internet (Bensch, 2007), control robotic assistive devices (Millán, 2004, Bell, 2008, Galán, 2008) and, to some extent, also restore lost motor function (e.g., by controlling a neuroprosthesis, Pfurtscheller, 2003; Müller-Putz, 2005a). Some of these achievements were not reached in isolated laboratory environments, but in patient homes or clinical settings. These promising first results show that the technology has evolved to a state where it may be ready to be tested and evaluated in real world environments.

The goal of this chapter is to introduce readers to the field of BCIs and to review basic principles and currently used methodologies. Practical examples are provided in order to illustrate the usage, the performance, and also the limitations of modern BCI systems. Due to the limited space available, we are unable to provide extensive details and have had to omit some important alternative approaches and associated references. The chapter emphasizes those approaches which have been extensively evaluated by our group and demonstrated to be useful in practical applications. We also discuss new trends and ideas, in order to stimulate further research in this compelling new area.

BACKGROUND

Figure 1 illustrates the basic steps involved in direct brain-computer interaction. To establish closed-loop interaction, the user's brain activity has to be first monitored and digitized (signal acquisition). Second, signal processing methods are applied to extract features of interest from the acquired signal and classification (or regression) methods are used to translate them into control commands for a device (pattern recognition and machine learning). The user perceives the initiated action and this sensory feedback closes the loop.

The following sections briefly review available recording technologies, brain signals used for operating BCIs, and commonly used pattern recognition and machine learning methods.

Signal Acquisition

Three different types of brain signals have been used in BCI research. First, electrical signals reflecting neuronal activity in the brain can be recorded in one of three ways: (i) electrodes placed on the scalp (electroencephalogram, EEG) (Birbaumer, 1999; Millán, 2003; Pineda, 2003; Pfurtscheller, 2006; Vaughan, 2006; Blankertz, 2006), (ii) electrodes placed on the surface of the cortex without penetrating the cortex (electrocorticogram, ECoG) (Miller; 2007, Schalk, 2008; Scherer, 2009), or (iii) electrodes placed within the cortex (intracortical single unit or multiunit recordings) (Maynard, 1997; Hochberg, 2006). Second, rather than measuring electrical activity, one can use magnetoencephalography (MEG) to

Figure 1. Basic steps involved in direct brain-computer interaction

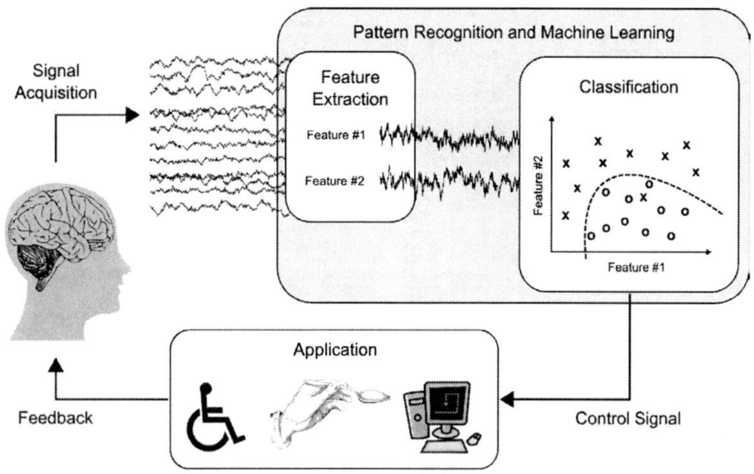

measure the magnetic fields associated with neuronal ionic currents using gradiometers (superconducting quantum interference devices, SQUIDs) in magnetically shielded rooms (Mellinger, 2007). Finally, one can also measure neuronal activity indirectly by measuring the corresponding changes in blood flow and blood oxygenation levels. One type of response, known as the blood oxygen level dependent (BOLD) response, is measured through functional magnetic resonance imaging (fMRI) (Weiskopf, 2004). A different method, known as near infrared spectroscopy (NIRS), measures the level of oxyhemoglobin (Coyle, 2007). While fMRI relies on detecting changes in the signals used to construct magnetic resonance images (MRI),, NIRS applies light in the near infrared spectrum and recalculates the oxygenation of the tissue by measuring the amount of absorption.

Recording techniques are typically classified as non-invasive (EEG, MEG, fMRI, NIRS) or invasive (ECoG and intracortical). Important characteristics for BCI applications are the spatial and temporal resolution of the recording technique. While changes in electric and magnetic fields can be detected within milliseconds, changes in blood oxygenation can be measured only in the range of several seconds. Invasive methods typically have a higher spatial and temporal resolution than non-invasive methods, but these gains are accompanied by increased medical risks for the user. Invasive methods are typically used only in animals or in surgical settings in human patients.

The Electroencephalogram (EEG)

Here, we focus on the non-invasive EEG, which currently represents the most common signal source for BCIs in humans. The popularity of EEG is primarily due to its non-invasive nature, low expense (compared to methods such as MEG and fMRI), portability, and wide availability.

EEG signals are potential differences recorded from electrodes placed on the scalp and reflect the temporal and spatial summation of electrical inputs to large groups of neurons lying beneath the recording electrode. The time resolution is in the range of milliseconds, signal amplitudes are usually within the range of $\pm 100\mu V$ (10^{-6} V), and the spatial resolution is in the range of 5 cm^2. The poor spatial resolution of EEG is caused by the different layers (meninges, cerebrospinal fluid, skull, scalp) between the source of the signal (the neural activity in the cortex) and the sensor placed on the scalp. These layers act as a volume conductor and effectively low-pass filter and smear the signal sources. Thus, EEG provides only a "bird's eye" view of brain activity and offers low spatial resolution.

Due to the small amplitude of the recorded signals, EEG is also very sensitive to noise and artifacts. Artifacts are signals that do not originate from the brain, but which may influence BCI output. The most frequent artifacts generated by the user are muscle activities (which can be measured using the electromyogram, EMG) and eye movements (measured via the electrooculogram, EOG). Figure 2(a) shows a typical EEG trace with EOG and EMG artifacts. The high amplitude EOG artifact in the figure is caused by blinking of the eyes while the large EMG disturbances are caused by clenching of the teeth. Artificial noise is usually due to nearby electronic devices (e.g., 60 Hz power line interference). Given that EEG is very sensitive to noise, measures for ensuring a high signal-to-noise ratio (SNR) are desirable. The level of expertise and care that goes into affixing the EEG sensors onto the scalp can have an important affect on impedances and SNR. Wet EEG sensors are most commonly used in BCI applications. These require scalp preparation and the use of electrolytic gels, slowing down the sensor placement process. Additionally, these wet EEG sensors also need to be re-applied frequently in order to maintain low impedances. Consequently, for the practical use of BCIs, it is advantageous to use a minimum number of EEG sensors. Dry electrodes that can be simply placed on the scalp without any scalp preparation or gel use are under development. Thus far, however, their signal quality appears to be inferior compared to wet electrodes.

Figure 2. EEG signals and oscillatory EEG features

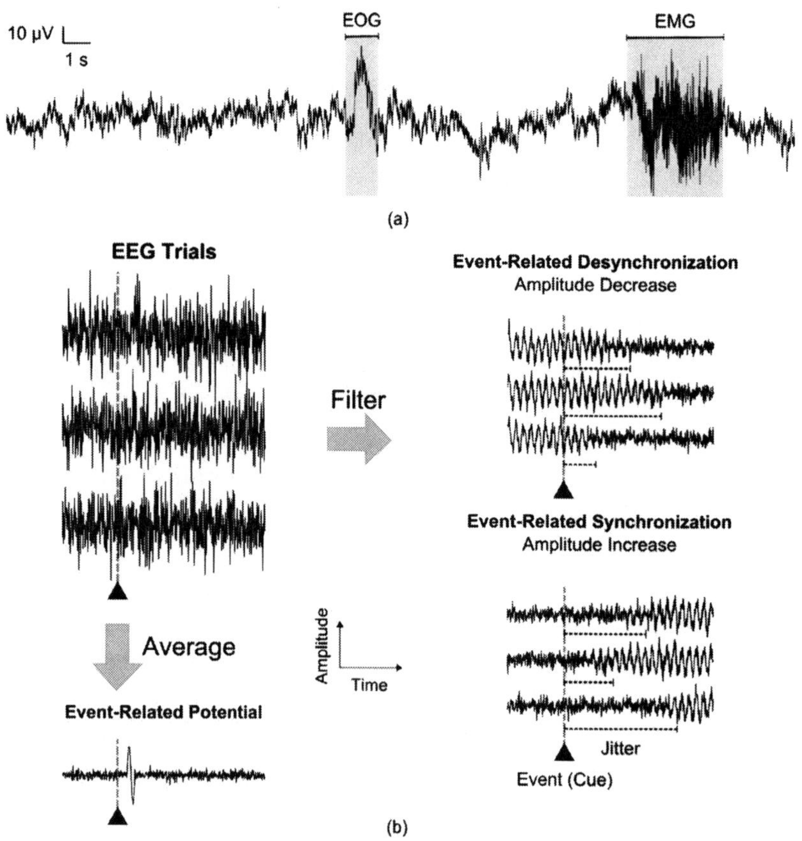

Evoked and Induced Oscillatory EEG Activity

Two types of EEG signals have been linked to cognitive function and have thus been used to operate BCIs: event-related potentials (ERPs) and event-related changes in the on-going oscillatory EEG activity.

ERPs are electrical potential shifts that are time-locked to perceptual, cognitive, or motor events. "Time-locked" here implies that the time between the event and the occurrence of the electrical potential shift is approximately constant. Therefore, ERPs represent the stereotyped temporal signature of macroscopic brain electrical activity. Due to the previously discussed poor spatial resolution of EEG, single ERPs are generally not visible to the naked eye. To make ERPs visible, the SNR has to be increased. This can be achieved by averaging the EEG recordings of a large number of trials (by repeating the event causing the ERP). Due to the constant response time, the average enhances ERPs and suppresses uncorrelated and random brain activity. The plots on the left hand side in Figure 2(b) illustrate this process. The dashed vertical lines indicate the time of event onset. Please note that the ranges of the y-axes are different for the individual curves but for ease of comparison, the amplitudes were normalized.

A number of different ERPs are used for BCI-based control. Internally-paced ERPs, i.e. ERPs which the user can intentionally generate, include slow cortical potentials (SCP) (Birbaumer, 1999), motor related potentials (MRPs) (Birch, 2003), and the "Bereitschaftspotential" (Blankertz, 2003). ERPs evoked by external stimuli, commonly called evoked-potentials (EPs), are auditory evoked potentials (AEPs) (Nijboer, 2008), the visual evoked potential (VEPs) (Sutter, 1992), its cognitive component the P300 (positive shift in the EEG signal about 300ms after stimulus presentation) (Donchin, 2000), steady-state VEP (SSVEP) (Cheng, 2002) and steady-state somatosensory EPs (SSSEP) (Müller-Putz, 2006). In the latter two cases, steady-state indicates that external stimuli are presented in such a rapid sequence that the resulting evoked brain responses are overlapping and thus reflect the stimulus frequency. The ability of users to perceive an external stimulus, however, potentially leads to residual muscle activity (e.g. gaze control to focus on distinctive light sources for (SS)VEPs) and may necessitate careful monitoring for artifacts. Practical BCIs are generally based on SSVEPs and the P300; the duration of the evoked responses is usually less than 500 milliseconds.

A second major class of EEG signals useful for BCIs are event-related changes of on-going oscillatory EEG activity. These usually occur in the form of event-related desynchronization (ERD) or event-related synchronization (ERS) (Pfurtscheller, 1999). The term ERD means that rhythmic components in the ongoing brain signal undergo a decrease in the amount of synchrony reflected by a decrease in amplitude in a specific frequency band. In contrast, the term ERS describes an enhancement of rhythmic activity evident in an increase in amplitude. Idealized examples are shown on the right hand side in Figure 2(b). After an event or cue-signal instructing the user to change his/her brain activity, amplitude changes in specific frequency components can be observed. The onset time of this behaviorally induced ERD and ERS (ERDS) response can however be different in each trial, i.e, non-phase-locked to the event (leading to phase-jitter). Therefore such ERDS responses are usually quantified in the spectral domain, i.e., by estimating the power spectrum.

The most commonly used mental task to induce ERDS is motor imagery (MI), i.e., the kinesthetic imagination of movements (Neuper, 2005). MI may be seen as the rehearsal of a motor act without the overt motor output; neural activity occurs, but the actual movement is blocked at some subsequent corticospinal level. MI and the preparation or programming phase of movement involve activation of very similar cerebral structures (Decety, 1996; Crammond, 1997). MI typically activates premotor and primary sensorimotor areas and results in ERD or ERS of "mu" (7-13 Hz) and "central beta" (13-30 Hz) rhythms in the EEG (Pfurtscheller, 1997). ERDS-based BCIs therefore rely on robust estimation of the power spectrum in these frequency ranges and the reliable detection of changes in the computed power spectrum, based on EEG data over a couple of seconds. Further details can be found in the Applications section.

Pattern Recognition and Machine Learning

Pattern recognition refers to methods and algorithms that map input patterns to appropriate categories or actions (Duda, 2001). Pattern recognition in EEG BCI systems typically consists of a feature extraction stage and a classification stage. Features are distinctive properties of input patterns that help in differentiating between several categories. Generally, spatial, temporal and spectral characteristics of ERPs and ERDS are used to obtain reliable features. The classifier then has the task of assigning labels to the input patterns based on these extracted features. The plot in Figure 1 entitled "Classification" shows a hypothetical example of a two class problem (class 'x' versus class 'o') based on two features (labeled #1 and #2). BCIs typically employ statistical classifiers, i.e., the categorization is based on the probability distribution of the features. Due to the poor spatial resolution of EEG and its inherent variability, it is desirable to extract features and train user-specific models for classification based on each user's EEG data. To this end, during an initial calibration phase, different mental activity patterns are collected and used to train user-specific classifiers. After training, the classifier are used to detect these patterns in the ongoing EEG. The non-stationarity of EEG, however, also requires training on the part of the user to be able to reliably generate the appropriate EEG patterns. Operating a BCI is thus akin to learning a new motor skill.

The best possible control can be achieved in the shortest possible time only by optimizing both feature extraction and classification. Training data sets are usually limited because data collection is time consuming and demanding for subjects. Careful selection of features can simplify pattern representation and decrease measurement costs (i.e., the number of electrodes), besides potentially yielding an increase in classification accuracy (Jain, 2000). A large number of features may result in perfect discrimination but require an inordinate amount of time to compute or overfit the data. On the other hand, an excessive reduction in the number of features may result in decreased performance. It is consequently crucial to find a feature-classifier combination that generalizes well (i.e., that achieves good performance on new and unseen data). Machine learning methods are used to automatically identify EEG patterns and features that are discriminative, and to optimize the signal processing parameters. Crucial for optimization is to ensure that only physiological meaningful features are selected.

Many different signal processing and pattern recognition methods have been used. Methods such as spatial filtering have been used to enhance the SNR of the EEG; these include Laplacian re-referencing (McFarland, 1997) or common spatial patterns (CSP) (Blankertz, 2006), principal component analysis (PCA) (Lugger, 1998), and independent component analysis (ICA) (Makeig, 2004; Naeem, 2006). Methods for feature extraction include band power measures (Scherer, 2007a), Fourier Transform (Müller-Putz, 2005b), Wavelet packet analysis (Graimann, 2004), (adaptive) autoregressive parameters (Schlögl, 1997), and phase measures such as the phase-locking value (Brunner, 2006) or bi-phase relationships (Darvas, 2009). For classification, linear and quadratic discriminant analysis (Vidaurre, 2007; Müller, 2003), support vector machines (Müller, 2003; Shenoy, 2008), artificial neural networks

(Peters, 1998), or hidden Markov Models (HMM) (Obermaier, 2001) have been investigated. Other machine learning algorithms that have been applied include methods inspired by evolutionary biology such as Genetic Algorithms (Scherer, 2004), clustering methods such as the distinction sensitive learning vector quantization (DSLVQ) (Pregentzer, 1999), and greedy search algorithms as the sequential forward floating selection (SFFS) (Leeb, 2007).

APPLICATIONS

In order to illustrate the differences between ERP and ERDS-based BCIs, we show two practical applications. The first application illustrates how an ERP (the P300) can be used to command a partially autonomous humanoid robot to perform a complex task such as walking to a specific location and picking up a desired object. The second application shows motor imagery based interaction with Virtual Environments and the internet-based program Virtual Google Earth. Both P300 and motor imagery induced oscillations have been successfully used in a number of other studies with able-bodied and disabled subjects (Piccione, 2006; Sellers, 2006; Vaughan, 2006; Pfurtscheller, 2003; Müller-Putz, 2005; Neuper, 2003).

P300-Based Control of a Robot

There is growing interest in intelligent robotic devices for assisting paralyzed and disabled individuals in performing various tasks in daily life. Our first application illustrates how the P300 can be used to select tasks (or goals) which can then be executed autonomously by a helper robot. As an example, if the user is thirsty and would like some water, a helper robot could be commanded to get a cup of water from the kitchen. To be able to autonomously perform this task, the robot requires prior knowledge of the environment and some amount of autonomy, i.e., it has to be able to navigate in the given environment, know the location of cups and water, and be able to manipulate objects.

A BCI system developed by our group (Bell, 2008) uses a semi-autonomous humanoid robot (Fujitsu HOAP-2) to interact with objects in the environment. The robot can autonomously move and possesses the ability to pick up and drop off objects. To be able to identify objects, the humanoid is equipped with cameras and computer vision algorithms.

The diagram in Figure 3 summarizes the experimental paradigm, The top panel shows images of the humanoid robot in action. The bottom row depicts the user's computer screen. First, from a predefined starting position the robot autonomously walks towards a table with a red object and a green object (image marked "1"). The user receives a live feed from the robot's cameras, thereby immersing the user in the robot's environment and allowing the user to select actions based on the objects in the image (screen marked "2"). Objects are found using computer vision techniques. The robot transmits the segmented images of the objects it sees (in this case, a red and a green object) and queries the user about which one to pick up (a binary classification problem). The selection is made by the user using a P300-BCI as described below. After picking-up the object selected by the user (image marked "3"), the robot asks the user which location it should bring the selected object to. Possible locations include a table on the left side and a table on the right side of the arena. Images of the possible locations are presented using an overhead camera (screen marked "4"). Again the selection of the destination is made by the user by means of the P300. Finally, the robot walks to the destination selected by the user and places the object on the table at the selected location (image marked "5").

The BCI above for controlling the humanoid robot uses a visually evoked potential known as P300, so named because it occurs about 300 ms after the user consciously attends to a changing

Figure 3. P300-based control of a humanoid robot

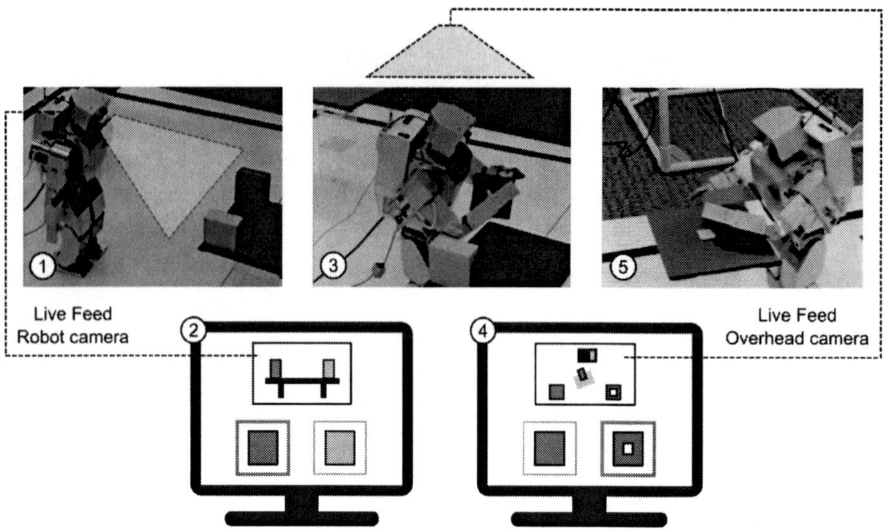

visual stimulus. The visual stimuli were the segmented images of objects captured by the humanoid's camera. Each time the robot expects new instructions, the images of the possible choices (objects in the camera image or images of destination locations) are presented to the user. These images are scaled and arranged as a grid on the screen. The lower part in Figure 3 schematically shows the visual stimuli presented to the user. In the upper half of the computer screen, the live feed of the humanoid's camera was presented. In the lower part, the segmented images were arranged for selection. To select the desired option using EEG, the user focuses his or her attention on the image of choice while the border of each image is flashed in random order every 250 ms. In order to focus the user's attention and robustly evoke the P300, subjects were asked to mentally count the number of flashes on their image of choice.

In order to calibrate the BCI system, an initial 10 minute data collection protocol was used. During this time, a 2 x 2 layout of four different images, arranged as a grid, was presented on the screen. Participants in the study were asked to attend to a pre-selected image while the borders around the images were flashed one at a time in random order every 250 ms (ten flashes overall per image). This procedure was repeated for each of the four image positions four times. Thirty-two EEG channels were recorded form electrodes placed over the entire head according to the 10-20 system (standardized electrode placement scheme). A linear classifier (a "soft-margin support vector machine") was trained to discriminate between the P300 response for the desired image versus other image flashes. For classification, data segments of 500 ms duration starting from the time of flash presentation were used. A spatial filter was used to transform the EEG into a signal which was maximally discriminative between the desired and the other images (further details can be found in Bell (2008)). This analysis allows the identification of the maximum number of repetitions for each image required to achieve stable classification (maximum 10 flashes). To detect the desired image in a multi-image scenario, each image flash was classified and the image with the highest number of hits after all flashes was selected as the user's choice. The results, based on nine able-bodied subjects, show that an accuracy of 95% can be achieved for discriminating between four classes.

The theoretical chance classification level for four classes is 25%. With the implemented rate of 4 flashes per second, the selection of one out of four options takes 5 sec, yielding an information transfer rate (ITR) of 24 bits min^{-1}.

The study demonstrates that P300-based BCI control can be achieved with a reasonably high accuracy within a relatively short training period. The ITR can be increased by increasing the number of images (or other command options); however, making one selection would still require a similar time window.

In the above study, the robot initiated communication whenever new instructions were required. Since the user is required to change brain state depending on an external cue, this operation mode is called cue-guided. The user, however, should ideally have the choice of interacting with the device at any given moment. For example, the user may want to interrupt the current instruction and to select a different object. To enable such "self-paced" communication and provide on-demand access to the controlled device, the BCI needs to constantly analyze the user's ongoing brain activity, not just during predefined time periods. One way to enable on-demand P300-based access would be to present control commands on the screen and flash them all the time. Unless the user is intentionally attending to the flashes, no P300 is evoked and thus, no control command will be selected. Another option would be to combine the P300 system with an ERDS-based BCI such as the one described below.

Sensorimotor Rhythm Based Control of Computer Applications

An alternative to using ERPs for BCI is to extract control signals by detecting ERDS events. The typical frequency range of ERDS in EEG-based BCIs is 8-30 Hz. In comparison, EOG artifacts have a maximum in the frequency range below 4 Hz and EMG at frequencies higher than 30 Hz. Consequently oscillatory EEG components used for BCI control are close to the range of the artifacts. The self-paced 3-class BCI described here (originally proposed in Scherer (2007a, 2008)) incorporates methods to reduce EOG artifacts and to detect EMG activity. Furthermore to reduce the complexity of the BCI, only three bipolar EEG channels, recorded from six electrodes, were used.

For the initial calibration of the ERDS-based BCI, 22-channel EEG during cue-guided left hand, right hand, foot and tongue motor imagery (MI) was recorded. For each class, 144 trials of 4 second length with several seconds of break in between were collected. Subject-specific oscillatory patterns, electrode locations, and the three most discriminative imagery tasks were identified by means of the distinction sensitive learning vector quantization (DSLVQ) method (Pregenzer, 1999). A committee of Fisher's linear discriminant analysis (LDA) linear classifiers (Duda, 2000) was trained for classification. To gain self-paced control, cue-guided feedback training was first performed until the 3-class classification accuracy was satisfactory, i.e., about 80% (33% corresponds to the theoretical random accuracy level).

Figure 4(a) shows the selected electrode positions and the classification performance achieved during feedback training for one subject. At second 0 ("Cue") the subjects was asked to move the feedback cursor from the center of the screen towards a target placed close to the left, the right or the bottom border by imagining left hand, right hand or foot movements, respectively. The plot shows the time course of the classification accuracy as a function of time. On average, 2.5 s after cue presentation, the classification accuracy was around 80%. During the cue-guided feedback training, not only were the parameters of the BCI adapted to the user's brain activity, but the brain also learned to reliably generate the requisite patterns. In the next step, to allow self-paced operation, an additional LDA classifier was trained to discriminate between motor imagery (the three tasks pooled together) and non motor imagery activity (MI and non-MI activity). For 3-class self-paced operation, we combined the output of the two classifiers: whenever motor imagery activity was detected by the MI/non-MI LDA, the committee vote was used as the BCI output signal.

Three subjects participated in this study. After a total training time of about 5 hours, the accuracy of the LDA committee classifier was higher than 80%. A cue-guided experiment with longer non-motor imagery periods (randomly between 7-17 seconds) resulted in a false positive detection rate, i.e., rate at which non motor imagery was classified as motor imagery, of about 17% (Scherer, 2008).

To allow subjects to voluntarily initiate, hold, release or switch between motor imagery tasks, a computer game-like virtual environment (VE) was implemented. Figure 4(b) shows a picture of a subject wearing an EEG electrode cap while interacting with the computer application. The screenshot on the upper-left hand side shows the VE which consisted of a meadow, a tree and several hedges. The task was to navigate through the virtual world, and find and pick up scattered objects (coins). For navigation, the three motor imagery patterns were translated into rotate to the left, rotate to the right (90 degree per second, respectively) and move forward (1 unit per second; size of the VE 30x30 units). The BCI transmitted the classification results every 20 milliseconds to the VE and the position of the virtual camera was modified accordingly. Subjects had three minutes time to move through the VE and collect the coins. An example trajectory is depicted in the map in Figure 4(b) (blue line). The locations of the coins are highlighted (yellow). From the trajectory, one can see that the subject was able to use the BCI to successfully navigate in the VE and accomplish the task. After the experiment, subjects reported that the BCI was detecting their intent correctly a majority of the time.

Figure 4. Motor imagery based control of computer applications. Adapted from (Scherer, 2007a)

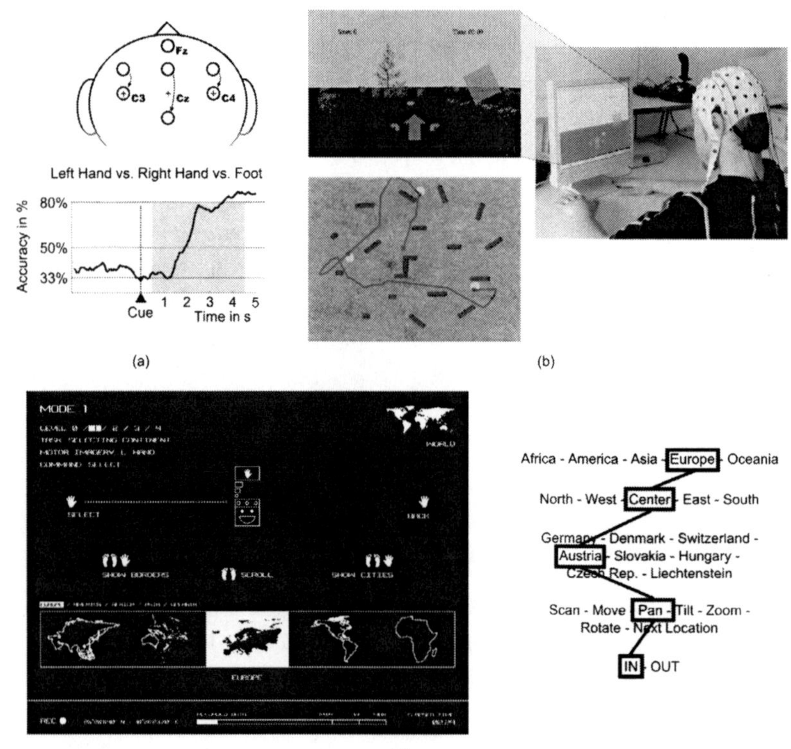

Three output classes are not enough to allow meaningful operation of standard software applications such as word processors and internet browsers. In order to be able to use the above presented 3-class self-paced BCI with the Google Earth virtual globe program (Google Inc., Mountain View, CA, USA), a special graphical user interface (GUI) was developed (Scherer, 2007a). Figure 4(c) shows the GUI. The user is represented by an icon positioned in the middle of the screen. Icons representing GUI control commands are arranged around the user and can be selected by moving the feedback cursor (bold line) over it. Available commands include 'Scroll', 'Select' and 'Back'. In the lower part of the GUI, control commands for Google Earth are listed. By browsing through the available menu options ('Scroll'), the desired menu entry can be selected ('Select'). Google Earth's virtual camera position is then repositioned accordingly. To minimize the number of BCI selections, the countries of the world were hierarchically grouped by continent and continental area. The diagram in Figure 4(c) shows the selections required to move the camera position over Austria and zoom in. Two hundred and one different options are available. Three selections were required to isolate the country of interest and to position Google Earth's virtual camera. To move to the desired location, the fourth command level provided commands for direct manipulation of the virtual camera. Wrong selections could be undone ('Back').

Since the geographical data has to be downloaded from internet databases (which takes time), correct detection of non-MI periods is important to avoid erroneous selections. After an additional training time of about 10 hours, one subject previously participating in the 3-class self-paced experiment successfully operated Google Earth in front of a public audience. The average time to select the desired country was about 20 seconds. Additional information along with multimedia material about the public demonstration (called "Brainloop") is available at http://www.aksioma.org/brainloop.

The results of the BCI described above demonstrate that voluntarily generated mental activity can be used to encode messages for artificial devices. The study, however, also shows that gaining control can be time consuming and that a lower number of classes can be differentiated compared to an ERP-based system. The advantage is that users autonomously can induce ERDS-patterns by mental activity at any time and communication is not tied to external stimuli.

The GUI developed for the Google Earth application shows that it is possible to overcome low ITRs by incorporating concepts from the fields of human–computer interaction and usability. A carefully designed user interface and judicious use of the BCI output may help overcome inaccuracies from misclassification, thereby helping reduce erroneous selections. A more detailed description on how interactions can be designed to explicitly take into account uncertainty and dynamics of control inputs can be found in Williamson (2009). Once the EEG patterns have been established and the BCI has been trained, we have found that the BCI can work reliably for long periods of time without the need for any updates. The Google Earth user's oscillatory patterns, for example, have been stable for two years. Such long-term stability of trained brain patterns significantly contributes toward the creation of reliable brain-computer communication.

FUTURE TRENDS

After approximately two decades of basic research, BCI systems have begun to move out of the laboratory and are finding their way into homes of patients and clinical environments. One very important issue is usability and the design of the non-invasive recording equipment. Currently available electrode caps and wet electrodes are not practical for daily application. Future recording devices will need to be more comfortable to wear and less expensive. In fact, the first generation of wireless recording devices with dry electrodes have started appearing on the market (e.g., Emotive Systems, San Francisco, CA, USA). The main area of application of these devices, however, is gaming and entertainment. Whether and to what extent these prove to be useful for BCI applications remains to be seen. Such novel recording devices are nevertheless an important step toward enhancing usability and increasing user acceptance of BCIs for daily use.

An additional factor that may increase user acceptance is reducing the training time required for ERDS-based BCIs. Promising preliminary results have been obtained using on-line adaptive classifiers (Vidaurre, 2006) or "general" features for BCIs (Vidaurre, 2009; Shenoy, 2008). These approaches are based on extracting features which work reasonably well for new users without the need for time-consuming parameter optimization and using classifiers that adapt on-line to brain patterns induced by mental activities. However, an overarching theory of co-adaptation of mind and machine remains to be developed. Such a theory would entail finding models that can predict changes in brain activity and adapt in sync with the human user to achieve the common goal of brain-based control. Developing such a theory and methods for co-adaptation remain active areas of BCI research.

From an applications point of view, there is a growing trend towards building BCIs which facilitate access to standard communication channels such as phone or email. As an example, as part of the Seventh Framework Programme, the European Union is currently funding BCI research focusing on improving the quality of life and autonomy of physically disabled individuals.

There is also considerable interest in leveraging BCI technology to accelerate functional recovery and rehabilitation after neural injury. Motor imagery, for example, can be used to enhance neural plasticity after stroke. Before therapeutic effects are perceivable by affected individuals, BCI methodologies can be used to monitor and provide feedback on cortical reorganization (Scherer, 2007b; Meng, 2009). First clinical trials of some of these methodologies are already in progress.

Advances in neuroscience and technology (Moritz, 2008; Ganguly, 2009) have lead to ambitious goals in BCI research, e.g., the restoration of lost motor or sensory function through neuroprostheses and neurally controlled prosthetic limbs. Since the information transfer rates of BCIs (especially non-invasive BCIs) can be quite low, there is considerable interest in investigating the neural mechanisms of motor control. For example, knowledge of neural control mechanisms and the biomechanical principles of the hand have led to artificial devices with human hand-like dexterity.

BCI technology has thus far primarily targeted paralyzed and disabled individuals. The performance of modern BCIs, however, has risen to a level where able-bodied individuals could benefit from the technology. Besides entertainment (e.g., BCI-operated games), there are potential applications for BCI technology in working environments where movements are constrained, as in the case of astronauts working in zero gravity environments (Rossini, 2009).

EEG-based BCIs are likely to remain the most widely used class of BCIs over the next several years owing to their affordability, portability, and non-invasive nature. Recently, there has also been increased interest in ECoG signals recorded from the surface of the brain. ECoG is typically recorded in patients who are being monitored prior to epilepsy surgery. Because ECoG electrodes do not penetrate the brain surface (they do penetrate the skull), they are not as invasive as intracortical implants that are placed inside the brain. ECoG allows electrical signals from several different brain areas to be recorded while at the same time providing temporal resolution in the millisecond range and a higher signal-to-noise ratio than EEG. First results suggest that BCI control signals can be accurately detected and that training periods can be decreased compared to EEG-based BCIs (Shenoy, 2008). More research, however, is needed to demonstrate the superiority of ECoG and other invasive technologies over non-invasive methods such as EEG, and questions regarding safety and long term-use have to be addressed.

The trend towards implantable and thus potentially wireless devices also raises the question of neurosecurity (Denning, 2009). In the future, this question may become especially important if the device is not only able to record brain activity, but also stimulate particular brain circuits (e.g., cognitive prosthetics).

CONCLUSION

This chapter introduced some of the basic concepts involved in brain-computer interfaces (BCIs) and reviewed two methods for non-invasive BCI control using EEG. Due to the non-stationarity of EEG, an important requirement to gain reliable control within a limited period of time is the co-adaptation of the human brain and the machine. As discussed above, the degree of adaptation required on the part of the user and the machine strongly depends on the type of EEG signal being used.

The results of the presented applications demonstrate that ERP-based BCIs are relatively accurate and require little training on the part of the subject. The drawback is the dependency on external stimulation. BCIs based on ERDS, on the other hand, allow on-demand self-paced control by the user. However, the speed of communication is lower, fewer classes can be discriminated, and the training period is longer. Combining ERP and ERDS-based control could be a potentially fruitful way of improving the performance and flexibility of non-invasive BCIs in the near future.

ACKNOWLEDGMENT

This work was supported by NSF grants 0622252 and 0930908, a Microsoft External Research grant, and the Packard Foundation.

REFERENCES

Bell, C. J., Shenoy, P., Chalodhorn, R., & Rao, R. P. N. (2008). Control of a humanoid robot by a noninvasive brain-computer interface in humans. *Journal of Neural Engineering, 5*(2), 214–220. doi:10.1088/1741-2560/5/2/012

Bensch, M., Karim, A. A., Mellinger, J., Hinterberger, T., Tangermann, M., & Bogdan, M. (2007). Nessi: An EEG-controlled web browser for severely paralyzed patients. *Computational Intelligence and Neuroscience, 2007. Article ID, 71863*, 1–5.

Birbaumer, N., Ghanayim, N., Hinterberger, T., Iversen, I., Kotchoubey, B., & Kübler, A. (1999). A spelling device for the paralysed. *Nature, 398*(6725), 297–298. doi:10.1038/18581

Birch, G. E., Mason, S. G., & Borisoff, J. F. (2003). Current trends in brain-computer interface research at the Neil Squire Foundation. *IEEE Transactions on Neural Systems and Rehabilitation Engineering, 11*(2), 123–126. doi:10.1109/TNSRE.2003.814450

Blankertz, B., Dornhege, G. Krauledat, M., Müller, K. R., Kunzmann, V., Losch, F., & Curio, G. (2006). The Berlin Brain-Computer Interface: EEG-based communication without subject training. *IEEE Transactions onNeural Systems and Rehabilitation Engineering, 14*(2), 147–152.

Blankertz, B., Dornhege, G., Schäfer, C., Krepki, R., Kohlmorgen, J., & Müller, K. R. (2003). Boosting bit rates and error detection for the classification of fast-paced motor commands based on single-trial EEG analysis. *IEEE Transactions on Neural Systems and Rehabilitation Engineering*, *11*(2), 127–131. doi:10.1109/TNSRE.2003.814456

Brunner, C., Scherer, R., Graimann, B., Supp, G., & Pfurtscheller, G. (2006). Online control of a brain-computer interface using phase synchronization. *IEEE Transactions on Bio-Medical Engineering*, *53*(12), 2501–2506. doi:10.1109/TBME.2006.881775

Cheng, M., Gao, X., Gao, S., & Xu, D. (2002). Design and implementation of a brain computer interface with high transfer rates. *IEEE Transactions on Bio-Medical Engineering*, *49*(10), 1181–1186. doi:10.1109/TBME.2002.803536

Coyle, S. M., Ward, T. E., & Markham, C. M. (2007). Brain-computer interface using a simplified functional near-infrared spectroscopy system. *Journal of Neural Engineering*, *4*(3), 219–226. doi:10.1088/1741-2560/4/3/007

Crammond, D. J. (1997). Motor imagery: never in your wildest dream. *Trends in Neurosciences*, *20*(2), 54–57. doi:10.1016/S0166-2236(96)30019-2

Darvas, F., Miller, K. J., Rao, R. P. N., & Ojemann, J. G. (2009). Nonlinear phase-phase cross-frequency coupling mediates communication between distant sites in human neocortex. *The Journal of Neuroscience*, *29*(2), 426–435. doi:10.1523/JNEUROSCI.3688-08.2009

Decety, J. (1996). Do imagined and executed actions share the same neural substrate? *Brain Research. Cognitive Brain Research*, *3*(2), 87–93. doi:10.1016/0926-6410(95)00033-X

Denning, T., Matsuoka, Y., & Tadayoshi, K. (2009). Neurosecurity: security and privacy for neural devices. *Neurosurgical Focus*, *27*(1), E7. doi:10.3171/2009.4.FOCUS0985

Donchin, E., Spencer, K. M., & Wijesinghe, R. (2000). The mental prosthesis: assessing the speed of a P300-based brain-computer interface. *IEEE Transactions on Bio-Medical Engineering*, *8*(2), 174–179.

Dornhege, G., Millan, J. R., Hinterberger, T., McFarland, D., & Müller, K. R. (Eds.). (2007). *Towards Brain-Computer Interfacing*. Cambridge, MA: The MIT Press.

Duda, R., Hart, P., & Stork, D. (Eds.). (2000). *Pattern Classification* (2nd ed.). New York: Wiley Interscience.

Galán, F., Nuttin, M., Lew, E., Ferrez, P. W., Vanacker, G., Philips, J., & Millán, J. R. (2008). A brain-actuated wheelchair: asynchronous and non-invasive Brain-computer interfaces for continuous control of robots. *Clinical Neurophysiology*, *119*(9), 2159–2169. doi:10.1016/j.clinph.2008.06.001

Ganguly, K., & Carmena, J. M. (2009). Emergence of a stable cortical map for neuroprosthetic control. *PLoS Biology*, *7*(7), e1000153. doi:10.1371/journal.pbio.1000153

Graimann, B., Huggins, J. E., Levine, S. P., & Pfurtscheller, G. (2004). Toward a direct brain interface based on human subdural recordings and wavelet-packet analysis. *IEEE Transactions on Bio-Medical Engineering*, *51*(6), 954–962. doi:10.1109/TBME.2004.826671

Hochberg, L. R., Serruya, M. D., Friehs, G. M., Mukand, J. A., Saleh, M., & Caplan, A. H. (2006). Neuronal ensemble control of prosthetic devices by a human with tetraplegia. *Nature*, *442*(7099), 164–171. doi:10.1038/nature04970

Jain, A. K., Duin, R. P. W., & Mao, J. (2000). Statistical pattern recognition: a review. *IEEE Transactions on Pattern Analysis and Machine Intelligence*, *22*(1), 4–37. doi:10.1109/34.824819

Leeb, R., Lee, F., Keinrath, C., Scherer, R., Bischof, H., & Pfurtscheller, G. (2007). Brain-computer communication: Motivation, aim, and impact of exploring a virtual apartment. *IEEE Transactions on Neural Systems and Rehabilitation Engineering*, *15*(4), 473–482. doi:10.1109/TNSRE.2007.906956

Lugger, K., Flotzinger, D., Schlögl, A., Pregenzer, M., & Pfurtscheller, G. (1998). Feature extraction for on-line EEG classification using principal components and linear discriminants. *Medical & Biological Engineering & Computing*, *36*(3), 309–314. doi:10.1007/BF02522476

Makeig, S., Debener, S., Onton, J., & Delorme, A. (2004). Minim event-related brain dynamics. *Trends in Cognitive Sciences*, *8*(5), 204–210. doi:10.1016/j.tics.2004.03.008

Maynard, E. M., Nordhausen, C. T., & Normann, R. A. (1997). The Utah intracortical electrode array: a recording structure for potential brain-computer interfaces. *Electroencephalography and Clinical Neurophysiology*, *102*(3), 228–239. doi:10.1016/S0013-4694(96)95176-0

McFarland, D. J., McCane, L. M. ,., David, S. V., & Wolpaw, J. R. (1997). Spatial filter selection for EEG-based communication. *Electroencephalography and Clinical Neurophysiology*, *103*(3), 386–394. doi:10.1016/S0013-4694(97)00022-2

Mellinger, J., Schalk, G., Braun, C., Preissl, H., Rosenstiel, W., Birbaumer, N., & Kübler, A. (2007). An MEG-based brain-computer interface (BCI). *NeuroImage*, *36*(3), 581–593. doi:10.1016/j.neuroimage.2007.03.019

Meng, F., Tong, K. Y., Chan, S. T., Wong, W. W., Lui, K. H., & Tang, K. W. (2009). Cerebral Plasticity After Subcortical Stroke as Revealed by Cortico-Muscular Coherence. *IEEE Transactions on Bio-Medical Engineering*, *17*(3), 234–243.

Millán, J. R., & Mouriño, J. (2003). Asynchronous BCI and local neural classifiers: an overview of the Adaptive Brain Interface project. *IEEE Transactions on Neural Systems and Rehabilitation Engineering*, *11*(2), 159–161. doi:10.1109/TNSRE.2003.814435

Millán, J. R., Renkens, F., Mouriño, J., & Gerstner, W. (2004). Noninvasive brain-actuated control of a mobile robot by human EEG. *IEEE Transactions on Bio-Medical Engineering*, *51*(6), 1026–1033. doi:10.1109/TBME.2004.827086

Miller, K. J., denNijs, M., Shenoy, P., Miller, J. W., Rao, R. P. N., & Ojemann, G. (2007). Real-time functional brain mapping using electrocorticography. *NeuroImage*, *37*(2), 504–507. doi:10.1016/j.neuroimage.2007.05.029

Moritz, C. T., Perlmutter, S. I., & Fetz, E. E. (2008). Direct control of paralysed muscles by cortical neurons. *Nature*, *456*(7222), 639–642. doi:10.1038/nature07418

Müller, K. R., Anderson, C. W., & Birch, G. E. (2003). Linear and nonlinear methods for brain-computer interfaces. *IEEE Transactions on Neural Systems and Rehabilitation Engineering*, *11*(2), 165–169. doi:10.1109/TNSRE.2003.814484

Müller -Putz, G. R., Scherer, R., Brauneis, C., & Pfurtscheller, G. (2005b). Steady-state visual evoked potential (SSVEP)-based communication: impact of harmonic frequency components. *Journal of Neural Engineering*, *2*(4), 123–130. doi:10.1088/1741-2560/2/4/008

Müller-Putz, G. R., Scherer, R., Neuper, C., & Pfurtscheller, G. (2006). Steady-state somatosensory evoked potentials: suitable brain signals for brain-computer interfaces? *IEEE Transactions on Neural Systems and Rehabilitation Engineering*, *14*(1), 30–37. doi:10.1109/TNSRE.2005.863842

Müller-Putz, G. R., Scherer, R., Pfurtscheller, G., & Rupp, R. (2005a). EEG-based neuroprosthesis control: a step towards clinical practice. *Neuroscience Letters*, *382*(1-2), 169–174. doi:10.1016/j.neulet.2005.03.021

Naeem, M., Brunner, C., Leeb, R., Graimann, B., & Pfurtscheller, G. (2006). Seperability of four-class motor imagery data using independent components analysis. *Journal of Neural Engineering*, *3*(3), 208–216. doi:10.1088/1741-2560/3/3/003

Neuper, C., Müller, G. R., Kübler, A., Birbaumer, N., & Pfurtscheller, G. (2003). Clinical application of an EEG-based brain-computer interface: a case study in a patient with severe motor impairment. *Clinical Neurophysiology*, *114*(3), 399–409. doi:10.1016/S1388-2457(02)00387-5

Neuper, C., Scherer, R., Reiner, M., & Pfurtscheller, G. (2005). Imagery of motor actions: differential effects of kinesthetic and visual-motor mode of imagery in single-trial EEG. *Brain Research. Cognitive Brain Research*, *25*(3), 668–677. doi:10.1016/j.cogbrainres.2005.08.014

Nijboer, F., Furdea, A., Gunst, I., Mellinger, J., McFarland, D. J., Birbaumer, N., & Kübler, A. (2008). An auditory brain-computer interface (BCI). *Journal of Neuroscience Methods*, *167*(1), 43–50. doi:10.1016/j.jneumeth.2007.02.009

Obermaier, B., Guger, C., Neuper, C., & Pfurtscheller, G. (2001). Hidden Markov models for online classification of single trial EEG data. *Pattern Recognition Letters*, *22*(12), 1299–1309. doi:10.1016/S0167-8655(01)00075-7

Peters, B., Pfurtscheller, G., & Flyvbjerg, H. (1998). Mining multi-channel EEG for its information content: an ANN-based method for a brain-computer interface. *Neural Networks*, *11*(7-8), 1429–1433. doi:10.1016/S0893-6080(98)00060-4

Pfurtscheller, G., & Lopes da Silva, F. H. (1999). Event-related EEG/MRG synchronization and desynchronization: basic principles. *Clinical Neurophysiology*, *110*(11), 1842–1857. doi:10.1016/S1388-2457(99)00141-8

Pfurtscheller, G., Müller, G. R., Pfurtscheller, J., Gerner, H. J., & Rupp, R. (2003). 'Thought'-control of functional electrical stimulation to restore hand grasp in a patient with tetraplegia. *Neuroscience Letters*, *351*(1), 33–36. doi:10.1016/S0304-3940(03)00947-9

Pfurtscheller, G., Müller-Putz, G. R., Schlögl, A., Graimann, B., Scherer, R., & Leeb, R. (2006). 15 years of BCI research at Graz University of Technology: current projects. *IEEE Transactions on Neural Systems and Rehabilitation Engineering*, *14*(2), 205–210. doi:10.1109/TNSRE.2006.875528

Pfurtscheller, G., & Neuper, C. (1997). Motor imagery activates primary sensorimotor area in humans. *Neuroscience Letters*, *239*(2-3), 65–68. doi:10.1016/S0304-3940(97)00889-6

Piccione, F., Giorgi, F., Tonin, P., Priftis, K., Giove, S., & Silvoni, S. (2006). P300-based brain computer interface: reliability and performance in healthy and paralysed participants. *Clinical Neurophysiology*, *117*(3), 531–537. doi:10.1016/j.clinph.2005.07.024

Pineda, J. A., Silverman, D. S., Vankov, A., & Hestenes, J. (2003). Learning to control brain rhythms: making a brain-computer interface possible. *IEEE Transactions on Neural Systems and Rehabilitation Engineering*, *11*(2), 181–184. doi:10.1109/TNSRE.2003.814445

Pregenzer, M., & Pfurtscheller, G. (1999). Frequency component selection for an EEG-based brain to computer interface. *IEEE Transactions on Bio-Medical Engineering*, *7*(4), 413–419.

Rossini, L., Dario, I., & Summerer, L. (Eds.). (2009). *Brain Machine Interfaces for Space applications: Enhancing astronaut's capabilities. International Review of Neurobiology* (*Vol. 86*). New York: Academic Press.

Schalk, G., Brunner, P., Gerhardt, L. A., Bischof, H., & Wolpaw, J. R. (2008). Brain-computer interfaces (BCIs): detection instead of classification. *Journal of Neuroscience Methods*, *167*(1), 51–62. doi:10.1016/j.jneumeth.2007.08.010

Scherer, R., Lee, F., Schlögl, A., Leeb, R., Bischof, H., & Pfurtscheller, G. (2008). Towards self-paced Brain-Computer Communication: Navigation through virtual worlds. *IEEE Transactions on Bio-Medical Engineering*, *55*(2), 675–682. doi:10.1109/TBME.2007.903709

Scherer, R., Mohapp, A., Grieshofer, P., Pfurtscheller, G., & Neuper, C. (2007b). Sensorimotor EEG patterns during motor imagery in hemiparetic stroke patients. *International Journal of Bioelectromagnetism*, *9*(3), 155–162.

Scherer, R., Müller, G. R., Neuper, C., Graimann, B., & Pfurtscheller, G. (2004). An asynchronously controlled EEG-based virtual keyboard: improvement of the spelling rate. *IEEE Transactions on Bio-Medical Engineering*, *51*(6), 979–984. doi:10.1109/TBME.2004.827062

Scherer, R., Schlögl, A., Lee, F., Bischof, H., Janša, J., & Pfurtscheller, G. (2007a). The self-paced Graz brain-computer interface: methods and applications. *Computational Intellignece and Neuroscience, 2007. Article ID*, *79826*, 1–7.

Scherer, R., Zanos, P. Z., Miller, K. J., Rao, R. P. N., & Ojemann, J. G. (2009). Classification of Contralateral and Ipsilateral Finger Movements for Electrocorticographic Brain-Computer Interfaces. *Neurosurgical Focus*, *27*(1), E12. doi:10.3171/2009.4.FOCUS0981

Schlögl, A., & Flotzinger, D., & Pfurtscheller. (1997). G. Adaptive autoregressive modeling used for single-trial EEG classification. *Biomedizinische Technik*, *42*(6), 162–167. doi:10.1515/bmte.1997.42.6.162

Sellers, E. W., & Donchin, E. (2006). A P300-based brain-computer interface: initial tests by ALS patients. *Clinical Neurophysiology*, *117*(3), 538–548. doi:10.1016/j.clinph.2005.06.027

Shenoy, P., Miller, K. J., Ojemann, J. G., & Rao, R. P. N. (2008). Generalized features for electrocorticographic BCIs. *IEEE Transactions on Bio-Medical Engineering*, *55*(1), 273–280. doi:10.1109/TBME.2007.903528

Sutter, E. E. (1992). The brain response interface: Communication through visually induced electrical brain responses. *Journal of Microcomputer Applications*, *15*, 31–45. doi:10.1016/0745-7138(92)90045-7

Vaughan, T. M., McFarland, D. J., Schalk, G., Sarnacki, W. A., Krusienski, D. J., Sellers, E. W., & Wolpaw, J. R. (2006). The Wadsworth BCI Research and Development Program: at home with BCI. *Neural Systems and Rehabilitation Engineering. IEEE Transactions on*, *14*(2), 229–233.

Vidaurre, C., Krämer, N., Blankertz, B., & Schlögl, A. (2009). Time domain parameters as a feature for EEG-based brain–computer interfaces. *Neural Networks*, *22*(9), 1313–1319. doi:10.1016/j.neunet.2009.07.020

Vidaurre, C., Scherer, R., Cabeza, R., Schlögl, A., & Pfurtscheller, G. (2007). Study of discriminant analysis applied to motor imagery bipolar data. *Medical & Biological Engineering & Computing*, *45*(1), 61–68. doi:10.1007/s11517-006-0122-5

Vidaurre, C., Schlögl, A., Cabeza, R., Scherer, R., & Pfurtscheller, G. (2006). A fully on-line adaptive BCI. *IEEE Transactions on Bio-Medical Engineering*, *53*(6), 1214–1219. doi:10.1109/TBME.2006.873542

Weiskopf, N., Mathiak, K., Bock, S. W., Scharnowski, F., Veit, R., & Grodd, W. (2004). Principles of a brain-computer interface (BCI) based on real-time functional magnetic resonance imaging (fMRI). *IEEE Transactions on Bio-Medical Engineering*, *51*(6), 966–970. doi:10.1109/TBME.2004.827063

Williamson, J., Murray-Smith, R., Blankertz, B., Krauledat, M., & Müller, K. R. (2009). Designing for uncertain, asymmetric control: Interaction design for brain-computer interfaces. *International Journal of Human-Computer Studies*, *67*, 827–841. doi:10.1016/j.ijhcs.2009.05.009

Wolpaw, J., Birbaumer, N., McFarland, D., Pfurtscheller, G., & Vaughan, T. (2002). Brain computer interfaces for communication and control. *Clinical Neurophysiology*, *113*(6), 767–791. doi:10.1016/S1388-2457(02)00057-3

KEY TERMS AND DEFINITIONS

Brain-Computer Interface (BCI): Communication system able to accept commands directly from the human brain without any muscle activity.

Classification: Assignment of labels to input patterns based on their extracted features.

Electroencephalogram (EEG): Bioelectrical brain activity recorded non-invasively from electrodes placed on the scalp.

Event-Related Desynchronization (ERD) and Synchronization (ERS): Phenomena reflecting sensorimotor brain activity resulting in an amplitude decrease (ERD) or increase (ERS) of oscillatory components. ERD and ERS are stimulus locked but not phase-locked to an event.

Feature Extraction: Transformation of input data into a set of features. Features are distinctive properties of input patterns that help in differentiating between the categories of input patterns.

Humanoid Robot: Autonomous robot whose design is based on the human body.

Motor Imagery (MI): Mental imagination of movements.

Neuroprosthesis: Devices that can substitute for a motor, sensory or cognitive capability that has been lost or damaged due to an injury or disease.

P300 Event Related Potential (ERP): An ERP is an electrical potential shift in EEG that is time-locked to a perceptual, cognitive, or motor event. A P300 ERP is an ERP that occurs about 300 ms after the user consciously attends to a changing visual stimulus.

Virtual Environment (VE): Computer-simulated environment mimicking the real (or an imaginary) world.

Chapter 16
Wireless Sensor Networks and Systems

Jaime Lloret
Polytechnic University of Valencia, Spain

Miguel Garcia
Polytechnic University of Valencia, Spain

Hugo Coll
Polytechnic University of Valencia, Spain

Miguel Edo
Polytechnic University of Valencia, Spain

ABSTRACT

Sensor networks are one of the most powerful technologies applied to control and supervising systems. They are present in almost all environments, so we can find them in different industrial, medical, security and/or home applications. In addition, the use of wireless technologies applied to sensor networks improves the final system. Examples given are the enlargement of the coverage area and the low deployment costs. Nowadays a combination of both items is used in many common implementations of a wide variety of applications. This chapter is focused on the use of sensor networks applied to disabled and elderly people. We will study the wireless technologies most used for this purpose and we will show a survey with the benefits when they are applied.

INTRODUCTION

Since sensors are able to collect data from the environment, sensor networks are used for many application areas. The most well known areas are habitat monitoring, fire detection, motion tracking, reservoir water controlling or intruders controlling (Xu, 2003). In order to control, monitor, tracking or detect something, a large quantity of sensor

DOI: 10.4018/978-1-60566-206-0.ch016

nodes that have to be able to detect the event being monitored (light, pressure, sound, heat, humidity, electro-magnetic field, proximity, location, etc.), is needed. Moreover, the data transmission to a base station, in order to take the appropriate action, must be taken into account. Wireless sensor networks have become very useful for our lives and they have started to be more and more common between us.

The appearance of micro-sensors has encouraged the development of wireless sensor networks in a wide range of applications due to the benefits given by their small size and the possibility of using them in any place because of the wireless technologies.

First of all, the main advantages are the easy installation and the high reduction of the deployment costs. Moreover, because of its physical architecture, these systems can cover higher extension than the wired ones, providing high scalability and being the perfect solution for open scenarios and natural and forest environments. Furthermore, it is fast and easy to make changes on the network once it has been installed. Their flexibility and adaptability are their main features.

This chapter is going to show and describe several wireless sensor networks that were used for disabled and elderly people. It will not be focused on the sensor or what it is measuring, but on the network of sensors, what types are set up and what benefits give a wireless sensor network to the disabled and elderly people.

WIRELESS TECHNOLOGIES

Four main wireless technologies are applied to wireless sensor networks. Depending on the environment where it is going to be used, the type of use, the infrastructure conditions and/or the coverage extension needed, one of them (or a combination of two of them) can result the best option to develop the system.

Bluetooth is an open specification for wireless networks which is based on radiofrequency. It operates in the Industrial Scientific Medical (ISM) frequency band (2.4 GHz) forming wireless personal area networks (WPAN) (IEEE Std 802.15.1-2005, 2005). It has low energy consumption and its cost is quite low. Bluetooth controls its interference, and the susceptibility to the interference, by using spread spectrum modulation. It uses a frequency-hopping spread spectrum signaling method (FHSS). Bluetooth was formalized in IEEE 802.15.1 standard in its version 1.2. This technology uses a small area network without infrastructure (piconets). Nodes share a physical channel with a clock and a unique sequence of jumps in the same piconet. In Bluetooth, different channels can coexist. While a master can only belong to one piconet, any other device can belong to several piconets at the same time. This overlap is denominated scatternet (dispersed network), although there are not defined routing capacities among them. This technology appeared to be used for the devices interconnection like computers, mp3, PDAs, etc. at a distance of about 10m, although lasts products in the market achieve 100m. of coverage radius. Furthermore, this coverage range can be longer with higher antenna gain and even longer distances can be gotten using signal repeaters.

ZigBee is a non-profit alliance with more than 100 members, where most of them are semiconductors manufacturers. ZigBee and IEEE 802.15.4 are standards-based protocols that provide the network infrastructure required for wireless sensor network applications (IEEE Std 802.15.4-2006, 2006). IEEE 802.15.4 defines the physical and MAC layers, and ZigBee defines the network and application layers. This technology is focused on creating low-rate wireless personal area networks (LR-WPAN). Its objective is to develop and to implement a low energy consumption and low cost wireless technology. It is presented as a very economic solution for Wireless Sensor Networks. It is also destined towards energy management, automation and remote control applications. ZigBee products work in a wide range of bands. Examples given are 2.4 Ghz, using the modulation OR-QPSK with expansion direct sequence spread spectrum signaling (DSSS), and 868Mhz in Europe or 915Mhz in North America, using the modulation BPSK with expansion DSSS. Its energy consumption is very low; it consumes 20 times less energy than IEEE 802.11 standard and its implementation is relatively simple. On the contrary, the typical coverage range of ZigBee is around 50m, although this value could increase, depending on the environment.

Radio-frequency identification (RFID) is a technology based on the use of an object (usually called RFID tag) that transmits the identity of an object or person (in the form of a unique serial number) to a receiver using radio waves (Finkenzeller, 2003). A typical RFID tag consists of a microchip with a little amount of memory and an antenna. The memory can store information of a product, a person or a shipment. On the other side, the reader retrieves the data stored on the RFID tag. The system operation is based on the transmission of a query signal and the reception and analysis of the RFID tag response by the receiver. At last, the information obtained is passed to the control system.

RFID tags can be classified in passive and active tags. Passive tags do not have power supplier to make its transmission, so it obtains the energy needed from the query signal. On the other hand, active tags have a small battery in order to supply the power to the tag. RFID operates in Industrial Scientific Medical (ISM) frequency band. There are several frequency ranges for this purpose and, unlike Bluetooth (that only operates in 2.4 GHz), there are RFID systems developed within the four main ISM operating frequency. So we can find systems with an operating frequency from a few KHz to microwaves band (Ward et al. 2006).

Inside the IEEE 802.11 standard (IEEE Std 802.11-2007, 2007), standard variants like IEEE 802.11a, IEEE 802.11b, IEEE 802.11g and IEEE 802.11n are included among others. The original standard also defines the CSMA/CA protocol as the access method. CSMA/CA is a carrier sense and multiple access method used to avoid collisions among the data frames. In Europe, the 2.4000–2.4835 GHz band is divided into 13 channels each of width 22 MHz but spaced only 5 MHz apart, with channel 1 centered on 2.412 GHz and channel 13 on 2.472 GHz to which Japan adds a 14th channel 12 MHz above channel 13. In the United States of America, only the first 11 channels can be used. The availability of channels is regulated by each country, constrained in part by the allocated radio spectrum to various services. IEEE 802.11b data is encoded using direct sequence spread spectrum signaling (DSSS) technology. It uses CCK (Complementary Code Keying) modulated with the QPSK technology to achieve a maximum raw data rate of 11 Mbit/s. IEEE 802.11a/g use orthogonal frequency division multiplexing (OFDM) methods with maximum 52 sub-carriers, achieving a maximum raw data rate of 54 Mbps. IEEE 802.11n is a new standard for wireless communications that presents a significant increase in the maximum raw to a maximum theoretical value of 600 Mbit/s. The current state of the art supports a PHY rate of 450 Mbit/s, with the use of 3 spatial streams at a channel width of 40 MHz. Furthermore, IEEE 802.11n uses MIMO (multiple-input multiple-output); this is the utilization of multiple transmitter and receiver antennas to improve the system performance. MIMO technology provides Spatial Division Multiplexing (SDM) that spatially multiplexes multiple independent data streams which are transferred simultaneously within one spectral channel of bandwidth. This causes the increasement of the data rate and coverage area, in contrast with the other variants. Basically, IEEE 802.11 can work in two ways; the ad-hoc mode, when the stations communicate to each other directly, and infrastructure mode, in which the stations access to the network through one or several access points. Its coverage can reach more than 300 meters. The effective overall coverage range of IEEE 802.11a is lower than that of IEEE 802.11b/g. In theory, IEEE 802.11a signals are absorbed more readily by walls and other solid objects in their path due to their smaller wavelength and, as a result, cannot penetrate as far as those of IEEE 802.11b.

In Table 1, a comparison of the four wireless technologies aforementioned is shown. The operation frequency bands are shown for each technology, coverage area, data rate, battery autonomy and main applications. We can see that there is a common frequency to all technologies, the band of 2.4 GHz. The use of this frequency allows different systems to be interconnected and to work together.

WLAN technology offers the best bandwidth and the highest coverage area, but the power consumption is extremely high compared with the rest of technologies. That is why WLAN is usually used in fixed installations, where the power supply is not result a problem.

RFID let us attach a passive tag to an object or person, so there is no power consumption in this part (the power is supplied by the reader signal). However, the tag has to be very close to the reader in order to send the information (most of RFID applications use the 13.56 MHz band, so the distance between tag and reader should be shorter than 1.5 meters).

Bluetooth and Zigbee are the most used technologies in wireless sensor developments. It is due to their low power consumption while they offer a reasonable coverage area. The first one has higher bandwidth and coverage area, while Zigbee consumes less energy.

However, when developing relatively wide area networks, the best option usually is a combination of Bluetooth, Zigbee or RFID and WLAN, so WLAN is used in fixed receivers or sensors located in all the rooms or chambers of the building and the rest of technologies are used in mobile sensor systems.

Table 1. Wireless technologies comparison table

	WLAN (IEEE 802.11)	Bluetooth (IEEE 802.15.1)	Zigbee (IEEE 802.15.4)	RFID
Frequency Bands	5 GHz (a/n) 2.4 GHz (b/g/n)	2.4 GHz	2.4 GHz 868/915 MHz	2.4 GHz 433 MHz 865/956 MHz 13.56 MHz 125-134 KHz
Raw Data Rate	11 Mbps (2.4 GHz in b) 54 Mbps (2.4 GHz in g or 5 GHz in a) 500 Mbps (2.4 GHz and 5 GHz in n)	1Mbps	250 Kbps (2.4 GHz) 40 Kbps (915 MHz) 20 Kbps (868 MHz)	100 Kbps (2.4 GHz) 30 Kbps (433 - 956 MHz) 25 Kbps (13.56 MHZ) < 1 Kbps (134 KHz)
Coverage Range	100m-300m-900m	10m-100m	30m-50m	10m (2.4 GHz) 5m (956 MHz) 100m (433 MHz) 1.5m (13.56 KHz) < 0.5m (134 KHz)
Battery Autonomy	Hours	Days	Years	Years (Active tags)
Best Applications	Internet Inside building	Computer and phone peripherals	Low-cost control and monitoring	Security and control

SENSOR NETWORK COMPONENTS

A sensor network is formed by sensor nodes, also called motes. Despite of what they are measuring with their sensing unit, a mote needs to process the data and to store it using a processing unit. Then, it also has to transmit the information to the network using the transmitter/receiver unit but taking care of how many energy is available in its power unit (Akyildiz et al. 2002; Khemapech et al. 2005). The processing unit has a processor, usually a microcontroller, a volatile memory and a non-volatile memory, if the data needs to be stored. In order to transmit information, some specific protocols for sensor networks have been proposed. When the information of many motes is coordinated using a protocol, the environment can be measured in great detail. The most well-known protocols will be discussed in the following section. Mote components can be seen in Figure 1.

One of the main issues in today's mote development are its power supply and its size.

A sensor network is a group of motes that cooperate to carry out a specific task. The precision of their tasks depends on the density of the scatter and on the coordination of the motes. In the past, sensor networks were formed by a small number of motes that were connected with a central station, but, nowadays, wireless sensor networks allow distributed networks providing more measurements and closer to the event.

In order to manage the hardware of a mote, an operative system is needed. It is responsible for making the mote to carry out its operations and tasks. Several operative systems have been developed for the motes such as Bertha, MagnetOS, LiteOS, TinyOS and so on.

The programming of sensors is quite complicated because they have a limited calculus capacity and very few resources. Several programming languages have been developed to program the motes. Some of them are nesC, Protothreads, DCL and so on.

Once we have introduced a brief description about motes and some information related with them, the next section describes the protocols used by them for communication.

WIRELESS SENSOR NETWORK PROTOCOLS

In order to enable the communication and data transfer between two sensor nodes, some rules and conventions are needed. A protocol defines the behavior of the nodes, their connections and how they exchange information over the medium. The communication process between motes and how the data from a mote moves through the network to another mote is implemented using communication layers. Each layer is reasonably self-contained so that the tasks assigned to each layer can be implemented independently. This enables the solutions offered by one layer to be updated without adversely affecting the other ones. The sensor has 4 layers. The three upper ones handle data transport issues. A wide variety of communication protocols exist for each one of

Figure 1. Mote components

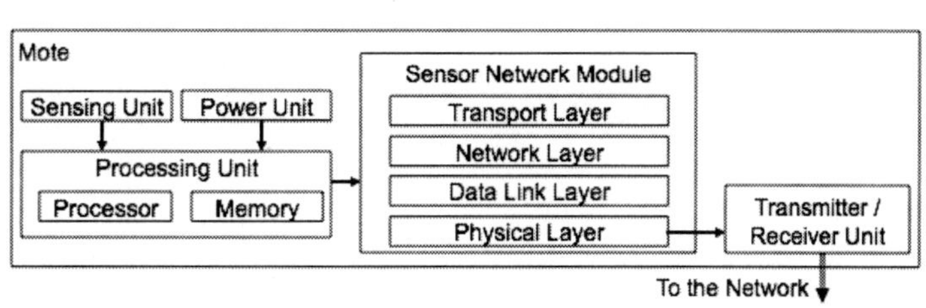

them. The following list gives a brief description of the sensor layers and some protocol examples are given:

1. Physical Layer: It is close to the physical network medium. In this layer is placed how the sensor node transmits to the medium and how receives from it. Wireless sensors use the air as the transmission medium, typically the frequencies of 433 MHz, 915 MHz and 2.4 GHz.
2. Data Link layer: It provides the functional and procedural means of transfering data between network sensor nodes and of detectinf and possibly correcting errors that may occur at the physical layer. Data link layer protocols deployed for wireless sensors are, IEEE 802.15, Bluetooth, ZigBee and RFID.
3. Network Layer: It provides the functional and procedural means of transferring variable length data sequences from a source to a destination through a path. Many routing protocols have been designed for ad-hoc and sensor networks they can be grouped in Pro-active Routing, Reactive Routing, Geographical Routing and so on.
4. Transport Layer: This layer becomes necessary if it is wanted to access the system from Internet or other external networks. As far as we know it is not any work published that discusses or proposes different mechanisms, to be applied in sensor networks exclusively, from the ones used in Internet.

WIRELESS SENSOR NETWORKS FOR DISABLED AND ELDERLY PEOPLE

Because wireless sensor networks have a wide variety of applications, they could be used to monitor, control or track any issue related with disabled of elderly people. In this section we are going to show several wireless sensor network implementations and architectures that are really deployed or proposed for them.

Home-Based Health Monitoring System

This kind of system is based on the installation of several wireless sensors placed inside the house (or in the closest surroundings), so the patient could be always localized. Furthermore, to have under medical control some patients without having a doctor at home is possible by wearing several sensors monitoring their health constants.

In 2006, Bo Sun Hwang et al. developed a monitoring system which was focused on the activities of an individual daily living inside a home (Hwang et al. 2006). Sensors communicate through the Bluetooth protocol. The system detects the movements of a subject and then his/her activity pattern and position in a home is analyzed by a tracking algorithm. The system can be used to monitor disabled and elderly people by means of the actigraph (activity graph) obtained from their system.

Another work was presented by HyungJun Kim et al. in 2006 (HyungJun et al. 2006). This time, they proposed a home-based monitoring system that is continuously and unobtrusively monitoring a patient's condition. The system is implemented using Zigbee technology.

A combination of health care and home automation system is shown by Paulo Bartolomeu Vasco Santos et al. in (Santos et al. 2007). This modular system can mount different subsystems depending on the patient needs. Its main advantage, in addition to be able of sensing several vital signals, is the possibility of automating the house in order to make it accessible for disabled people. It is useful for quadriplegic people. For example, the system can open or close the door when the patient is going to pass through it.

A. Wood et al. presented ALARM-NET, a wireless sensor network for assisted-living and residential monitoring, in (Wood et al. 2006). It integrates environmental and physiological sensors in a heterogeneous architecture in order to determine circadian activity rhythms of the residents.

In 2007, Yaw-Jen Lin et al. presented a ubiquitous monitor system integrated with biosensors and Radio Frequency Identification (RFID) technology (Lin et al. 2007). Patients wear a light weight and small size unit with a RFID tag dotted with memory and three sensors. The sensors measure the pulse rate, blood oxygen saturation and temperature. The building has many RFID readers installed and connected to the control centre, so when a patient pass close to a reader, the tag sends the data allocated in its memory. The system was deployed to improve the activity of daily living of the disabled and elderly people and to detect the emergencies or accidents. It can be sued to enhance the quality of care.

Motion Caption Systems

There are two ways to deply motion caption systems. The first one is installing sensors in the building with motion detection or micro cameras. The second option is to place movement sensors in the patient clothes or attached to his/her body (called wearable sensors), so they get the information directly from the body and transmit it to the receivers sited on the house.

It is possible to determine what activity is doing the patient and detect if he/she has any problem by analyzing his/her motions. In this case, the control centre will attempt to contact with the patient (usually by phone), sending medical assistance when the patient ask for it or when he/she does not answer the phone.

Marjorie Skubic presented in (Skubic, 2007) a multidisciplinary project to investigate the use of thre sensors technology to provide early identification of problems in mobility and cognition. The system helps the residents to manage illnesses and impairments, and stay as healthy and independent as possible. It uses an event-driven video sensor network, which identifies the residents' features, and a reasoning component that fuses sensor and video data and analyzes patterns of the behavioral activity.

F. Brunetti et al. presented a system in (Brunetti et al. 2006) for motion caption and assessment in biomechanics using a wireless inertial sensors network using the IEEE 802.15.4 protocol. The platform expands the frontiers of movement analysis for motion caption. This technology can be applied to a movement study and to wearable robotics like an artificial leg, artificial hand, etc.

Using the same IEEE 802.15.4 protocol, Chao Chen et al. designed a movement and position control system in (Chen et al. 2009). It is based on the use of wearable wireless sensor systems dotted with accelerometers. The system recognizes the speed and angle of the patient movements and his/her position. By analyzing those data, the control system can detect if a person has fallen and, in case of it, it launches an alarm signal.

Nuri F. Ince et al. presented a healthcare service in home setting to elderly and cognitively disabled people in (Ince et al. 2008). It is based on the installation of several fixed sensors that locate the patient at home and, by working together with wearable sensors, collect data to determine what bathroom activities are being done.

Health Body Area Network

The implementation of a Health Body Area Network (HBAN) consists on the attachment of several sensors to check vital statistics and other parameters (depending on the application needs) from the patient in order to have a real-time control.

According to that, Chris Otto et al. presented in (Otto et al. 2006) a system which is able to control the main vital statistics and the intensity and duration of rehabilitation exercises that the patient has to made at home. But, the most important contribution of the proposal is the possibility of having this control wherever the patient is placed. It is possible because of the combination of ZigBee (or Bluetooth) and a mobile phone or personal digital assistant (PDA) GPRS/3G data network connection.

In (Huan-Bang et al. 2007), Huan-Bang Li et al. propose the body area networks as a potential technology to provide high quality of life and comfort for the people. They overviewed some possible application areas and usage models such as medical and healthcare applications and applications for supporting persons with disabilities. They proposed Zigbee and Bluetooth as the wireless technology for the sensors.

An application to rehabilitation centers is presented by Bartosz P. Jarochowski et al. in (Bartosz et al. 2007). In this case the patient wear a personal node placed on a belt clip or incorporated into an arm-band. This node has all the information about the patient's session rehabilitation exercises. He/she can obtain some type of information, such as his/her statistics. The machine can adjust the duration and intensity of the exercise to the medical prescription automatically. It is done by installing receivers on all the exercise machines of the centre which are in communication with the personal node that each patient wears. At the end, the information about all the session is sent to the medical control centre. Then, it is analyzed by the doctors and the planning for the next session is charged on the personal node if it is needed.

Position Estimation

There are several position detection and location tracking systems based on wireless sensor networks. Generally, they are based on the receiver that gathers the signal from the transmitter, which is placed in the patient. There are other systems that are use different signals sent by a group of transmitters to several receivers placed on the building. They are very useful to locate people with Alzheimer or to locate disabled people with very little motion.

Two examples of this kind of systems using the Zigbee technology were presented by Li-wei Chan et al. in (Li-wei et al. 2006) and by A. Marco et al. in (Marco et al. 2008). The last one is the result of a project partially supported by the European Union and by the Spanish Ministry of Science and Technology.

Another proposal was presented by the same authors of this paper in (García et al. 2007), but, we used the WLAN technology instead of ZigBee. The paper shows two approaches where wireless sensors could find their position using the WLAN technology. The scenario is an indoor environment that contains walls, interferences, multipath effect, humidity and temperature variations, etc., and both approaches are based on the Received Signal Strength Indicator (RSSI). Both Indoor Position Systems are developed taking into account real measurements of the signal variations. Then, we compared our proposals with other systems in existence in (Lloret et al. 2009). It was not proposed only for disabled and elderly people, but it can be used for it.

Later, the same authors proposed a new stochastic approach in (Lloret et al. 2009). It is based on the combination of deductive and inductive methods (in order to provide accurate measurements in hard environments). Wireless sensors could find their position using IEEE 802.11b/g standard inside the floor of a building. The system uses the deployed wireless access network that is also used for internet access and data transfer. Our goal was to reduce the training phase in an indoor environment; but, without loosing precision. Finally, we compare the measurements taken from our proposal in a real environment with the measurements taken from other developed systems providing the best results. The system proposed can be used for disabled and elderly people in order to estimate their position.

Table 2. Technologies used in home-based health monitoring systems

Reference	WLAN	Bluetooth	ZigBee	RFID
B. S. Hwang et al. (Hwang et al. 2006)		X		
HyungJun Kim et al. (HyungJun et al. 2006)			X	
V. Saaantos et al. (Santos et al. 2007)			X	
A. Wood et al. (Wood et al. 2006)	Not defined			
Yaw-Jen Lin et al. (Lin et al. 2007)				X

Assisted Displacements

Wireless Sensor Networks can be applied to deploy systems oriented to help disabled people in order to move on their own in a safe way.

One of the most used applications to assist the displacements is the wheelchair. It consists of a range of sensors mounted with the objective to avoid collisions. A good survey about intelligent autonomous wheelchairs to provide navigation feedback and obstacle detection was presented by T. Gomi et al. in (Gomi et al. 1998). But none of the sensor systems presented used a wireless sensor network, only wired. Another solution was presented by J. L. Sevillano et al. in (Sevillano et al. 2009). In case of indoor scenarios, their proposal is to set up a detection system based on cameras on the ceiling of the different plants of the building. Using this system, the wheelchair does not need to carry a lot of equipment. Thus, it is cheaper and more battery saver.

A. Mpitziopoulos et al. presented in (Mpitziopoulos et al. 2008) a system to help blind people to walk around the city. The system detects possible obstacles on the street and looks for an alternative path in order to arrive to the desired destination.

ANALYSIS OF THE USE OF WIRELESS TECHNOLOGIES

Once we have shown a wide variety of networks and systems and their possible applications, let us analyze the technologies from the point of view of the implementation. Tables from 2 to 6 show the technologies used in each system. They are referenced in order of appearance.

Table 2 shows the technologies used in Home-Based Health Monitoring Systems. In this sort of applications, WLAN technology was the only one that was not used. In case of reference (Wood et al. 2006), the system is presented without telling what technology was used. This is because they only presented a theoretical model.

Table 3 presents the technologies used in Home-Based Health Monitoring Systems. As we can see, in this case, there is a preference in using ZigBee instead of Bluetooth. The authors of ref-

Table 3. Technologies used in motion caption systems

Reference	WLAN	Bluetooth	ZigBee	RFID
M. Skubic (Skubic, 2007)	X			
F. Brunetti et al (Brunetti et al. 2006)			X	
C. Chen and C. Pomalaza-Ráez (Chen et al. 2009)			X	
J. L. Sevillano et al. (Ince et al. 2008)	Not defined			

Table 4. Technologies used in health body area network

Reference	WLAN	Bluetooth	ZigBee	RFID	Other
Chris Otto et al. (Otto et al. 2006)		X	X		3G/GPRS
Huan-Bang Li et al. (Huan-Bang et al. 2007)		X	X		
B. P. Jarochowski et al. (Bartosz et al. 2007)			X		

Table 5. Technologies used in position estimation

Reference	WLAN	Bluetooth	ZigBee	RFID
Li-wei Chan et al. (Li-wei et al. 2006)			X	
A. Marco et al. (Marco et al. 2008)			X	
M. Garcia et al. (García et al. 2007) and J. Lloret et al. (Lloret et al. 2009)	X			
J. Lloret et al. (Lloret et al. 2009)	X			

erence (Ince et al. 2008) do not define the type of technology used because it was a theoretical work.

Table 4 shows the technologies used in Health Body Area Network. References (Otto et al. 2006) and (Huan-Bang et al. 2007) were deployed to be used by Bluetooth or ZigBee. In (Otto et al. 2006), a 3G or GPRS connection is used in addition to Bluetooth or ZigBee.

Table 5 shows the technologies used for position estimation. These applications are deployed with ZigBee. The systems presented by the same authors of this chapter used WLAN technology.

Finally, in Table 6, we can see the technologies used in assisted displacements.

Figure 2 shows the percentage of usage of each wireless technology for disabled and elderly people. Information gathered show that ZigBee is the widest deployed technology. This is due to its extremely low power consumption. When power supply is not so limited, Bluetooth is a good alternative. WLAN become the best technology when the system needs to cover a wide area and when the power supply is not a problem.

CONCLUSIONS AND FUTURE WORK

This chapter has demonstrated the benefits of the wireless sensor networks and systems for disables and elderly people. We have shown in this chapter that there are four main wireless technologies applied to sensor networks. There are many works that use them to develop different control and helping systems for disabled and elderly people. Although there are many proposals, most of them are theoretical and their implementation in real

Table 6. Technologies used in assisted displacements

Reference	WLAN	Bluetooth	ZigBee	RFID
T. Gomi and A. Griffith (Gomi et al. 1998)	No applicable			
J. L. Sevillano et al. (Sevillano et al. 2009)			X	
A. Mpitziopoulos et al. (Mpitziopoulos et al. 2008)	Not defined			

Figure 2. Percentage of use of wireless technologies

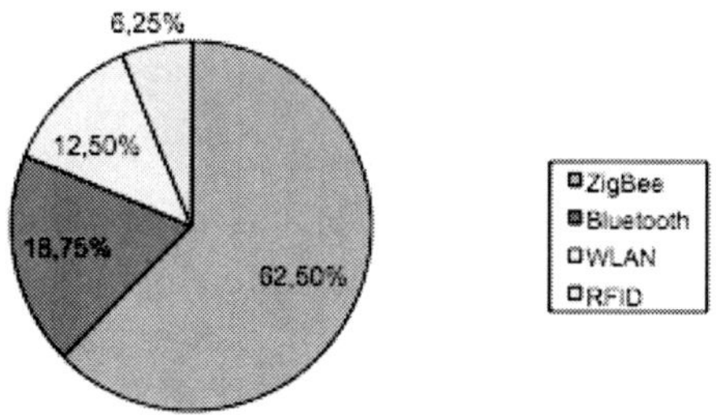

environments is not as high as desired. It is maybe due to their low commercialization.

Zigbee is the most used technology for disabled an elderly people. It is given because this technology does not consume too much power, so it is the best option for wearable devices. But, when it is needed to cover higher distances and monitor wide areas, and the power can be supplied without proplems, WLAN is the best technology.

In a near future, the main goal is to make these technologies more accessible by enhancing the wireless sensor networks in order to obtain a global remote healthcare system. In this way, we consider that future researches should implement groups of sensors (Lloret et al. 2007) to make life easier for disabled and elderly people.

REFERENCES

Akyildiz, I. F., Su, W., Sankarasubramaniam, Y., & Cayirci, E. (2002, August). A survey on sensor networks. *IEEE Communications Magazine*, 102–114. doi:10.1109/MCOM.2002.1024422

Brunetti, F., Moreno, J. C., Ruiz, A. F., Rocon, E., & Pons, J. L. (2006). A new platform based on IEEE802.15.4 wireless inertial sensors for motion caption and assessment. *28th Annual International Conference of the IEEE Engineering in Medicine and Biology Society. EMBS '06* (pp. 6497-6500). New York, USA.

Chan, L., Chiang, J., Chen, Y., Ke, C., Hsu, J., & Chu, H. (2006, May). *Collaborative localization: enhancing wifi-based position estimation with neighborhood links in clusters*. Paper presented at the 4th International Conference on Pervasive Computing (Pervasive 2006), Dublin Ireland.

Chen, C., & Pomalaza-Ráez, C. (2009, February). *Monitoring Human Movements at Home Using Wearable Wireless Sensors*. Paper presented at the Third International Symposium on Medical Information & Communication Technology, Montreal (Canada).

Finkenzeller, K. (2003). *RFID handbook: fundamentals and applications in contactless smart cards and identification* (2nd ed.). West Sussex, UK: Wiley.

Garcia, M., Martinez, C., Tomas, J., & Lloret, J. (2007, October). *Wireless Sensors self-location in an Indoor WLAN environment*. International Conference on Sensor Technologies and Applications (SENSORCOMM 2007), Valencia (Spain).

Gomi, T., & Griffith, A. (1998). Developing intelligent wheelchairs for the handicapped. In Mittal et al. (Eds.), *Assistive technology and AI* (LNAI 1458, pp. 150-78).

Hwang, B. S., Choi, J. M., & Park, K. S. (2006, October). *A novel method for unobtrusive measurement of indoor activities using sensor-based monitoring system*. The International Special Topic Conference on Information Technology in Biomedicine (ITAB 2006), Ioannina, Greece.

IEEE. (2005). IEEE Std 802.15.1-2005 (Revision of IEEE Std 802.15.1-2002) (pp. 0_1-580).

IEEE. (2006). IEEE Std 802.15.4-2006 (Revision of IEEE Std 802.15.4-2003) (pp. 0_1-305).

IEEE. (2007). IEEE Std 802.11-2007 (Revision of IEEE Std 802.11-1999) (pp. C1-1184).

Ince, N. F., Min, C., Tewfik, A. H., & Vanderpool, D. (2008). *Detection of Early Morning Daily Activities with Static Home and Wearable Wireless Sensors*. Journal on Advances in Signal Processing.

Jarochowski, B. P., Shin, S., Ryu, D., & Kim, H. (2007). Ubiquitous Rehabilitation Center: An Implementation of a Wireless Sensor Network Based Rehabilitation Management System. In *Proceedings of the 2007 International Conference on Convergence Information Technology* (pp. 2349-2358). Washington, DC: IEEE Computer Society.

Khemapech, I., Duncan, I., & Miller, A. (2005, June). A survey of wireless sensor networks technology. In *Proceedings of the 6th Annual PostGraduate Symposium on the Convergence of Telecommunications, Networking & Broadcasting*. Liverpool, UK.

Kim, H., Jarochowski, B., & Ryu, D. (2006). A Proposal for a Home-Based Health Monitoring System for the Elderly or Disabled (LNCS 4061, pp. 473-479).

Li, H.-B., Takizawa, K., Zhen, B., & Kohno, R. (2007, July). Body Area Network and Its Standardization at IEEE 802.15.MBAN. *16th IST Mobile and Wireless Communications Summit* (pp. 1-5). Budapest, Hungary.

Lin, Y.-J., Su, M.-J., Chen, S.-J., Wang, S.-C., Lin, C.-I., & Chen, H.-S. (2007, April). A Study of Ubiquitous Monitor with RFID in an Elderly Nursing Home. *International Conference on Multimedia and Ubiquitous Engineering (MUE'07)* (pp. 336-340). Seoul, Korea.

Lloret, J., Garcia, M., Boronat, F., & Tomás, J. (2009, June). The Development of Two Systems for Indoor Wireless Sensors Self-location. *Ad Hoc & Sensor Wireless Networks: An International Journal*, *8*(3-4), 235–258.

Lloret, J., Garcia, M., & Tomas, J. (2007, June). *A Group-Based Architecture for Wireless Sensor Networks*. International Conference on Networking and Services (ICNS'07). Athens (Greece).

Lloret, J., Tomás, J., Garcia, M., & Cánovas, A. (2009, May). Hybrid Stochastic Approach for Wireless Sensors Self-Location in Indoor Environments. *Sensors (Basel, Switzerland)*, *9*(5), 3695–3712. doi:10.3390/s90503695

Marco, A., Casas, R., Falco, J., Gracia, H., Artigas, J. I., & Roy, A. (2008). Location-based services for elderly and disabled people. *Computer Communications*, *31*(6), 1055–1066. doi:10.1016/j.comcom.2007.12.031

Mpitziopoulos, A., Konstantopoulos, C., Gavalas, D., & Pantziou, G. (2008). Hazard Monitoring for Visually Impaired People Enabled by Wireless Sensor Networking Technology. In *Proceedings of the 1st international conference on Pervasive technologies related to assistive environments* (Vol. 282, Article 21).

Otto, C., Milenković, A., Sanders, C., & Jovanov, E. (2006). System architecture of a wireless body area sensor network for ubiquitous health monitoring. *Journal of Mobile Multimedia*, *1*(4), 307–326.

Santos, V., Bartolomeu, P., Fonseca, J., & Mota, A. (2007, July). *B-Live - A Home Automation System for Disabled and Elderly People*. Paper presented at the International Symposium on Industrial Embedded Systems. SIES '07. Lisboa (Portugal).

Sevillano, J. L., Cascado, D., Cagigas, D., Vicente, S., Luján, C. D., & Díaz del Rio, F. (2009, May). *A Real-Time Wireless Sensor Network for Wheelchair Navigation*. Paper presented at the 7th IEEE/ACS International Conference on Computer Systems and Applications. Rabat (Morocco)

Skubic, M. (2005). *Assessing Mobility and Cognitive Problems in Elders*. AAAI 2005 Fall Symposium, Workshop on Caring Machines: AI in Eldercare. Arlington, Virginia, November, 2005.

Ward, M., van Kranenburg, R., & Backhouse, G. (2006). *RFID: Frequency, standards, adoption and innovation*. JISC Technology and Standards Watch.

Wood, A., Virone, G., Doan, T., Cao, Q., Selavo, L., Wu, Y., et al. (2006). *ALARM-NET: Wireless Sensor Networks for Assisted-Living and Residential Monitoring* (Tech Rep CS-2006-11). Department of Computer Science, University of Virginia.

Xu, N. (2003). *A survey of sensor network applications, Survey Paper for CS694a*. Computer Science Department, University of Southern California. Retrieved from http://enl.usc.edu/~ningxu/papers/survey.pdf

KEY TERMS AND DEFINITIONS

Ad-Hoc Network: An ad-hoc network is a local area network (LAN) that is built spontaneously as devices connect and based on the communication between all the members without the need of a network controller to coordinate the flow of messages in the network.

Frequency-Hopping Spread Spectrum: FHSS is a method of transmitting radio signals by rapidly switching a carrier among many frequency channels. In order to synchronize the transmitter and the receiver a pseudorandom sequence known by both is used. Bluetooth has been designed to operate in noisy radio frequency environments. That noise produces interferences in the system, being allocated in some random frequencies. By switching among frequencies the impact of noise results highly decreased.

IEEE 802 Standard: An IEEE 802 standard is a group of rules that specifies how to implement a local or metropolitan area network. That rules are determined by the Institute of Electrical and Electronics Engineers (IEE), and there are many different standards, each one defining one communications system. So, IEEE 802.11 standard is dedicated to wireless local area networks (WLAN) and 802.15 defines wireless personal area networks.

Industrial Scientific Medical (ISM) Frequency Bands: The ISM radio bands are a group of frequency ranges originally reserved internationally for the use of RF electromagnetic fields for industrial, scientific and medical purposes other than communications. Due to the initial potential use of these frequencies, all equipments must be protected from interferences at ISM bands. This interference protection is the reason for which nowadays several of these frequencies are used by unlicensed communications devices, like cordless phones.

Piconet: Also called Bluetooth personal area network, a piconet is a network of devices connected ad hoc using Bluetooth technology. A piconet is formed when at least two devices connect, and can support up to eight devices.

Routing Protocol: A routing protocol is a set of rules which function is to determinate what is the correct way and order for information to be sent in a computer network. As a computer software, it is executed and the transmitter obtain as a result in which direction data have to be sent in order to arrive to the desired receiver (the data can go through several equipments before get the destination).

Scatternet: A group of independent and non-synchronized piconets that share at least one common Bluetooth device.

Chapter 17
Model-Based Approaches for Scanning Keyboard Design:
Present State and Future Directions

Samit Bhattacharya
Indian Institute of Technology Guwahati, India

ABSTRACT

Many individuals with speech and motor disorders face problems in expressing themselves in an easy and intelligible way. An array of Augmentative and Alternative Communication (AAC) devices and techniques is used to alleviate their problems. One of the commonly used computer based AAC systems is the scanning keyboards. A scanning keyboard refers to an on-screen keyboard operated with a scanning input method. There are many ways to place alpha-numeric characters on the keyboard interface. Therefore, it is necessary to compare alternative layouts to determine the best one in terms of user performance. Usually, layouts are compared by testing prototypes with physically disabled users. This approach is problematic since it is difficult to get physically disabled users or collect data from those users. An alternative approach is to use models to compute user performance, which can serve as the basis of layout comparison as well as automatic design space exploration. Several of these models and design space exploration algorithms are reported in the literature. A review of these works is presented in this chapter. The chapter is concluded with a discussion on the limitations of the existing works and the issues that can be taken up for further research.

INTRODUCTION

Speech and writing are two of our primary means of communication. However, there are many individuals who face problems in expressing themselves in an easy and intelligible way using either of these means, due to their physical disabilities. Their problems arise because of the non-functional or partially functional body parts, which are responsible for producing speech and

DOI: 10.4018/978-1-60566-206-0.ch017

motor actions. Such disabilities include Cerebral Palsy, Muscular Dystrophy, Friedrich's Ataxia, Quadriplegia and spinal cord injuries with characteristic symptoms of tremor, spasm, poor motor co-ordination, restricted limb movement, reduced muscle strength, slurring of speech or no speech at all. Similar symptoms are also seen among the elderly able-bodied population afflicted with Parkinson's disease, strokes and arthritis. Computer based *Augmentative and Alternative Communication* (AAC) systems and techniques are developed to assist these people in their day-to-day communications (Beukelman & Miranda, 1998).

AAC systems are used as writing tools by persons who fail to control their extremities and also as communication prosthesis by those having speech disorders. The generation of text in both of these cases is a necessary activity. Text generation with computers requires the use of the *direct* input devices like mouse or keyboard. Many individuals with severe motion impairments, however, lack sufficient mobility to reach for these devices or sufficient motor control to switch accurately and efficiently between them. The *scanning keyboards* provide an alternative interface for text generation to them. In this chapter, model-based approaches for *efficient* scanning keyboard design are discussed. The term *efficient* here refers to designs that allow users to achieve high text entry rate with high accuracy. The chapter is organized as follows.

In the next section, a survey on AAC systems is presented. The survey is followed by a detailed discussion on scanning keyboards, including the challenges faced by the scanning keyboard designers. The different model-based approaches are discussed next along with the strengths and weaknesses of each approach and the scope for future research.

SURVEY OF AAC SYSTEMS

There exists wide variation in the physical, cognitive and linguistic abilities of individuals who need AAC. In order to cater to diverse user requirements, different AAC systems and techniques have been developed. The simplest of these techniques include attention calling bell, communication through *yes* or *no*, gestures and message cards. The most sophisticated among these non-electronic means of augmentative communication are the *communication boards*. A communication board can contain alphanumeric characters, words, icons, symbols, phrases or sentences (Worah, 2001). In order to convey a message, users of such boards "point" (with fingers or head-mounted pointers) to the appropriate items present on the board. In addition to these non-electronic techniques, many computer-based AAC systems are also used. Computer-based systems can be classified depending on the nature of the input as the (a) non-text based and (b) text based.

In the non-text based AAC systems, communicative messages are composed with the selection of icons or images from the system interface. An example is the "MinSpeak" system (Albacete et al., 1998), where *ambiguous* icons (i.e. each icon having multiple meanings associated with it) are used as input. In order to form a communicative message, users select two or more of these icons in sequence, which is converted to a textual and/or spoken message. In the "Picture WordPower" by Nancy Inman (http://www.inmaninnovations.com/), messages are constructed with unambiguous icons. Each icon corresponds to a linguistic item. A user needs to select a sequence of these icons following the syntactic word ordering of English to form a message. Another system that uses unambiguous icons is the "iconCHAT" by Patel et al. (2004). In order to compose a message with "iconCHAT", a user needs to first select the verb, and then specify the agent, object, and various other verb-dependent message components. A similar approach was reported by Bhattacharya and Basu (in press) to implement "Sanyog", an iconic system in Indian languages. Apart from icons, symbols and sign languages are also used for non-text based AAC[1].

As opposed to the non-text based AAC systems, textual units such as characters, words or phrases are used to compose messages in the text-based AAC systems. The non-text based systems are primarily developed for individuals who lack the sophisticated grammatical knowledge for composing complex linguistic constructs like complex sentences or paragraphs, such as children, adults with cognitive retardation and neo-literates. For users having the required linguistic abilities, the text based systems are preferred as those offer more flexibility in creating novel and spontaneous texts that are essential for having a natural communication.

A concern for the designers of the text-based systems is the communication rate that a user can achieve. It is observed that persons who need to use AAC usually have low spoken communication rate (less than 8 *words per minute* (WPM) in some cases (Beukelman & Miranda, 1998)), compared to those without any communication impairments (ranging from 150 to 250 WPM (Goldman-Eisler, 1986)). On the other hand, while skilled typists can achieve text entry rates in the range of 30-40 WPM, speech and motion impaired users can only output at best 10-15 WPM using a keyboard (Copestake, 1997). The text entry rate of AAC users drops further if alternate input methods (e.g. scanning and access switches) are used. However, alternate input methods are a necessity for many AAC users due to their physical disabilities (Johansen & Hansen, 2002).

In order to balance the trade-off between the text entry rate and the alternate input methods, the size of the input textual unit is varied resulting in a range of text-based AAC systems. At one end of this range are the *character level* text entry systems, where text is composed from individual characters. Scanning keyboards are examples of character level text entry systems. Soft keyboards operated with *eye trackers* (Hansen et al., 2004) or other types of alternate direct input methods are also used as character-level text entry systems. Text entry rate of AAC users of soft keyboard based systems were reported to vary between 0.5 to 5 WPM (Instance et al., 1996; Vanderheiden, 1988). To increase the text entry rate, several *rate enhancement techniques* were proposed and augmented with soft keyboards. These included *prediction* (Garay-Vitoria & Abascal, 2006) of next characters or word, *abbreviation expansion* (Lesher & Moulton, 2005) and *ambiguous keyboards* (Lesher et al., 1998a). Such augmented soft keyboards were reported to have higher text entry rates (6-8 WPM, (Lesher et al., 1998b)).

Another group of character-level text entry systems developed for AAC users are the *gesture* driven systems. In these systems, *continuous gestures* are used to input characters. The *trackball EdgeWrite* (Wobbrock & Myers, 2006) is an example of such systems, having a text entry rate of 6-8 WPM. The *Dasher* system (Ward & Mackay, 2002), however, was reported to have a high text entry rate of 25 WPM with eye tracking input method.

In order to improve the rate of text entry, other text entry methods with higher level of *input units*, such as words and phrases were proposed. The *Compansion* system (Demasco & McCoy, 1992), for example, was designed to process and expand a group of un-inflected content words into a full phrase or sentence. Copestake (1997) reported a similar system, called *Cogeneration*. Depending on the vocabulary organization, users of Compansion systems can achieve text entry rates in the range of 10-15 WPM. *Storage and recall* of larger text passages, including phrases, sentences and paragraphs within an AAC system was proposed to obtain even higher rate of text entry. In addition to simple storage and recall systems, *conversational modeling* was also tried. In AAC systems that attempt to model conversational situations, *scripts* (Dye et al., 1998), *schemata* (Carpenter et al., 1997) and *frames* (Higginbotham et al., 1999) are stored along with phrases and sentences for recall and use within conversational settings. The reported rate of communication with such systems was relatively high (e.g. 64 WPM with the TALK system (Todman, 2000)).

Although the text entry rate increases as the unit of input becomes larger, character level text input continues to be needed within higher order AAC systems (word level and storage and recall based) for the creation of novel and spontaneous statements during conversation (Arnott, 2005). It is also needed to support off-line writing tasks, including the composition of essays, stories, letters and messages. Hence, there is a continuing need in AAC for design of improved character-level text entry methods with alternate inputs. Being a character-level text input method widely used by AAC users, design of efficient scanning keyboards is therefore a necessary and important area of research.

SCANNING KEYBOARDS

The core component of a scanning keyboard is a *soft* keyboard (Trewin & Arnott, 2007; Venkatgiri, 1999). The keys are laid out spatially in rows and columns on the keyboard interface. Users select the keys from the interface to compose text. The keys are selected using a scanning input method.

As opposed to direct selection, scanning input methods are called *indirect* or *sequential* selection methods (Venkatgiri, 1999). In scanning input, the interface elements are periodically and successively highlighted. This process is called *scanning*. The scanning methods implemented on soft keyboards are often called the *matrix scanning* (Steriadis & Constantinou, 2003). In such scanning, the screen is assumed to represent a matrix. The items present on the screen are individual cells of that matrix. The most general form of matrix scanning is a 3-level scan, often called the *block-row-item* scan. In a 3-level scan, the on-screen items are grouped into *blocks*. Each block comprises of a set of *rows* of items. The system initially starts a block level scan. During this process, the block that contains the desired item is selected by the user. Once a block is selected, the system begins a row level scan inside the block. During the row level scanning, the row in which the desired item lies is selected. Then the items of the selected row are scanned. When the scanning reaches the desired item, the item is selected. Other two variants of the 3-level scanning are the 2-level (or *row-item*) scanning and the 1-level (or *item*) scanning. Each matrix scanning method is implemented in either of the two ways, namely (a) *auto* scanning and (b)*guided* scanning. In auto scanning, a highlighter moves automatically through on-screen elements, pausing at each element for a pre-defined time delay called the *scan period*. When the highlighter pauses on the desired element, users activate an *access switch* to select the element. In guided scanning, both the tasks of moving the highlighter (called *navigation*) and selecting a highlighted element are performed through activation of access switches, requiring more than one access switch to operate such interfaces.

Access switches are specially designed devices that require lesser motor control to operate than mouse or keyboard. Any active body part of a user including hand, foot, mouth or head can be used to operate such switches. In order to cater to users with various types and degrees of disabilities, switches of different shapes and sizes are developed. Some of these switches are shown in Figure 1. The switch activation depends on the type of access switch. For example, in case of a press switch (Figure 1(a)), switch activation implies putting pressure on the switch surface. The switch shown in Figure 1(b) can be activated by lips.

Figure 2 illustrates a scanning keyboard in which a 2-level scanning is used to operate a QWERTY-like soft keyboard. Selection of the letter `F' from this interface is carried out in two steps. In the first step shown in Figure 2(a), rows of the keyboard are scanned. When the row containing `F' is highlighted, the row is selected by activating an access switch. In the second step

Figure 1. Different types of access switches

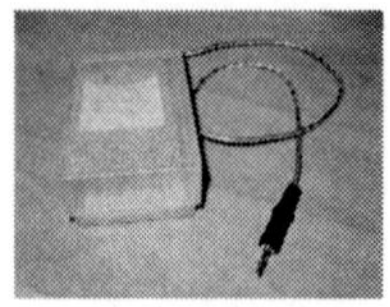

(a) Press switch

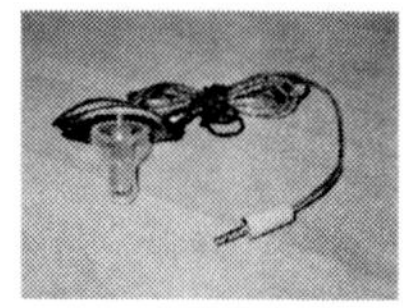

(b) Lip switch

shown in Figure 2(b), the items in the row are scanned. When `F' is highlighted, it is selected.

Design Issue

Use of the sequential access makes text entry with scanning keyboards very slow. Typical entry rates for such keyboards vary between 0.5-5 WPM. Moreover, disabled users are found to make significant amount of errors during text entry with such keyboards (Bhattacharya et al., 2008b), which further affects their text entry rate.

Both the keyboard layout as well as the scanning input method determines the speed and accuracy of text entry with scanning keyboards. There can be *k*! possible layouts for a keyboard with *k* keys. Moreover, scanning can be implemented in any one of the six different ways (i.e. 3-level, 2-level and 1-level scanning, each of which can be implemented either as auto scanning or guided scanning) for each of these possible layouts. The variations in both the layouts and the input methods result in a large *design space* for scanning keyboards. For example, a 27 letter scanning keyboard has 27! possible layouts. Taking into

Figure 2. Example of a scanning keyboard

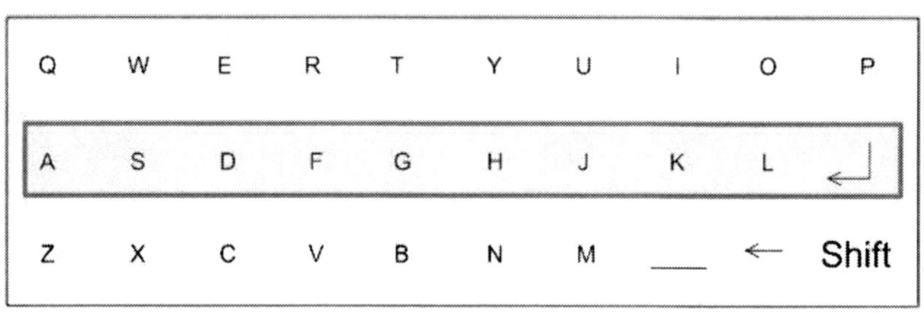

(a) First step: row scan

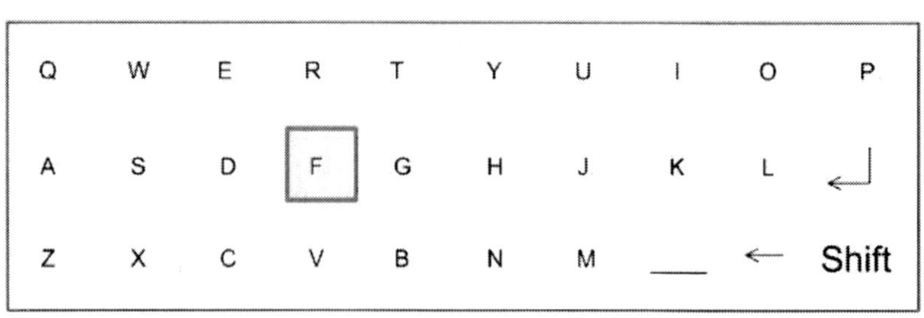

(b) Second step: item scan

account the six different scanning input methods, the total size of the design space becomes 6×27! or approximately 6.5×10^{28}. The challenge to a designer of scanning keyboards is to choose an appropriate design from this large design space.

Need for Model-Based Approach

In order to search for a suitable design from the design space, designers often rely on their experience and intuition. Even for an experienced designer, experience rarely leads to a single design. Consequently, designers implement prototype systems and evaluate them with real users. However, with AAC systems such an approach has the following two problems.

a. It is difficult to find sufficient number of disabled users for evaluation. In many developing countries like India, social conditions prevent many disabled users from revealing their identities and hence participate in the design process. Also, lack of exposure to computers in the disabled community in these countries compounds this problem.
b. Collection of sufficiently large usage data for analysis is also problematic. The problem arises due to the disabilities of the users who can not work continuously for a long stretch of time. Sometimes it takes several months to collect data.

As a result, designers have to rely on a limited amount of usage time to test their systems. These difficulties point to the necessity of working towards an automated design approach, which helps to make efficient use of the limited usage data. In the literature related to scanning keyboard design, works which attempted to replace or reduce user testing in the design cycle using automated or semi-automated design techniques can be found. These works are broadly of the following two types.

a. *Model based evaluation techniques*: In this group of works, *performance models* were employed to evaluate designs. Performance models are cognitive-psychological behavioral models of the users, which could *compute* user performance for a given design. For text entry systems, user performance is commonly measured in terms of the *rate of text entry*. The design approach works as follows. Given a set of design alternatives, performance models compute text entry rate for each design in the set. The designs are then compared on the basis of the computed text entry rates, in order to determine the best among the set.
b. *Automatic exploration of design space*: The above approach was developed primarily to identify the best design in a given set of design alternatives, assuming that the alternatives are limited in number. In other words, the approach is suitable when a small subset of the design space is present. However, it is also possible to find out a *good* design by exploring the entire space of alternative designs. A number of design space exploration algorithms were reported in the literature to achieve this objective. All these algorithms used performance models to compare designs during the exploration of the design space.

These two approaches are discussed in details in the following sections.

PERFORMANCE MODELS FOR SCANNING KEYBOARDS

The performance models reported in the literature that are relevant to scanning keyboard design are of the following three types.

a. Models to compute the performance of AAC users of soft keyboards.

b. Models to compute the performance of a scanning keyboard user.
c. Models to compute the performance of soft keyboard users having no disabilities.

These models and their role in the design of scanning keyboards are discussed next.

KLM/GOMS Models

KLM (acronym for **K**eystroke **L**evel **M**odel) and its successor GOMS (acronym for **G**oals, **O**perators, **M**ethods and **S**election rules) are two predictive user modeling techniques widely used in the field of human computer interaction (John & Kieras, 1996). KLM/GOMS models allow designers to perform quantitative analysis of system behavior from a description of the system, making it possible to identify design problems or compare designs.

Both of these techniques were applied to model performance of AAC users. Development of GOMS models for evaluation of soft keyboards for disabled users was reported by Horstmann and Levine (1990). Koester and Levine (1997) used KLM for the same purpose. Any KLM/GOMS analysis consists of the following stages.

1. A prototype of the system is conceptualized/designed.
2. A typical task is described using the corresponding *modeling language*. The description consists of the steps to be taken to carry out the given task. For KLM analysis, the description is a linear sequence of basic steps known as the *primitives*. A hierarchy of *goals* is used to describe the task in GOMS. At the lowest level of the goal hierarchy are the primitives.
3. A quantitative analysis of the task description is performed using pre-determined values of the primitives.

Model by Rosen and Goodenough-Trepagnier

Rosen and Goodenough-Trepagnier (1981) developed a model to compute performance of soft keyboard users, with particular emphasis to users with motor disorders. In subsequent discussions, this model is referred to as the RG model. Three parameters were used to develop the RG model, which are described below.

Linguistic cost ***c***, measured in average number of language units per word. For a device in which selections are made from alphabetic characters, each character represents a language unit. Other possible language units might be phonemes, morphemes, graphemes or complete words depending upon the specific communication aid and its implementation. The objective of choosing a particular language unit in a given design problem is the reduction of *c*.

Average number of motor acts per language unit ***m***. A sequence of motor acts may be required to select a language unit. As an example, encoding the 26 letters, space and period so that they can be generated using only 10 keys will require multiple keystrokes for at least some of the characters.

Average time per act ***t***. In a traditional keyboard, this is the time per keystroke. If instead the characters are displayed on a monitor and a joystick is used to move a cursor, it becomes the average time to "acquire and shoot" a target. In a scanning input system, it is the average scan time plus the average switch activation time per selection.

From these three parameters, average time required to form a word t_w was calculated using Eq. 1.

$$t_w = c \times m \times t \qquad (1)$$

Equation 1 represents text entry tasks without reference to any specific input method. An extension to the RG model was proposed by Damper

(1984), to make the model applicable to scanning keyboards. In the extended RG model, the average time to compose a word (t_w of Eq. 1) was calculated with Eq. 2.

$$t_w = \frac{c}{r}\sum_{i=1}^{K} p_i(s_i + 1) \tag{2}$$

In Eq. 2, r is the *scan rate* (i.e. number of scan periods per second), p_i is the probability of occurrence of the ith character present on the interface (calculated from a corpus of text) and s_i is the number of *scan steps* (i.e. shifting of highlighter) required to select the ith character starting from a pre-determined or *home* position. K is the total number of keys present on the interface. From Eq. 2, the communication rate of scanning keyboard users in WPM was measured as $1/t_w$.

Soukoreff-MacKenzie Model

Soukoreff and MacKenzie (1995) proposed a model, often called the FD model (MacKenzie & Soukoreff, 2002; Zhai et al., 2002), to evaluate soft keyboards used on small sized mobile devices like PDAs. The model did not consider any physical disabilities on the part of a user and it was assumed that the user would select keys from the interface with finger (touch) or stylus movement. Following components were considered to develop the model.

Visual search time: To select a character from a keyboard interface, the user first needs to locate the corresponding key on the interface. The time to locate a key is called the *visual search time* and is denoted by *RT*. In the FD model, *RT* was calculated using the Hick-Hyman law (Hick, 1952; Hyman, 1953) shown in Eq. 3, where a and b are constants and K is the total number of keys present on the interface.

$$RT = a + b\log_2 K \tag{3}$$

Movement time: In addition to locating the character, the user also needs to move finger or stylus from the current location to select the key. The time to make a manual movement from one key to another (movement time) was calculated using the Fitts' law (Fitts & Peterson, 1964) shown in Eq. 4 where MT_{ij} is the movement time from the source to target key, a' and b' are constants, d_{ij} is the Cartesian distance between the two keys and w_j is the width of the target key.

$$MT_{ij} = a' + b'\log_2\left(\frac{d_{ij}}{w_j} + 1\right) \tag{4}$$

Digraph probability: In the FD model, the probability of occurrence of character pairs or *digraphs* was considered. The digraph probability was calculated from a text corpus by Eq. 5, where $freq_{ij}$ is the digraph frequency and DP_{ij} is the digraph probability of characters k_i and k_j. K is the total number of individual characters present on the interface.

$$DP_{ij} = \frac{freq_{ij}}{\sum_{i=1}^{K}\sum_{j=1}^{K} freq_{ij}} \tag{5}$$

From DP_{ij} and MT_{ij}, the mean movement time MT_m for a given layout was calculated with Eq. 6.

$$MT_m = \sum_{i=1}^{K}\sum_{j=1}^{K} DP_{ij} \times MT_{ij} \tag{6}$$

Using Eq. 3 and Eq. 6, the user performance for a soft keyboard was calculated in *characters per second* (CPS). Two categories of users were assumed to calculate performance; *novice* and *expert*. The novice users were assumed to take non-zero time to visually locate characters on an interface. Their performance was represented by Eq. 7(a). On the other hand, the expert users were assumed to have complete familiarity with the interface layout and hence have a *zero* visual search time. Thus, an expert user's performance was represented by Eq. 7(b).

$$CPS_{FD}(Novice) = \frac{1}{RT + MT_m} \quad (7a)$$

$$CPS_{FD}(Expert) = \frac{1}{MT_m} \quad (7b)$$

Model by Bhattacharya et al.

Bhattacharya et al. (2008c) reported models for computing text entry rate for auto and guided scanning keyboards. The models assumed that each key on the keyboard is assigned a location. For 3-level scanning, the location is of the form <b,r,c> where *b* denotes the block in which the key is located, *r* denotes the row holding the key and *c* denotes the location of the key itself. Similarly, each key on 2-level and 1-level scanning keyboards are assigned locations of the form <r,c> and <c>, respectively.

The time required to select a key k_j after another key k_i was called the *focus movement and selection time*, denoted by FT_{ij}. Expressions to compute FT_{ij} were reported for both auto and guided scanning, which are shown in Eq. 8(a) and Eq. 8(b). In Eq. 8, *FOC*() represents *system overhead time* or the time a user waits for an element to be highlighted after activation of the access switch, T_{SO} is the total system overhead time, *T* is the scan period, *X* represents the distance between keys and *A* and A' are constants. The quantity T_{GS} represents the average switch activation time of a user, which was theoretically found to be 478 ms. The values of *X*, *A*, *A'* and T_{SO} for different scanning methods are shown in Table 1, assuming source and target key locations to be <b,r,c> and <b',r',c'> for 3-level scanning, <r,c> and <r',c'> for 2-level scanning and <c> and <c'> for 1-level scanning. The quantities *B*, *R* and *C* denote total number of blocks, rows and items on the corresponding interfaces, respectively.

$$FT_{ij} = T_{SO} + (X + A).T. \quad \textbf{(8a)}$$

$$FT_{ij} = +(X + A')(T_{GS} + FOC()) \quad \textbf{(8b)}$$

FT_{ij} was used to compute the average key selection time FT_m for the entire layout. Equation 9(a) was proposed for the purpose, where DP_{ij} is the digraph probability of the source and target keys and *K* is the total number of keys present on the interface. Using this average key selection time, the text entry rate in characters/second (CPS) was computed. Equation 9(b) was proposed to compute text entry rate for auto scanning keyboard users and *expert* users of guided scanning keyboards. In order to compute text entry rate for *novice* users of guided scanning keyboards, Eq. 9(c) was proposed, where *RT* is the same as in Eq. 3.

$$FT_m = \sum_{i=1}^{K}\sum_{j=1}^{K} DP_{ij} \times FT_{ij} \quad \textbf{(9a)}$$

$$CPS = \frac{1}{FT_m} \quad \textbf{(9b)}$$

$$CPS = \frac{1}{RT + FT_m} \quad \textbf{(9c)}$$

Model for User Errors

All the above models were designed to compute user performance in terms of text entry rate. An important assumption made by all these models was that, the interaction was error-free. In other words, user will always make the correct selection from the interface. Although it simplified the

Table 1. The parameter values of Eq. 8 for different scanning methods.

	3-level	2-level	1-level
X	(b'+r'+c')-b, b≤b' B+(b'+r'+c')-b, b>b'	(r'+c')-r, r≤r' R+(r'+c')-r, r>r'	c'-c, c≤c' C+c'-c, c>c'
A	-0.5, b≤b' B-0.5, b>b'	-0.5, r≤r' R-0.5, r>r'	-0.5, c≤c' C-0.5, c>c'
A'	1, b≤b' B+1, b>b'	1, r≤r' R+1, r>r'	1, c≤c' C+1, c>c'
T_{so}	3.FOC()	2.FOC()	FOC()

computation, this is not a very realistic assumption. Studies have shown that scanning keyboard users are prone to make errors (Bhattacharya et al., 2008b). It is therefore necessary to incorporate the effect of errors in the computation of text entry rate.

A relevant model in this regard was reported by Bhattacharya et al. (2008a). In the model, the following two types of errors made by the users were considered.

- The "timing error" (TE), that is, the user fails to activate the access switch when the desired element is highlighted.
- The "selection error" (SE), that is, the user selects a wrong element.

A measure, called the "ErrorProneness" or *EP*, was proposed to quantify the effect of errors on user performance. Each keyboard has an *EP* value associated with it, which was defined as the joint probability of TE and SE for the keyboard.

In order to compute *EP* with respect to the design characteristics, namely the layout and the scanning input method, the concept of "focus distance" was proposed. The focus distance f_{ij} between two keys (k_i, k_j) was defined as "the number of shifting of highlighter and switch activations required to select k_j after k_i". A set of expressions, shown in Table 2, was derived and reported by Bhattacharya et al. (2008a) to compute f_{ij} on the basis of the locations of k_i and k_j in terms of their block, row and item numbers.

Each scanning keyboard is associated with a range of focus distances. As the first step of *EP* computation, the mean focus distance for the keyboard, f_{mean}, is computed with Eq. 10 where f_{ij} is the focus distance of any key pair (k_i, k_j) and DP_{ij} is the digraph probability of the key pair. *K* is the total number of keys on the interface.

$$f_{mean} = \sum_{i=1}^{K}\sum_{j=1}^{K} f_{ij} \times DP_{ij} \qquad (10)$$

EP was defined as the joint probability of error in selecting two keys in succession having a focus distance f_{mean}. It was found that TE and SE probabilities were statistically independent. Therefore, *EP* was defined as the TE probability for f_{mean} denoted as $P_{TE}(f_{mean})$ multiplied by an average value representing SE probability denoted by p_{se}. In the formulation of the above model, it was assumed that both the errors would occur *always*, between the selections of two keys. Hence, the notion of joint probability was used. A more general case was reported in Bhattacharya (2009, chapter 5, pp. 104-105), where either of the two or both may occur. In that case, *EP* was defined as the probability of making TE or SE or both for f_{mean}. Using this definition and using the facts that (a) TE and SE are independent and (b) SE probability is given by p_{se}, Eq. 11 was proposed to compute *EP*.

$$EP = p_{se} + (1 - p_{se}) \times P_{TE}(f_{mean}) \qquad (11)$$

Table 2. Expressions to calculate focus distance between keys for the three scanning methods.

	Focus Distance	Remarks
3-level	$[(b_j + r_j + c_j) - b_i + 1], b_i \le b_j$ $[B + (b_j + r_j + c_j) - b_i + 1], b_i > b_j$	$k_i < b_i, r_i, c_i >$ $k_j < b_j, r_j, c_j >$ B = total number of blocks
2-level	$[(r_j + c_j) - r_i + 1], r_i \le r_j$ $[R + (r_j + c_j) - r_i + 1], r_i > r_j$	$k_i < r_i, c_i >$ $k_j < r_j, c_j >$ R = total number of rows
1-level	$[c_j - c_i + 1], c_i \le c_j$ $[C + c_j - c_i + 1], c_i > c_j$	$k_i < c_i >$ $k_j < c_j >$ C = total number of items

The distribution of TE probabilities with respect to focus distance was found to be governed by Eq. 12 where f represents the focus distance. f_{min} and f_{max} in Eq. 12 are the minimum and maximum values for the range of focus distances associated with a keyboard. The TE probability at f_{min} is denoted by p_{min}. f_c in Eq. 12 denotes the *critical* focus distance that separates the two regions (exponential decay and growth) of the distribution. The TE probability at f_c is represented by p_c. λ_0 and λ_1 denote the decay and growth rates, respectively.

$$P_{TE}(f) = \begin{Bmatrix} p_{min.} e^{\lambda_0 (f - f_{min})}, \text{when } f_{min} \le f \le f_c \\ p_{c.} e^{\lambda 1 (f - f_c)}, \text{when } f_c \le f \le f_{max} \end{Bmatrix} \quad (12)$$

In Bhattacharya et al. (2008a), the empirically estimated values of the parameters in Eq. 12 and the p_{se} values for the three scanning methods were reported. These values are shown in Table 3 where $R_f = f_{max} - f_{min} + 1$.

Bhattacharya et al (2008a) also reported a method to use the error model in evaluating scanning keyboards. In their method, set of scanning keyboard layouts was taken as input. Two values were computed for each of these layouts; an error-free text entry rate using Eq. 9 and the *EP* using Eq. 11. The layouts were then compared taking into account both of these measures.

DESIGN SPACE EXPLORATION ALGORITHMS

Getschow et al. (1986) proposed an algorithmic approach to systematically explore the design space. The work was based on a "greedy" algorithm that placed alphabetical letters in the *most easily accessible* positions according to the letter's frequency. That is, the letter with the highest frequency was placed at the most easily accessible position, the letter with the second highest frequency was placed at the second most easily accessible location and so on. However, the approach did not consider many arrangements that could be substantially better. This was because the algorithm did not consider the placement of letters with respect to each other.

The opposite approach to the simple greedy algorithm is an exhaustive algorithmic search of the design space that calculates the efficiency of each and every combination of letter arrangement. However, the complexity of an exhaustive search is O(K!), where *K* is the total number of keys. This is too large even for modern computing devices. Several other algorithms were proposed in the literature that tried to balance this trade-off, by reducing the search complexity while at the same time, increasing the number of alternatives examined. These algorithms are discussed in the following subsections.

Table 3. Parameter values for TE and SE distributions.

Scanning type	Parameter values
3-level	$p_{\min} \approx 0.95, p_c \approx 0.5$ $f_c \approx f_{\min} + \lfloor R_f / 2 \rfloor$ $\lambda_0 = \frac{1}{\lfloor R_f / 2 \rfloor} \ln 2, \lambda_1 = \frac{1}{(R_f - 1) - \lfloor R_f / 2 \rfloor} \ln 2$ $p_{se} \approx 0.25$
2-level	$p_{\min} \approx 0.5, p_c \approx 0$ $f_c \approx f_{\max}$ $\lambda_0 = \frac{1}{(R_f - 1)} \ln 2$ $p_{se} \approx 0.15$
1-level	$p_{\min} \approx 0.75, p_c \approx 0.05$ $f_c \approx f_{\min} + \lfloor R_f / 3 \rfloor$ $\lambda_0 = \frac{1}{\lfloor R_f / 3 \rfloor} \ln 15, \lambda_1 = \frac{1}{(R_f - 1) - \lfloor R_f / 3} \ln 5$ $p_{se} \approx 0.05$

Adaptive Evolutionary Search

Levine and Goodenough-Trepagnier (1990) described the "adaptive evolutionary search", to find the best design from the design space. The algorithm was applied to design the following three types of keyboards. Each of these keyboards had 26 letters of the English alphabet, the *space* character and the period.

a. Soft keyboards with single character per key.
b. Soft keyboards with multiple characters per key.
c. Soft keyboards with encoded representation of the characters.

Performance models for each of the above keyboard types were developed from Eq. 1. In the proposed search algorithm, initially a set of random solutions or keyboard arrangements was generated, evaluated and ranked. For evaluating solutions, performance models were used. This initial set formed generation *zero*. The best of these arrangements were selected and allowed to reproduce. Reproduction consisted of *replicas* that vary from their *parent* due to random switching of character locations, assignment patterns and so on. In this way, offsprings were generated forming generation *one*, and the process was repeated for subsequent generations. The result of the repeated cycles of selection and reproduction was the evolution of designs exhibiting *improved* performance.

Dynamic Simulation Method

In this approach (Zhai et al., 2002), "dynamic" model of soft keyboards was developed. In the modeling technique, a soft keyboard was represented as a spring connecting all possible pairs of keys present on the interface. To construct the initial spring, the keys were placed randomly with spaces between them. The elasticity of each spring was proportional to the digraph probability between the two keys, so that keys with higher digraph probability would be pulled together with greater force. In addition, viscous frictions were assumed to be present between the keys and between the keys and their environment. The steady state when all keys were pulled together formed a candidate design.

The final positions of the keys might not be at the minimum tension state because some keys could block others from entering a lower energy state. In order to reduce the deadlock or local minimum states, two methods were proposed. In one of them, experiments were carried out with different initial states. In the other method, an extended segment (a *strut*) was incorporated in each spring. The strut held the keys apart, so that other keys could be pulled through these gaps to reach a lower level of tension. The length of the strut was manually adjusted in the dynamic simulation process. At the end of each simulation cycle, the strut length was reduced to *zero*. So, all the keys were pulled against each other, forming a layout of a soft keyboard.

The movement efficiency of the design was then calculated according to Eq. 6 and compared with known results. When unsatisfactory, the layout could be *stretched* out to serve as another initial state for the next iteration of the same process. The iteration was repeated until a satisfactory layout was formed.

Fitts'-Digraph Energy and Metropolis Method

In this method, Eq. 6 was defined as the "Fitts'-Digraph energy" and a "Metropolis" algorithm, which is a "Monte Carlo" method used widely to search for the minimum energy state in statistical physics, was proposed to search the design space of soft keyboards (Zhai et al., 2002).

The algorithm performed a *random walk* in the soft keyboard design space. In each step of the walk, the algorithm picked a key and moved it in a random direction by a random amount to reach a new configuration. The level of Fitts'-Digraph energy in the new configuration was then calculated. The decision to retain the new configuration, as the starting position for the next iteration, was taken depending on a Metropolis function shown in Eq. 13. In Eq. 13, *W(O-N)* is the probability of changing from configuration *O* (old) to configuration *N* (new), ΔE is the change in energy, *k* is a coefficient, and *T* is the temperature that could be interactively adjusted.

$$W(O-N) = \begin{Bmatrix} e^{-\frac{\Delta E}{kT}} & \text{if } \Delta E > 0 \\ 1 & \text{if } \Delta E \le 0 \end{Bmatrix} \quad (13)$$

An existing good layout, stretched over a larger space, was used as an initial state. In addition to the automatic random walk process, interactive *annealing* that is commonly used in the Metropolis searching process, was also applied. The annealing process involved bringing the temperature (*T* in Eq. 13) through several up and down cycles. When the temperature was brought up, the system had a higher probability of moving upward in energy and jumping out of local minima. When the temperature was brought down, the system descended down to a lower energy level. This annealing process was repeated until no further improvement was seen.

Genetic Algorithm Approach

A GA approach to soft keyboard design was proposed by Raynal & Vigouroux (2005). In the proposed approach, each layout was treated as an individual and represented as a sequence of character locations. The initialization of the first population consisted of placing the character keys randomly on the interface. The algorithm was designed to produce a layout with an optimal performance, where optimality was defined as the highest text entry rate. Equation 9(b) was used to predict text entry rate of each individual in a population. The predicted text entry rates were subsequently used for selection from the population. Hence, Eq. 9(b) was used as the fitness function.

In order to converge quickly, the crossover was carried out on the *worst* individuals' part. It may be noted that an individual's part was a character represented by its location. To determine crossover regions, performance of a part *i* denoted by PP_i was defined as in Eq. 14.

$$PP_i = \sum_{j=1}^{K} DP_{ij} \times MT_{ij} \tag{14}$$

Using this definition, the maximum performance for each character *i*, PP_i^{max} was calculated. To obtain PP_i^{max}, the character was placed at the center position on the interface. The remaining characters were placed on the closest positions according to the digraph frequency. Finally, Eq. 14 was applied to the resulting individual. Moreover, for each individual I_n of the current population, performance of each character, PP_i^{In} was calculated using Eq. 14.

From PP_i^{max} and PP_i^{In}, a measure called the *improvement potential* (IP_i^{In}), defined as in Eq. 15, was calculated for each character *i* in the individual I_n. The measure corresponded to the difference between the maximum performance of a character and its performance on the individual I_n, weighed by the unigram character frequency p_i.

$$IP_i^{I_n} = \frac{PP_i^{\max} - PP_i^{I_n}}{p_i} \tag{15}$$

The improvement potential measure was used to sort the characters in the individual. Then a random number of crossovers were performed between the characters which had the highest improvement potential. Mutation was implemented by swapping the locations of two characters. The algorithm involved a random number of mutations in each population.

DISCUSSION

Several performance models and design space exploration algorithms are reviewed in the preceding sections. A pertinent question is, are all these models equivalent? If not, which one of them is the most suitable to design scanning keyboards? A comparative study of these models is presented in the following to answer this question.

The KLM/GOMS models require that a task description be created for each alternative design for comparison. For a scanning keyboard, a typical task consists of inputting a string of characters. User performance may vary depending on the nature of the input string (i.e. number of characters present in the string, frequency distribution of characters in the string etc.). Since it is not possible to evaluate the user performance for all possible character strings, it may be necessary to take a carefully chosen large sample of strings such that the possibility of wrong prediction is reduced. However, task descriptions are constructed manually which is a tedious and time consuming process. The problem is particularly severe for scanning keyboards having a large number of design alternatives. To address the limitations of KLM/GOMS based approaches, it is therefore desirable that the models do not take task description as input. The RG model and the FD model are found to satisfy this condition.

Although scanning input methods were considered in the Damper's extended RG model (Damper, 1984), it was assumed in the model that after every selection, the highlighter would return to a *home* position. The *unigram* probabilities of Eq. 2 reflect this assumption. As a consequence, the model can be used to compute performance of keyboards in which each on-screen location requires a fixed and pre-determined number of scan steps for its selection.

The above assumption made in the Damper's extended RG model is a special case for more general scanning input methods, where the number of scan steps required to select an element is dependent on the previous selection. Unigram probabilities are not suitable to model such general cases and n-gram statistic with $n \geq 2$ is necessary. Moreover, the Damper's model considered auto scanning input methods only. Consequently, the scan rate used in the model was sufficient to represent the user. In guided scanning, however, the user has to manually shift the highlighter among on-screen elements, which involves visual search. Thus, in order to apply the Damper's model to compute user performance for general types of auto and guided scanning, it is necessary to carry out the following enhancements to the model.

a. Replace unigram probabilities with n-gram statistics for $n \geq 2$.
b. Incorporate visual search component in the model.

The FD model computes performance taking into account digraph probabilities (i.e. n=2) and also has a visual search component. Thus, the FD model is better suited to model both auto and guided scanning input methods. However, as far as scanning keyboards are concerned, it has the following limitations.

Addressing scanning interaction: Use of scanning and access switches implies that the movement (of finger or stylus) time component in the FD model is not applicable for scanning keyboards. To incorporate scanning interaction, the motor movement time in the FD model should be replaced with a component that calculates *highlighter* movement time, i.e. the time to move the highlighter from the source to the target key. Also, it is necessary to estimate and incorporate the access switch activation time in the model, to make the model prediction more accurate.

Consideration of user errors: Since it has been found that errors affect the performance of scanning keyboard users significantly, it is important that the model takes into account the effect of errors. The FD model does not do so.

Improving visual search time prediction: The Hick-Hyman law was used to compute the visual search time component of the FD model. Sears et al. (2001) demonstrated that the Hick-Hyman law does not model visual search behavior of soft keyboard users properly. Further, no work has been done till date to study the effect of the *visual cue* (i.e. the highlighter) on visual search strategy of scanning keyboard users. Hence, it is necessary to work on and improve the visual search time prediction component of the FD model.

In the models by Bhattacharya et al (2008a; 2008c), the first two of the above issues have been addressed. Hence, among all the models reviewed, the models by Bhattacharya et al., when used together as reported in Bhattacharya et al. (2008a), are most suitable for scanning keyboard design.

On the other hand, the design space exploration algorithms were based on the models that did not account for scanning input. The Damper's (1984) extended RG model was not used in any of the algorithms. Moreover, all the algorithms considered a single objective, namely, the text entry rate maximization. The text entry rates were computed without taking the effect of errors into account. None of the existing design space exploration algorithms reviewed in Section 5, therefore, is suitable for scanning keyboard design. In Bhattacharya (2009, Chapter 6), a multi-objective simulated annealing algorithm was reported that explores the scanning keyboard design space on the basis of two objectives, namely, (a) the maximization of the error-free text entry rate and (b) the minimization of the *EP*. Obviously, this approach is more suitable in the context of scanning keyboard design, as it accounts for the effect of user errors in the design process. The experiments carried out to demonstrate the efficacy of the approach had shown promising results. As a consequence, it may be asserted that multi-objective design space exploration algorithms are more suitable for scanning keyboards. Investigations may be carried out to determine the *best* algorithm, considering different multi-objective optimization techniques that include evolutionary search, ant colony optimization, particle swarm techniques and so on, in addition to the simulated annealing approach.

CONCLUSION

Scanning keyboards are systems meant to enable severely speech and motor impaired individuals communicate with the outside world with less time and effort. The objectives of reducing time and effort are important for the physically disabled users. Consequently, evaluating a design to ascertain if the objectives are met is integral to the design process. The major issue in scanning keyboard design with the traditional approach is the problems in testing designs with physically disabled users. The works reviewed in this chapter present an alternative to the traditional method, in which models and algorithms are employed in design. Since the use of models and algorithms reduces the need for extensive user testing in the design cycle, the works are capable of addressing the difficulties faced by scanning keyboard designers.

The two components of the approach are performance modeling and design space exploration algorithms. The state of the art of the scanning keyboard performance models is quite developed with one major limitation to be addressed, which is to develop an appropriate visual search prediction model for the users of guided scanning keyboards. On the other hand, development of design space exploration algorithms for scanning keyboards is an activity still in its nascent stage. Considering its multi-objective nature, it is important to investigate different multi-objective optimization techniques to develop an efficient scanning keyboard design space exploration algorithm.

REFERENCES

Albacete, P. L., Chang, S. K., & Polese, G. (1998). Iconic language design for people with significant speech and multiple impairments. In Mittal, V. O., Yanco, H. A., Arnois, J., & Simpson, R. (Eds.), *Assistive Technology and Artificial Intelligence, Application in Robotics, User Interface and Natural Language Processing* (pp. 12–32). LNAI.

Arnott, J. L. (2005). Text entry in augmentative and alternative communication. In *Proceedings of Efficient Text Entry*. Retrieved from http://drops.dagstuhl.de/opus/volltexte/2006/519/pdf/05382.ArnottJohn.P%aper.519.pdf

Beukelman, R. D., & Mirenda, P. (1998). *Augmentative and Alternative Communication* (2nd ed.). Baltimore, MD: Brookes Publishing Co.

Bhattacharya, S. (2009). *Models and algorithms for design of scanning keyboards.* Unpublished doctoral dissertation, Dept. of Computer Science and Engineering, Indian Institute of Technology Kharagpur, India.

Bhattacharya, S., & Basu, A. (in press). Design of an Iconic Communication Aid for the Individuals with Speech and Motor Impairments in India. *Assistive Technology*. Rehabilitation Engineering and Assistive Technology Society of North America (RESNA). *Press.*

Bhattacharya, S., Basu, A., & Samanta, D. (2008a). Computational Modeling of User Errors for the Design of Virtual Scanning Keyboards. *IEEE Transactions on Neural Systems and Rehabilitation Engineering, 16*(4), 400–409. doi:10.1109/TNSRE.2008.925073

Bhattacharya, S., Samanta, D., & Basu, A. (2008b). User Errors on Scanning Keyboards: Empirical Study, Model and Design Principles. *Interacting with Computers, 20*(3), 400–418. doi:10.1016/j.intcom.2008.03.002

Bhattacharya, S., Samanta, D., & Basu, A. (2008c). Performance Models for Automatic Evaluation of Virtual Scanning Keyboards. *IEEE Transactions on Neural Systems and Rehabilitation Engineering, 16*(5), 510–519. doi:10.1109/TNSRE.2008.2003377

Carpenter, T., McCoy, K., & Pennington, C. (1997). Schema-based organization of reusable text in aac: user-interface considerations. In *Proceedings of RESNA '97 Annual Conference* (pp. 57-59). Pittsburgh, PA, USA.

Copestake, A. (1997). Augmented and alternative nlp techniques for augmentative and alternative communication. *Proceedings of the ACL workshop on Natural Language Processing for Communication Aids* (pp. 37-42). Madrid, Spain.

Damper, R. I. (1984). Text composition by the physically disabled: A rate prediction model for scanning input. *Applied Ergonomics, 15*, 289–296. doi:10.1016/0003-6870(84)90201-1

Demasco, P., & McCoy, K. F. (1992). Generating text from compressed input: an intelligent interface for people with severe motor impairments. *Communications of the ACM, 35*(5), 68–79. doi:10.1145/129875.129881

Dye, R., Alm, N., Arnott, J. L., Harper, G., & Morrison, A. (1998). A script-based aac system for transactional interaction. *Natural Language Engineering, 4*(1), 57–71. doi:10.1017/S1351324998001867

Fitts, P. M., & Peterson, J. R. (1964). Information capacity of discrete motor responses. *Journal of Experimental Psychology, 67*, 103–112. doi:10.1037/h0045689

Garay-Vitoria, N. & Abascal, J. (2006). Test prediction systems: A survey. *International Journal on Universal Access in the Information Society. Special issue on User-Centered Interaction Paradigms for Universal Access in the Information Society, 4*(3), 188–203.

Getschow, C. O., Rosen, M. J., & Goodenough-Trepagnier, C. (1986). A systematic approach to design a minimum distance alphabetical keyboard. In *Proceedings of RESNA (Rehabilitation Engineering Society of North America) 9th Annual Conference*, Minneapolis, MN.

Goldman-Eisler, F. (1986). *Cycle linguistics: Experiments in spontaneous speech.* New York: Academic Press.

Hansen, J. P., Torning, K., Johansen, J. A., Itoh, K., & Aoki, H. (2004). Gaze typing compared with input by head and hand. In *Proceedings of the 2004 symposium on Eye tracking research and applications* (pp. 131-138). San Antonio, Texas, USA.

Hick, W. E. (1952). On the rate of gain of information. *The Quarterly Journal of Experimental Psychology, 4*, 11–36. doi:10.1080/17470215208416600

Higginbotham, D. J., Wilkins, D. P., & Lesher, G. W. (1999). Frametalker: a communication frame and utterance-based *augmentative* communication device. In *Proceedings of RESNA 99 Annual Conference* (pp. 40–42). Long Beach, CA., USA.

Horstmann, H. M., & Levine, S. P. (1990). Modeling of user performance with computer access and augmentative communication systems for handicapped people. *Augmentative and Alternative Communication, 6*, 231–241. doi:10.1080/07434619012331275514

Hyman, R. (1953). Stimulus information as a determinant of reaction time. *Journal of Experimental Psychology, 45*, 188–196. doi:10.1037/h0056940

Instance, H. O., Spinner, C., & Howarth, P. A. (1996). Providing motor impaired users with access to standard graphical user interface (GUI) software via eye-based interaction. In *Proceedings of 1st European Conference on Disability, Virtual Reality and Associated Technology*, UK.

Johansen, A. S., & Hansen, J. P. (2002). Augmentative and alternative communication: The future of text on the move. *Proceedings of the seventh ERCIM workshop on User Interface for All* (pp. 367–386). Paris, France.

John, B. E., & Kieras, D. E. (1996). The GOMS family of user interface analysis techniques: Comparison and contrast. *ACM Transactions on Computer-Human Interaction, 3*(4), 320–351. doi:10.1145/235833.236054

Koester, H. H., & Levine, S. P. (1997). Keystroke level models for user performance with word prediction. *Augmentative and Alternative Communication, 13*, 239–257. doi:10.1080/07434619712331278068

Lesher, G. W., & Moulton, B. J. (2005). An introduction to the theoretical limits of abbreviation expansion performance. In *Proceedings of the RESNA 2005 Annual Conference*.

Lesher, G. W., Moulton, B. J., & Higginbotham, D. J. (1998a). Optimal character arrangements for ambiguous keyboards. *IEEE Transactions on Rehabilitation Engineering, 6*, 415–423. doi:10.1109/86.736156

Lesher, G. W., Moulton, B. J., & Higginbotham, D. J. (1998b). Techniques for augmenting scanning communication. *Augmentative and Alternative Communication, 14*, 81–101. doi:10.1080/07434619812331278236

Levine, S. H., & Goodenough-Trepagnier, C. (1990). Customised text entry devices for motor-impaired users. *Applied Ergonomics, 21*, 55–62. doi:10.1016/0003-6870(90)90074-8

MacKenzie, I. S., & Soukoreff, R. W. (2002). Text entry for mobile computing: Models and methods, theory and practice. *Human-Computer Interaction, 17*, 147–198. doi:10.1207/S15327051HCI172&3_2

Patel, R., Pilato, S., & Roy, D. (2004). Beyond linear syntax: An image-orientation communication aid. *Assistive Technology Outcomes and Benefits, 1*(1), 57–67.

Raynal, M., & Vigouroux, N. (2005). Genetic algorithm to generate optimized soft keyboard. *Proceedings of CHI'2005* (pp. 1729-1732), Oregon, USA.

Rosen, M. J., & Goodenough-Trepagnier, C. (1981). Factors affecting communication rate in non-vocal communication systems. In *Proceedings of the 4th Annual Conference on Rehabilitation Engineering* (pp. 194–196).

Sears, A., Jacko, J. A., Chung, J. C., & Moro, F. (2001). The role of visual search in the design of effective soft *keyboards. Behaviour & Information Technology, 20*, 159–166. doi:10.1080/01449290110049790

Soukoreff, W., & MacKenzie, I. S. (1995). Theoretical upper and lower bounds on typing speed using a stylus and soft keyboard. *Behaviour & Information Technology, 14*, 370–379. doi:10.1080/01449299508914656

Steriadis, C. E., & Constantinou, P. (2003). Designing human-computer interfaces for quadriplegic people. *ACM Transactions on Computer-Human Interaction, 10*, 87–118. doi:10.1145/772047.772049

Todman, J. (2000). Rate and quality of conversations using a text-storage aac system: Single-case training study. *Augmentative and Alternative Communication, 16*(3), 164–179. doi:10.1080/07434610012331279024

Trewin, S., & Arnott, J. (2007). Text entry when the movement is impaired. MacKenzie, I. S. & Tanaka-Ishii, K. (Eds), *Text Entry Systems: Mobility, Accessibility, Universality*, chapter 14, pages 289–304. Morgan Kauffmann.

Vanderheiden, G. C. (1988). Overview of the basic selection techniques for augmentative communications: Past and future. In Bernstein, L. F. (Ed.), *The vocally impaired: Clinical practice and research* (pp. 5–39). Philadelphia: Grine and Stratton.

Venkatagiri, H. S. (1999). Efficient keyboard layouts for sequential access in augmentative and alternative communication. *Augmentative and Alternative Communication*, *15*, 126–134. doi:10.1080/07434619912331278625

Ward, D. J., & Mackay, D. J. (2002). Fast hands-free writing by gaze direction. *Nature*, *418*(6900), 838. doi:10.1038/418838a

Wobbrock, J. O., & Myers, B. A. (2006). Trackball text entry for people with motor impairments. In *Proceedings of CHI '06* (pp. 479–488). Quebec, Canada.

Worah, S. (2001). *My Stamp Book*. Kolkata, India: Indian Institute of Cerebral Palsy.

Zhai, S., Hunter, M., & Smith, B. A. (2002). Performance optimization of virtual keyboards. *Human-Computer Interaction*, *17*, 89–129. doi:10.1207/S15327051HCI172&3_4

KEY TERMS AND DEFINITIONS

Access Switches: Specially designed input devices for motor-impaired computer users.

Augmentative and Alternative Communication (AAC): Augmentative and alternative communication is any method that supplements or replaces speech and writing when these are temporarily or permanently impaired and inadequate to meet all or some of a person's communication needs

Design Space Exploration: The process of searching for a good design among all the designs in the design space.

Design Space: The set of all possible designs.

Model-Based Design: Automated design techniques where performance models and design space exploration algorithms are used to design a system.

Performance Models: Computational model of user performance.

Scanning Keyboards: Soft keyboards operated using an input method that involves scanning and access switches.

Scanning: Scanning is the technique of periodic highlighting of on-screen elements.

Soft Keyboards: Soft keyboards are on-screen keyboards, i.e. the keys are laid out spatially on the computer screen.

Text Entry Rate: Number of characters/words entered per second/minute (CPS/WPM). This metric is used to measure performance of character-level text entry systems.

ENDNOTE

1 See for example http://www.evertype.com/standards/by/bliss.html containing links to works on the use of Bliss symbols for AAC.

Section 5
Experiences and Applications

Chapter 18
Projects from the Orange Foundation in Favour of People with Obstacles to Communication

Verónica Pensoosi
Orange Foundation, Spain

Blanca Villamía
Orange Foundation, Spain

Manuel Gimeno
Orange Foundation, Spain

INTRODUCTION

"The spoken word is a mighty lord, and for all that it is insubstantial and imperceptible it has superhuman effects. It can put an end to fear, do away with distress, generate happiness, and increase pity". These lines from Gorgias, one of Plato's dialogues, sum up the power of the word, considered as one of the main vehicles (although it is important to emphasise that it is not the only one) through which people can transmit their thoughts, and communicate with each other. In fact, it could even be affirmed that the truly essential factor is not even the spoken word, but instead the power of the individual to contact their equals, sharing their 'inner world', their ideas and their needs, in order to feel part of a collective and to express themselves.

However, there are several groups of people with obstacles to communication who have greater difficulties both in using the spoken word, and in finding alternative communication systems that allow them to connect with others on an equal footing. This tends to lead to a feeling of isolation and frustration, as well as the impossibility of becoming integrated into society.

DOI: 10.4018/978-1-60566-206-0.ch018

Being sensitive to this problem, the Orange foundation focuses its efforts, although not exclusively[1], on promoting communication by these social groups, fostering the creation of links between people through a series of tools that make communication possible, resorting to alternative methods when necessary, adapting the type of language to the needs of people with functional diversity. An example is the use of pictograms, which have proved to be useful for people with Autism Spectrum Disorders (ASD).

Also, the Orange Foundation especially values technological projects that offer interesting and novel solutions for people suffering from exclusion as a result of congenital or acquired disabilities. With this aim in mind, the Orange Foundation supports applied research, promoting innovative Research and Development projects, and frequently working with universities on applied research products, with the firm belief, in the words of Johan Wolfgang Goethe, that "Knowing is not enough; we must apply. Willing is not enough; we must do."

Furthermore, in order to ensure the usability of the projects from the Orange Foundation, the testing of results is essential, from the design stage onwards. The Orange Foundation firmly believes that the close collaboration between the target group and the team experimenting on the different prototypes ensures that the definitive development of the project responds to the user's needs.

Specifically, the Orange Foundation, created in 1998, promotes projects aimed at improving the quality of life of people with different types of disability. However, after its integration in the France Télécom Group in 2005, the work of the Foundation has become increasingly focused on six clearly defined areas in line with the work of the group's foundations in different parts of the world: autism spectrum disorders, visual disabilities, hearing disabilities, the fight against illiteracy, the education of girls in developing countries, and vocal music.

With this approach in mind, we will now present some of the projects of the Orange Foundation, organised under the following headings: 1) Visual technologies for visual thinkers: projects aimed at people with autism; and 2) Communicating, learning and playing with technology: projects aimed at reducing the digital divide.

VISUAL TECHNOLOGIES FOR VISUAL THINKERS: PROJECTS AIMED AT PEOPLE WITH AUTISM

The world of autism is complex, and a good way of understanding it might be to listen to the words of people with autism spectrum disorders who have been able to describe their inner world, such as Temple Grandin, a professor of animal science at an American university, who has Asperger's Syndrome. "I think in images. Words for me are like a second language. I translate spoken and written words into colour films, with a soundtrack and everything, which pass through my head like a videotape. When someone talks to me, their words are immediately translated into images."

A number of scientific studies[2] have confirmed that people with ASD activate especially those areas of the brain that evoke visual and spatial images, which causes difficulties in conceptualising abstract ideas. Therefore, the methods that are most widely used today with people with autism are also highly visual, such as the TEACCH Programme and the PECS (Picture Exchange Communication System).

In this case, at the end of 2006 the Orange Foundation and the Autism and Learning Difficulties Group of the Robotics Institute of the University of Valencia, Spain, began to collaborate in order to design a series of technological solutions that could be of use for people with ASD, through the following projects:

AZAHAR

The aim of the Azahar project is to develop a series of applications for communication, entertainment and planning purposes which, when implemented through everyday tools such as the mobile phone or computer, help to improve the quality of life and independence of people with autism. The project focuses on applications that help to improve communication; spatial-temporal structuring, fostering the anticipation and prediction of future activity; and leisure and entertainment.

The project, supported by the Avanza Plan of the Spanish Ministry of Industry, Tourism and Trade, began in 2007 with a planned duration of two years, to focus on the development of ten applications.

- Clocks and learning the concept of time: the TIC-TAC Application
- Alternative Expressive Communication System (SAC): the Hola Application
- Video and/or voice calls
- Messages between mobile phones
- Photo album
- Visiting card (Summarised personal guide)
- SOS request
- MP3 player
- Alerts, alarms, reminders and notifications
- Digital radio on the mobile phone.

As an example, we will describe the TIC-TAC application, which responds to a real difficulty suffered by people with autism: understanding the abstract concept of time. This issue was well explained by Theo Peeters, founder of the Center for Training Professionals in Autism: "People with autism tend to have difficulty in 'going beyond the literal'. So how are they going to understand what 'invisible time' is? They have very serious and understandable difficulties with time, which cannot only be explained by a low level of development."

Figure 1. Different TIC-TAC situations

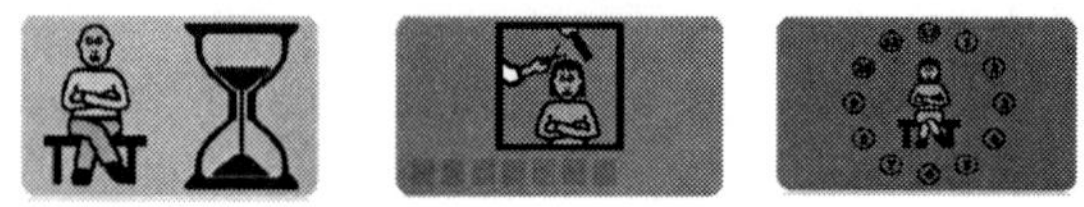

In order to address this need, the TIC-TAC application consists of a series of assistive methods to make time visible, audible and tangible, making it possible to show the duration and passage of time through different sensory modalities (visual, auditory and tactile), accompanying this representation with pictograms or images that identify the activity underway, and the standby situation. The TIC-TAC instrument is designed to be used in waiting periods, leisure time, working time, and in situations of sensory overload. A series of examples are shown in Figure 1.

The other nine applications have been designed with similar criteria. Once all of the different applications that make up AZAHAR have been completed, it will be possible to download them for free from the website of the Orange Foundation http://www.fundacionorange.es/ and execute them on the following devices:

- Mobile devices: mobile phones using Windows Mobile and the Symbian operating system with touch screens have been chosen, to avoid the complexity of buttons. Also, Java technology has been used.
- Portable devices: personal computers, touch-sensitive blackboards, touch-sensitive monitors, tablet PCs, Ultra Mobile Personal Computers (UMPC) or PDAs.

THE PICTOGRAM ROOM PROJECT

The starting point of the Pictogram Room project is to reflect on the pictograms, which have proved to be effective as communication and learning instruments for people with autism. As a result, pictograms are increasingly used for people with ASD, the majority of whom learn to handle them; but do they really understand what is shown on each pictogram? On consulting teachers of pupils with ASD, these often indicate that even a slight change to the pictogram is enough for pupils with autism to no longer be able to understand it.

Based on these premises, the Pictogram Room project uses a room with Augmented Reality to teach autistic people to understand the pictograms, focusing especially on those with lower intellectual abilities. The project assumes that with the help of Augmented Reality, the possibility of using pictograms superimposed over real objects may help people with autism to see the connection between the real image and the pictogram in real time.

Augmented Reality makes it possible to present, in a visual manner, a series of educational activities aimed at improving the learning process of people with autism in the areas of knowledge in which they have greater limitations, offering the following advantages:

- It provides a tangible presence and a representation of the body.
- It permits predictable situations.
- It makes it possible to make internal processes and states explicit (for example, through thought bubbles).
- It makes it possible to highlight specific aspects of reality.
- It makes it possible to insert computer-generated graphic information (images, photos, etc.) in real situations.
- It facilitates the processes of generalisation.
- It allows activities to be individualised to a significant extent.

In particular, Pictogram Room is complemented with the design of a solid educational methodology aimed at teaching the following skills to people with autism who have reached lower levels of cognitive development, and with major limitations:

- Communication through gestures or signs;
- Anticipation;
- Mental flexibility;
- The meaning of one's own activity;
- Self-awareness;
- The ability to imitate;
- The capacity for abstraction and imagination.

This is a project developed by the Orange Foundation in collaboration with the Autism and Learning Difficulties Group of the Robotics Institute of the University of Valencia, Spain, and Weimar University in Germany. The experimental evaluation of the developments also involves the collaboration of two users' associations: the Ávila Autism Association, and the Burgos Autism Association. The project, which began at the end of 2007, is expected to last for three years. The technological development of the Pictogram Room project is supported by the Avanza Plan of the Spanish Ministry of Industry, Tourism and Trade.

SUPPORTIVE VIEWS (WWW.MIRADASDEAPOYO.ORG)

Miradas de Apoyo (Supportive Views) is a web portal designed by the ADAPTA Foundation, whose dissemination is supported by the Orange Foundation and the Caja de Ahorros del Mediterráneo. It is the result of combining the knowledge and methodologies of traditional Person Centred Planning (PCP) with the possibilities offered by new technologies.

PCP has been extensively developed in the USA, Australia, Canada and the United Kingdom, and is currently expanding throughout all of Europe. It is a system based on an essential central idea that proposes a new approach towards people with disabilities, no longer considering them as a passive subject who receives help, but instead an active subject who chooses their own destiny. In PCP, the person towards whom the support is focused must be the centre and the protagonist of the process, taking control of their own life. The process consists of creating a circle of support around a disabled person, who becomes the main focus of the actions.

Against this backdrop, the Supportive Views website is an instrument of commitment and dedication for a support group that is formed around a person, with the aim of improving their quality of life. Supportive Views offers a personalised space for each support group, for its participants, and especially for the person at its centre. Each group can personalise its sections, their names, images, tabs, and in general any important aspect of the website. Also, each supervisor responsible for the website can allow or restrict different types of access, in order to protect the privacy of the person at its centre.

The Supportive Views website was launched in July 2009, and can be reached at the following address: www.miradasdeapoyo.org

COMMUNICATING, LEARNING AND PLAYING WITH TECHNOLOGY: PROJECTS AIMED AT REDUCING THE DIGITAL DIVIDE

Today, at the start of the twenty-first century, advanced societies are witnessing the incorporation of Information and Communications Technologies (ICT) into the daily lives of their inhabitants. Technological change is occurring at a ferocious pace, requiring individuals to have an enormous ability to assimilate and adapt to these new possibilities. This undoubtedly has highly positive consequences, but also involves a series of risks or negative aspects, including what is known as the 'Digital Divide' which marks the difference, whether between individuals, groups, or geographic areas, in terms of access, use and skills with regard to ICT.

The Orange Foundation strives to reduce the digital divide by promoting projects that make technology available for users with functional diversity, in order to make their lives easier and to extend the possibilities for communication, learning and entertainment to other social groups at risk of exclusion, such as the elderly or people with intellectual disabilities, through the development of the following projects.

IN-TIC PROJECT

Assistive systems or products for information, communication or indication are applications or instruments designed for people with functional diversity, intended to provide access and ensure the usability of ICT regardless of the physical, mental or sensory needs and capacities of these groups. In particular, the In-TIC project makes it possible for people with functional diversity to improve their personal autonomy in two ways:

- Using computers, thanks to an assistive system that makes it possible to personalize a series of functions and programmes.
- Having personalised access to mobile devices, with the possibility of using them as a means of communication.

Essentially, the In-TIC project provides accessibility (the opportunity to use ICT) and usability (interacting with ICT) through interfaces or keyboards that can be adapted to the specific characteristics or needs of each person, which vary depending on their abilities and the difficulties they have to overcome. For example, there are differences between people with physical or sensory disabilities who have problems with the input devices used with the computer (such as the mouse or keyboard), and people with sensory disabilities who have difficulties with the output

Figure 2. In-TIC personalized keyboard

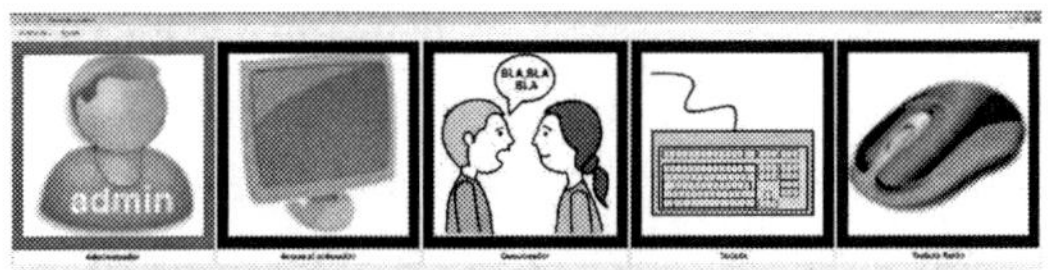

peripherals (screen, loudspeakers, printer), or people with intellectual disabilities who do not have problems in accessing computers, but instead in their use. As a result, the virtual keyboards or screens can be designed by professionals based on the specific abilities of each user, simplifying the use of the computer, as shown in Figure 2.

By creating and configuring virtual keyboards, users are enabled to interact with desktop computers, laptops and tablet PCs, access the Internet, communicate and execute certain applications, games, etc. As a result they are able to become more self-sufficient, participating in an active and more independent life. They are able to enjoy new types of entertainment, participation and training, also facilitating their communication and interpersonal relations.

The features for personalisation and adaptation, the different possibilities for accessing the computer, and the integrated communicator for mobile telephones and PCs, combined with its free distribution, make In-TIC a unique and innovative assistive product for groups of people with functional diversity.

This project has been promoted by the Orange Foundation and developed by the IMEDIR Group from the University of A Coruña in collaboration with ASPACE (the Association of Parents of Persons with Cerebral Palsy), and the Red Cross. The PC application is currently available in Spanish, Galician and English, and is compatible with the Windows operating system. It can be downloaded from www.intic.ud.es or en www.fundacionorange.es. The application for mobile devices using the Windows Mobile operating system is currently under development, with plans for its release in 2010.

EDAD PROJECT

As part of its work dedicated to inclusion and in order to respond to these needs, the Orange Foundation, together with the research team from the Education Psychology Department of the Complutense University of Madrid (UCM), decided to work on the development of the EDAD Project (Dynamic Stimulation and Digital Literacy). It was created with the premise that the use of ICT in learning does not only mean that the students (in this case, the elderly) learn how to use computers, but also that they use technological tools as a cognitive instrument for developing mental processes: the aim is not to learn about technology, nor to learn from technology, but instead to learn with technology. In this case, the project has a double objective: to promote the use of technological systems for the social integration of the elderly, and to use the potential of technology as a system for cognitive rehabilitation and the prevention of intellectual deterioration.

The elderly are a group that is usually marginalised from the Information Society, despite the fact that they form an increasingly important part of our population, have a large amount of free time at home, and can benefit from ICT to access information, process administrative documentation, or make on-line purchases from their home, contact family and friends, transmit their know-how and enrich their leisure activities. ICT also allow them to remain active at work or in their community.

Apart from promoting the use of new technologies amongst the elderly, the EDAD course has a series of added values:

- The course is not limited to teaching computer literacy, as it incorporates a system for cognitive rehabilitation and the prevention of intellectual deterioration through a series of 'mental gymnastics' exercises.
- The on-line course is free, and can be accessed by individuals or group classes;

the latter method is the most advisable for bringing the elderly into contact with ICT.

- The EDAD project has designed a solid teaching methodology that focuses on the student's skills and provides training in different stages, adapted to the abilities of the elderly (developing motivation, emotional and analytical intelligence, etc.)
- The adapted design of the Moodle platform ensures that it can be navigated easily by the elderly.
- The course includes the possibility of training trainers to assist the teachers who want to offer the course.
- The course forms a part of an educational research project led by the Complutense University of Madrid, with the participation of the universities of Granada and Valladolid, focusing on the social integration and prevention of intellectual deterioration amongst the elderly through the use of technological systems.

Since it began in 2006 with several pilot groups, the project has become extensively widespread, and currently involves hundreds of users and dozens of teachers throughout all of Spain, also thanks to a collaboration agreement with the Regional Government of Castile-León through CEDETEL, and with the Principality of Asturias, through the CTIC Foundation.

CITI PROJECT

The CITI Project (Intellectual Competence and Information Technologies) came about as a result of the BIT project (Computer and Technology Bases), a pioneering project in the world, that began in 1999 with the support of the Orange Foundation in collaboration with the Down Syndrome Foundation of Madrid and the Carlos III University of Madrid. The aim is to create a methodology capable of training people with Down's syndrome and other special educational needs in the use of computers and other technologies. The final objective of the BIT project is to promote the integration of this community at social, educational and employment level. Apart from the different courses that have been offered, the project has included the creation of the CD 'The Thinking Ark' (Learning, Resolving, Understanding, Applying), which contains different multimedia activities aimed at strengthening the cognitive skills of this social group.

After analysing the potential of mobile devices and their widespread use amongst the intellectually challenged, it was decided to create CITI, a game for mobile phones that includes a series of educational games aimed at such users. The purpose of these activities is to improve cognitive processes such as attention, memory, orientation and reasoning, amongst others.

The CITI project is one of the first computer games designed with and for people with intellectual disabilities. The game is set in an imaginary city with various, real-life situations: the park, cultural centre, home and shopping centre. It is available from www.fundacionorange.es or by sending an SMS to 7551 with the word 'Citi'.

Due to the success and acceptance of the game, and the improvements in cognitive skills observed in the evaluation process carried out with a pilot group of people with intellectual disabilities, it was considered opportune to develop CITI for PC, thereby ensuring that the application would reach the highest possible number of users. It will shortly be available to download from the websites of the Orange Foundation and the BIT Project.

This project has been developed in collaboration with the Down Syndrome Foundation of Madrid, and with the support of the Avanza Plan of the Spanish Ministry of Industry, Tourism and Trade.

CONCLUSION

This chapter has presented a solution based on a recommender system to address the technological challenges to support the needs of people with intellectual disabilities towards their work integration and independent life, in the scope of the CISVI and AMI4Inclusicion research projects.

Personal autonomy can be supported with recommendations offered within the mentoring process, both in two complementary scenarios: (1) facilitating the mentoring work for human mentors, and (2) reproducing some of this support and offering it dynamically when certain actions of the users are detected in the environment. The first scenario (facilitating the mentoring work for human mentors) is applied in the research direction that promotes the labour integration of people with cognitive disabilities. The second one (reproducing some of this support and offering it dynamically when certain actions of the users are detected in the environment) is applied to support independent life.

The recommender system offers (1) a general system for the mentor to "configure" adaptations or helps adjusted to the needs of one particular user, in the form of recommendations, (2) direct recommendations to the mentor and the user in their own activities, and (3) help to the mentor to detect troubles and possible next actions for the user.

REFERENCES

Barrera, C., Santos, O. C., Gutierrez y Restrepo, E., Boticario, J. G., Moranchel, J., Roldán, J. R., & Casas, R. (2009). Empowering disabled people: e-learning challenges for independent life. In *Proceedings of the 3rd Workshop Towards User Modeling and Adaptive Systems for All: Modeling and Evaluation of Accessible Intelligent Learning Systems* (TUMAS-A 2009) held in conjunction with AIED 2009 (pp. 38-44).

Blochl, D., Rumershofer, H., & Wob, W. (2003). Individualized e-learning systems enabled by a semantically determined adaptation of learning fragments. In *Proceedings of the 14th International workshop on Database and Expert Systems Applications* (pp. 640-645).

Brown, I., & Brown, R. (2003). *Quality of Life and Disability. An Approach for Community Practitioners*. Jessica Kingsley Publishers.

Down syndrome online (n.d.). Retrieved from http://www.down-syndrome.org/about/

Drachsler, H., Hummel, H. G. K., & Koper, R. (2007). Personal RS for learners in lifelong learning: requirements, techniques and model. *International Journal of Learning Technology*. eInclusion@EU project (2004, October). D1.1 Analytic Framework - eInclusion and eAccessibility priority issues. Retrieved from http://www.einclusion-eu.org/Document.asp?View=TRUE&MenuID=77#_ftnref62

KEY TERMS AND DEFINITIONS

Accessible Lifelong Learning (ALL): Focuses on access to education and lifelong learning which are both more and more mediated through ICT.

e-Inclusion: Approach to preventing digital exclusion, i.e prevent that disadvantaged people and disadvantaged groups could be left behind in the development of the information society.

Independent Living: Ability to perform the activities of daily life with no or little help from others.

Information and Communication Technologies (ICT): Use of electronic computers and computer software to convert, store, protect, process, transmit, and securely retrieve information.

Mentor: Someone who oversees the career and development of another person through teaching, advising and providing psychological support.

Radio Frequency Identification (RFID): An portable storage system that uses an object (tag) applied to a product for the purpose of identification and tracking using radio waves.

Recommender Systems: Systems that guide people to interesting materials or services based on information from other people, providing recommendations based on opinions/behaviours of others.

ENDNOTES

1 In the case that concerns us, the description of the work of the Foundation will focus on R&D projects aimed at improving the quality of life of the disabled, and fighting against digital illiteracy. For more detailed information on other projects of the Foundation, visit its website: http://www.fundacionorange.es.

2 Kana RK, Keller TA, Cherkassky VL, Minshew NJ, Just MA. Sentence comprehension in autism: thinking in pictures with decreased functional connectivity. Brain. 2006;129(Pt 9):2484–2493
Gaffrey MS, Kleinhans NM, Haist F, Akshoomoff N, Campbell A, Courchesne E, Muller RA. Atypical participation of visual cortex during word processing in autism: An fMRI study of semantic decision. Neuropsychologia. 2007;45(8):1672-84.

Chapter 19
Occupational Therapists' Perceptions about the Non-Use of Recommended Assistive Technology (AT)

Patricia M. Wielandt
University of Alberta, Canada

ABSTRACT

First this chapter will present an overview about assistive technology (AT). Next factors identified in the literature and thought to influence AT use will be presented. The second part of the chapter will present the findings extracted from a larger three-phase study, which aimed to obtain occupational therapists' perceptions about AT non-use. Drawing from their experiences therapists identified the client-, AT-, intervention-focused factors which they had found to influence use. Some of these factors were similar to those identified in the literature, with therapists offering additional perspectives about the role these issues actually played in affecting AT use. In addition, therapists highlighted other important factors, not previously identified as influential or which had received little attention. Overall results showed support for a client-centred approach during the provision of AT. Suggestions were made to incorporate the Matching Person with Technology (MPT) model into current practice to guide the AT provision process.

INTRODUCTION

Over the past forty or so years a substantial collection of literature has accumulated surrounding the topic of assistive technology (AT) use. This indicates not only various health professionals' collective concerns about the non-use of recommended AT, but it also highlights the complexities involved in the AT provision process. Indeed to ensure a successful AT outcome there must be an exact match between the clients' needs, the activity to be undertaken and the environment in which the activity will occur.

DOI: 10.4018/978-1-60566-206-0.ch019

In earlier studies researchers used the term 'compliance rate' when measuring the frequency of AT use. Currently, the term 'compliance' is not used and instead we use the terms 'AT use' and 'AT non-use'. Most of the reviewed studies had multi-diagnostic sample sizes which ranged from 8 to 502 subjects, used a wide variety of definitions for AT use, had different follow-up timeframes, with some larger studies surveying use in an extensive range of AT (Wielandt & Strong, 2001). Interestingly, there was no literature located which examined AT non-use from the perspective of the health professionals who provide AT for clients. Obtaining therapist perspectives would be useful and could add to the body of knowledge surrounding AT non-use. The purpose then of this research was to gain an understanding of occupational therapists' perceptions about AT non-use, which was then compared and contrasted with the available literature.

BACKGROUND

An integral part of the occupational therapy management of individuals with disability or dysfunction is assisting them in the successful completion of personally relevant activities of daily living (ADL). Such a goal may be achieved by programs designed to increase relevant performance components, activity adaptation and/or environmental modifications. Recommending AT is a frequently used element of therapeutic interventions designed to modify the person's environment to facilitate optimal activity engagement.

AT is usually recommended to enhance the client's level of independence and promote the safe completion of essential daily tasks. Often though the use of recommended AT makes it possible for the person to engage in activities away from their home and within their community. This then has a markedly positive effect on their subjective wellbeing and provides them with a real sense of achievement (Mann, 2001; Schemm & Gitlin, 1998). Additionally, AT plays a pivotal role in the rehabilitation process by improving a client's functional capabilities and assisting them in the transition from rehabilitation to home (Wielandt, 2003).

In spite of the many positive outcomes associated with owning AT, there are diverse rates of AT use reported in the literature, ranging from 35% (Garber & Gregorio, 1990) to 100% (McGrath, Goodman, Cunningham, McDonald, Nichols & Unruh, 1985). In a recent study Scherer and Craddock (2002) reported that approximately 30% of obtained AT is either abandoned or discarded within the first year.

In order to understand AT non-use various researchers have identified many factors (positive and negative influences), which have usually been based on the client's rationale for non-use (Wielandt, 2003). These predominant factors can be arranged into three distinct groups: client-, AT- and intervention-focused. Client-focused factors include socio-demographics, diagnosis and perceived benefits of the AT itself. Influences in the AT-focused group involve functionality and aesthetic quality. Intervention-focused factors surround elements of the service delivery model including assessment, AT selection and training.

Client-Focused Factors

Various demographic factors including the client's age (Caudrey & Seeger, 1983; Edwards & Jones, 1998; Forbes, Hayward & Agwani, 1993; Geiger, 1990; Haworth & Hopkins, 1980; Sonn & Grimby, 1994), gender (Edwards & Jones, 1998; Haworth, 1983; Haworth & Hopkins, 1980; Sonn & Grimby, 1994) and living situation (Edwards & Jones, 1998; Geiger, 1990; Sonn & Grimby, 1994) have been found to influence the use of AT. Certain diagnoses also appear to be connected to AT use and these include polio (Grynbaum, Kaplan, Lloyd & Rusk, 1963), lower limb amputations (Gitlin, Schemm, Landsberg, & Burgh, 1996), rheumatoid arthritis (Haworth, 1983), spinal cord injury (Shipham, 1987) and stroke (Prangrat, Mann & Tomita, 2000). Clients' perceptions regarding AT has also been associated with use, with positive perceptions about the usefulness of AT more likely resulting in the item being used (Gitlin et al.,1996; Tyson & Strong, 1990) compared to when it elicits feelings of embarrassment (Mann, Hurren & Tomita, 1993; Neville-Jan, Piersol, Kielhofner & Davis,1993) or makes the client feel like 'an invalid' (Kaplan, Grynbaum, Rusk & Anastasia, 1996, p.401).

AT-Focused Factors

Features of the AT can positively affect use when it enhances the client's functional capabilities (Dunn et al, 1998; George, Binns, Clayden & Mulley, 1988; Keating, McLean & Quinsey, 1989; Kohn, Enders, Preston & Motloch 1983; Page, Gale, Fitzgerald & Feeney, 1980; Riemer-Reiss & Wacker, 2000). Conversely, AT thought of as difficult or uncomfortable were not used (Dunn et al., 1998; Kaplan et al., 1966; Page et al., 1980). Furthermore the aesthetic qualities of the AT have been linked to use (Caudrey & Seeger, 1983; Chamberlain, Thornely, Stowe & Wright, 1982; Kohn et al., 1983; Korpela, Seppanen & Koivokko, 1993; McGrath et al., 1985; Neville-Jan et al., 1993). Interestingly two studies with high rates of AT use also reported having elevated AT appearance approval ratings in their respective work (Caudrey & Seeger, 1982; McGrath et al., 1985).

Intervention-Focused Factors

The use of a client-centred approach when recommending AT was identified as having an association with actual use (Kohn et al., 1983; Korpela et al., 1993; Markley & Shepperd, 1990). Elements of this approach involve working collaboratively with the client and their family or significant others during the entire AT provision process (Chen, Mann & Tomita, 2000; Kohn et al., 1983; Stowe, Chamberlain, Thornely & Wright, 1982). Also, encouraging clients and families to voice their opinions about the AT were highlighted as important aspects of a client centred intervention. Further, conducting extensive assessments of the client's physical abilities (George et al., 1988; Kohn et al., 1983; Seeger & Fisher, 1982) as well as their home environment (Neville-Jan et al., 1993; Stowe et al., 1982; Thornely, Chamberlain & Wright, 1977) was identified as being related to AT use, as all of this information would ensure an accurate match of the AT with the clients' physical and contextual requirements (Clemson & Martin, 1996; Coghlan, Robinson, Newmarch & Jackson, 1980; Finlayson & Havixbeck, 1992; Garber & Gregorio, 1990; Gitlin et al., 1993; Page et al., 1980; Shipham, 1987).

Furthermore, the role of adequate AT training was seen as important in preventing AT non-use (Chamberlain et al., 1982; Cowan & Turner-Smith, 1999; Gitlin et al., 1993; Mann et al., 1993, Neville-Jan et al., 1993). Some studies with high AT usage rates, highlighted this association by reporting that subjects in their studies had been most satisfied with the AT instruction provided to them (Caudrey & Seeger, 1983; Finlayson & Havixbeck, 1992; Keating et al., 1989; McGrath et al., 1985).

In the past AT was recommended using the medical model of rehabilitation which focused on the client's diagnosis and resultant dysfunction with a broad ultimate goal of functional independence Gitlin & Levine, 1992; Scherer, 2002; Smith, 1995; Tewey, Barnicle & Perr, 1994). Often it appeared that AT recommendations were made on the basis of the client's diagnosis and their functional limitations only (Wielandt, 2003). However, with the emergence of the social model of rehabilitation, attention has now shifted from the clients' disabilities towards to the environmental and societal barriers that preclude them from actualising their potential (Craddock & McCormack, 2002).

Within this newer model of service provision it is vital to consider the clients' opinions and expectations regarding intervention outcomes (Scherer, 2003). This approach is more client-driven and means that clients' beliefs, attitudes and values will need to be considered in the AT provision process and that 'it is no longer acceptable to point to technological solutions before the prospective users' goals are fully defined and the individuals' needs and preferences are apparent' (Scherer, 2002, p.3). Gaining clients' opinions about their intended AT use was seen as the acquisition of useful information (Gitlin et al., 1996), which can act as a means to individualising the intervention and ensuring that clients' perceptions of the proposed AT are considered (Smith, 1995).

According to Scherer (2002) clients now require interventions that acknowledge the human perspective of AT use, where their perceptions are sought and acknowledged, where client-collaboration is considered the norm and where expected AT outcomes include autonomy, maximal activity engagement and participation both at home and within the context of wider society. Scherer (2003) further suggested the need to evaluate the outcome of AT use and examine the current modes of AT service provision in order to more adequately meet client requirements. She also signalled to health professionals that AT provision methods would have to change markedly in order to ensure an individualised approach.

Understanding the issues that influence AT use is of paramount importance to therapists if they are to provide an intervention which results in better health outcomes for their clients. Whilst the literature identifies many factors that appear to influence AT use, only two studies using focus group methodology (Angelo, Buning, Schmeler & Doster, 1997; Gitlin & Burgh, 1995) examined the occupational therapy process when providing AT.

The results that are presented next in this chapter are extracted from a larger three-phase study undertaken in Australia. The overall purpose of this study was to identify predictors of AT use following discharge from rehabilitation. Initially a review of the medical and health behaviour literature regarding general medical compliance was undertaken to ascertain the extent of the topic. Next a comprehensive review of the AT literature (1963-2003) was conducted to identify the predominant factors that influenced use (Wielandt & Strong, 2000). The first phase of the study included using focus groups to gain occupational therapists' perspectives about AT non-use and will be reported on next in this chapter. The second phase of the larger study was essentially a clinical audit to determine the current rate of recommended AT use (Wielandt, McKenna, Tooth & Strong, 2001) Additionally clients' rationale for AT non-use was also sought in this phase. Factors identified in both of the literature reviews and from the occupational therapy 'experts' in the first phase were examined and then triangulated with information from clients who had been recommended AT. This informed the final phase of the study where logistic regression analysis was performed to explore the predictive relationship of factors identified in the two previous phases, in relation to AT use (Wielandt, McKenna, Tooth & Strong, 2006).

METHODS

Procedure and Participants

This phase of the larger study used a qualitative research design incorporating focus group interviews. This method of data collection is advantageous for participants as it permits the natural exchange of attitudes, opinions and perceptions (Allison & Strong, 1994; Krueger, 1994; Lau, 2000). Participants were occupational therapists working at the two metropolitan hospitals in Australia, who had previously agreed to attend a focus group held at their place of employment. Ethical approval was obtained from the University of Queensland's Behavioural and Social Sciences

Ethical Research Committee and the ethical review committees of the two hospitals involved in this phase of the research. Written and verbal information about the study was provided to participants, with written informed consent obtained from them prior to their participation. Focus groups ran on average for 70 minutes and were audio-taped for later transcription.

Measures

To focus and direct the thinking of participants, six open-ended questions were formulated based on the findings from literature reviews the researcher had conducted and discussions with clinicians with experience in AT provision. These questions included: 'when you are prescribing equipment, what factors do you consider?'; 'what factors do you think influence patient's use of prescribed equipment?'; 'do your patients use their equipment as you have recommended? and could you tell me about your experiences of this?'; 'what do you think are the reasons for patient non-use of recommended equipment?'; 'at what stage of the occupational therapy intervention process have you noticed non-use of equipment by patients?'; when non-use of equipment occurs what do you think occupational therapists can do about this?' All of the questions were arranged from general to specific, and thus organised into a focused sequence that was logical to the participants.

Data Analysis

Manual thematic analysis was undertaken, with transcripts being read several times to gain a comprehensive impression of the data, as well as to identify the major themes. Thematic coding and categorisation occurred where all data pertinent to each identified theme was scrutinized. To establish analytical themes checking and comparing of each item with the rest of the data took place. Triangulation was achieved by using field notes, focus group transcripts, participant checking and an independent colleague check.

Terminology

It should be noted that in this Australian study the terms 'equipment' and 'patient' were used instead of 'AT' and 'client'.

FOCUS GROUP FINDINGS

Characteristics of the Participants

A total of 17 occupational therapists (from a possible 18) working in the two hospitals participated in the two focus groups (11 in one group, and 6 in the other). Sixteen participants were women. The mean age was 27.3 years with a range of 22 to 37 years. The participants had been practising occupational therapists for an average of 5.2 years, ranging from 4 months to 16 years. Their clinical caseloads included rehabilitation (N=10), general surgery/cardiac conditions (N=5), hand conditions (N=1) orthopaedic surgery (N=1).

The findings from the focus groups will be presented using categories identical those to developed when reviewing the AT literature for the predominant factors affecting AT use.

Overall, participants identified some of the well-known client-, AT- and intervention- focused factors mentioned in the literature (and presented earlier in this chapter), which they perceived to influence AT use. However, they also highlighted other factors which had not been mentioned in the literature or had at least not received as much attention.

Client-Focused Factors

Whilst the influence of gender, living arrangements, and perceived need on AT use is well established, focus group participants were able to offer additional insights surrounding these client-focused factors.

Gender

Some participants advised that from their experience that women tended to use AT more than their male counterparts.

Elderly men don't seem to be willing to use equipment in many cases, as much as what the women do and ...that might be a case of them thinking that their wife can help them out.

Elderly males were possibly brought up to believe that they should be able to cope with anything and why should they need to be helped.

These perceptions appear to be referring to the influence of clients' generational attitudes and values regarding AT use, which were not identified in the literature.

Living Arrangements

Whilst home visits were considered essential by participants in ensuring AT use, some participants mentioned the importance of ascertaining family members' perceptions of the AT.

Some people are really aware of other family members and if there is only one toilet in the house and an over-toilet frame needs to be used, well they often decline to use it because of the perceived inconvenience to others.

Also the patient maybe too frail to take a shower and we recommend they use a bath board, non-slip mat and hand held hose so they are safe when showering. But if others in the home complain about the extra equipment in the bathroom then we find the patient often stops using it as they don't want to upset others that are caring for them.

From these comments the influence of family is evident and it would be prudent to include all family members during AT selection, as well as during a home visit to avoid any negative influences occurring. No literature was located regarding family influence of AT use.

Perceived Benefit of AT

In accordance with the AT literature participants identified the importance of gauging the clients' perceptions about the benefits of the recommended AT. They then went on to describe the usefulness of pre-surgery clinics for increasing client awareness of the benefits of AT. One participant encapsulated the group conversation well with the following:

In pre-op(erative clinics) we have people who will have a joint replacement, they know what they are in for, they know what the equipment is like, they have trialled the equipment and they are only too keen to arrange the hiring of it before they even come to hospital. So awareness of what they need for a full recovery has made a big difference to their compliance.

In another scenario, another participant commented that when she encountered clients who did not agree with her AT recommendations, she believed they just needed a period of time at home to get a clearer picture of what their actual AT requirements were.

I think in rehab though what you generally find is, the need for the person to go home and see how they manage and then they come back (to the out-patient clinic) and then they are usually a lot more accepting of equipment, which had been previously recommended.

Given the importance placed upon clients' perceptions in the literature, these comments are particularly useful in illustrating the different methods that can be used to facilitate client's perceived usefulness of the recommended AT. Interestingly Moy (1995) recommended that therapists always consider the client's perceived need first, before recommending AT, as this information was essential in determining whether AT would in actual fact be used.

The additional client-focused factors participants perceived to influence AT use included: cultural appropriateness, acceptance of illness, presence of anxiety and/or depression and client motivation.

Cultural Appropriateness

The group's conversations surrounding client's perceived usefulness of AT led to a discussion by participants about the need to consider cultural differences when recommending AT. Participants suggested that therapists must be sensitive to the cultural appropriateness of recommending AT for clients from various ethnic backgrounds. Recommending AT in instances where it is considered more appropriate for family to assist with various ADL tasks may lead to AT non-use.

People from other cultures often don't do things for themselves (when they have an illness/disability)... they prefer or expect that others do tasks for them.

It is easy to offend the patient's families as well.... so make sure you are familiar with the cultural norms for that patient.... before you even talk about equipment... because you don't want to upset them.

Whilst the influence of ethnicity was not mentioned in the AT literature, it is mentioned elsewhere regarding culturally appropriate occupational therapy services. With several authors suggesting that therapists need to ensure that AT not only assists the client with functional tasks but that it also assists in all of their culturally defined social roles (Blakeney, 1991; Robinson 1987; Small & Grose, 1993).

Acceptance of Illness or Diagnosis

When discussing the importance of perceived benefits participants highlighted that client acceptance of their illness or disability was pivotal in influencing recommended AT use. They likened the client's experience to that of the grieving process whereby they need to come to terms with the changes to their identity and lifestyle before the need for AT could be accepted.

There is a bit a struggle with the acceptance... you have people with problems who you can't really talk to (about equipment).... and say how this can be really preventive. But they consider that they are not that bad enough to use it yet.

They don't want to know about equipment... it is like they are still grieving and are not ready to talk about that just yet. They just don't want to even think about it. They are just not ready.

We have a lot of patients who are often in denial and think that they will get back to their full functional level, that they were at before... and often you can see that they won't, but they are in complete denial, so they are often the ones we have difficulty with in prescribing equipment... because of the acceptance thing.

Acceptance of (their) disability... accepting that this is your ultimate stage... if they are not at that point of accepting... not ready... then they are not at that point that they are to be interested (in equipment)... they are going to think about things for a while.

Another participant advised that she found it difficult to discuss with clients the need for AT soon after their diagnosis had been made. She advised at this stage clients were usually not ready to consider using AT as they were still coming to terms with the impact of the illness or disability on their life.

Every disability in the really early stages.... no matter even though you are trying to prescribe equipment and have it out to them as soon as possible.... that is not what they are interested in early.... It is too early to accept it. They are not ready.

Whilst little information about a client's adjustment to disability exists in the AT literature, it is considered to be an essential element that needs to be assessed prior to recommending AT (Galvin & Scherer, 1996).

Anxiety and Depression

Discussion by participants regarding the difficulties experienced by clients whilst adjusting to their illness or disability led both sets of focus group participants to mention that anxiety and/or depression in their experience could negatively impact AT use. It was suggested that the presence of such conditions had the potential to interfere with the client's ability to recall AT training sessions and this in turn could lead to AT non-use.

We do have patients who are really scared about dislocating their new hip and that interferes with their progress. I found that if I taught an anxious patient how to adjust an over-toilet frame, they don't seem to remember much. Like you try to explain to them and they are saying 'yes' but if you ask them five minutes later to demonstrate how to adjust the item they can't remember.

In rehab I have found that when patients are depressed... like when they are really in the pits (depressed), they aren't able to take things in. They don't remember anything you have shown or told about the equipment. It is a waste of time for them and us.

Whilst not identified in the AT literature as a factor influencing use there is limited information available regarding psychological distress causing difficulty for clients in recalling all aspects about their therapeutic intervention (Glazer et al., 2002; Kautzmann, 1991; Kutner, Zhang, McClellan & Cole, 2002).

Client Motivation

The concept of motivation was also frequently mentioned when the focus groups discussed client readiness to use AT and was perceived by them as an indicator of whether AT would be used or not.

There is no point in prescribing it (equipment); if they have no intention to use it...you need to take that into consideration.

You need to get an idea of their motivation, whether they will use it or not, when you suggest equipment for them.

Look at the patients themselves whether they are interested in resuming those tasks once they get home... I would not try to force something on them.

Limited evidence was located in the AT literature regarding the role of motivation and AT use. In the medical literature clients with reduced psychological health were seen as less likely to undertake recommended treatments (Coons et al., 1994; Cremniter, Payan, Meidinger, Batista & Fermanian, 2001) and were considered at risk of being non-compliant as their motivation levels affected their understanding of the treatment regimen (Shapiro et al., 1995). Further, Kemp (1993) suggested that motivation is one of the most important issues affecting rehabilitation and adaptation to disability.

AT-Focused Issues

The prevalence of AT characteristics such as functionality and aesthetic appeal affecting client's use of AT has been extensively documented. However, the influence of AT availability and costs when purchasing AT has not received as much attention.

AT Functionality

Focus group participants, in keeping with the literature, advised that when client's considered AT to be useful it was more likely to be used.

It is like people with hoists and things……… they need to get something out of it….. it must either help them or their careers.

I think that how the therapist educates the patient about the equipment can really influence the use of it. Then they can see how useful (it is) for themselves.

"Also if they are told it is complicated and difficult to use they are not likely to try to use it, so you need to demonstrate to them how easily they can use the equipment.

Like if they can see it is helpful and they can complete activities without help from others, then it is seen as worthwhile.

Such comments underscore the need to ensure that a dedicated part of the AT provision process be devoted to educating clients, through the use of demonstrations and hands-on practice experiencing AT use. During this process the client will be able to gain an understanding through active experience with the AT of its usefulness. No prior identification of this useful strategy was located in the literature.

AT Aesthetic Appeal

Participants mentioned that AT use could be very much affected by how it actually looked and this particular feature of the AT this was most important to consider during AT provision.

I often find that patients don't use equipment … if they do not like how it looks.

How equipment (grab rails) looks is important… patients worry…. is it going to mark the house… or indicate to others that someone with a disability lives there? Also they worry will it affect the resale value of their property.

Often smaller items like dressing sticks and long-handled combs are not used because of how they look with those wooden handles for instance.

From these comments it seems it would be far-sighted of therapists to ascertain clients' perceptions about the aesthetic qualities of the recommended AT, ahead of provision, in order to avoid AT non-use later. Perhaps also by therapists offering a selection of the different styles of AT, clients may be able to choose an item that best fits their aesthetic requirements. No literature was found to support these perceptions.

Availability

Having ready access to recommended AT including its timely delivery were highlighted as influencing use by focus group participants.

I actually consider what equipment we have got available here for loan; it is no use recommending something, which is not available.

If you are ordering equipment from the Home Medical Aids Scheme when it is going to be arrive… months down the track? If that is the case then patients will have been making do without it …then you may find when the equipment finally arrives…. they may not want use it as they have coped alright without it.

Sparse evidence was located in the literature about the possible relationship between AT availability and AT use. However, Galvin and Scherer

(1996) recommended that a comparison of AT services be made, prior to selection, between the various suppliers to ensure that the clients' delivery requirements are met. Following an audit Wilson, McCracken and Cummings (1999) found that subjects in their study waited on average 39 days for the delivery of AT and this had negatively influenced AT use.

Costs

The costs associated with purchasing recommended AT was also considered by some participants to affect its use. They indicated that the majority of clients they worked with were in receipt of some form of social security benefits and having a fixed income often precluded them from buying recommended AT.

I think one of the big factors is the cost of the equipment, and how many pieces of equipment (are needed).... it can sometimes be restrictive.

Sometimes... they just have no money to pay for equipment.... but we try to look at low cost options like hiring, or having the family try and borrow from elsewhere.

The costs of AT... it is a huge concern for a lot of patients.... sometimes they decide to take the cheaper option... (buying something they can afford) and that might not be the most optimal.

The issue of cost identified by the participants in this study was acknowledged by Scherer (1998) as being an important factor to be explored with clients, prior to AT selection, so that they were aware of all up-front costs, as well as expenses required in the future. Furthermore, Moy (1995) suggested that therapists recommend AT that suit the clients' requirements, including financial needs.

Intervention-Focused Factors

Participants identified the importance of using a client-centred approach during the AT provision process as described in the literature. They also provided information about other intervention-focused factors, not as well documented, that from their experience influenced AT use and these included: the provision of written materials during AT training, the trialling of AT and incorporating a follow-up into the AT provision process.

Client-Centred Approach

The use of a client-centred approach when prescribing AT was seen by participants as a means of encouraging clients to use their AT. They suggested that all of the client- and AT-focused factors that had been identified during the focus group could actually be discussed with the client during the AT provision process.

Such an approach was thought to produce a more accurate picture of clients' needs, as their values, beliefs and opinions could be heard and acknowledged during this process.

It makes a big difference when they are actually involved in the problem solving process... of getting to decide what equipment... or what pieces of equipment ... if they can have a say in it.

If they are involved in problem solving with you... they use the equipment... it was part of their decision too... it's like they own the decision.

When clients' opinions were not acknowledged participants reported that they became disinterested in the prescribed AT and often discarded it.

Sometimes when we make recommendations (without collaborating)... you can tell they are not going to even buy it (equipment), you can tell they don't agree with you. It depends on their comments (about the equipment)...you can pick that up very easily.

Provision of Written Information on AT

The provision of written information to clients which contains information about the correct use of AT, details of suppliers and the associated costs was considered important by participants.

Something we started here a few years ago, we started to give written information about equipment, so they actually have fairly mainstream information about OT equipment.... on that A4 sheet is where they can purchase it, the costs and bit of a blurb about what it actually does... providing them with written material tends to increase compliance.

Providing clients with written information about the AT was also seen as a means of encouraging continued use of AT after discharge.

what also helps is that they have got literature that they can take home and have good look at and digest whilst they wait to come in (for surgery) and maybe having seen the equipment here and using some (equipment) at home as well.

There was no evidence in the literature that this recommended strategy had previously been considered as a factor which could influence AT use.

Trialling AT

Clients trialling AT whilst still in hospital was also seen by participants as useful in promoting AT use. This then increased the likelihood that AT would be used at home after discharge.

And you give them opportunities too if they are able to trial equipment rather than just hear about (it).... it might be different. To trial the equipment in hospital may help them use it in the end.

A trial period to get used to the equipment... to build up their confidence. That will make them more likely to use it.

Sometimes equipment can be quite fiddly to actually use ... and they think it is going to be too hard and time consuming to use it... so trialling gives them some experience with it.

Furthermore, the trialling of AT in hospital allowed the therapist to evaluate the client's ability to cope as well as the adequacy of the AT. This assisted the therapist to then prescribe the most appropriate item of AT.

In rehab you almost always trial the equipment first....before prescribing it....to make sure it is going to be beneficial...make sure it is what they want.

With patients needing equipment...I trial self care equipment with them.

If they have had the use of a certain piece of equipment while in hospital, they are familiar with how it is used.

Another element of trialling identified by participants was the practice of issuing AT prior to surgery, which encouraged the client to become competent in its use before surgery. This was seen as an important factor which affected AT use after discharge to home.

Getting used to the equipment before surgery... so they are confident using it before they come in for surgery and they know it works for them.

Similarly, having clients attend an outpatient clinic before surgery for AT training appeared to have a positive affect on AT use after discharge.

One thing that really helps... is the pre-admission clinic for total hip replacements... so that we can educate them about what kinds of equipment they might need... and they have a couple of weeks to get organised.

We show them the wards and the bathrooms and the equipment they will use in here....so they know what to expect. We show them how to adjust an over-toilet seat and then we get them to demonstrate how to use it...they need to know that because we want them to get this equipment before they have surgery and become familiar using it at home... essentially trialling it before they come in here for the operation.

The literature yielded little evidence regarding the possible relationship between the trialling of AT and actual use.

Follow-Up

Although post-discharge follow-up was not part of the focus group participant's current routine practice many commented that it would be helpful in reducing the incidence of AT non-use.

It would be better if we could catch up with them after discharge....to iron out any problems that might have occurred since discharge.

You would find out...if it's being used or not, and if not then you have the chance to find out why... so you could find out about patient's (reasons) as why it's not being used

The need to follow-up on clients issued with AT after being discharged to home was not identified in the AT literature as influencing use. However several AT provision models (Bains Assistive Technology System (BATS) (Bain, 1997); Human Activity Assistive Technology (HAAT) (Cook & Hussey, 2002); Matching Persons with Technology (MPT) (Scherer, 1998), consider that follow-up was an essential component of the provision process, as client's needs and priorities may have changed (Bain, 1997; Scherer, 1998), or unnoticed mechanical problems may have occurred (Cook & Hussey, 2002). Furthermore, other authors advocated the use of post-discharge home visits as an ideal opportunity to work through any problems which may have arisen since the client was discharged (Egan, Warren, Hessel & Gilewich, 1992; Gitlin, Miller & Boyce, 19999; Smith, 1988).

Overall results from the focus groups identified the need for occupational therapists to use a client-centred approach during AT provision process. Drawing from their experiences with AT provision, participants identified the factors that they had found to influence AT use. Some of these factors were similar to those located in the existing AT literature with participants offering additional perspectives about the role these issues play in influencing AT use. Furthermore participants mentioned several other important factors which had either not been previously identified in the AT literature as influential or had received sparse attention.

The client-focused factors identified included gender, living arrangements, perceived benefit of the AT, cultural appropriateness of the AT, and client's acceptance of illness/disability, the presence of anxiety and/or depression, and client motivation levels. Clients' perceptions regarding AT functionality and aesthetic appearance together with AT availability (including the timeliness of delivery) and purchase costs comprised the AT-focused factors that were highlighted.

Participants also suggested using a client-centred approach, the provision of written materials about AT, the trialling of AT either at home or in hospital and the inclusion of a follow-up phase during AT provision as the intervention -focused factors which appear to influence AT use.

The findings of this research have important implications for the provision of AT by occupational therapists. Factors identified in the AT literature as well as those highlighted by participants in this study need to be incorporated to provide the basis for a set of best practice guidelines regarding AT provision.

As previously mentioned there is little information available concerning the process that occupational therapists use when recommending AT. Furthermore, no particular practice model appears to be used by occupational therapists to guide them during the AT provision process. Understanding the issues that influence AT use is essential if better health outcomes for clients are expected. Therapists, informed by the numerous AT utilisation studies that have been undertaken have been aware for a number of years that some clients reject or discard their recommended AT. There is however little evidence regarding research into strategies to avoid or minimise AT non-use.

The use of the MPT model (Scherer, 1998) would be appropriate in guiding the AT provision process, as it considers activity- environment- client-AT factors and therefore ensures an accurate match between clients' needs and the recommended AT.

The MPT process commences with the identification of the precise needs and aims of AT use, thereby highlighting the nature of the task or occupation to be undertaken upfront (Wielandt et al., 2006). Next the model concentrates on factors surrounding the milieu or environment where the AT will be used, client personal and psycho-social attributes, including requirements and opinions, and characteristics of the AT such as suitability, functionality and appearance (Scherer, Sax, Vanbiervliet, Cushman & Scherer, 2005). Another useful feature of this model is its ability to accurately measure a client's predisposition to AT use. Overall the MPT model could easily be incorporated into current occupational therapy practice as it promotes a collaborative intervention style where the therapist and client formulate strategies to prevent AT non-use occurring throughout the AT provision process (Wielandt, 2003).

FUTURE TRENDS

During this study it became apparent that a client-centred approach to AT provision is required in order to reduce incidents of non-use, thereby permitting clients to experience the intended benefits of AT use. It is suggested that a clinical trial could be conducted to determine whether the use of the MPT model assists occupational therapist to identify potential problems with AT use during the provision process. Such a study could also evaluate the strengths and limitations of incorporating this model in the clinical setting. Furthermore, subsequent to best practice principles for AT provision being developed, as recommended in this study, research needs to be conducted to evaluate these guidelines using a controlled trial methodology.

CONCLUSION

The purpose of the study was to gain an insight into occupational therapists' perceptions about the non-use of AT and to compare and contrast these with those identified in the available literature. Findings lend support for the use of a client-centred approach during AT provision. Previously using the medical model of rehabilitation, an overall goal for occupational therapy clients would have been to attain functional independence during activities of daily living. This approach focused on the client's diagnosis and the subsequent functional limitations. It did not allow for the consideration of clients' perceptions surrounding their illness, the AT and the ensuing interventions. However with the current shift of focus in rehabilitation towards a more social model of rehabilitation service provision, it may be useful to integrate these findings with information from the literature about the factors which influence AT use and develop a set of best practice principles to ensure a client-centred approach. Furthermore, it is recommended that occupational therapists consider incorporating the MPT model into current practice, as this model provides extra particulars about client's perceptions, AT characteristics and milieu details not usually identified during routine AT provision. This proposed formulation of best practice principles and the suggestion to frame AT provision around the MPT model could be useful in minimising non-use so that clients are able to experience optimal activity engagement and participation in wider society without any limitations.

REFERENCES

Allison, H., & Strong, J. (1994). Verbal strategies used by occupational therapist in direct client encounters. *The Occupational Therapy Journal of Research, 14*(2), 112–129.

Angelo, J., Buning, M. E., Schmeler, M., & Doster, S. (1997). Identifying best practice in the occupational therapy assistive technology evaluation: an analysis of three focus groups. *The American Journal of Occupational Therapy., 51*(10), 916–920.

Bain, B. K. (1997). Evaluation. In Bain, B. K., & Leger, D. (Eds.), *Assistive technology: an interdisciplinary approach* (pp. 17–31). New York: Churchill Livingstone.

Blakeney, A. B. (1991). The impact of culture on patient education. *Occupational Therapy Practice, 2*(3), 12–20.

Caudrey, D. J., & Seeger, B. R. (1983). Rehabilitation engineering service evaluation: a follow-up survey of device effectiveness and patient acceptance. *Rehabilitation Literature, 44*(3-4), 80–85.

Chamberlain, M. A., Thornely, G., Stowe, J., & Wright, V. (1981). Evaluation of aids and equipment for the bath II: a possible solution to the problem. *Rheumatology and Rehabilitation, 20*, 38–43. doi:10.1093/rheumatology/20.1.38

Chen, T. Y., Mann, W. C., Tomita, M., & Nochajski, S. (2000). Caregiver involvement in the use of assistive devices by frail older persons. *Occupational Therapy in Research, 20*(3), 179–199.

Clemson, L., & Martin, R. (1996). Usage and effectiveness of rails, bathing and toileting aids. *Occupational Therapy in Health Care, 10*(1), 41–59. doi:10.1300/J003v10n01_04

Coghlan, J. K., Robinson, C. E., Newmarch, B., & Jackson, G. (1980). Lower extremity bracing in paraplegia: a follow up study. *Paraplegia, 18*, 25–32.

Cook, A. M., & Hussey, S. M. (2002). *Assistive technologies: principles and practice*. St Louis, MO: Mosby Inc.

Coons, S. J., Sheahan, S. L., Martin, S. S., Hendricks, J., Robbins, C. A., & Johnson, J. A. (1994). Predictors of medication non-compliance in a sample of older adults. *Clinical Therapeutics, 16*(1), 110–117.

Cowan, D., & Turner-Smith, A. (1999). The user's perspective on the provision of electronic assistive technology: equipped for life? *British Journal of Occupational Therapy, 62*(1), 2–6.

Craddock, G., & McCormack, L. (2002). Delivering an AT service: a client-focused, social and participatory service delivery model in assistive technology in Ireland. *Disability and Rehabilitation, 4*(1,2,3), 160-170.

Cremniter, D., Payan, C., Meidinger, A., Batista, G., & Fermanian, J. (2001). Predictors of short-term deterioration and compliance in psychiatric emergency patients: a prospective study of 457 patients referred to the emergency room of a general hospital. *Psychiatry Research, 104*(1), 49–59. doi:10.1016/S0165-1781(01)00293-1

Dunn, R. B., Weaver, L. Y., Lucero, Y., Langbeing, F., Fehr, L., Johnson, P., & Riedy, L. (1998). Follow up assessment of standing mobility device users. *Assistive Technology, 10*(2), 84–93.

Edwards, N. I., & Jones, D. A. (1998). Ownership and use of assistive devices amongst older people in the community. *Age and Ageing, 27*(4), 462–46.

Egan, M., Warren, S. A., Hessel, M., & Gilewich, G. (1992). Activities of daily living after hip fracture: pre and post discharge. *Occupational Therapy in Research, 12*, 342–356.

Finlayson, M., & Havixbeck, K. (1992). A post-discharge study on the use of assistive devices. *Canadian Journal of Occupational Therapy, 59*, 201–207.

Forbes, W. F., Hayward, L. M., & Agwani, N. (1993). Factors associated with self-reported use and non-use of assistive devices among impaired elderly residing in the community. *Canadian Journal of Public Health, 84*(1), 53–57.

Galvin, J. C., & Scherer, M. J. (1996). An outcomes perspective of quality pathways to the most appropriate technology. In J.C. Galvin & M.J. Scherer. *Evaluating, selecting and using appropriate assistive technology* (pp.1-26). Gaithersburg, MA: Aspen Publication.

Garber, S. L., & Gregorio, T. L. (1990). Upper extremity assistive devices: assessment of use by spinal cord injured patients with quadriplegia. *The American Journal of Occupational Therapy., 44*, 126–131.

Geiger, C. M. (1990). The utilization of assistive devices by patients discharged from an acute rehabilitation setting. *Physical & Occupational Therapy in Geriatrics, 9*, 3–25.

George, J., Binns, V. E., Clayden, A. D., & Mulley, G. P. (1988). Aids and adaptations for the elderly at home: underprovided, underused and undermaintained. *British Medical Journal, 296*, 1365–1366. doi:10.1136/bmj.296.6633.1365

Gitlin, L. N., & Burgh, D. (1995). Issuing assistive devices to older patients in rehabilitation: an exploratory study. *The American Journal of Occupational Therapy., 49*, 994–1000.

Gitlin, L. N., Levine, R., & Geiger, C. (1993). Adaptive device use by older adults with mixed disabilities. *Archives of Physical Medicine and Rehabilitation, 74*, 149–152.

Gitlin, L. N., & Levine, R. E. (1992). Prescribing adaptive devices to the elderly: principles for treatment in the home. *International Journal of Technology & Aging, 5*(1), 107–120.

Gitlin, L. N., Miller, K. S., & Boyce, A. (1999). Bathroom modification for frail elderly renters: outcomes of a community-based program. *Technology and Disability, 10*, 141–149.

Gitlin, L. N., Schemm, R. L., Landsberg, L., & Burgh, D. (1996). Factors predicting assistive device use in the home by older persons following rehabilitation. *Journal of Aging and Health, 8*, 554–575. doi:10.1177/089826439600800405

Glazer, K. M., Emery, C. F., Frid, D. J., & Banyasz, R. E. (2002). Psychological predictors of adherence and outcomes among patients in cardiac rehabilitation. *Journal of Cardiopulmonary Rehabilitation, 22*, 40–46. doi:10.1097/00008483-200201000-00006

Grynbaum, B. G., Kaplan, L. I., Lloyd, K. E., & Rusk, H. A. (1963). Methodology and initial findings in a follow-up study of spinal cord dysfunction. *Archives of Physical Medicine and Rehabilitation, 44*, 208–215.

Haworth, R. J. (1983). Use of aids during the first three months after total hip replacement. *British Journal of Rheumatology, 22*, 29–35. doi:10.1093/rheumatology/22.1.29

Haworth, R. J., & Hopkins, J. (1980). Use of aids following total hip replacement. *British Journal of Occupational Therapy, 43*, 398–400.

Kaplan, L. I., Grynbaum, B. G., Rusk, H. A., Anastasia, T., & Gassler, S. (1966). A reappraisal of braces and other mechanical aids in patients with spinal cord dysfunction: results of a follow-up study. *Archives of Physical Medicine and Rehabilitation, 47*, 395–405.

Kautzmann, L. N. (1991). Facilitating adult learning in occupational therapy patient education programs. *Occupational Therapy Practice, 2*, 1–11.

Keating, W., McLean, D., & Quinsey, K. (1989). Survey of appropriate provision and usage of prescribed equipment- the client's perspective. *Australian Journal of Occupational Therapy, 36*(3), 131–135. doi:10.1111/j.1440-1630.1989.tb01210.x

Kemp, B. J. (1993). Motivational issues in the use of technology by older persons: a model and recommendations. *Technology and Disability, 2*(1), 65–70.

Kohn, J., Enders, S., Preston, J., & Motloch, W. (1983). Provision of assistive equipment for handicapped persons. *Archives of Physical Medicine and Rehabilitation, 64*, 378–381.

Korpela, R., Seppanen, R. L., & Koivokko, M. (1993). Rehabilitation service evaluation: a follow-up of the extent of use of technical aids for disabled children. *Disability and Rehabilitation, 15*(3), 143–150. doi:10.3109/09638289309166005

Krueger, R. A. (1994). *Focus groups: a practical guide for applied research*. Newbury Park, CA: Sage Publications.

Kutner, N. G., Zhang, R., McClellan, W. M., & Cole, S. A. (2002). Psychosocial predictors of non-compliance in haemodialysis and peritoneal dialysis patients. *Nephrology, Dialysis, Transplantation, 17*, 93–99. doi:10.1093/ndt/17.1.93

Lau, A. (2000). *A quality of life study on non-institutionalised elderly stroke survivors in Hong Kong*. Unpublished Doctor of Philosophy thesis. Brisbane: The University of Queensland.

Law, M., & Mills, J. (1998). Client-centred occupational therapy. In Law, M. (Ed.), *Client-centred occupational therapy* (pp. 1–18). Thorofare, NJ: Slack Inc.

Mann, W. C. (2001). Technology. In Bonder, B. R., & Wagner, M. B. (Eds.), *Functional performance in older adults* (2nd ed., pp. 429–446). Philadelphia: F.A. Davis Company.

Mann, W. C., Hurren, D., & Tomita, M. (1993). Comparison of assistive device use and needs of home-based older persons with different impairments. *The American Journal of Occupational Therapy., 47*(11), 980–987.

Markley, V. J., & Shepperd, J. A. N. (1990). Corset supply and the Hastings corset shop. *British Journal of Occupational Therapy, 53*(4), 155–157.

McGrath, P. J., Goodman, J. T., Cunningham, J., MacDonald, B. J., Nichols, T. A., & Unruh, A. (1985). Assistive devices: utilisation by children. *Archives of Physical Medicine, 66*, 430–432.

Moy, A. (1995). Equipment-help or hindrance? In Bumphrey, E.E. (Ed.), *Community practice: a text for occupational therapists and others involved in community care* (pp.111-121). Padstow, Cornwall: T.J. Press Ltd.

Neville-Jan, A., Piersol, C. V., Kielhofner, G., & Davis, K. (1993). Adaptive equipment: a study of utilization after hospital discharge. *Occupational Therapy in Health Care, 8*, 3–18. doi:10.1300/J003v08n04_02

Page, M., Galer, M., Fitzgerald, J., & Feeney, R. J. (1980). Problems of the selection, provision and use of aids. In Bray, J., & Wright, S. (Eds.), *The use of technology in the case of the elderly and disabled* (pp. 119–123). Westport, CT: Greenwood.

Prangrat, T., Mann, W. C., & Tomita, M. (2000). Impact of unilateral neglect on assistive device use. *Technology and Disability, 12*, 53–69.

Riemer-Reiss, M. L., & Wacker, R. R. (2000). Factors associated with assistive technology discontinuance among individuals with disabilities. *Journal of Rehabilitation, 66*(3), 44–50.

Robinson, L. (1987). Patient compliance in occupational therapy home health programs: sociocultural consideration. *Occupational Therapy in Health Care, 4*(1), 127–137. doi:10.1300/J003v04n01_11

Schemm, R. L., & Gitlin, L. N. (1998). How occupational therapists teach older patients to use bathing and dressing devices in rehabilitation. *The American Journal of Occupational Therapy., 52*(4), 276–282.

Scherer, M. (2003). *The importance of assistive technology outcomes*. January 2003 Article of the month. Retrieved February 12, 2003 from http://www.ebility.com/articles/at.shtml

Scherer, M. J. (1998). *The Scherer MPT model: matching people with technologies*. Webster, NY: Author.

Scherer, M. J. (2002). Editorial. The change in emphasis from people to person: Introduction to the special issue on assistive technology. *Disability and Rehabilitation, 24*(1/2/3), 1- 4.

Scherer, M. J., & Craddock, G. (2002). Matching Person & Technology (MPT) assessment process. *Technology & Disability: Special Issue on Outcome Measures, 14*, 125–131.

Scherer, M. J., Sax, C., Vanbiervliet, A., Cushman, L., & Scherer, J. (2005). Predictors of assistive technology use: The importance of personal and psychosocial factors. *Disability and Rehabilitation. Assistive Technology, 27*(21), 1321–1331.

Seeger, M. S., & Fisher, L. A. (1982). Adaptive equipment used in the rehabilitation of hip arthroplasty patients. *The American Journal of Occupational Therapy., 36*, 503–508.

Shapiro, P. A. (1995). Psychosocial evaluation and prediction of compliance problems and morbidity after heart transplantation. *Transplantation, 60*(12), 1462–1466. doi:10.1097/00007890-199560120-00016

Shipham, I. (1987). Bath aids – their use by a multi-diagnostic group of patients. *International Rehabilitation Medicine, 8*(4), 182–184.

Small, L. M., & Grose, J. (1993). A cultural perspective on rehabilitation and modality use with elder persons- a pilot study. *Physical & Occupational Therapy in Geriatrics, 11*(3), 71–80.

Smith, R. (1988). Quality assurance in equipment ordering for the spinal cord-injured client. *The American Journal of Occupational Therapy., 42*(1), 36–39.

Smith, R. (1995). A client centred model for equipment prescription (client values and roles, effective use of adaptive equipment). *Occupational Therapy in Health Care, 9*(4), 39–52. doi:10.1300/J003v09n04_04

Sonn, U., & Grimby, G. (1994). Assistive devices in an elderly population studied at 70 and 76 years of age. *Disability and Rehabilitation, 16*(2), 85–92. doi:10.3109/09638289409166017

Stowe, J., Thornely, G., Chamberlain, M. A., & Wright, V. (1982). Evaluation of aids and equipment for bathing survey II. *British Journal of Occupational Therapy, 45*, 92–95.

Tewey, B.P., Barnicle, K. & Perr, A.(1994). The wrong stuff. *Mainstream*, October, 19-23.

Thornely, G., Chamberlain, M. A., & Wright, V. (1977). Evaluation of aids and equipment for the bath and toilet. *British Journal of Occupational Therapy*, *40*, 243–246.

Tyson, R., & Strong, J. (1994). Adaptive equipment: Its effectiveness for people with chronic lower back pain. *The Occupational Therapy Journal of Research*, *10*, 111–121.

Wielandt, T. (2003). *The identification of the factors which influence the post-discharge use of prescribed adaptive equipment.* Unpublished Doctor of Philosophy thesis. Brisbane: The University of Queensland.

Wielandt, T., McKenna, K., Tooth, L., & Strong, J. (2001). Post-discharge use of bathing equipment prescribed by occupational therapists: What lessons to be learned? *Physical & Occupational Therapy in Geriatrics*, *19*(3), 47–63.

Wielandt, T., McKenna, K., Tooth, L., & Strong, J. (2006). Factors that predict the post-discharge use of recommended assistive technology (AT). *Disability and Rehabilitation. Assistive Technology*, *1*(1-2), 29–40. doi:10.1080/09638280500167159

Wielandt, T., & Strong, J. (2000). Compliance with prescribed adaptive equipment: A literature review. *British Journal of Occupational Therapy*, *63*(2), 65–75.

Wilson, J., McCracken, E., & Cummings, Y. (1999). Assistive devices: an audit of waiting times. *British Journal of Occupational Therapy*, *62*(6), 269–271.

KEY TERMS AND DEFINITIONS

Assistive Technology (AT): Any item, piece of equipment or product system whether acquired commercially off the shelf, modified or customised, that is used to increase, maintain or improve functional capabilities of individuals with disabilities.

Bain Assistive Technology System (BATS): Examines the needs of the consumer, the environment in which AT is used, the characteristics of the AT and the task to be undertaken. All elements are considered to be integral.

Client-Centred Approach: Involves a flexible collaborative therapeutic intervention with all stakeholders and includes personalised interventions that have a focus on the person-environment-occupation relationship.

Human Activity Assistive Technology (HAAT) Model: Considers the person, the activity to be completed, aspects of the AT and the context in which this interaction takes place.

Matching Persons to Technology (MPT) Model: Involves consideration of the needs of the person, their environment where AT will be used and characteristics of the AT itself before recommending AT to ensure a correct interface and decrease chances for non-use.

Medical Model: Treatment focuses firmly on the person's illness or disability and subsequent dysfunction and limitations. Traditionally therapeutic interventions are aimed at improving the person's functional independence.

Occupational Therapy: Use of meaningful occupation to assist people who have disabilities in achieving a healthy and balanced lifestyle and to enable an inclusive society so that all people can participate to their potential in daily occupations of life.

Social Model of Rehabilitation: Emphasizes a collaborative therapeutic intervention that addresses both the importance of a person's engagement in meaningful activity as well as facilitating their participation in wider society.

Chapter 20
Sensors and their Application for Disabled and Elderly People

Jesus Tomas
Polytechnic University of Valencia, Spain

Jaime Lloret
Polytechnic University of Valencia, Spain

Diana Bri
Polytechnic University of Valencia, Spain

Sandra Sendra
Polytechnic University of Valencia, Spain

ABSTRACT

Over the years, several systems have been developed in order to improve the quality of life of the disabled and elderly people. Moreover, many systems and devices have been deployed based on their necessities. All of these systems integrate sensors, in order to carry out their functions, and they combine the electronic field, for the sensing systems, and the mechanic field, for their mobile parts. In this paper, we will classify the sensors and their basic principles. The signals gathered by them usually have very low values, thus operational amplifiers are employed frequently to amplify these signals. Finally, we will show the most well known sensor applications for disabled and elderly people. It will be very useful for researchers that need to integrate sensors in their deployment.

INTRODUCTION

New technologies are a valuable instrument to mitigate the disabled and elderly people problems. When we speak about the disability concept (Ferreira, 2007), we refer to the fault of capacity or difficulty to carry out an activity that is considered as normal.

There are some statistical studies published that give the number of people that suffer some kind of disability. It is really surprising; according to the Statistical National Institute (INE), 8.5%

DOI: 10.4018/978-1-60566-206-0.ch020

(3,847,900 people) of the Spanish people declare to have some disability. In addition, more than 1.3 million need some kind of help to carry out the basic activities in their daily life. More than 60,000 are children and adolescents (INE, 2008).

The illnesses that can affect and hinder the disabled people to accomplish their daily activities can be classified according to their nature. We distinguish the following ones:

- Sensory illnesses, that mainly affect the visual and auditory system and frequently it can reduce the tact sense.
- Physical illnesses, that it usually affects the movement and body coordination, organic illnesses.
- Metabolic and viral illnesses and cardiopathies among others are included
- Mental and psychiatric illnesses.

The use of new technologies to develop devices for disabled and elderly people is being quite important. Our purpose, along the following pages, is to present different types of sensors and the way to process and amplify their signals. We will also show some commercial references in order to introduce the reader to the topic and analyze the circuits needed to sense the environment to facilitate the live for disabled and elderly people.

The rest of the document is structured as follows. Section 2 defines the sensor and shows the type of data that can be sensed and a classification according to their utility. The operational amplifier and the main topologies and structures of instrumentation amplifiers, which are employed in sensors, are explained in Section 3. Section 4 shows some works about devices for disabled and elderly people. Lastly, future works and conclusions are shown in section 5.

WHAT IS A SENSOR?

A sensor is a device, formed by sensitive cells, that transforms physical or chemical magnitudes (instrumentation variables) in useful signals to measure or control systems (electric magnitude). The instrumentation variables depend on the type of sensor and they can be temperature, distance, acceleration, inclination, displacement, pressure, humidity, pH, etc. The electric magnitude can be a value of electric resistance, an electric capacity, a voltage, an electric current, etc. A transducer and a sensor are different devices and they should be differentiated. A transducer is a device that transforms a physical magnitude into a different physical magnitude (such as mechanical energy or electric energy). A transducer can be a microphone that transforms an audio wave into an electric signal. A sensor is a device that provides an output signal, given by a specific physical quantity. The input value is called measure magnutude and it causes an answer in the sensor. An example is a linear variable differential transformer (LVDT), which converts a position into an electric signal (Nyce, 2004). Therefore a sensor can be considered as a transducer and vice versa. All sensors can be classified and included inside of one of the groups shown in Table 1.

Frequently, the signals obtained from the sensors are not useful to be processed and it is necessary additional circuits, as the Wheatstone bridge, or signals conditioner circuits, based on amplifiers, in order to adapt the voltage levels from the rest of the circuit. Most of these sensors offer us analog output signals and, in many cases, we need to adapt these signals in order to work with digital control devices like PCs.

It will be necessary to use an analog to digital converter. Figure 1 shows an example with all circuit blocks needed.

A sensor converts a magnitude without electric characteristic into electric signals, due to its physical effect. It can be: resistance, capacity,

Table 1. Sensors clasification

Criterion	Type	Description
Energy contribution	Modulator	The output energy comes from an external source
	Generator	The output energy is given by the input
Output signal	Analogical	The output varies in a continuous mode
	Digital	The exit varies discontinuously
Operation mode	Defection	The measured magnitude causes a physical effect in some parts of the device
	Comparison	It tries to stay the defection to zero, applying opposed effects to the one generated by the magnitude

inductance, magnetism, charges and electric field, piezoelectric effect and Hall effect (Fraden, 2003).

Charges and Electric Fields Based Sensor

In dry climate, the separation of electric charges appears due to the objects movement. This phenomenon receives the name of triboelectric. Two types of electric charges should be differenced (positive and negative charge). The same types of charges are repelled, while opposite charges are attracted. For covenant, the lines of electric field usually move from positive to negative potentials, and the density of the field lines represents the magnitude of electric field.

Three types of materials can be differentiated: conductive, where the electrons circulate freely through the material, insulator, where the electrons can not circulate, and the semiconductors material. The last one is a mixture among the conductive and insulator material, and their electric behaviour depends on the doping applied. The main semiconductors are the Silicon (Si) and Germanium (Ge). They are usually doped with atoms of Boron (B), Aluminum (Al) or Gallium (Ga) for P doping, where the majority carriers are the holes, and Arsenic (As), Antimony (Sb) and phosphorus (P) for N doping, where the majority carriers are the electrons.

Expression 1 relates the intensity of electric field $\left(\vec{E}\right)$ with the attraction or repulsion $\left(\vec{F}\right)$ that a punctual charge $\left(q_0\right)$ can suffer.

Figure 1. Block diagram of sensor

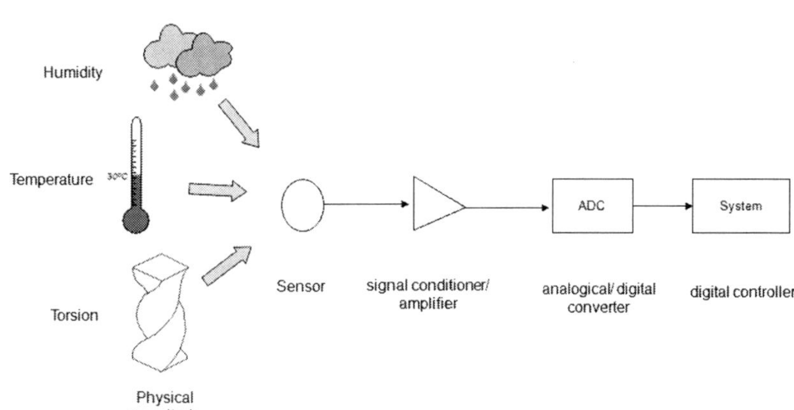

Figure 2. Piezoelectric crystal in direct mode and converse mode

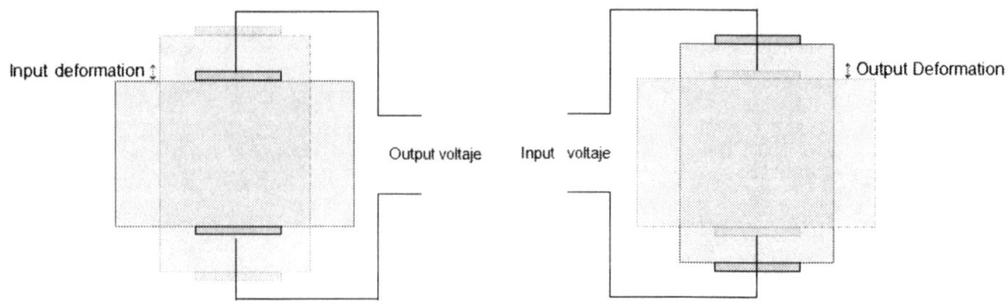

$$\vec{E} = \frac{\vec{F}}{q_0} \quad (1)$$

Where $\vec{E}$ and $\vec{F}$ are vectors with the same direction and sense.

Capacitive Sensor

In a capacitive sensor, the capacity between two or more conductors, in a dielectric medium (generally liquid or air) is measured. The conductive capacity is the property of acquiring electric load when it is subjected to an electric potential with regard to another in neutral state. A capacitor is a device formed by two conductive or armours, in badges or sheets, separated by a dielectric material. When the capacitor is subjected to a difference of potential it acquires an electric load. The capacity is measured in Farads (F).

Expression 2 shows that the capacity directly depends on the badges area, the dielectric proprieties and it is inversely proportional to the separation among the badges

$$C = \varepsilon_0 \cdot \varepsilon_r \cdot \frac{A}{d} \quad (2)$$

Where:

ε_0: dielectric of the vacuum
ε_r: Relative permittivity of the dielectric material among the badges
A: the effective area of the badges
d: distance between the badges

The capacitive sensors are usually used to measure the proximity, people or vehicles detection. They are also used to measure the pressure, liquids level, detection of the ice and even to detect the material properties (Baxter, 1997).

Piezoelectric Effect Based Sensor

The piezoelectricity is a phenomenon given in some crystals. When the crystal is subjected to a mechanic tension, acquire an electric polarization in all its volume, appearing a voltage and electric loads in its surface (direct effect). On the contrary, when a voltage is applied, the crystal acquires a deformation (converse effect). It can be seen in Figure 2. The piezoelectric effect is usually reversible: when stopping to subject the crystal to an external voltage or electric field, it recovers its original form.

The piezoelectric material can be natural or made of synthetic crystals which does not have a symmetry centre. When a compression or a shear is applied, a dissociation of the gravity centre is performed and positive or negative loads are caused.

Elementary dipoles and loads with opposed sign appear in the faced surfaces.

Two groups of materials can be distinguished: crystals, that have piezoelectric character in a natural way, and the crystals called ferroelectrics, which present piezoelectric properties after being subjected to a polarization.

The equations that model the behaviour of the piezoelectric materials are given by expressions 3 and 4:

$$D = \varepsilon \cdot E \tag{3}$$

$$S = s \cdot T \tag{4}$$

Where, D is the electric displacement, ε is the permittivity, E is the electric field, S is the deformation and T is the tension. These two equations can be combined giving the relationship between the load and the deformation. They are given by expression 5 and 6:

$$\{S\} = [s^E]\{T\} + [d^T]\{E\} \tag{5}$$

$$\{D\} = [d]\{T\} + [\varepsilon^T]\{E\} \tag{6}$$

Where d represents the piezoelectric constant of the material, the superscript E indicates that the magnitude is measured under electric field constant or zero, and the superscript T indicates that it is a transpose of matrix form.

The sensors based on piezoelectric crystals, usually are used to force measures, torsion, tension, pressure of a fluid or acceleration, among others (Gautschi, 2001).

Induction and Magnetism Based Sensor

The inductive sensors are a kind of sensors that are used to detect ferrous metallic materials. They are used for positioning applications and to detect the presence of metallic objects in a certain situation (control of presence or of absence, detection in passing, jam, positioning and count).

The voltage value V generated in a reel of N spires due to the magnetic field B and the reel area A is given by expression 7:

$$V = -N\frac{\partial(B \cdot A)}{\partial t} \tag{7}$$

The inductive sensors of proximity are formed by an internal reel. A magnetic field, is generated when a current circulates through the reel. If a metal object is close to the magnetic field, this object will be detected.

The detecting circuit recognizes the impedance changes of the sensor reel. When the detecting circuit detects that the impedance changes, it sends a signal to the amplifier placed at the exit that will change its state. When the metal is not detected, the magnetic field oscillates with a regular width.

Resistive Sensor

In a conductive material, the electrons circulate freely through it. All the conductive materials are not equals; some of them present bigger resistance to electrons movement than others. This is resistance to the electric current.

Expression 8 shows the resistance R in a metallic conductor that is connected to a voltage V and it is crossed by a current I.

$$R = \frac{V}{I} \tag{8}$$

The resistance can be expressed as a function of the material type as it is shown in expression 9.

$$R = \rho\frac{l}{a} \tag{9}$$

Where, ρ is the material resistivity, l the longitude of the metallic piece and a is their traverse section.

Hall Effect Based Sensor

The Hall Effect consists on the appearance of an electric field in a conductive matter when it is crossed by a magnetic field. It is called Hall field (E_H). When a conductive or semiconductor material, located in a magnetic field, is crossed by an electric current with a speed **v**, a magnetic force appears in charge carriers that stray it and group it to a side of the conductor or semiconductor material.. Bound to the electric field, the Hall tension appears.

The force $\vec{F}$ that exercises a subjected particle q_0 to a magnetic field $\vec{B}$ and it is moved to a speed $\vec{v}$ is given by expression 10.

$$\vec{F} = q_0 \cdot \vec{E} + q_0 \cdot \vec{v} \times \vec{B} \tag{10}$$

This field causes the appearance of an electric force $\vec{F}_e$ at the same direction, but in opposed sense of the electric field generated by the battery (F_m). When the two forces arrive to a balance state, the situation given in expression 11 is performed.

$$F_e = F_m \rightarrow q_0 \cdot E = q_0 \cdot v \cdot B \rightarrow E = v \cdot B \rightarrow \frac{V_H}{d} = v \cdot B \rightarrow V_H = v \cdot B \cdot d \tag{11}$$

Where d is the width of the material piece.

The Hall Effect sensors measure magnetic fields (Teslameter), electric currents intensity or to elaborate proximity detectors, among other applications (Ramsden, 2006).

The sensors can be classified according to the magnitude sensed or controlled (Fraden, 2003), (Baxter, 1997). In this classification we will only take into account those sensors that can be applied directly to help disabled and elderly people.

Sensors of Gravity Based on Pendulous Sensors (Inclinometer)

The inclination can be measured using the sensor ADXL202 manufactured by Analog devices. It is an accelerometer of two axes, low consumption, digital output and it is integrated in a monolithic chip. An accelerometer is a sensor that measures the movement and the vibrations, in its dynamic measurement mode, and the inclination (with regard to the gravity), in its static mode. This sensor has many advantages, due to its small size, solid integration, and easy connection with the microcontroller.

The market offers devices with several mechanical solutions, many of them are based on a free weight on a viscous medium. There are sensors based on the viscous liquid movement and an electric conductive inside a cavity. The mobile parts in many cases are submerged in oil in order to avoid oscillatory movements of the pendulum. The sensors can be based on many properties such as capacitive, electrolytic, piezoelectric, magnetic effect and resistive variation.

Sensors of Gravity Based Mercury Contacts

They are used to measure the inclination, although it is not possible to obtain intermediate values. It indicates an open or closed contact. The mercury contacts use to be a glass cylinder which contains two contacts. These sensors can be employed as warning system (e.g. the case of a person that falls on the floor). The sensor can be connected to a mobile phone or PDA that can call to a programmed number.

Sensors of Pressure, Force and Displacement Based on Strain Gauges

The Strain gauges are based on the electric resistance variation according to the deformation, in a conductive thread calibrated, or in resistances built with semiconductor tracks. They are also used, combined with springy or deformable pieces, to detect indirect efforts.

In gauges of thread, the resistance is formed by a thread prepared in zigzag form on an elastic support, with a preferable direction. When the gauge is deformed in the preferable direction, a lengthening of the thread and a decrease of their section is generated, and, therefore, a variation in their resistance is registered. The gauge should have a high resistance (between 100 and 1000 ohms) in order to measure enough resistance variations, and it has to work with a very low consumption, in order to avoid the Joule effect. The measure of deformations requires a laborious calibration, and the amplification is usually carried out using differential methods with three threads. The semiconductor gauges have more sensibility than the thread gauges because the phenomenon of resistance variation given by the deformation is joined to a piezoelectric effect. But, this phenomenon depends on the temperature extremely and it always forces to compensate the results thermally. This hinders the calibration.

Force Sensors

This type of sensor bases its operation on strain gauges. These devices transform a force, traction or a compression, in variations of electric resistance. It let us measure the force applied to an object.

Pressure Sensors

There is a broad range of pressure sensors in the industry. Mostly of them are aimed to measure the fluid pressure on a membrane. Motorola MPX2100 series devices are a small size piezoresistances that are made of pressure-sensitive silicon. They perform a voltage change which is directly proportional to the pressure applied to them. The sensor consists of a monolithic silicon diaphragm to measure the effort and a thin film resistor network integrated on a chip. The chip is set, calibrated and temperature compensated by laser.

In electronic sensors, the pressure acts on an elastic membrane and it measures the bending. In order to detect it, various physical principles can be used. It could be inductive, capacitive, piezoresistive, optical, monolithic (with extremely small electronic modules, fully connected), ohmic (through strain gauges) or Hall effect, where a permanent magnet attached to the membrane causes a change on the Hall potential.

These sensors are useful for prosthetic systems, especially for picking up objects.

Sensors of Proximity

Proximity sensors are necessary when you need to determine the position of an object, without any contact with it. They may be linear (displacement sensors) or switch, where the switching between two states indicates a particular position. Proximity sensors, commonly used in industry, are the inductive and the capacitive ones.

Inductive proximity sensors are based on the damping phenomenon that occurs in a magnetic field due to the induced currents (Foucault currents) by nearby materials, but this material should be metallic.

The capacitive sensors detect changes in the parasitic capacitance between the detector and the object whose distance was measured. They are used to measure distances of metallic and nonmetallic objects, such as wood, liquid and plastic materials.

Ultrasonic Sensors

The sensor emits ultrasonic pulses that are inaudible by the human ears. The impulses travel at the speed of sound and reach an object, then the waves are reflected and captured again by the ultrasonic receiver. A controller is built to deliver a burst of pulses and, then, starts counting the time it takes to get the echo. This time is proportional to the distance to the object. These devices are capable of detecting transparent objects like glass and plastics. However, in very turbulent air environments, with high noise, it can not be used because of its dependence on the medium.

Optical

The photocells are optical sensing elements. The same device can hold the emitter and the detector of the light beam, which is reflected on the object. They usually work with frequencies in the infrared band. The advantages of such detectors are: their immunity to electromagnetic interference, large detection distances, high response speed, color identification and detection of small objects. There is an improvement of the optical sensors that uses optical fiber. The main disadvantage is that it can not detect transparent objects.

When a proximity detector is needed, several factors must be considered. The detections of short distances (< 50 mm) can be accomplished with inductive or capacitive sensors. The election depends on the metallic nature of the material. For longer distances (> 50 mm), the use of ultrasonic or optical sensors is necessary. Proximity sensors can be installed in wheelchairs or blind systems in order to alert the users of the proximity of an object.

Sensors of Humidity

There are several types of humidity sensors. Resistive humidity sensors consist of a thin sheet of a polymer capable of absorbing water, where two contacts are printed in a conductive material, woven metal or coal. When the amount of water in the polymer changes, the electrical resistance through the polymer varies, thus this parameter is measured.

We can also find capacitive humidity sensors, where the permittivity of the dielectric changes when it is in contact with other values of humidity.

Sensors of Acidity

An ISFET (Ion Sensitive Field Effect Transistor) is an electronic-chemical sensor that reacts to any change in the pH. When the ion concentration changes (the basic pH or acid pH properties change), the quantity of ions that passes through the membrane and is deposited on the transistor gate, varies. This occurs when the sensor is in contact with the substance to be tested and varies the current that flows through the transistor.

This device is based on MOSFET transistors and it is formed by the following elements:

- A gate or membrane usually made of Si_3N_4, Al_2O_3 and Ta_2O_5.
- Source and drain areas for the substance.

This type of sensor is often used in chemical, food and ecology industry. Both humidity sensors could be used as warning system for urine detection.

Temperature Sensors Based on NTC and PTC Thermistor

A thermistor is a resistor whose value varies with the temperature. There are two types of thermistors: NTC (Negative Temperature Coefficient), which resistive value decreases when the temperature increases, and PTC (Positive Temperature Coefficient), whose electric resistance value increases when the temperature increases.

In electronics, it is important to know the temperature of the devices and systems used for sensing. It is important to protect the circuits from overheating and to avoid reaching dangerous levels of warming.

Temperature Sensors Based on RTD

RTD (Resistance Temperature Detector) sensors are based on the join of a conductive of platinum and other metals. They are used to measure the temperatures by contact or immersion. It is used when semiconductors or other sensitive materials can not be used. Its operation is based on the dilation phenomenon. That is, when the temperature rises, the metal expands and increases the electrical resistance.

Temperature Sensors Based on Bimetal

If an object is formed by two or more metals joined, it is called bi-metallic object. It is not a mixture or alloy of two metals. It is a device consisting of several layers of different metals. Trimetal and tetrametal are objects made for three and four separate metals respectively. Bimetal thermostats convert a temperature change in a mechanical movement. They are formed by two layers of metals with different thermal expansion coefficients and by temperature variations tend to bend toward the side of lower coefficient of expansion.

This property is used in power circuit breakers, where the current through the bimetal heats it. It opens the circuit to limit the peak current.

Integrate Circuits for Temperature

There are a wide variety of integrated circuit temperature sensors. These sensors are grouped into four main categories: output voltage, output current, output resistance and digital output. In voltage, we find LM35 (in °C) and LM34 (in K) from National Semiconductor Corporation. Currently, one of the most well known sensors is the AD590 from Analog Devices Inc. The resistance output sensors are less common (there are some from Phillips and Siemens).

Pirosensors (Remote Flame Sensors)

There are sensors that can determine the presence of a fire at a certain distance. It is based on the detection of a range of ultraviolet light (very sensitive in the range of wavelengths from 185 nm to 260 nm). E.g. a sensor built with UVTron bulb manufactured by Hamamatsu Photonics can detect a match into a sunny room 5 meters away. A wide variety of remote flame sensors can be found. Some of them detect ultraviolet light. Others detect infrared light.

This type of sensor is often used to detect gas-fueled flames and liquid fuel as the main component of fire alarms or monitors combustion burners, etc…

Light Sensors Based on Photodiode

The photodiode is a semiconductor diode formed by a PN junction where the semiconductor is exposed to a light through a crystal cover (with a lens form). It is especially sensitive to the incidence of visible light or infrared. All semiconductors are sensitive to the light, but the photodiodes are designed to achieve the maximum sensitivity.

In a PN junction, the current flows from the P crystal to the N crystal. It is called direct polarization. There is not any current flowing in the opposite direction. In the photodiode, the current that varies with the changes of the light, is circulating in opposite direction to the one given by the PN junction. That is, the photodiode should be inversely polarized in order to work properly and it should record an increment of the current when the diode is excited by the light.

The silicon photodiodes are built to be sensitive to the visible light (wavelength up to 1.1 μm) or germanium to be sensitive to the infrared light (wavelength up to approximately 1.8 μm), although there are devices with other semiconductor materials.

Sensors of Light Based on Photorresistance

A photoresistance or LDR (light-dependent resistor) is an electronic component whose resistance decreases when the incident light intensity increases.

The electrical resistance value of an LDR is low when light strikes and very high when it is dark (1 MΩ or more in the dark and 100 Ω in bright light). A LDR is a high resistance semiconductor such as cadmium sulfide (CdS). If the light has high frequency, photons are absorbed by the semiconductor which gives enough energy to the bound electrons to jump into the conduction band. The resulting free electron, and its hole, conducts electricity, thereby the resistance decreases.

The resistance values vary with the delay (tenths of seconds). It is different going from dark to bright than from bright to dark. For this reason, the LDR is not usually used in applications where the light signal varies rapidly.

LDRs are manufactured in various types and they can be found in many consumer items such as cameras, security alarms or on/off street lighting systems.

Sensors of Light Based on Phototransistor

The phototransistors are very similar to the regular transistors. They are composed by a semiconductor material, forming two PN junctions. They have three external connections: collector, base and emitter. Its packaging usually contains a small opening to allow the light penetration in order to produce the photoelectric effect. Its collector current flow can be controlled by the base current. The phototransistor current conduction is controlled by the current given when the light enters through the small opening.

Phototransistors have very short response time and it can respond quickly to very quick light changes. Because there is an amplification factor involved, the phototransistor delivers quite much electric current variations in response to the changes of the light intensity. The phototransistors are more sensitive to the light than the LDRs.

Sensors of Light Based on Photocells

A photocell performs a direct conversion of the light energy into electrical energy. This phenomenon is called photovoltaic generation. Some materials can absorb and emit photons of light electrons; it is the photoelectric effect. The result of this effect is an electric current that can be used to supply energy to the circuits.

Photovoltaic cells or solar cells are composed by the same semiconductor materials that are used in the microelectronics industry. A thin semiconductor wafer, with a specific treatment, generates an electric field that is positive on one side and negative on the other. When light energy falls into it, the electrons are beaten and torn from the atoms of the semiconductor material. The uprooted electrons form an electric flow that provides energy.

Photovoltaic cells are often used to obtain solar energy and to charge batteries. A sensor based on a photoelectric cell is capable of activate a circuit with its own energy provided by the presence of the light. Moreover, due to their size, fragility and price, the photoelectric cells are not considered the most desirable option to be used as a detector of light signals.

Sensors of Light Based on CCD Cells

CCD devices (Charge-Coupled Device) are integrated circuits that have an array of light sensitive cells. They are a large number of sensitive items that are packaged in a small area. They handle a large amount of image information.

The integrated circuit comprises a set of capacitors electrically coupled that are aligned each other. It can transfer their charge using methods based on electric fields. The light-sensitive elements are the capacitors, which are loaded or unloaded depending on the light that crash to them. These features make the CCD a key element for the development of existing video cameras and

Figure 3. Internal diagram of an operational Amplifier

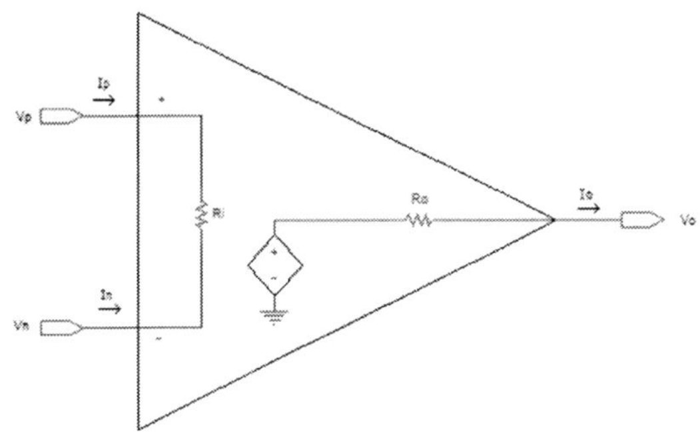

Figure 4. Transfer function of operational amplifier

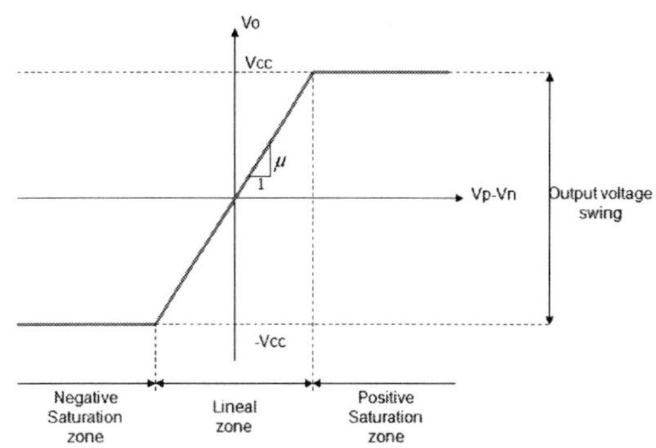

photographic extremely miniaturized with high image quality. They are also used for some types of sensors that read visual information such as scanners, readers, faxes, classifiers letters, binders of documents, etc.

SIGNAL CONDITIONER SYSTEMS

As it has been previously said, the signals coming from the sensors usually have very small values that can not be directly used. For this reason, the basic topologies used in the amplification circuits, and the combination of them to obtain bigger benefits, are shown in this section.

The Ideal Operational Amplifier

The operational amplifier is the main active lineal device given in the technology of the Integrated circuits. Figure 3 shows an example. It is a general purpose device which works with signals from 0 Hz to a frequency defined by the manufacturer. It was initially made to do mathematical operations (addition, subtraction, etc.) in analogical computers, in the 40's. The operational amplifiers have a differential input and a very high gain. Their operation features are determined by the feedback elements and their distribution regarding to the feeding values and their inputs.

The first operational amplifiers used a basic component: the vacuum valve. The vacuum valves were mainly an electronic component employed to amplify, to modify or to commute electric signals by means of the control of the electrons movement in the vacuum space. They are used in very low pressure or in presence of special gases. This element is considered the predecessor of the electronics, because it facilitated the advance of the electronics, during the second of half of the 20th century.

The most distinctive feature of an operational amplifier is its transfer function. The relationship among the input voltage (positive input V_p and negative input V_n) and the output voltage (V_o) is given by the transfer function.

Figure 4 shows that the function is divided in a lineal area, where the output signal is proportional to the difference among its two inputs, and two saturation areas. The slope of the straight line is denominated amplifier gain (open loop gain) and it is represented by μ.

The behaviour of the lineal area is represented by expression 11.

$$Vo = \mu \cdot \left(Vp - Vn\right) \quad (11)$$

When the output value *Vo* is bigger than feeding voltage $\pm Vcc$, the output will be limited by these values minus some small internal losses.

The relationship between the input and the output of an operational amplifier directly depends on the connected elements and on its location regarding to the positive input, the negative input and the output terminals. The following pages will show the basic topologies of amplification systems and their expressions (Thomas, 1984).

Non Inverter Amplifier

In this topology the input signal V_in is applied to the non inverter input. The other input has connected two resistances that give us a gain value. It can be seen in figure 5a. The relationship between the input and the output signal is shown in expression 12.

$$V\_out = \frac{R1 + R2}{R2} \cdot V\_in \qquad (12)$$

Where the quotient $\frac{R1 + R2}{R2}$ is the gain factor. This value is positive and indicates that the output signal is equal to the input signal multiplied by this factor.

Inverter Amplifier

The main characteristic of the circuit shown in figure 5b is that the input signal and the feedback loop are applied to the inverter input. The non inverter input is connected to the earth.

Expression 13 shows the relationship between the input and output signals.

$$V\_out = -\frac{R2}{R1} \cdot V\_in \qquad (13)$$

Figure 5. Basic structures

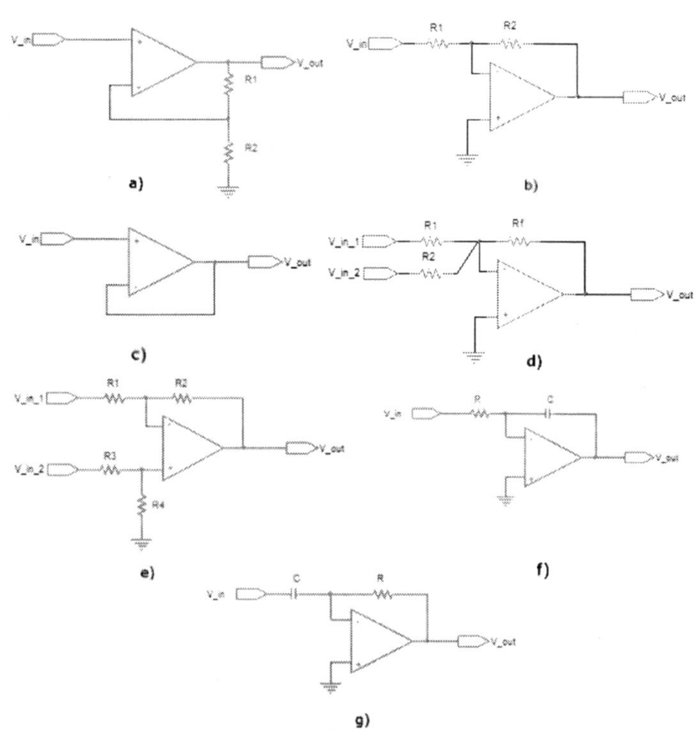

Where the quotient $-\frac{R2}{R1}$ is the gain factor. As we can see, this value is negative and indicates the difference of signs among the signals signs.

Voltage Follower

A voltage follower is a transparent system that does not carry out any change between the input and output signal. This type of circuit is usually used in coupled circuit, because it presents null output impedance. It is shown in figure 5c. The system only has a feedback loop between the output and input terminals, thus, $V\_out = Vn$. Because the entry is directly connected to the non inverter input and *Vp=Vn*, the relationship between the input and output is represented by expression 14.

$$V\_out = V\_in \tag{14}$$

Where the gain factor is 1.

Adder Amplifier

The adder circuit is shown in figure 5d. It has two inputs connected to the negative terminal and the positive input is connected directly to the earth.

As we can see in expression 15, the output signal is a pondered sum of the two inputs, multiplied by a gain.

$$V\_out = -\frac{RF}{R1}\cdot V\_in\_1 - \frac{RF}{R2}\cdot V\_in\_2 \tag{15}$$

This circuit can be seen as two overlap configurations of the inverter amplifier. It is a circuit of multiple entrances and two different gains $-\frac{RF}{R1}$ and $-\frac{RF}{R2}$. Because the gains are negative, the name of this system is called inverter adder amplifier.

Differential Amplifiers

The differential amplifier also has two inputs, as figure 5e shows. One of them is connected to the negative terminal and the other one to the positive one.

The relationship between the input and output signals can be represented by expression 16 and it can be obtained by means of circuit analysis, like the overlapping technique.

$$V\_out = \frac{R4}{R3+R4}\cdot\frac{R1+R2}{R1}\cdot V\_in\_2 - \frac{R2}{R1}\cdot V\_in\_1 \tag{16}$$

Differentiator Amplifier

A differentiator amplifier carries out the derived calculation of the input wave signal. It is seen in figure 5f.

The output wave form has an opposite sign because the input signal is made in the inverter terminal. Expression 17 shows the relationship between the input and the output signals.

$$V\_out(t) = -R\cdot C\cdot\frac{\partial V\_in(t)}{\partial t} \tag{17}$$

Where $V\_out(t)$ and $V\_in(t)$ are time dependent functions.

Integrator Amplifier

An integrator amplifier carries out a special sum called integration, where the output voltage is proportional to the area located under the wave giveb by the input signal. It is shown in figure 5g.

Its behaviour is shown in figure 6, the area located under the output curve in a given moment is equal to the input signal value multiplied by the lapsed time, that is, $V\_out = V\_in\cdot t$.

Expression 18 shows the relationship between the input and the output signal:

Figure 6. Integrator amplifier behaviour

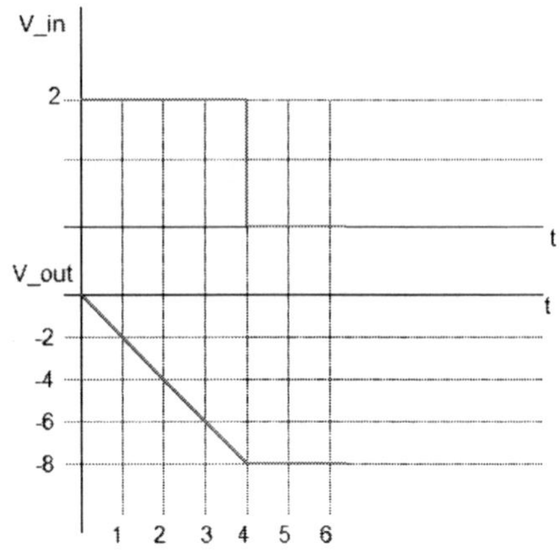

$$V\_out(t) = -\frac{1}{R \cdot C} \cdot \int_t V\_in(t) \cdot \partial t + V\_initial \quad (18)$$

Where $V\_out(t)$ and $V\_in(t)$ are time dependent functions. In some cases this circuit can be used as filter.

In electro-medicine and in many industrial applications, very low signals are measured (microvolts or some millivolts). These signals are very susceptible to be affected by big signals coming from different noise sources (such as motors, illumination tubes, etc). In order to obtain these measurements, instrumentation amplifiers with an appropriate common mode rejection ratio (CMRR) have to be used.

An instrumentation amplifier (Pallás, 2003) is an electronic device created with operational amplifiers. It is designed to have high input impedance and a high CMRR. It is able to achieve important amplifications, with very low noise and with simple or double power. It also has low thermal derives, low consumption and low output variation even close to the limit of its power.

Model of Instrumentation Operational Amplifier Based on Two Operational Amplifiers

The scheme shown in figure 18 is a basic design of the instrumentation amplifiers. Both inputs, $V1$ and $V2$, are connected to the non inverters inputs of the operational amplifiers without any additional connection of refuelling.

The resistances follow the relationship shown in expression 19.

$$\frac{R4}{R3} = \frac{R2}{R1} \quad (19)$$

The circuit is formed by two cascade stages, but none of them follows the basic structures shown previously. The global gain can be adjusted by the external resistance R_g, without the modification of the circuit features.

The relationship between their terminals is given by expression 20.

$$V\_out = Vd \cdot \left(1 + k + \frac{R2 + R4}{Rg}\right) \quad (20)$$

Figure 7. Instrumentation amplifier based on two operational amplifiers

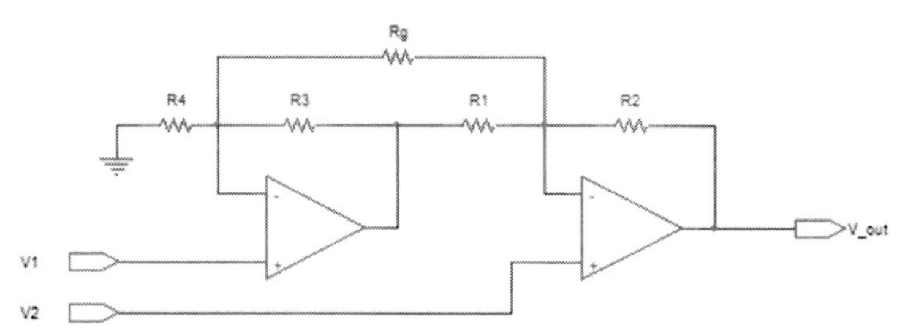

Where $Vd = V2 - V1$ and $k = \frac{R4}{R3} = \frac{R2}{R1}$.

An improvement of this system is a model of instrumentation amplifier based on three operational amplifiers.

Model of Instrumentation Operational Amplifier Based on Three Operational Amplifiers

In Figure 19, the classic design, used by most of the instrumentation amplifiers, is shown. In this model, the two inputs are connected to the non inverters inputs of the operational without having any additional feedback connection.

The resistances used in the output stage are chosen taking into account that the difference among them should be minimum (around ±0.1%).

This model let us have a CMRR of at least 54 dB which is adapted for every purpose. The first stage consists of two operational amplifiers as a preamplification system. The third operational is an operational amplifier in differential mode with unitary voltage gain. The global gain of the system can be adjusted by the resistance R2.

The expression 21 shows the relationship between their input signals and their output.

$$V\_out = -V1 \cdot \left(\frac{R3}{R2} \cdot E_{R2} \cdot E_{R1} + \frac{R1 + R2}{R2} \cdot \frac{R5}{R4} \right) + V1 \cdot \left(\frac{R3 + R2}{R2} \cdot E_{R2} \cdot E_{R1} + \frac{R1}{R2} \cdot \frac{R5}{R4} \right) \tag{21}$$

Where $E_{R1} = \frac{R4 + R5}{R4}$ and $E_{R2} = \frac{R7}{R6 + R7}$.

This type of circuit is not usually mounted with discreet elements; the manufacturers use to provide the complete circuit integrated in a single chip. Examples given are INA125 or INA124, by Texas Instrument.

SENSORS APPLICATIONS FOR DISABLED PEOPLE AND ELDERLY PEOPLE

There are many devices developed to attend disabled people with mobility problems. These systems allow them to carry out many daily activities, improving their quality of life. In case of children, sensors can help to improve their cognitive, physical and social development (Bulter, 1986). Among all the systems that can be read in the literature, we have highlighted the most sophisticated ones.

Bio-Mechanical Prosthesis

The feet and hands have several functions. With the hands, people can grab, manipulate and explore objects; the feet help us to stay erect, to walk or to maintain the balance. When a person lacks of these body parts, he/she is reduced of some of

Figure 8. Instrumentation amplifier based on three operational amplifiers

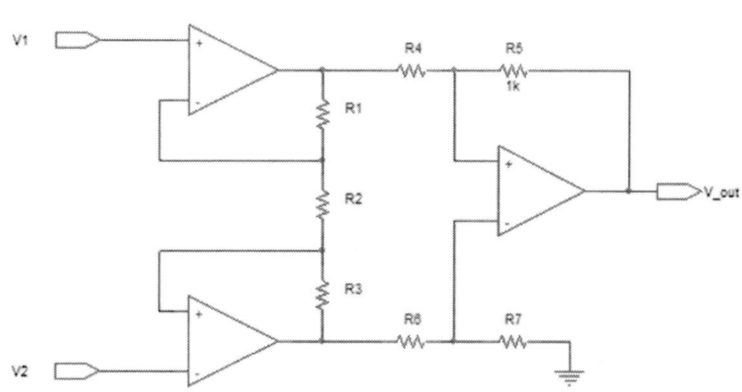

capacities to carry out a normal life. The bio-mechanical prosthesis are electronic devices with the appearance of a part of the human extremity (arm, hand, leg), endowed with an articulation system, similar to the human ones. They let the person catch and manipulate objects with precision, without breaking them. They are the most developed systems in the last years.

We can find many works related with the development of bio-mechanical prosthesis. One of them is presented by M.C. Carrozza et al. in (Carrozza, 2003). They present an artificial hand to replace an amputated member. It incorporates the main functions that a person would carry out in a normal situation. Their paper present the production process and the experiments carried out to its characterization. The prosthesis hand is formed mainly by an artificial muscle-skeletal system. It also contains a position system and forces the sensors to their correct manipulation. It has an embedded system for the device control that reacts to the received stimuli, and a machine/human interface that converts the stimuli coming from the central nervous system, to the prosthesis. It is a system formed by three fingers (thumb, index and medium) that allow catching objects with different size, texture and forms. The set of sensors are placed in the index and medium fingers, and they are connected with the thumb by a differential system. The signals obtained are transmitted directly, by the wired system, to the mobile parts of the prosthesis, what allows grabbing the objects with different form. The strength used to catch an object is proportional to the elastic properties sensed by the strength sensor. The signals obtained by this sensor are used to know the movements for the fingers. The experiments and tests carried out show that the device was able to sustain objects, making a force of 18 N.

Another work included in the prosthesis field is presented by D. J. P. Cotton et al. in (Cotton, 2007). They present a prototype of a group of sensors that can be integrated in hand prosthesis. It is a wired system that is formed by a force sensor and a temperature sensor. They are installed in the prosthesis fingertips. Also, the strength sensor system is divided in two sensors; one is the static strength, to measure the strength executed to an object, during the process of catching it, and a sensor that measures the dynamic strength and operates as a vibration sensor. All of them are built following the thick-film technology, taking advantage of the piezoresistive effect, the piezoelectric effect, the thermal-resistive effects and the thick-film properties. Many of strength sensors are built as a Wheatstone bridge with at least 4 sensors. The prosthesis usually uses a half of the Wheatstone bridge, but this can generate an incorrect result. They propose to place both sensors along the fingertips, but in different positions. When the resistance changes are measured in both sensors, the strength value is obtained. It is independent of their position. The other strength sensor is a slip sensor. It is based on the piezoelectric proprieties of the lead-zirconate-Titanate (PZT). It returns a load that is proportional to the fingertips surface vibration level. When an object is caught, it should not move. If the object moves, it means that it is slipping from his hand. The prosthesis must act to avoid the fall. Lastly, the temperature sensor is a thermistor. It checks if the temperature is adequate for the prosthesis, avoiding its damage. Their test demonstrated that the prosthesis would be able to wear a weight of 10.8 N.

Wheelchairs

The conventional motorized wheelchairs are often systems equipped with an electric motor powered by batteries, which is controlled by a joystick. D.A. Sanders et al. present a motorized wheelchair for disabled people in (Sanders, 1997). It is equipped with a system for detecting doorways. The system consists of two transmitters and two proximity receivers. The proximity sensors are based on ultrasonic devices. They are cheap and robust. The main objective of this unit is to avoid the collision with objects and obstacles, gently directing the chair out of the path where the object is located. The sensor system examines the front area of the wheelchair and identifies the door edges. The chair will choose the direction based on the outputs of both sensors. If sensors are not activated, the chair is in an area without objects. When one of them is activated, it means that the chair is approaching to an object. Moreover, if both sensors detect the object at the same distance, it may indicate that the chair is close to a door. If both sensors detect an object, the wheelchair will reduce the speed and change the path to a place without obstacles. The wheelchair lets the disabled people move freely at home, without worrying to crash with objects and obstacles.

Another work related with a wheelchair is shown in (Mazo, 2001). The authors show a wheelchair that can operate in different modes depending on the degree of disability of the user. This system is called SIAMO. It is based on a distributed control system. It has a control system, a navigation system, a human/machine interface and an environment detection system. The interesting parts for us are those that integrate sensing systems, such as human/machine interface and environment detection system. The human/machine interface is responsible for transforming orders from the user input, given by electrical stimuli, to the system. The exchange of commands and status information between the vehicle and the user is adapted according to the particular needs of the user (level and type of disability). The control alternatives are a linear control command, the joystick and several buttons, tactical control screen, voice commands (speech processing), control through breathing and control through eye movements. There are micro-cameras in front of the user to capture the images from the eyes. These images are processed and some orders are generated according with them. The cameras base their measurements on the shape formed between the two eyes and mouth. The direction is determined by two factors: the orientation of the head, which determines the overall direction, and the eyes guidance. The authors pay special attention to important issues such as visualizing the environment to prevent falls, accidents, and to facilitate tracking. SIAMO system uses mainly 2 types of sensors. The first one is based on ultrasonic sensors, which are used to detect obstacles around the chair while it is moving. The other detectors are infrared sensors and they are used to detect unevenness and a ladder. There are 2 possible approaches: the first one is based on an Infrared emitter and a position sensitive device (PSD) detector, the second one is a laser transmitter and a CCD camera as detector. All these sensors in the wheelchair let the disabled people have greater freedom and provide them a degree of autonomy.

Communications Based on Ryes Movements

People that can not communicate their emotions have a high rate of disability. It affects the whole body mobility due to possible brain damage or degenerative diseases (like multiple sclerosis). Communications based on the eye movement have been developed for this people. K. Grauman et al. present a prototype called "Blink Link" where the user is able to generate the clicks of a mouse by blinking eyes. This system lets the user to work with computer programs, video games or control programs (Grauman, 2001). Depending on the length of the blinks, the system is able to distinguish between voluntary and involuntary ones, and it only considers valid long blinks to generate mouse clicks, while short ones are discarded in the process of capturing the stimuli. The authors have used a color video camera, equipped with a CCD sensor. It works at a ratio from 27 to 29 frames per second. The camera captures images of the user's face, and renders the image. Depending on the movements of their eyes, the device generates different outputs. This device lets the user to write messages with a keyboard in the same screen. The keyboard has alphanumeric characters (A-Z and 0-9) and through the movement and blinking eyes, the users can access to the program. It also has the ability to store preprogrammed messages associated with a specific sequence of flashes longer and shorter which allows sending messages faster. There are alternatives to this method such as devices for monitoring the head movements, switches operated by hand and chin, mouth-operated joysticks or cameras oculographic estimators, among others. But the presented system does not require user's physical mobility, which is an advantage over other methods.

H. Lim et al. presented a communication system based on eye blinking in (Lim, 2005). This device is suitable for people with a high rate of disability. The detection system is based on an infrared light emitting diode as a sender, and an infrared receiver. The infrared LED emits a beam of light that is reflected on the eye surface, and this reflection is captured by the detector. The eye acts as a kind of mirror and, when the person closes it, the beam is not reflected from the eye and the system does not detect light.

The program used contains alphanumeric characters (A-Z and 0-9), and additional functions such as sending help messages. It also contains a notepad window to write messages. In order to communicate the system with the PC that runs the programs, it uses Bluetooth technology.

This system has the advantage that it does not require the use of the hands or the chin, like many others, because sometimes the paralyses that may suffer some people are total.

Sensors for Medical Applications

Although next works are used for all people, they may be mostly interesting for disabled people.

Between the related works, we can find a programmable implantable system, based on the CMOS technology, to measure intraocular pressure (Stangel, 2001). The system is composed by a capacitive pressure sensor array. Moreover, it has a temperature sensor, based on the temperature behavior of the MOS transistors when they work in weak inversion. The implantable component allows intraocular pressure and temperature measurements in remote mode. The outdoor unit and the implanted system are inductively coupled to exchange information and supply. This system allows the collection of measurements from the eye for a long period of time without the need of disturbing the patients. It lets the doctor to detect diseases and eye abnormalities as glaucoma. Other systems may be used for the same purpose, but in many cases they require surgery which leads to increase the risk given by a suregery.

There is a patent in (Wurzel, 1988) that presents a cardiac prosthesis, designed for total heart replacement or cardiac care applications with an integrated pressure sensor. Its purpose is to control blood pressure. Blood pressure is the pressure strength exerted by circulating blood on the walls of blood vessels. This prosthesis consists of two chambers separated by a membrane, which function is to pump blood throughout the body. There is a set of valves that control the entry and exit of blood as a function of the hemodynamic parameters as blood pressure. Although, there are other techniques for measuring blood pressure, they are considered invasive because they require the insertion of a catheter using surgery. The non-invasive technique proposed by the authors is a sensing system integrated in the prosthesis. It is a membrane located in the path that follows the blood inside the prosthesis. The proposed device is a strength-to-voltage transducer based on piezoelectric properties, which provides a voltage value proportional to the strength of the blood exerted on the sensor. This voltage is processed and displayed on an external display, and, depending on this value, signals are generated to act on the mechanical heart, providing information on the amount of blood pumped and the frequency.

CONCLUSION AND FUTURE TRENDS

In this document we have described the most well known sensors that can be used to develop sensor systems for disabled and elderly people. We have also shown the main circuits that can be used to develop simple sensors for disabled and elderly people. A researcher can use this study in order to develop a new sensor device for a specific purpose.

We have shown many developed systems to help disabled and elderly people, but their prices are too high. May be this study will facilitate the comprehension of developing sensors in this area.

There are new research lines working on optical sensors. They can be used in many applications. The sensor developers are improving the systems in existence while trying to reduce the production costs.

REFERENCES

Baxter, L. K. (1997). *Capacitive sensors: Designs and applications*. New York: IEEE Press.

Butler, C. (1986). Effect of powered mobility on self-initiated behaviours of very young children with locomotor disability. *Developmental Medicine and Child Neurology*, *28*(3), 325–332. doi:10.1111/j.1469-8749.1986.tb03881.x

Carrozza, M. C., Vecchi, F., Sebastiani, F., Cappiello, G., Roccella, S., Zecca, M., et al. (2003). *Experimental analysis of an innovative prosthetic hand with proprioceptive sensors. IEEE International Conference on Robotics and Automation (ICRA '03)* (Vol.2, pp. 2230-2235). Taipei. (Taiwan)

Cotton, D. J. P., Chappel, P. H., Cranny, A., White, N. M., & Beeby, S. P. (2007). Thick-film force and slip sensors for a prosthetic hand. *IEEE Sensors Journal*, *7*(5), 752–761. doi:10.1109/JSEN.2007.894912

Ferreira, M. A. V., & Velázquez, E. D. (2007, October). La discapacidad: una modalidad inexplorada de exclusión social. In *Proceedings of III Congreso Nacional sobre Universidad y discapacidad. XII Reunión del Real Patronato sobre Discapacidad*. Zaragoza (Spain).

Fraden, J. (2003). *Handbook of modern sensor: Physics, designs, and applications* (3rd ed.). New York: Springer Science.

Gautschi, G. (2001). *Piezoelectric sensorics: force, strain; pressure, acceleration and acoustic emissions sensors, materials and amplifiers*. Berlin: Springer –Verlag.

Grauman, K., Betke, M., Gips, J., & Bradski, G. R. (2001). Communication via eye blinks – detection and duration analysis in real time. In *Proceedings of the 2001 IEEE Computer Society Conference on Computer Vision and Pattern Recognition (CVPR 2001)* (Vol.1, pp. 1010-1017). Kauai Marriott (Hawaii)

Lim, H., & Singh, V. K. (2005). Design of healthcare system for disable person using eye blinking. *Fourth Annual ACIS International Conference on Computer and Information Science (ICIS '05)* (pp. 551-555). Las Vegas (USA)

Mazo, M., García, J. C., Rodríguez, F. J., Ureña, J., Lázaro, J. L., & Espinosa, F. (2001). An integral system for assisted mobility. *IEEE Robotics & Automation Magazine*, *8*(1), 46–56. doi:10.1109/100.924361

National Statistics Institute (NIE). (2008). Retrieved from http://www.ine.es/prensa/np524.pdf

Nyce, D. S. (2004). *Linear position sensors: Theory and applications*. New Jersey: Wiley-Interscience John Wiley & Sons, Inc.

Pallás, R. (2003). *Señales y acondicionadores de señal* (4th ed.). Barcelona: Marcombo S.A.

Ramsden, E. (2006). *Hall-effect sensors: theory and applications* (2nd ed.). Oxford: Elsevier.

Sanders, D. A., Stott, I. J., Goodwin, M. J., Tewkesbury, G. E., Cawte, H. & Poland, G.A. (1997) Computer systems and strategies to assist a disabled person in navigating a powered wheelchair through a doorway. *IEEE Colloquium on Computers in the Service of Mankind: Helping the Disabled* (Digest No.: 1997/117, pp.7/1-7/4).

Stangel, K., Kolnsberg, S., Hammerschmidt, D., Hosticka, B. J., Trieu, H. K., & Mokwa, W. (2001). A programmable intraocular CMOS pressure sensor system implant. *IEEE Journal of Solid-state Circuits*, *36*(7), 1094–1100. doi:10.1109/4.933466

Thomas, R. E., & Rosa, A. J. (1984). *Circuits and signals: an introduction to linear and interface circuits*. New York: Wiley-Interscience John Wiley & Sons, Inc.

Wurzel, D. (1988). Cardiac prosthesis having integral blood pressure sensor. Temple University of the Commonwealth System of Higher Education. 623/3 (United States Patent), 4781715, 1 November 1988.

KEY TERMS AND DEFINITIONS

Bio-Mechanical Prosthesis: Artificial extension that replaces or provides a missing body part for various reasons.

Common Mode Rejection Ratio (CMRR): It measures the tendency of the device to reject input signals common to both input leads

Instrumentation Amplifier: Electronic device used to adjust a signal within limits

Operational Amplifier: It is an electronic circuit used mainly for analog signal processing.

Physical Disability: The fault of capacity or difficulty of people to carry out an activity considered as normal.

Piezoelectric Crystal: Natural and synthetic crystals without center of symmetry that generate a voltage value when a force is applied to him due to the dissociation of the symmetry centers of the charges contained

Semiconductor Material: The ability of a material to conduct current is directly proportional to the number of free electrons in the material

Sensor: Device, formed by sensitive cells, that transforms physical or chemical magnitudes in useful signals for a measure or control system.

Transducer: Device that transforms a physical magnitude into a different physical magnitude, such as, mechanical energy into electric energy.

Chapter 21
Telegerontology®: A New Technological Resource for Elderly Support

José C. Millán-Calenti
University of A Coruña, Spain

Ana Maseda
University of A Coruña, Spain

ABSTRACT

One of the priorities of a modern society must be to offer all individuals the possibility to access all resources available. In this sense, there are still great differences even among well-developed countries when it comes to facing shortages in two important groups, elderly people and disabled people, even more so in the case of elderly people who are also disabled. The amazing progress of remote ICT applied to this field has meant spectacular advances, some of which will be described in this chapter. We will also devote one section to future tendencies and finally, we will focus on the system called Telegerontology®, which apart from including the basic principles of accessibility and usability, also includes those of gerontology attention, i.e., the capacity to assess the patient before the intervention.

INTRODUCTION

As the number of elderly people grows progressively and medical advances increase life expectancies, it is foreseen that the percentage of elderly people over 65 will raise from 7.3% in year 2000 to 16.2% by 2050, while 37.7% of the Japanese population, 24.1% of British, 21.0% of the EEUU population and 30% of Europeans will be older than 65 (United Nations, 2007). The growing number of elderly people also increases the dependence and/or pathologies associated with aging such as Alzheimer's disease (AD) or depression. These people need support from caregivers and there is a social and economical pressure for staying at home as long as possible. This phenomenon increases the need of help from their family and professional carers. For family carers to assume the role of caregivers is a serious

DOI: 10.4018/978-1-60566-206-0.ch021

undertaking that increases the risk of psychological, social and financial burden.

Similar to the aging phenomenon, the development of the information and communication technologies (ICT) make their application possible in different social and sanitary areas and with different objectives, like the one we are dealing with, focused on providing on-line services to the elder environment, both his/her own home or a residence. Moreover, since elderly disabled people constitute a large group, another aspect to take into account would be to have the technology to minimize their deficits.

In order for elderly people and remote control devices to interact efficiently, it is necessary to consider the elderly characteristics as well as the accessibility and usability of the devices. In a large percentage of cases, elderly people report good health, despite the elderly representing the largest group of people with disability. One important element when approaching the use of ICT addressed to the disabled population would be to assess elderly people capacities which, in principle, would be enough to interact with the machine; that is, the capacity to see, the capacity to listen, to communicate and to carry out different tasks. In Spain (INE, 2008), the total disability rate per thousand inhabitants is 302.7; 349 per thousand when referring to women and 240.7 when referring to men. This figure goes up to 514.6 per thousand for people over the age of 80. With regard to disabilities that may interfere in the interaction with the ICT, 91.4 per thousand present with visual disability or limitation; 103.5 per thousand with hearing limitation; 59.9 per thousand with communication limitation and 50.1 per thousand present with some disability in knowledge application and task development (Table 1). Furthermore, women represent a higher rate than men and it is common to find individuals presenting with several disabilities at the same time.

Disability in the elderly population will be an extra handicap in the use of ICT; hence the development of devices fulfilling the "accessibility" and "usability" criteria is necessary to reach the highest number of users. Accessibility is a term that refers to the guarantee that any resource, no matter what its origin, is available to all people, disabled or otherwise (Berners-Lee & Fischetti, 1999); while "usability" is a measurement to know how much a product can be used by some people to reach certain objectives (Nielsen, 1993). It is clear that both terms can be used with several meanings in different situations but in this case we are referring to the use of ICT; that is, any device we design no matter to whom it is addressed, and more over if it is addressed to disabled elderly people, must fulfill the accessibility and usability premises. In our case, and since we refer to the ICT application as reaching the interaction between a remote control and a user via Internet, we would need to know how a remote assistance device addressed to elderly people with or without disability would be, in order to fulfill the aforementioned premises. The answer is not an

Table 1. Elderly people with some disability of limitation with regard to the use of new technologies, by gender. Rate per thousand (Source INE, 2008)

	Total	Men	Women
Total for all disabilities	302.1	240.7	349.0
Vision	91.4	71.2	106.5
Hearing	103.5	94.1	110.5
Communication	59.9	48.9	68.0
Learning, knowledge application and task development	50.1	35.2	61.3

easy one and the ideal device still doesn't exist, but what we can state for now is that the elements to be used by the end user would be as easy and intuitive as possible.

As far as the hardware is concerned and regarding the remote assistance system, it will vary depending on the system features, but in general, the necessary elements will be a computer (set-box), a screen, a pointing device (mouse or mouse emulator), web cam, microphone and audio, and the necessary devices for other types of measurements such as biomedical parameters or domotic control. With regard to the software, it must adapt to the system features providing a friendly interface. The control centre and user environment must be connected via Internet.

Since many of the aspects referred to accessibility and usability are dealt with in another chapter of this book, we will now describe the aspects related to the devices included in Telegerontology® and for that, we will make a short summary of the main remote assistance devices existing in the market from its beginning; then, we will present the system called Telegerontology® explaining its architecture and features and finally a presentation of some of the projects which, based on their innovations and interest, may contribute to the development of this field of knowledge.

BACKGROUND

Independently from other devices used with more or less efficiency, the start-up of the remote assistance in the socio sanitary field goes back to the 1960s, when different countries started to use the first tele-alarm equipment. In general, when speaking about tele-alarm, we refer to a transmitter device the elder wears (normally a bracelet or pendant) equipped with a switch that, when pressed, emits a signal to the control centre. Obviously, tele-alarm systems have further developed from the early ones, like the above mentioned which sets a telephone call to a prefixed number answered by a telephone operator, to the most sophisticated ones where the signal is emitted from any device having that capacity, both if the user presses the switch or the device detects a specific situation (long immobility, fall, crossing the limit area, etc.) generating a hearing/visual/mixed signal that makes it easier for the receptor to locate the transmitter.

Tele-care is a system similar to the above but, in this case, the reception of an alarm signal will start up a number of different welfare services. We are more interested in the services based on the ICT than in those related to direct attention. In general, the name of tele-care refers to the provision of remote social services.

The Tele-care allows elderly people and/or those with disability, who live alone and in risk situation to get in touch (by phone) with the assistance centre. At the beginning, tele-care had an eminent social content and included immediate support via telephone; the mobilization of resources in emergency situations; monitoring of users via periodic calls and the agenda as a reminder for drug intake or tasks, among its services.

When Dr. Khalid Mahmud in 1993 founded American Tele-care and tested a blood pressure meter inside an aluminum box connected to a videophone, we were probably witnessing the birth of telemedicine or telehealth. Nowadays, telematic stations are able to carry out remote registers of several parameters such as blood pressure, pulse, heart and lung sounds, oxygen saturation, weight, blood sugar, lung capacity and volume, cognitive screening and drug intake control, among other functionalities.

Several systematic revisions (Barlow, Singh, Bayer, & Curry, 2007; Botsis & Hartvigsen, 2008) have verified the importance of the tele-care systems addressed to elderly people living in their own homes, particularly when suffering chronic pathologies like diabetes, heart failure, cognitive impairment, chronic obstructive pulmonary disease, chronic wounds or mobility disabilities. End users reported great satisfaction although would prefer a combination of both home tele-care and conventional health-care delivery. With regards to diabetes in particular, Chan et al. (2005) observed a 100% compliance with the program in their study of diabetic people. Significant reductions in total calorie intake as well as body mass index were achieved. Miyauchi et al. (2003) proposed a system able to control patient movements when walking, running or at his/her position at a specific moment. The system, equipped with an accelerometer, can detect sudden changes in the position (such as falls) and set off an alarm.

The possibilities of telemedicine are huge and, nowadays, it is possible to send almost any kind of information via the Internet to be assessed or interpreted by other professionals. It is also possible to establish diagnosis or to perform operations without being in direct contact with the patient. Pervasive home monitoring is set to play an important role in maintaining the independence and improving the quality of life for elderly people at a lower cost (Rajasekaran, Radhakrishnan & Subbaraj, 2009).

The development of computerized applications of cognitive stimulation has also benefited elderly people. These applications consist of a number of sequential activities that attempt to stimulate the different brain functions. Some need a digital support (CD, DVD…) to be run while others are executed via the Internet; moreover, some of them are feedback applications registering the results while others do not register anything. We understand that a good computerized application of cognitive stimulation should include a system to assess the cognitive level of the user in order to periodically, assess and adapt the activities to the detected level. On the other hand, the assessment via cognitive stimulation applications would allow us to do a longitudinal monitoring of the users. Alternatively (or complementary, depending on the case), those telemedicine systems equipped with a videoconference would take advantage of the resources and establish tele-surgeries with specialists (Guilfoyle et al., 2002), carry out psychometric tests (Tyrrell, Couturier, Montani, & Franco, 2001) or establish therapeutic procedures (Arnaert & Delesie, 2001).

An example of some cognitive stimulation applications currently commercialised is Gradior, developed by the Fundación Intras in 1999. It is based on the traditional stimulation method consisting of the systematic and repetitive application of tests and exercises, previously selected by the therapist according to the necessary level of difficulty. The advantage of this method is the possibility to do a neuropsychological assessment simultaneously, which makes it possible to know the user's evolution through time. The program emits positive and negative reinforcements according to the given answers, avoiding feelings of frustration and motivating the user to continue with the tests. Gradior was designed to be used in a care centre under the supervision of a therapist. In order to beat these care limitations, a new project named TeleGradior was developed after the agreement between the Fundación Intras and Telefónica. The Fundación ACE and Edu@migos developed SmartBrain, a system that allows the patient to interact with the cognitive stimulation program via the internet or a CD-ROM. When using an internet connection, the therapist can remotely define the therapies and check the results. SmartBrain does not assess the results of the activities so the user's longitudinal monitoring is not possible. The German company Schuhfried commercialises various products focused on the psychological assessment and the cognitive training such us the Vienna Test System of computerized psychological diagnosis with more than 80 tests; Cogniplus, of cognitive training adapted to the user's deficit; and RehaCom, software of cognitive rehabilitation consisting of different levels of difficulty. Cogniplus and RehaCom need a specific panel, which makes their use more limited. Two programs, CogniFit Personal Coach and MindFit are commercialised under the name CogniFit, Personalised Brain Fitness Programs. CogniFit Personal Coach is a cognitive training application which adapts to the user's capacity while MindFit is a CD program developed to assess, exercise and improve the daily necessary cognitive skills like short and long term memory, work memory, visual and hearing memory, task schedule and attention, decision-making and hand-sight coordination. The IBM Thinkable is the IBM contribution in the field of cognitive intervention. The program is addressed to professionals working with people suffering from memory loss. Other commercialised products that do not focus exclusively on the cognitive training try to cover wider areas, such as ElderGames, for example, which aims to investigate the therapeutic game effects on elderly people from the positive results obtained in younger subjects; or Brain Training, which is a videogame in which the activities display as the player solves the games (Table 2).

As seen above, the offer for cognitive intervention applications is large but, in our opinion, any application addressed to elderly people and/or with therapeutic objectives within the cognitive field should fulfill a number of requirements, described in Table 3.

TELEGERONTOLOGY®

Concept

The aim of Telegerontology® is to be a new resource of gerontology support that takes advantage of the ICT development in the online caring environment. Its objective is the remote caring of elderly people so that both the hardware devices, programs and interfaces have been designed to fulfill the accessibility and usability standards.

Telegerontology® is included in the so-called "Apoyo Gerontológico a Domicilio" resources (*Home Gerontology Support*) (Millán-Calenti, 2006) which take, as a starting point, the necessity of an assessment of the user's needs previous to intervention. In order to do so, Telegerontology® must be able to obtain the results of the user-machine interaction and it is this particularity that makes this technology different from others.

Among its functionalities, Telegerontology® includes five basic services: tele-alarm, tele-rehabilitation, professional at home, an application of cognitive tele-stimulation and different health contents. Determination of biomedical parameters and control of domotic elements are in the process of integration.

Table 2. Main applications of cognitive stimulation

Company	Product Name	Web Page
Fundación Intras	Gradior Telegradior	http://www.intras.es/
Fundación Ace Educ@migos	Smartbrain	http://www.smartbrain.net/smartbrain/previo_en.html
Schuhfried	Vienna Test System Cogniplus RehaCom	http://www.schuhfried.at/en/home.html
CogniFit (Personalised Brain Fitness Programs)	CogniFit Personal Coach MindFit	http://www.cognifit.com/home1
IBM	Thinkable	http://www.ibm.com/es/es/
Eldergames	ElderGames	http://www.eldergames.org/
Nintendo	Brain Training	http://www.touchgenerations.com/esES/games_DS_TGP/brain_training/overview_brain_training.php

Table 3. Minimum requirements for a computerized application of cognitive stimulation

Requirements	Features
Design	Simple. Avoiding the necessity of continuous supervision by the therapist
Dynamics	Possibility to include more activities at any time
Economics	Facilitate its use to all groups of people, regardless of economical level
Time to carry out the activities	Adapted to the level of difficulty of each activity
Reinforces	Always in positive
Failure options	Restrict the number of allowed failures according to the level of difficulty
Answer options	Each activity will have several answer options based on the level of difficulty; avoid random answers when including only two answer options
Procedure	Simple and intuitive
Instructions	Via auditory and visual channel
Images	Use photos instead of drawings
Icons	Simple and easy to understand
Interaction mode	Use an adapted, ergonomic design and easy comprehension device

The required equipment to operate Telegerontology® is a control centre, one or several remote controls and software communicating both via Internet (Figure 1).

Architecture

The objective of Telegerontology® is to put professionals and users in different locations in contact; users could be at their homes, institutions, sanitary premises, etc. and the professionals in a control centre or any other physical premise. In order for the professionals to efficiently develop their activity, they need to have access to the information contained in the user's medical record and be able to communicate between themselves. All information will be stored in a server located in the care centre or by "housing" in a service supplier.

Figure 1. Architecture Telegerontology® system

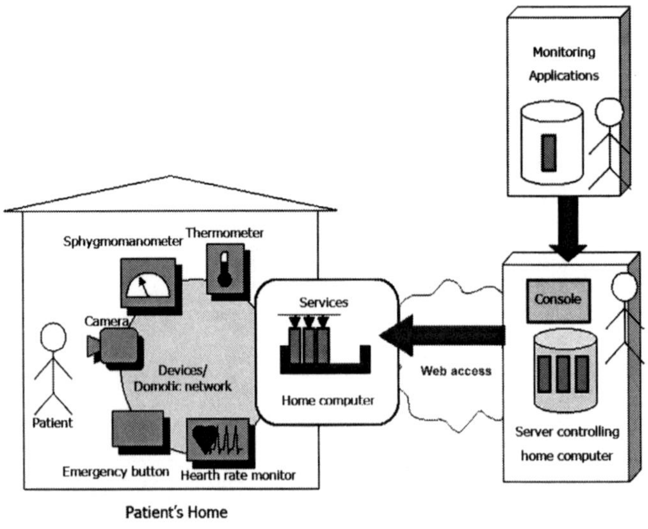

Internet is the means used to connect the control centre and the end users due to its wide distribution and its increasingly affordable price.

The equipment to be installed at the user's home will be an emergency button, one camera to supervise the user's state and establish videoconferences, various devices to monitor the patient's vital signs and a computer that will integrate all these services and use a broad band access (ADSL, HDLC…). This basic installation will grow rapidly both in number and the types of devices, due to the new developments and according to each patient's needs. For this reason, the software integrating the computer functionality is modular and as independent as possible. The system is divided into services and each service is directly pluggable within the general container.

The servers, control centre and Call-Centre for user's attention are located in the Data Centre as well as the therapies recording and emission rooms and the offices for the support personnel. If necessary, the Call-Centre could be relocated to somewhere else. The system could integrate connected units of mobile attention to go to the remote centre in certain situations such as the installation of the necessary equipment.

Figure 2 shows a diagram of the Telegerontology® architecture.

Control Centre

The functioning philosophy of Telegerontology® establishes a Socio-sanitary centre as the perfect place to locate the Control Centre because they will provide most of the Telegerontology® contents: transmission of physical or cognitive rehabilitation sessions and professional at home sessions, apart from getting the emergency calls and the results of the users-devices interaction.

Thanks to the technologies used, both the caring part and the alarms reception have an identical physical structure and hardware/software requirements. The software does not require installation as it runs from the servers; this way, all working

Figure 2. Telegerontology® Architecture Diagram

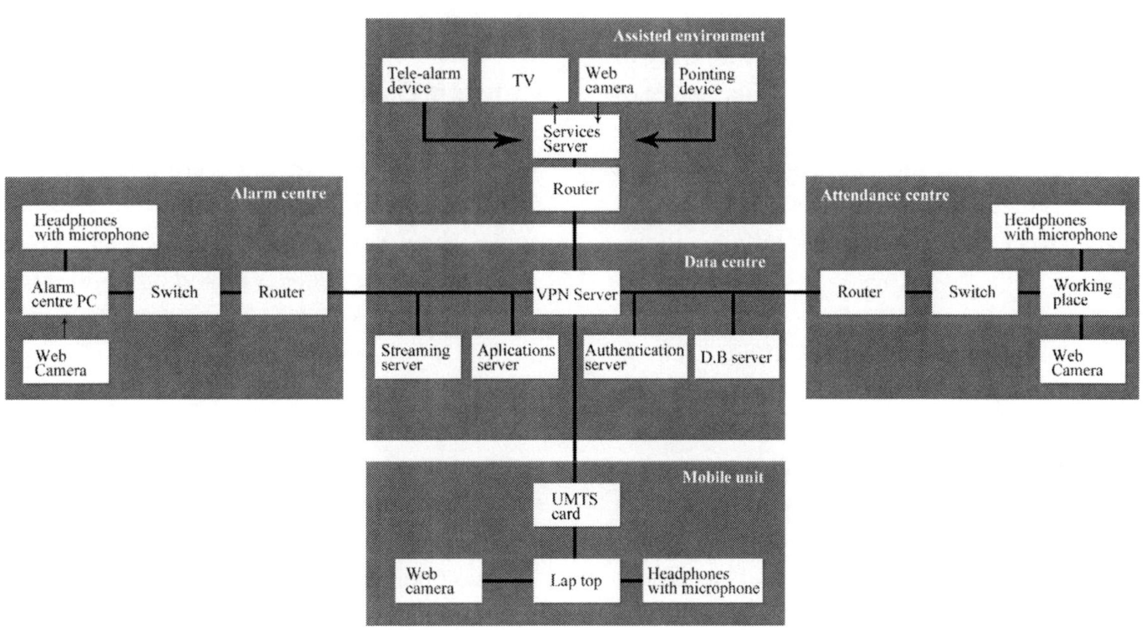

places are available for all functions. If necessary, it is possible to install working places in different locations with the sole restriction of having a control centre. This characteristic enables a simple and fast growth.

Hardware requirements for each location are a router (which routes to the external IP); a switch for data interconnection among different equipment; a PC assistance/alarm working place consisting of one multimedia computer from which the telegerontology staff interacts with the patients and with the management applications of the assistance centre; a web cam, headphones and a microphone.

This equipment will run the following software: a web browser to interact with the applications and general web contents deployed in the applications´ servers of the assistance centre or other prefixed locations; Messenger to allow therapists to receive videoconferences from the users´ homes or from other therapists and to send instant messages; and an alarm application for reception of users' alarms.

Data Centre

In an initial stage, servers can be located in the control centre, but as the number of users grow and consequently, the needs of band width, it will be necessary to locate them in the Data Centre of a telecommunications company. As the number of users grows, servers should evolve towards a server farm with a Hot-Site Back Up.

The Data Centre would consist of the following elements:

- VPN server to connect the different remote equipment as if they were located in the same net.
- Database server to store all management information. Access to this information is only possible through the different applications and following the necessary safety rules.
- Management applications server to provide functionality to the management of gerontology records.
- Server for the cognitive stimulation application which provides the necessary activities for the assessment and diagnosis of patients, monitoring all the results.
- Server with useful contents or information for the end user.
- Instant message server that communicates the connected users to Messenger and to other instant message applications.
- Tele-alarm server to relieve and store the help requests made through the panic button.
- VOD or video server under demand.
- Videoconference server consisting of a videoconference call control system.
- Drivers´ server where all different necessary drivers would be stored to interact with the domotic and biomedical devices.
- Biomedical data server, responsible for the reception and processing of the medical data.
- GSM server, responsible for the communication with the GSM service supplier who will send the location data.

Remote Centre

We will refer to Remote Centre as each of the devices located outside the Control Centre, which means, those devices located at the user's home, social centers, residences or any other premises.

A complete Remote Centre would consist of the following devices:

- Screen, (a normal TV set or a computer screen)
- Web cam, microphone and headphones
- Service terminal integrating all the other components and providing the necessary computer safety

- Pointing device allowing interaction with the installed software at the Service Terminal. Its present shape is a wireless pad
- Router providing functionality to route to the external IP network
- Wireless Tele-alarm device
- Biomedical devices providing measurements and control of the patients′ vital signs, sending this information to the computer to be stored in the assistance centre
- Domotic devices allowing control and supervision of the user's home conditions
- Locating device providing technological support to locate the user

On the other hand, the service terminal will run the following software:

- The user's interface mediates between the user and the different services showing the adapted visual components
- A Web browser allowing the interaction with applications and general web content
- Terminal administration providing remote access
- Multimedia: allows reception, visualization and sending of multimedia content
- Tele-stimulation, implementing cognitive tele-stimulation activities
- Tele-alarm, sending alarm signal when the user presses the emergency button within the signal range
- Biomedical devices, allowing data transfer from the devices
- Domotic interfaces, controlling home devices and facilitating different activities, providing the user with certain safety by means of emergency detection devices.

Main Components

The Services' Terminal is composed of a VIA EPIA Motherboard that integrates a VIA C7-D processor without a fan, a 512Mb DDR2 RAM memory module and a 2Gb Compact Flash card connected to the IDE interface. A 12V input DC – DC power supply providing all the necessary energy allowing its connection to an external adapter or to a 12V battery without requiring forced cooling. Thanks to this configuration the Terminal can work occupying a small amount of space and without producing any noise.

The Terminal's Operating System Distribution had been developed based on *Ubuntu* Dapper fitting the necessary requirements and totally adapted to the Terminal's Hardware to improve performance. To avoid damaging the Compact Flash Card the Operating System works entirely in memory being loaded from an image in the compact flash by a "shoehorn" specially developed for this distribution. The Distribution includes a SSH server that allows Terminal's remote administration.

The Terminal's Graphical User Interface (GUI from now on) uses the SWT components allowing the dynamic load of services which are the pieces of software that really provide end user's functionality.

The Server-Terminal's Communications protocol is built on top of a Web Service, creating a session in the server with the first call in which the Terminal's and User's identifying data is maintained.

On top of the GUI, the cognitive stimulation application and a videoconferencing system that sends audio and video feeds using RTP have been built, as well as a streaming Video On Demand software.

Another service integrated into the GUI is a Web Browser (Firefox) configured to maximize accessibility allowing access to third party web sites.

The System integrates all kind of domotic devices, especially those security and safety oriented, such as smoke detectors, presence detectors, etc. These devices communicate wirelessly with the same protocol and frequency as the tele-alarm one.

A wireless pointing device (GeroPad®) has been developed and tested in a field study with over sixty users (Figure 3).

The alarm reception application allows attending alerts originated by the domotic devices or by the user itself. It has been developed taking advantage of technologies such as Java with SWT (allowing its execution in any environment), Java Web Start (allowing the execution in any Java-enabled computer without installation) and Web Services (providing communication between the Clients and the Server). Once a user-generated alert is processed, the System tries to launch a videoconference between the Users's Home and the professional attending the alert; once this videoconference is established the professional has all the information related to the User: call history, basic health information and the User's current location.

An Instant Messaging System, called GeroMessenger, allows the professionals working in the Tele-care Centre to share information, coordinate their actions and videoconference with the Users.

The administration application of the cognitive stimulation software (Telecognitio®) allows cognitive stimulation activities suitable for this software to be created and to review the User's cognitive state.

In the Tele-care centre a complete clinical, social and interaction history of the user is stored, in particular the information from areas most affecting elderly people. The clinical history management software simplifies the communication between different professional profiles attending the Users, taking into account both legal and privacy issues; It also helps researchers to exploit the data efficiently.

There are a lot of biomedical data acquiring devices in the market, but most of them don't offer the possibility of connecting to a computer system. Those that have this connection cost too much to be used in this project and use a proprietary protocol that forces a new driver to be developed for each one. In general, all devices are very complex, needing the user intervention to make the measurement and to transmit the data to the host computer. This is why the decision to develop a biomedical data measurement devices line that complies with the accessibility standards and at a small cost has been made.

Connection to the mainly used domotic nets is intended to create "ambient intelligence", and thus, control the User's environment increasing safety, security and comfort.

To reduce maintenance costs, it is necessary to develop a remote configuration and administration software tool which allows changing key parameters in the system. This software (being targeted to non-technical personnel) would be web based.

The tele-alarm device is basically a wireless button adapted to the User's needs allowing its installation as a pendant, a wrist watch and/or in a belt clip. Once the button is pushed, if the User is inside the Terminal's range, a videoconference is initiated between the User's home and the Tele-care Centre. In situations where the User is outside of the home, the tele-alarm device would send a signal directly to the Tele-care centre showing the User's location.

Figure 3. Designed pointing device

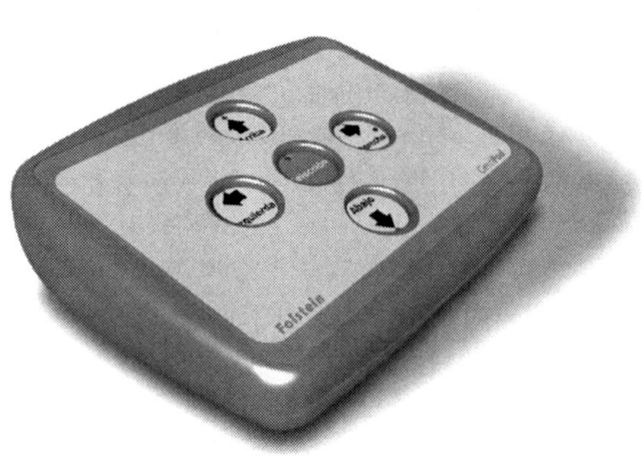

FUTURE TRENDS

The development of communication and information technologies (ICT) is unstoppable and thus, very difficult to foresee where it can take us. In the Telemedicine field, some projects stand out due to their innovating character like the Advance care and alert portable telemedical MONitor (AMON), whose objective was to develop and validate a bracelet device able to monitor data related to the heartbeat, blood pressure, 2 channel EKG, oxygen saturation, resistance and skin temperature and send it to a control centre via GSM/UMTS. Distance Information Technologies for home care (CHS) tried to develop a telemedicine system with a coordination clinic centre and units at the patients´ homes equipped with a personal computer including measurement devices for vital signs. It was particularly addressed to patients with diabetes mellitus, heart failure or trauma. The aim of the Remote Monitoring of Diabetic Feet (Diafoot) project is the design of a preventive system for remote monitoring of the feet of diabetics. According to this aim, a wireless sensor insole has been built, which is able to measure plantar pressure while the patient leads his/her normal life. Measured data are continuously sent to the Diabetic Foot Unit at Hospital, where a team of specialists analyze this information. Quite innovating was the device developed by Universal Remote Signal Acquisition for Health (U-R-Safe) which opens new possibilities for the textile and clothing field. Some recommendations have already been made (Meinander & Honkala, 2004). The concept is to have the elderly person wear medical measuring devices to register EKG, oxygen saturation, pulse, breathing, falls and once all data is collected, send it via Ultra Wide Band (UWB) when the elderly person is at home or via the wireless public Network (GPRS, UMTS and/or GEO satellites) when the elderly person is away from home. The system presents some kind of "intelligence" that allows it to discern when a potentially dangerous situation has occurred and consequently, forwards an alarm to the monitoring centre without the patient's intervention. Kishimoto et al. (2009) proposed a wearable computer for monitoring the physical conditions of elderly people and patients through an EMG and an accelerometer. Confident Information Environment for the Independent Living of People with Severe Disabilities (Confident) proposed the development of a system for the assistance of people with severe disabilities in all daily activities. The system includes a wireless handheld device that monitors vital signs and home environment sensors, a PDA with GPRS connection for the professional to consult the patient clinical record and a coordination centre. Supporting Independently Living Citizens (SILC) is focused on the development of an intelligent alarm system equipped with a range of biometric sensors programmed to trigger an alarm call automatically when a critical situation is detected. Biometric sensors monitor the heart pulse rate including the variation of the pulse and body temperature among others. It has the possibility to do electrocardiograms by connecting the terminals to the handheld device and also includes Bluetooth communication between the sensors and the control base, which connect with a service centre via telephone. It can also transfer the monitored vital sign data and the patient's voice. A wearable system supporting services to enable elderly people to live well, independently and at ease (ENABLE), intends to develop a system to help elders and their carers with the activities of daily living. Problems of everyday living to be addressed include: using the phone; raising the alarm in emergency to get help; being monitored for health conditions, a fall, or sign of distress, with automatic rising of alarm if necessary (Table 4).

On the other hand, there is another group of projects which, besides integrating telemedicine elements, try to develop the Smart-Home concept, i.e., homes equipped with different sensors which can anticipate different situations, particularly emergency situations and automatically send alarms to a control centre where the suitable resources can be activated. The SOPRANO project (http://www.soprano-ip.org) aims to design systems, which assist elderly people to cope with everyday life in greater comfort and safety. The main activities have focused on the investigation of the mental and communicative capacities of an elderly sample, on providing homes with sensorial and cognitive capacities to help the user and on allowing any user–independently of the sensorial disorder, to communicate with a remote centre. The concept of combining the smart house sensor technologies with an external provider in cases of emergency is shared with the EMERGE project (http://www.emerge-project.eu). EMERGE Supports elderly people with emergency monitoring and prevention. EMERGE start-point is the assumption that humans are bio-psycho-social beings whose character is to follow typical behavior, especially elderly people, so that the innovation is to algorithm this behavior in order to detect deviations from typical behavior patterns. The approach is to use sensors to monitor activity, location and vital data. Final del formulario

NETCARITY (http://www.ikerlan.es/site_preview/NETCARITY.php) seeks to advance ambient intelligence technologies by the integration of micro and nano systems in a networked wireless/wired multi-sensing environment with plug-and-play capabilities and intelligent decision making for an effective detection of critical situations and support of task completion. The MPOWER project (http://www.sintef.no/Projectweb/MPOWER) aims to simplify and speed up the task of developing and deploying services for persons with cognitive disabilities and the elderly. The platform will, in particular, support the integration of smart house and sensor technology, the interoperability between profession and institution specific systems, and a secure and safe information management, including both social and medical information. In the PERSONA project (http://www.igd.fraunhofer.de/igd-a1/projects/persona/index.html), the goal is to go forward in the Ambient Intelligence paradigm by the harmonization of Ambient Assisted Living (AAL) technologies and concepts. The system can detect specific emergency situations; call the doctors, firemen and safety people as well as automatically turn on/off electrical appliances, lights, cooker or TV set. The goal of SHARE-IT (http://www.cosy.informatik.uni-bremen.de/shareit/project.html) is to develop a scalable, adaptive system of add-ons to sensor and assistive technology so that they can be modularly integrated into an intelligent home environment to enhance the individual's autonomy. The system will be designed to inform and assist the user and his/her caregivers through monitoring and mobility help. The focus is on add-ons to be compatible with existing technologies and to achieve an easier integration into existing systems. Scalability is meant to include or remove devices from the system in a simple, intuitive way.

Robotics is another field where good results regarding companion or facilitating elements at home are being reached. Do you imagine a Robot, humanoid or not, accepted by elderly people which could be a companion and a caregiver at the same time? Obviously, it is not easy to imagine but undoubtedly such a robot will be a reality in a near future. In any case, independently from the robotics development in the area of elderly care, Galindo, Gonzalez, & Fernández-Madrigal (2006) propose the human-robot-integration concept, and their opinion is that human support would help the interaction with the robot.

The first companion Robots were designed to emulate animals, particularly dogs, as they are considered the animal companion par excellence. In principle, these robots include multiple modes and simple programming systems. They have sensors to avoid hitting obstacles, can move different parts of their body independently and are normally remote-operated. Aibo, a robo-dog manufactured by the multinational Sony, was presented in 1999. It can learn, entertain or recognize the owner's voice and gestures, among other functions. Within the EU FP7, a consortium of 16 entities from 8 European countries are involved in the CompanionAble project (http://www.companioAble.net), whose objective is to provide the synergy of Robotics and Ambient Intelligence technologies and their semantic integration to provide for a care-giver's assistive environment. This will support the cognitive stimulation and therapy management of the care-recipient. This is mediated by a robotic companion (mobile facilitation) working collaboratively with a smart home environment (stationary facilitation). Another group of American researchers from the University of Illinois and Rush University (both in Chicago), have developed a Robot (RISQ technology) able to receive oral and gesture orders, even tactile orders, which can communicate with the patient, no matter his/her language problem. The Chinese from the Harbin Institute of Technology have developed a more or less 1.5 m height robot able to look for food and medicines, detect water or gas leaks, send images and even sing and play. Riken and Tokai Rubber Industries (http://www.riken.go.jp/engn/index.html) have developed a robot, named RIBA (Robot for interactive Body Assistance) capable of safely lifting and moving a human patient of up to 61 kg from a bed to a wheelchair and back. In order to carry out this delicate function, RIBA is equipped with tactile great precision sensors and a body encased in a soft exterior of urethane foam.

As seen in the above mentioned examples, prototypes are being developed in a number of different fields. Regarding Telegerontology®, while waiting for the so-called "broad band" to really be available everywhere, tries to include other domotic elements such as blinds, doors, lights and a wide range of sensors for biomedical determination apart from those already functioning like the temperature, pulse, blood pressure or oxygen saturation controls. In a near future, Telegerontology® could be able to incorporate its functionalities to a carer-robot to facilitate the elderly to stay at their own homes and so, delaying institutionalization.

CONCLUSION

The aging of the population, together with the decrease in the number of traditional caregivers of dependent people has launched the exhaustive search for new resources to somehow allow elders to live in their own home as long as possible. In this sense, ICT development tries to look for technical solutions to create real intelligent homes with the help of numerous sensors to detect and report any change in the house conditions or its inhabitants. Besides the Smart-Home concept, we must emphasize the great advance in Robotics, meaning the creation of real humanoids that in a near future will be able to emulate many of the functions currently assumed by the caregivers, "humans" in this case.

It is unpredictable where progress may take us, but in any case, from our point of view and independently from any support that machines can provide, a human being must be behind any device and obviously, behind the patient.

REFERENCES

Arnaert, A., & Delesie, L. (2001). Telenursing for the elderly. The case for care via video-telephony. *Journal of Telemedicine and Telecare*, *7*(6), 311–316. doi:10.1258/1357633011936912

Barlow, J., Singh, D., Bayer, S., & Curry, R. (2007). A systematic review of the benefits of home tele-care for frail elderly people and those with long-term conditions. *Journal of Telemedicine and Telecare*, *13*(4), 172–179. doi:10.1258/135763307780908058

Berners-Lee, T., & Fischetti, M. (1999). *Weaving the Web: The Original Design and Ultimate Destiny of the World Wide Web by Its Inventor*. San Francisco: Harper.

Botsis, T., & Hartvigsen, G. (2008). Current status and future perspectives in tele-care for elderly people suffering from chronic diseases. *Journal of Telemedicine and Telecare, 14*(4), 195–203. doi:10.1258/jtt.2008.070905

Chan, W., Woo, J., Hui, E., Lau, W., Lai, J., & Lee, D. (2005). A community model for care of elderly people with diabetes via telemedicine. *Applied Nursing Research, 18*(2), 77–81. doi:10.1016/j.apnr.2004.11.002

Galindo, C., Gonzalez, J., & Fernández-Madrigal, J. (2006). Control architecture for human-robot integration: application to a robotic wheelchair. *IEEE Transactions on Systems, Man, and Cybernetics. Part B, Cybernetics: A Publication of the IEEE Systems. Man, and Cybernetics Society, 36*(5), 1053–1067. doi:10.1109/TSMCB.2006.874131

Guilfoyle, C., Wootton, R., Hassall, S., Offer, J., Warren, M., Smith, D., & Eddie, M. (2002). Videoconferencing in facilities providing care for elderly people. *Journal of Telemedicine and Telecare, 8*(S3), 22–24. doi:10.1258/13576330260440745

INE. 2008. *Encuesta de Discapacidad, Autonomía Personal y Situaciones de Dependencia 2008 (EDAD 2008)* [Disability, Independence, and Dependency Situations Survey (EDAD 2008)] Retrieved September 30, 2009, from http://www.ine.es/jaxi/menu.do?L=0&type=pcaxis&path=%2Ft15/p418&file=inebase.

Kishimoto, M., Yoshida, T., Hayasaka, T., Mori, D., Imai, Y., Matsuki, N., Ishikawa, T., & Yamaguchi, T. (2009). An internet-based wearable watch-over system for elderly and disabled utilizing EMG and accelerometer. *Technology and health care-European Society for Engineering and Medicine, 17*, 121-131.

Meinander, H., & Honkala, M. (2004). Potential applications of smart clothing solutions in health care and personal protection. *Studies in Health Technology and Informatics, 108*, 278–285.

Millán-Calenti, J. C. (2006). *Principios de Geriatría y Gerontología* [Principles of Geriatric Medicine and Gerontology]. Madrid: McGraw Hill-Interamericana.

Miyauchi, K., Yonezawa, Y., Maki, H., Ogawa, H., Hahn, A., & Caldwell, W. (2003). A new microcomputer-based safety and life support system for solitary-living elderly people. *Biomedical Sciences Instrumentation, 39*, 179–182.

Nielsen, J. (1993). *Usability engineering*. New York: Academic Press.

Rajasekaran, M. P., Radhakrishnan, S., & Subbaraj, P. (2009). Elderly patient monitoring system using a wireless sensor network. *Telemedicine Journal and e-Health, 15*(1), 73–79. doi:10.1089/tmj.2008.0056

Tyrrell, J., Couturier, P., Montani, C., & Franco, A. (2001). Teleconsultation in psychology: the use of videolinks for interviewing and assessing elderly patients. *Age and Ageing, 30*(3), 191–195. doi:10.1093/ageing/30.3.191

United Nations. (2007). *World Population Prospects: The 2006 Revision*. Retrieved September 30, 2009, from http://www.un.org/esa/population/publications/wpp2006/WPP2006_Highlights_rev.pdf.

KEY TERMS AND DEFINITIONS

Accessibility: The guarantee that any resource, by any means, is able to be reached or acquired by everybody, with or without disability.

Geropad®: Pointing device, conventional mouse emulator which, equipped with four directional buttons and one central "enter" button allows to navigate through the Telegerontology® contents, thanks to its ergonomic design and usability.

Robotics: Science and technology robots; it includes different disciplines such as electronics, computing, artificial intelligence or control engineering and deals with the robot's design, manufacture and applications.

Smart-Homes or Home Automation: The automated control of household appliances and features in residential dwellings, particularly through electronic means.

Tele-Care: The remote care provided to the elderly living at home and to keep them living there.

Telegerontology®: Online Home Gerontological Support resource addressed to the elderly with the capacity to carry out a remote assessment.

Telemedicine: Medical care provided at a distance where medical information is transferred using Internet or other networks for the purpose of remote medical diagnosis, consultation and treatments.

Usability: Measurement to know how much a product can be used by some people to reach certain objectives.

Chapter 22
Experience Using Information and Communication Technologies with Elderly People

Laura Nieto
University of A Coruña, Spain

Betania Groba
University of A Coruña, Spain

Francisco Servia
University of A Coruña, Spain

ABSTRACT

The elderly show very low rates of access to and use of the new technologies in comparison with their significant weight in the overall population. It is essential to establish alternatives which respond to their needs and promote the access to and use of ICTs among all citizens on equal conditions. This chapter describes an experiment conducted with new technologies in the Red Cross Elderly Day Care Centre in A Coruña, using the In-TIC software and a specific methodology for intervention with elderly individuals. Three different lines of action were followed: initial evaluation of the users participating in the project; intervention by means of digital literacy and therapeutic stimulation sessions with the ICT; and final re-evaluation and data collection. The results obtained provide proof of an improvement in the users' cognitive abilities, the acquisition of computer knowledge and skills, and the satisfaction of the elderly with regard to new technologies.

DOI: 10.4018/978-1-60566-206-0.ch022

INTRODUCTION

Information and Communication Technologies (hereinafter, ICTs) are increasingly pervasive in our society, and in the majority of our everyday activities. Access to and use of ICTs provides citizens with a broad range of possibilities in terms of leisure, access to information, interaction, communication, training, etc. (Villar, 2003; Grande, Pereira, Mato & Pazos, 2008), as well as an enormous quantity of resources, making it possible to improve or even increase individuals' level of participation in activities which are significant for them, thus enabling them to comply with the social demands of the community to which they belong, and attain suitable levels of occupational performance.

Taking into account the continuous developments in the field of new technologies in recent years, one could say that the society in which we live has progressed along the path towards the so-called Information Society (Villar, 2003; Grande, Pereira, Mato & Pazos, 2008), a new social scenario characterised by the massive diffusion of computing, telematics and audiovisual communication media (Pousada, Groba, Orozco, Martinez, 2008). Promoting and facilitating the access to and use of ICTs for as many people and in the most egalitarian way possible is essential if individuals are to be able to respond to both their own vital needs and to the requirements and demands of the environments in which they live.

Nonetheless, we constantly come across situations in which there is no real access to ICTs and, hence, to this new society which is taking shape before our very eyes. This is true of many handicapped or elderly individuals who, faced with this process of innovation and technological development, find themselves in a situation of exclusion. This phenomenon is referred to as the digital divide, a term which defines the inequality arising as a consequence of certain groups of citizens' lack of integration into the new technologies (Grande, Pereira, Mato & Pazos, 2008), and consequently, into the so-called Information Society.

The Elderly and New Technologies

As mentioned above, this affects a fairly significant proportion of the population, particularly, individuals with low educational, training or economic levels, the people with disabilities and the elderly.

More specifically, "the elderly appear among the groups with the lowest levels of knowledge of and access to the new resources supplied by the new technologies" (Villar, 2003). Nevertheless, the proportion of this population group within the population as a whole is increasing steadily in practically all countries, a phenomenon to which Spanish society is not immune (Miranda, 2004). In accordance with the figures from the National Statistics Institute of Spain, obtained from the municipal census published on 1 January 2008, individuals over 65 years of age account for 16.54% of the total population. At the current moment, it is estimated that this percentage has reached 16.7% (current population estimates, as of 1 April 2009, calculated on the basis of the 2001 Population and Housing Census) and it is believed that this will continue to increase, approaching 30% by 2060 (long-term population projections obtained on the basis of the 2001 Population and Housing Census). (Instituto Nacional de Estadística, 2008a; Instituto Nacional de Estadística, 2001).

Evidently, the elderly represent a significant proportion of the population in our society; nonetheless, their access to and use of ICTs in general, and more specifically of computers and the Internet, is very low. In 2008, the percentage of individuals aged between 65 and 74 who at some time had used computer was 16.2%, while for the rest of the population (individuals between 16 and 74 years of age) the figure was 67.4%; the percentage for those who had access the Internet sometime during that year was 10.6%, while for the remainder of the population the figure was 61.7% (Instituto Nacional de Estadística, 2008b).

Figure 1. Percentage of individuals who used a computer or the Internet at some time in 2008

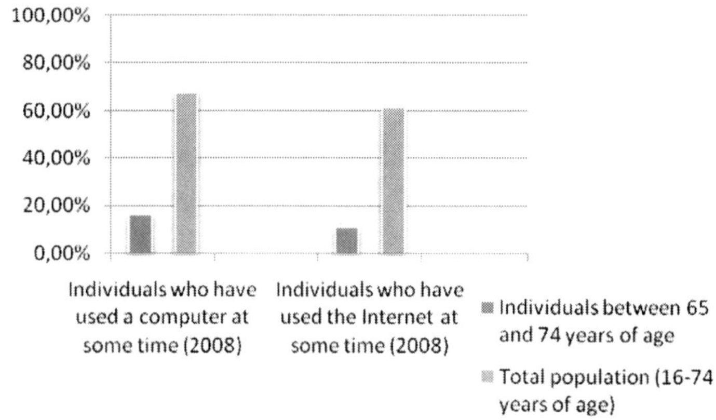

The abovementioned data are represented below, in Figure 1.

Thus, "the statistical data point to the fact that the elderly use technology to a lesser degree than the rest of the population" (Miranda, 2004), in spite of the benefits and possibilities it can offer them (communication and interaction with their surroundings, inter-generational exchange of knowledge and experience, exercising of cognitive functions, involvement in new forms of leisure and entertainment, etc.).

Access to and use of ICTs also constitutes an inherent right of all human beings, "without distinction of any kind, such as race, colour, sex, language, religion, political or other opinion, national or social origin, property, birth or other status", as stipulated in the Universal Declaration of Human Rights (United General Assembly, 1948), as well as in other national and international conventions, regulations and legislations.

Consequently, one of the challenges of this new Information Society is, clearly, to encourage the access of the elderly and other social groups in a situation of exclusion to ICTs, thus favouring their social integration and improving their personal autonomy, their quality of life and their level of health.

Digital Training Experiments

One of the principal obstacles that the elderly encounter when accessing resources and possibilities offered by the new technologies, is the lack of computer training and know-how, on both theoretical and practical levels (Villar, 2003).

Consequently, one of the lines of action to be followed is, unquestionably, training in computer literacy, which goes beyond mere technological instruction. This could be defined as a series of "educative actions aimed at the development of technical, social and ethical abilities relating to the use of ICTs", thus insisting on the opportunities that ICTs can provide for the development of individuals who are critical, active, reflective and capable of transforming the society in which they live (Travieso & Planella, 2008).

In this regard, numerous projects are being conducted on both national and international levels. In Spain, there are increasing numbers of computer services targeted specifically at the elderly, promoted from both the public and private sectors: Universities for the Elderly, associations, foundations, etc. (Gómez del Castillo, 2003). Among the recent educative endeavours worthy of special mention are those carried out in eight centres for the elderly in Barcelona (Villar, 2003), in the "Aula de Mayores" in the Universities of Murcia

(Gómez & Navalón, 2000) and of Extremadura (Corcho & Corcho, 2004), along with the initiatives promoted by the La Caixa Foundation (Obra Social Fundación La Caixa, 2007) and the Orange Foundation (Orange Foundation, 2009).

MAIN FOCUS OF THE CHAPTER

This chapter describes the experiment conducted with new technologies in the Red Cross Elderly Day Care Centre in A Coruña, using In-TIC software and a specific methodology for intervening with the elderly, both designed by the Medical and Radiological Diagnosis Information Technology Centre (IMEDIR) of the University of A Coruña.

This experiment was originally conceived as a Digital Literacy training project. Nonetheless, with the passing of time, additional objectives have been proposed regarding the therapeutic possibilities that ICTs may offer the elderly.

The final objective is to develop the support system, the In-TIC software, and make it available to individuals with functional diversity by means of a personalised intervention methodology, with the aim of facilitating interaction with the virtual setting and access to ICTs in equality of opportunity with all other citizens, reflecting the inherent right of all individuals to access the Information Society and to enjoy accessible, usable technologies.

MATERIAL AND METHODS

The In-TIC project is an initiative developed by the IMEDIR Centre; it is based fundamentally on the principle of the inclusion of the handicapped and the elderly into ICTs and in the Information Society.

In a society such as ours, where the population is ageing at an increasingly significant rate, it is becoming necessary to establish new alternatives to respond to the needs of citizens, and in this case, these are intervention alternatives addressing the needs of the elderly.

Participants

The principle of equal opportunities in access to ICTs was put into practice by making ICTs available to the elderly through the experiment in a day care centre for the elderly:

Red Cross Elderly Day Care Centre in A Coruña

This day care centre in A Coruña attends to 35 elderly individuals, suffering from problems of different degrees at a cognitive, physical, sensorial and/or social level; hence, the majority of them are individuals with functional diversity who have difficulties on an occupational level in some activities of their daily life, in their leisure activities or in their social participation.

The project was conducted integrally within the Day Care Centre, counting on the continual collaboration between the staff therein and the personnel of the IMEDIR Centre, with the project having been designed and implemented from its inception by three occupational therapists from the latter. Participating in the experiment were 11 users of the day care centre, divided into three groups. Two computer literacy sessions per week were carried out along with therapeutic stimulation of each one of the three groups.

Inclusion Criteria

- For the inclusion of users in the project, the following criteria were established:
- Aged 65 or over.
- Initial motivation for participating in the experiment.
- Presence of stable cognitive abilities, taking into consideration the scores obtained in one of the evaluation scales employed (MOCA, which will be explained below in

this chapter). A score of 15 out of 30 was set as the threshold for inclusion in this project.

Characteristics of the Users Participating in the Project

Table 1 shows the characteristics of said users in terms of sex, age, prior computer knowledge, difficulties perceived in handling ICTs and motivation for taking part in the project.

In summary, a total of nine women and two men took part, with a mean age of 79. In general, the users had no prior computer knowledge, but all of them demonstrated motivation for participating in the project.

Methodology

In order to implement the project, three differentiated lines of action were followed:

Evaluation

The first line of action consisted of a study and analysis of similar projects, such as the Orange Foundation's Edad project or the La Caixa Charity Relief's Computer Workshops. This first line of action also included a study and analysis of the support technology on the market regarding the access to and use of new technologies by the elderly.

During this stage, we also evaluated the different prior abilities and knowledge of the users

Table 1. Characteristics of the users participating in the experiment

Partici-pants	Sex*	Age	Prior computer knowl-edge	Difficulties handling ICTs**			Motiva-tion
				Cognitive	Sensorial	Physical	
User 1	*F*	*88*	*1*	*3*	*2 Visual*	*1*	*4*
User 2	*F*	*83*	*1*	*1*	*3 Visual*	*4*	*4*
User 3	*F*	*67*	*1*	*3*	*2 Visual* *2 Auditiv.*	*2*	*4*
User 4	*M*	*71*	*1*	*4*	*2 Visual*	*1*	*2*
User 5	*F*	*65*	*1*	*2*	*3 Visual*	*3*	*3*
User 6	*F*	*68*	*2*	*1*	*3 Visual*	*4*	*4*
User 7	*M*	*90*	*1*	*2*	*4 Visual*	*3*	*2*
User 8	*F*	*79*	*1*	*3*	*2 Visual*	*3*	*3*
User 9	*F*	*86*	*1*	*3*	*2 Visual*	*1*	*3*
User 10	*F*	*77*	*1*	*4*	*2 Visual*	*2*	*3*
User 11	*F*	*92*	*1*	*4*	*2 Visual*	*3*	*4*

It is used a rank from 1 to 4 for three items of the table
(Prior computer Knowledge; Difficulties handling ICTs and Motivation), being:
(1) None, (2) Little, (3) Moderate and (4) A lot

* SEX: F: Female M: Male
**Cognitive: it refers to the score obtained in Montreal Cognitive Assessment:
(1) Score 26-30; (2) Score 21-26; (3) Score 18-21 (4) Score <18
**Sensorial and Physical: it refers to score obtain in evaluations designed by the IMEDIR Centre.

participating in the study, using different evaluation tools.

Intervention

The second line of action consisted of implementing the project through computer literacy and therapeutic stimulation sessions using ICTs, each with duration of between 45 and 60 minutes. To do so, and based on the data gathered in the initial phase, the process was focused on:

Adapting Computer Equipment.

Designing virtual environments adapted to the users through the creation of In-TIC software interfaces.

Advising Users on the Use of Different Systems for Accessing ICTs.

Conducting digital literacy and therapeutic stimulation activities using a methodology designed specifically for that purpose.

Encouraging the learning of activities that support the occupational performance of activities in users' everyday lives.

Re-Evaluation and Collection of Data

The third, and final, line of action was based on the collection of data. It was carried out at the end of the intervention on the basis of recorded sessions, which were conducted by the occupational therapists who implemented the intervention and on the basis of different standardised instruments as well as interviews with users and with the professionals involved in the project.

The retrieved information will serve to establish results concerning the project and its functionality, whether or not there is an increase in the abilities evaluated, as well as the participants' perception of the ICTs and the possibilities that they offer to the elderly individuals involved in an equal opportunities project.

Material

Evaluation

The material used for the study and analysis of similar projects and other assistive technology available for the elderly was obtained on the basis of a bibliographic review of different documents in databases such as Dialnet, EMBASE, CINAHL, Pubmed and CSIC.

A number of different instruments were used during the evaluation period. For the evaluation of the users' cognitive abilities and skills, the scale used was the Montreal Cognitive Assessment (MOCA). This includes the following items: visuospatial/executive capacity, naming, memory, attention, language, abstraction, delayed recall and orientation. The total score for this scale is 30 points.

For the evaluation of prior computer knowledge and interests with regard to this matter, the Prior Computer Knowledge Questionnaire and the Needs and Demands Survey were employed, both designed by the IMEDIR Centre. The Prior Computer Knowledge Questionnaire comprises 25 items, evaluating the recognition of the components of a computer system, the identification of icons, the performance of different actions with the computer and the use of applications and programmes, among others. The Needs and Demands Survey comprises 26 questions and gathers personal data and information on computer resources which the individual has available.

Intervention

The material used for the intervention consisted of the In-TIC software along with an intervention methodology, structured into 5 blocks and 25 didactic units, developed specifically for the elderly.

The In-TIC software (Integration and accessibility of individuals with functional diversity in the use of Information and Communication Technologies) is a support system for the access to and use of ICTs, which allows the virtual environment to be personalised and simplified as far as possible using virtual keyboards.

The application has been developed based on the principles of equal opportunity in access to ICTs and on Universal Design or Design for All guidelines, whose objective is to arrange the environment in a way that enables everybody to perform equally and as independently as possible, and to integrate the different needs of individuals in installations which may be used by anybody (The Center for Universal Design, 1997). In this case, these principles are put into practice in compliance with the requirements established by the Spanish regulations for desktop applications (UNE 139802:2003. Computer Applications for people with disabilities. Computer accessibility requirements. Software).

The methodology comprises a set of 5 blocks and 25 didactic units which aim to familiarise users with the use of computers and the Internet. In turn, each of the didactic units is made up of different sessions. This is a methodology which is suited and adapted to the needs, capabilities, potentialities and interests of the elderly.

The didactic units are structures as indicated below:

- Block I, titled Introduction to the computer and its handling, is made up of four didactic units: Introduction to the computer, Using the mouse, In-TIC and Knowledge integration.
- Block II, titled Windows applications, is divided into five units: The text editor, Word; The graphic editing program, Paint; The calculator; The media player; and Knowledge integration.
- Block III, titled Internet and its possibilities, comprises the following didactic units: Introduction to the Internet, Web Browsers, Searching for images with Google, Searching for videos with Youtube, E-mail, The press and the radio on the Internet, and Knowledge integration.
- Blocks IV and V are made up of different activities from everyday life, from leisure activities to the social participation of users. The content developed in the first three blocks and the abilities and skills acquired enable users to perform the activities in the final two blocks. The aim thereof is to highlight, on one hand, the possible use of ICTs as a therapeutic stimulation tool in the intervention in different areas of occupational performance and, on the other hand, the opportunities they may provide to improve the quality of life and autonomy in said areas.
    - Block IV contains different didactic units related to basic activities and instrumental activities in daily life (hereinafter, BADL and IADL, respectively): Temporal and spatial orientation, Handling the euro and Doing the shopping. The first two present different therapeutics stimulation activities through ICTs. The final didactic unit proposes an activity aimed at showing users how they can apply the abilities and knowledge acquired throughout the course to a daily task, such as doing the shopping. It is left to the professional's judgement to decide whether or not it is necessary to undertake all the didactic units in this block, based on the cognitive and functional level of the users and their performance in these occupational areas. In some cases, the professional may go straight to Block V, if it is considered that the performance of the members of the group

with regard to the BADLs and IADLs is adequate.

- Block V, titled Leisure and social participation, comprises six didactic units: Leisure through ICTs, The microphone, The webcam, Working with a blog, Making a souvenir video and Open Day. The aim of these is to provide a final touch for the entire learning experience, showing, on one hand, the possible application of ICTs in significant leisure and social participation activities and, on the other, the preparation of a memento of the course, with the contribution of each one of the users.

Re-Evaluation and Collection of Data

Data collection was carried out with different measuring instruments used to register quantitative and qualitative variables, and which collect information on the different aspects that form part of the project as a whole.

For the re-evaluation, we used both the Montreal Cognitive Assessment (MOCA), which establishes to what extent the cognitive abilities were affected, and the Prior Computer Knowledge Questionnaire, designed by the IMEDIR Centre, with the aim of verifying the level of the users' knowledge of new technologies after having participated in the experiment.

Lastly, and with the aim of evaluating and analysing the qualitative aspects of the process of the project, the Satisfaction with the In-TIC Project Survey was conducted; interviews with each one of the users taking part were also carried out, and discussion groups were formed among them, using to this end a semi-structured interview template and recordings, and subsequently transcribing and analysing the accounts.

RESULT

Of the data collected, a number of different results are worthy of mention; these can be structured into two different levels.

On the quantitative level, a comparative study and analysis of the data from the MOCA scale and from the Prior Computer Knowledge Questionnaire were conducted (see Table 2). With regard to cognitive abilities, in 64% of cases an improvement was observed in relation to the overall score for the scale. More specifically, in the majority of cases the scores for visuospatial/executive capacity, attention and delayed recall have increased. In the remainder of cases, said abilities were maintained, and a slight deterioration was observed only in some individuals. On the other hand, the comparison of data from the Prior Computer Knowledge Questionnaire provides relevant results: in 90% of cases abilities for the independent handling and use of the computer were acquired in at least 15 of the 25 items included in the scale.

On a qualitative level, relevant results have been obtained regarding the participants' perception of ICTs and their impact on their health. The Satisfaction Survey showed a mean score of 4 out of 5 for personal satisfaction with the project and of 3 out of 5 for the perception of increased quality of life, personal autonomy and independence in activities in daily life. Finally, a number of different categories arose from the interviews and discussion groups, and of which worthy of special mention are independence, learning, difficulties and health, as recurring issues which the participants identify themselves when analysing their interaction with ICTs.

Based on the above, it can be said that, by way of general results for this project, improvements were obtained in the users' cognitive abilities, the acquisition of computer knowledge and skills, and the satisfaction of the elderly with regard to new technologies. Moreover, it was observed that, in those participants who showed the greatest

Table 2. Comparison of the initial and final scores obtained on the MOCA scale

Participants	Initial MOCA score	Final MOCA score
User 1	18/30	19/30
User 2	26/30	29/30
User 3	18/30	19/30
User 4	15/30	Not evaluable
User 5	21/30	26/30
User 6	27/30	25/30
User 7	24/30	21/30
User 8	18/30	21/30
User 9	18/30	19/30
User 10	16/30	19/30
User 11	17/30	17/30

motivation when starting the project, their continuance therein and their attendance of sessions was greater.

As we have seen, the events of the last few months have shown results, but also certain needs. The preliminary results clearly show that there is interest and motivation towards interaction and communication through ICTs on the part of the elderly. Nonetheless, it is essential to find the way of preparing and empowering users in order for them to acquire control over their own actions. The enormous quantity of information and knowledge equates to a challenge, and as such, opens new paths to be explored.

DISCUSSION AND CONCLUSION

The study conducted contains a series of limitations or difficulties with regard to contextual factors and the setting in which the project is carried out.

On one hand, an intervention specifically adapted to elderly is proposed, using material that had not previously been tested in other contexts, given that this is an "in-house" design. For said intervention, a methodology has been followed, and which in turn has a number of limitations, such as, availability of space and materials, absence of support products which would enable the accessibility and usability of ICTs by the elderly, the influence of the cultural and social setting when designing and preparing the didactic units.

On the other hand, there are information biases in the evaluation and re-evaluation of the participants in the project, particularly in the evaluation of cognitive abilities, due to the fact that users simultaneously receive stimulation from other therapies in the day centre, and due to the existence of age-related cognitive deterioration, which is not pathological, but which may have a bearing on the analysis proposed. Moreover, the small size of the sample studied should also be taken into account, as it precludes the reaching of definitive conclusions at present.

Nevertheless, a review of similar studies shows that, in general, interventions are aimed primarily at the handling of operating systems and computer programmes, and not at the real application of this knowledge in daily life or the satisfaction of users' needs or expectations.

Therefore, the methodology developed does not focus solely on the digital literacy and technological training of the target users. The contents dealt with throughout the project are particularly linked to occupations which are significant for the individual, and the application of the knowledge acquired in the performance of everyday activities through ITCs. Also, the new technologies incorporate the aspects of therapeutic intervention, the aim of which is to improve the quality of life of the individual and to increase his/her independence and autonomy.

Additionally, the experiment carried out can be characterised as being fully personalised, allowing all kind of adaptations to the needs, capacities and potentialities of the elderly and the true rate of learning. The benefits for the individuals participating in the project are numerous: promotion of cognitive and psychomotor activity, maintenance or improvement of certain mental functions, establishment of social links, involvement in new forms of leisure activities, encouragement to integrate into a new, constantly developing society, and the involvement of elderly individuals in activities which are significant for them through ICTs.

Thus, understanding the concept of health as the state of complete physical, mental and social well-being, and not only as the absence of illnesses, in line with the current definition proposed by World Health Organisation (World Health Organisation, 2001), after having conducted this experiment, we can assert that ICTs have an impact on the health of elderly individuals if they are used as a tool to empower them as individuals to control their actions in their life projects. Hence the need arises to promote initiatives facilitating the use of ITCs to the elderly and other social groups with functional diversity, thus encouraging their participation as citizens and their occupational performance.

In light of all the above, the aim is to ensure that the integration of elderly individuals into society and into their surroundings increases constantly, along with their quality of life and the state of health, understanding that in our new paradigm of health, "attaining a complete state of physical, psychic and social well-being on an individual level is not enough; rather, there must also be contextual conditions which allow this well-being to translate into to the recognition of the essential rights of individuals, reflected in the full, decent and significant participation of citizens within society, and in conditions of equality" (Emeric, 2008, pp. 30-41).

ACKNOWLEDGMENT

This work has been carried out with funding from the Orange Foundation. La Caixa Foundation and Mapfre Foundation have also contributed to making this project possible.

It is also acknowledged the cooperation and involvement of Ruben Grande, occupational therapist, who designed the scales and assessment questionnaires and led to the launching of the project with the elderly in Red Cross Day Care Centre.

Finally, it is needed to appreciate the work carried out by the Red Cross Elderly Day Centre of A Coruña and, specially, to all the people who have taken part in this experience, because it could not have been carried out without their support.

REFERENCES

Center for Universal Design. (1997). The Principles of Universal Design. Retrieved May, 2009, from http://www.design.ncsu.edu/cud/about_ud/udprinciplestext.htm.

Corcho, P. I., & Corcho, P. A. (2004). Informática para mayores. Una experiencia en la universidad de Extremadura. *Revista Latinoamericana de Tecnología Educativa*, 3, 529-534. Retrieved September, 2009, from: http://campusvirtual.unex.es/cala/editio/index.php?journal=relatec&page=index

Emeric, D., & Hernández, L. (2008). Nuevas Tecnologías y Participación Social. *Revista Informativa de la Asociación Profesional Española de Terapia Ocupacional*, *47*, 30–41.

Gómez, J. A., & Navalón, C. (2002). La experiencia de la "alfabetización informacional" en el Aula de Mayores de la Universidad de Murcia. *Revista Investigación Educativa.*, *20*(2), 469–486.

Gómez del Castillo, M. T. (2003, October). *Enseñanza de Internet para Personas Mayores.* Paper presented at II Congreso la Educación en Internet e Internet en la Educación, Madrid, Spain.: 2003.

Grande, R., Pereira, J., Mato, V., & Pazos, A. (2008). Accesibilidad de las personas mayores a las tecnologías de la información y la comunicación: Situación actual en España. In Pereira, J., Martínez, L.A., Fuertes, J.L., & Vázquez, J.M. (Eds.), *Tecnologías de la Información y las Comunicaciones en la Autonomía Personal, dependencia y accesibilidad* (pp. 93-114). Santiago de Compostela: Fundación Alfredo Brañas.

Instituto Nacional de Estadística (INE). (2001). Censo de Población y Viviendas (Population and Housing Census). *On-line database.* Retrieved September 2009, from http://www.ine.es

Instituto Nacional de Estadística (INE). (2008a). Padrón Municipal de Habitantes (Municipal Census of Inhabitants). *On-line database.* Retrieved September 2009, from http://www.ine.es

Instituto Nacional de Estadística (INE). (2008b). Encuesta sobre Equipamiento y Uso de Tecnologías de la Información y la Comunicación en los hogares (Survey on Equipment and Use of Information and Communication Technologies in Households). *On-line database.* Retrieved September, 2009, from http://www.ine.es

Miranda de Larra, R. (2004). Los mayores en la Sociedad de la Información: situación actual y retos de futuro. Madrid, España: Fundación AUNA.

Obra Social Fundación La Caixa. (2007). Taller de Iniciación a la Informática (Beginners' Computer Workshop). Retrieved September 2009, from http://portal.lacaixa.es/clubestrella/talleres/presentacion _es.html

Orange Foundation. (n.d.). Proyecto EDAD. Retrieved October, 2009, from http://www.fundacionorange.es/ fundacionorange/proyectos/proyecto_edad.html

Pousada, T., Groba, B., Orozco, K., & Martínez, M. (2008). Las Tecnologías de la Información y Comunicaciones como recursos educativos para alumnos con necesidades educativas especiales. In Pereira, J., Martínez, L.A., Fuertes, J.L., & Vázquez, J.M. (Eds.), *Tecnologías de la Información y las Comunicaciones en la Autonomía Personal, dependencia y accesibilidad* (pp. 399-418). Santiago de Compostela: Fundación Alfredo Brañas.

Travieso, J. L., & Planella, J. (2008). La alfabetización digital como factor de inclusión social: una mirada crítica. *UOCPapers*, 6, 1-9. Retrieved May 2009, from http://www.uoc.edu/uocpapers/

United Nations General Assembly. (1948). Universal Declaration of Human Rights. Retrieved September, 2009, from http://www.un.org/es/documents/udhr/

Villar, F. (2003). Personas mayores y ordenadores: valoración de una experiencia de formación. [from http://www.segg.es/page/revista/espanola /de/geriatria /y/gerontologia]. *Revista Espanola de Geriatria y Gerontologia, 38*(2), 86–94. Retrieved September 2009.

World Health Organization. (2001). *International Classification of Functioning, Disability and Health.* Geneva: World Health Organization.

KEY TERMS AND DEFINITIONS

Elderly: Old people; seniors or senior citizens. The boundary between middle age and old age cannot be defined exactly because it does not have the same meaning in all societies. In western societies it is considered old population or older people those who are 65 years old or older; being this threshold arbitrary, but generally accepted. United Nations considers the threshold of the older population over 60 years old.

Health: Health is a state of complete physical, mental and social well-being and not merely the absence of disease (World Health Organization).

ICT/ICTs: The Information and Communication Technologies are a set of technologies, components and techniques related to the media and the processing and transmission of information.

Information Society: Phase of social development characterized by the capacity of its members to obtain and share any information instantly from anywhere in the preferred form and also characterized by the technological development.

In-TIC: In-TIC (Integration and accessibility of individuals with functional diversity in the use of Information and Communication Technologies) is a software or a support system for the access to and use of ICTs for people with functional diversity, which allows the virtual environment to be personalised and simplified as far as possible using virtual keyboards.

Personal Autonomy: The ability to control, manage and take his own initiative, personal decisions about how to live according to the rules and preferences, and to develop the basic activities of daily living.

Quality of Life: The perception an individual has about his place in existence, in the context of culture and value system in which they live and in relation to their objectives, expectations, norms and their concerns (World Health Organization).

Chapter 23
Experiences Using Information and Communication Technologies with Children Affected by Cerebral Palsy

Thais Pousada
University of A Coruña, Spain

Miriam Piñeiro
ASPACE Coruña, Spain

Yolanda Vizcaya
ASPACE Coruña, Spain

ABSTRACT

Intervention using the New Technologies in children suffering from Infantile Cerebral Palsy (ICP) is aimed at attaining or promoting individual abilities of each user. To this end, all possible means and resources are facilitated to enable them to access communication and thus to attain higher levels of social integration and individual advancement for their personal development. One such resource is In-TIC, assistive software for the creation of virtual keyboards customised to the capabilities of each individual user. The experience gained from the application of this software, in combination with assistive hardware, has made it possible to facilitate and improve the access to and use of computers for children suffering from infantile cerebral palsy in the ASPACE Coruña Centre.

INTRODUCTION

Infantile Cerebral Palsy encompasses a range of chronic diseases arising from a lesion or defect in the development of the immature brain; i.e. it is fundamentally a neuromotor disorder (Madrigal Muñoz, A, 1998). It is characterised by alterations in the neuromuscular, musculoskeletal and sensory systems, being the direct result of the physiopathology, or of indirect compensations,

DOI: 10.4018/978-1-60566-206-0.ch023

and which thus limit activity (Piñeiro, M, Vizcaya, Y, Pérez, MJ, 2008).

In addition to affecting motor capacities, ICP is frequently accompanied by sensory, cognitive, communicative, perceptive and behavioural disorders and/or epilepsy (Confederación ASPACE, 2007). In addition to these purely physiological and anatomical complications, the symptomatology in this type of illness may have a series of consequences in the principal contexts of the individual, particularly in the social and cultural ones. This disorder is one of the most common causes of disability in infancy (Chia-Ling Chen et al., 2006).

Among the secondary difficulties, which are particularly relevant for contextualising the subject matter of the present chapter, we should point out the associated communication and learning disorders, and the effects on primary motor capacities.

The communication problems of individuals affected with ICP may be due to a low intellectual level (which hinders the development and acquisition of basic communicative patterns) and/or to difficulties in the articulation of words (dysarthria) (Madrigal Muñoz, A, 1998). Some users are capable of verbal communication, in some form (Confederación ASPACE, 2007), while others benefit from assistive technology through the use of augmentative and alternative communication systems (AACSs), such as communicators, tablet PCs or specific proprietary software.

ASPACE Coruña is the Association of Parents of Persons with Cerebral Palsy, a non-profit-making organisation working in the local setting, whose mission is to promote the establishment of rehabilitation and pedagogical centres and institutions for the recovery, teaching and psychological/educational treatment of children suffering from ICP who are affected physically and/or psychologically (ASPACE Coruña, 1978).

ASPACE Coruña has been present in this field for over 30 years, working constantly with a group of individuals suffering from infantile cerebral palsy and their families.

This organisation offers its services and treatments to individuals suffering from ICP within centre itself, which houses specialised installations. All users of this resource have serious sensory and intellectual handicaps. In practical terms, the 91 users of the centre all suffer from a significant reduction in their personal autonomy as, owing to a diminution in their organic and functional capacity, they are totally dependent for satisfying their basic needs. In the majority of cases, this dependence approaches 99%, as borne out by their disability certificates.

A New Technologies Department has recently been established in the ASPACE Coruña Centre, the principal aim of which is to provide users with the possibility of acquiring, promoting or improving linguistic, communicative, learning and socialisation abilities, all through the use of assistive technology, specific hardware and modern computer tools.

The core theme of this chapter deals with the experiences derived from the application of In-TIC software with users of the ASPACE Coruña Centre, and with the development of a work dynamics in the New Technologies Department. The principal aim is to provide access to and use of computers and of the most dynamic AACSs to the affected individuals.

BACKGROUND

Children with severe physical handicaps require special devices to help them perform their everyday activities, such as personal hygiene, travel, communication, controlling their environment and the use of computers (Hawley MS, Cudd, P.A. and Cherry, A.D, 1994). Consequently, this gives rise to the need for many different types of assistive technology, a basic tool for promoting the personal autonomy of these users.

Many children suffering from ICP have significant handicaps in the motor structures of their upper limbs, due to which they have severe difficulties in performing learning activities, above all those based on writing (Chia-Ling Chen et al, 2006).

Moreover, and as has already been mentioned, a high percentage of children with ICP are affected quadriplegically and suffer from associated communication disorders, having great difficulty in transmitting their wishes, thoughts and needs, due either to alterations in the development of language or to difficulties in speech, generally associated with severe motor problems (Piñeiro, M; Vizcaya, Y; Pérez, MJ; 2008). The impact on speech may result in the users' isolation, since this is one of the basic forms of interacting with the environment and modifying it in accordance with our needs. In the majority of cases, this isolation hampers their integration into the habitual settings with which they interact, giving rise to an attitude of dependent passiveness among users (Marcos Rodrigo, JM; 2009).

Until the appearance of communicators, and modern computer software, the communicative responses of these users was limited to moving their eyes towards the object or symbol desired, or to nodding/shaking their heads in response to their interlocutors. In this case, they can use their residual voluntary movements to communicate with their family, friends and healthcare professionals (Betke, Gips and Fleming, 2002). Although functional, this system is insufficient to cover the users' communication expectations.

On the other hand, the low cognitive performance of this community gives rise to learning problems. These may be slight, moderate or serious, and they take the form of slowness of certain tasks, such as reading, drawing, adding or subtracting, owing to the fact that the corresponding area in the brain is damaged. If the problem is not related to the child's general intelligence, it is called "a language specific problem", which is particularly common in individuals suffering from ICP (Confederación ASPACE, 2007).

Assistive technology is an important resource, currently at the height of its development, for helping and supporting these types of users in making full use of their voluntary movements to access computers.

More specifically, Information and Communication Technologies (ICTs) are consolidating themselves as fundamental sources of assistance for individuals with some type of disability. ICTs thus have a great deal of potential; they provide an extensive range of instruments to help these individuals mitigate or overcome some of their limitations (Miranda de Larra, R; 2007).

Assistive devices can be highly useful in helping to perform different everyday activities, including the use of computers, along with the act of communication and social participation (Murphy et al, 1995). In the case of communication disorders, many assistive devices take advantage of these new technologies to become true augmentative or alternative communication systems. Thanks to the latest technological advances, there are many dynamic communicators (programmable and with good voice output) and specific software packages on the market to enable the computer to be used as an AACŞ (Martine and Connolly, 2008). This chapter will show how a dynamic communication tool, In-TIC, has been developed through open source software.

Regarding the educational and learning needs associated to a cognitive deficit, Muntaner (2005) points out that the new technologies provide an ideal support for collaborating and encouraging learning faced with the diversity of children suffering from some sort of disability. These may be either an element for motivating and activating the learning process itself, or an educational support, which opens up a wide range of intervention possibilities for any student.

Table 1. Advantages of the application of ITCs in the education system

Author	*Proposed advantages*
Cabero, 2002	- Support in overcoming difficulties derived from operational deficit - Increased autonomy - Optimisation of synchronic and non-synchronic communication - Individualised training - Reduction and elimination of marginalisation and exclusion - Facilitation of social/labour integration - Increase in leisure activities - Time savings in the acquisition of abilities and skills - Opening up of the scientific and cultural world - Reduction of the feeling of academic and personal failure
Pérez and Beltrán, 2004	- Access - Independent exploration - Interactivity - Collaborative learning - Efficiency - Teacher productivity - Collection and representation of knowledge
Toledo, 2006	- New options for the participation and execution of learning and teaching tasks - Promoting abilities of children with disabilities - Access to information, to interaction and to participation in On-line activities - Opportunities in the educational process through digital e-learning alternatives - Increased motivation and self-esteem - Positive feedback

Thus, in the educational setting, ICTs may be of great help as a medium for accessing the curriculum, as promoters of school learning, as educational reinforcers, or as a means of individualising education. A number of different authors (Cabero, 2002; Pérez and Beltrán, 2004; Toledo, 2006) have studied, analyzed and prepared the recommendations concerning the use of ICTs as resources in the education system in general.

Lastly, and before presenting the characteristics of the experiment in the ASPACE Coruña Centre, mention should first be made of the problem of the so-called "digital divide". This concept has been defined as "the distance between those who make effective use of information and communication tools and those who, due to their functional diversity, cannot" (Gutiérrez, 2001). This refers to the inequality of possibilities existing in accessing information, knowledge and education through the new technologies (Cabero, 2004).

Technological development that is excessively rapid, and which does not consider the specific needs of individuals with functional diversity, may have the opposite effect of that witnessed to date: i.e. if, in their working framework, development companies and manufacturers fail to consider adapting devices to the operational shortcomings of this community, they will contribute, indirectly, to increasing their limitation in related activities and restricting their social participation. As a result, the distance or digital divide between those who make effective use of technology and those who have more difficulties will grow, adversely affecting their integration into the Information Society.

Accordingly, the basic "Design for All" regulations, which promote accessibility of ICTs for communities at risk of social and digital exclusion, must be incorporated into the creation, planning and development stages of new products and services.

EXPERIENCES USING INFORMATION AND COMMUNICATION TECHNOLOGIES WITH CHILDREN AFFECTED BY CEREBRAL PALSY

Material and Methods

Having contextualised the content of the present chapter, we now go on to describe the experience and the work carried out to date in the New Technologies Service of the ASPACE Coruña Centre, through the intervention with the In-TIC program.

The In-TIC application is assistive software which enables individuals with functional diversity to access and use computers by using different virtual interfaces or keyboards. The programme is divided into an interface creation environment (which healthcare and educational professionals use to design dynamic virtual keyboards which will be specific and personalised to the capabilities of each user) and an interaction environment, designed for end users (Grande, R et. al, 2008). These interfaces allow individuals who have problems accessing the computer operating system to use a number of different applications, such as the Office suite or Internet Explorer. Figures 1 and 2 show the different dynamic virtual keyboards of the In-TIC program.

Participants

The target population of the project comprises individuals diagnosed with infantile cerebral palsy, with difficulties in communication, in social relationships, in basic and instrumental activities of daily life and in learning.

Figure 1. Personalised keyboard for accessing the computer

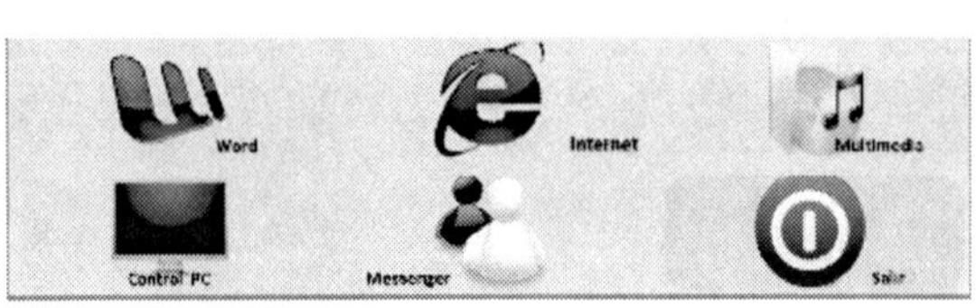

A small, representative sample was chosen, from among the 91 users of the ASPACE Coruña Centre, with the aim of applying the process described below, as an experimental activity.

Consequently, those users who had potential psychomotor capacities for the use of the computer and the AACSs, and who demonstrated an interest in the new technologies were selected.

The project was carried out with 18 users from the ASPACE Coruña Centre, divided into two groups:

- 12 individuals from the educational centre, who were thus under 22 years of age.
- 8 participants from the day centre, who were over 22 years of age.

Evaluation Process

One of the principal characteristics of In-TIC's usability is its compatibility with any hardware or assistive device for accessing the computer.

It is important to take into account that each user has certain individual capacities and specific needs, and that these requirements can be compensated using one ore more of the numer-

Figure 2. Virtual keyboard for using a word processor

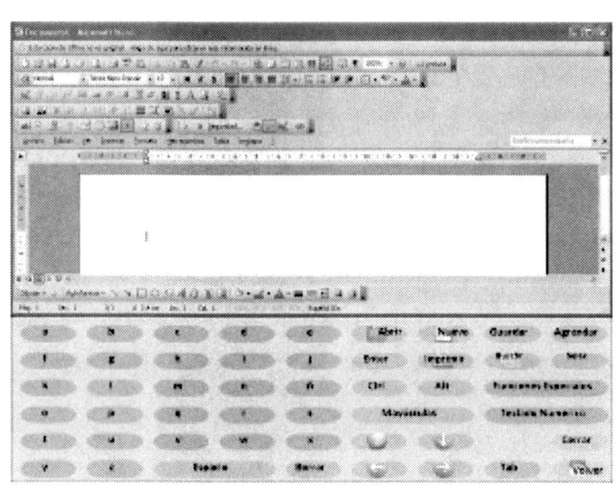

ous different examples of assistive technology. The New Technologies Department at ASPACE has a number of different assistive devices, the most important being head trackers for interface control (Harwins, WS and Jackson, RD, 1990; Chen et al, 2003), eye control devices (Gravil, N et. al, 1985; Park KS and Lee, KT, 1996), pressure switch-activated interfaces (Berardinis, LA, 1996; Gerpecheide, G, 1998), webcams (Betke, M; Gips, J; Fleming, P, 2002), signalling devices and different types of adapted mouse devices (trackball, joystick, etc.).

To ensure a perfectly integrated person-PC interaction, it was necessary to carry out an evaluation process prior to the design of specific templates and training for users in the use of the computer.

This prior phase consisted of applying a questionnaire, prepared in-house (designed by the work team comprising occupational therapists, speech therapists and computer programmers), to each of the participating users. The aim was to assess those capabilities considered necessary to access and operate the computer; these included sensory abilities and sensory processing (visual and auditory), motor capacities, cognitive abilities, linguistic abilities, reading-writing abilities and psycho-social abilities.

Table 2 shows the items in this questionnaire, divided into the aforementioned categories, with different sub-sections. The interviewer (member of the team) awarded one of the following scores to each item:

1 = The user has the ability
2 = The user has the ability, but with problems executing or maintaining it
3 = The user does not have the ability

Once the questionnaire had been applied to the 18 participants, the assistive devices most suited to their capacities and functional needs were selected.

Additionally, during the sample evaluation and selection process other data of interest for the presentation of the present work and the configuration of our interventions were obtained. In Figure 3, it can be seen that 73. 66% of the population in the ASPACE Coruña Centre needs support in communication: Augmentative or Alternative Communication Systems and assistive technologies:

- 56.42% of users have communicative intention, due to which they would require some assistive product[1] for communicating.
- 50.96% of the population of ASPACE requires some sort of Augmentative or Alternative Communication system (AACS)[2], or assistive device in order to operate the computer, to communicate or to access the Information Society.
- 30.94% already have the capacity to communicate via oral language, although they require assistive devices to access the computer.
- 26.34% had no possibility of being able to communicate, either via oral language, or with alternative resources or assistive products.

Training in the Use of Selected Assistive Devices

The majority of users participating in the project (15) had no prior experience in the use of the assistive devices which had been selected for them.

Consequently, the work team drew up a work plan with the aim of providing suitable training in the handling of these products.

Thus, a methodology divided up into six sections (two per week) was proposed, in which the following aspects were worked on:

- Demonstration of the selected assistive device.
- Explanation of its operation and type of connection with the computer.

Table 2. Evaluation questionnaire for determining assistive devices for accessing the computer

Sensory and sensory processing skills			
Visual capacity	Has the Ability		
	Yes (1)	With difficulty (2)	No (3)
Recognition of objects			
Recognition of real images			
Recognition of drawing representing objects			
Visual tracking			
Auditory capacity	Has the Ability		
	Yes (1)	With difficulty (2)	No (3)
Auditory attention			
Auditory discrimination			
Perception of conversation at medium volume			
Motorskills			
Motor skills	Has the Ability		
	Yes (1)	With difficulty (2)	No (3)
Fine motor skills			
Coarse motor skills			
Hand-eye coordination			
Bilateral coordination			
Cognitive capacities	Has the Ability		
	Yes (1)	With difficulty (2)	No (3)
Attention level			
Memory			
Sequencing			
Problem resolution			
Language skills	Has the Ability		

Figure 3. communicative situation in ASPACE Coruña

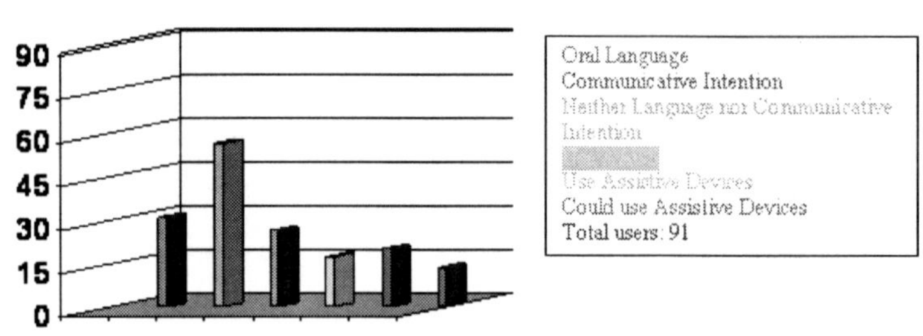

Figure 4. Selection of virtual keyboards

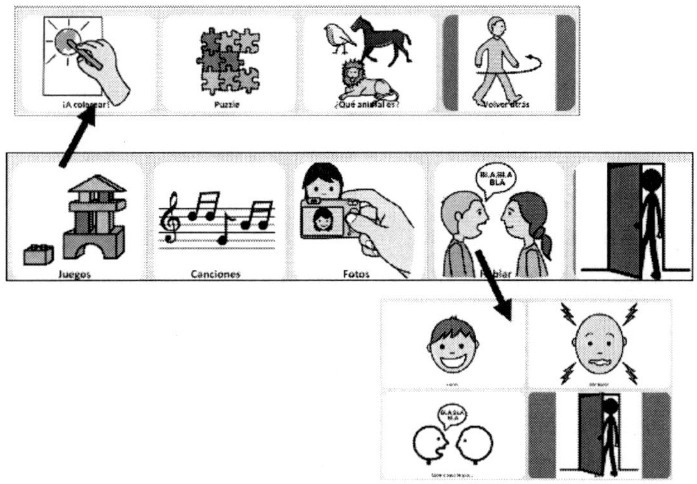

- Practical demonstration by the professional of the functions that the assistive device can perform.
- Use of specific software to encourage training in the use of the assistive device: http://www.vedoque.com/juegos/muevelamano.html and http://www.isftic.mepsyd.es/w3/eos/MaterialesEducativos/mem2001/raton/index.html
- Unguided operation of the assistive device, without assistive software.

Design of Specific Virtual Keyboards

At the same time as the previous phase was implemented, the occupational therapists and the speech therapist in the work team were designing the interfaces or specific virtual keyboards with In-TIC, in line with each user's needs when interacting with computers.

Using the In-TIC creation environment, the professionals were able to configure and modify the virtual keyboards which, with maximum levels of personalisation, would make it possible to access and operate certain programs on the computer.

Each keyboard comprises a set of buttons (as can be seen in Figure 4), each one of which can be configured in terms of both appearance and function.

Worthy of note among the functions with which the buttons have been programmed are navigation between keyboards, opening the Web browser, opening a specific program or representing an augmentative communication system.

During this process, the work team was supported by the teachers and psycho-pedagogues at the centre, who provided advice on the possible images, activities and texts to be included in the specific keyboards, thus making a contribution to complementing the learning process of those users at school age.

User Interaction with the PC via the Specific Keyboards

Finally, the intervention process was performed on the selected sample using the In-TIC software.

After the training phase in the use of assistive devices, users were now prepared to operate and interact with the virtual keyboard, designed specifically for them.

Since then, individualised sessions in the new technologies department have been proposed, in which, twice a week, each user is able to operate the computer and use different programs in a manner that is simple, convenient and adapted to their individual possibilities.

During the first two weeks, after each session, the users notified the professionals of any possible improvements that could be included into the virtual keyboards in order to facilitate the use of specific options in the programs used.

During this period, the modifications proposed by the users were incorporated into the keyboards - an additional option provided by In-TIC.

Subsequent to this trial process, users are currently continuing with their sessions in the New Technologies Department; these enable them to operate the ICTs and to access the Information Society independently, thanks to a combination of the assistive devices for accessing the computer and the In-TIC software.

Results

The results of implementing the In-TIC Project in the ASPACE Coruña Centre have been satisfactory, insofar as the objectives proposed have been attained. That is to say, a functional interaction with the new technologies for persons suffering from ICP has been obtained, by evaluating their requirements and personalising the manner of access as far as possible.

We now go on to describe the experience of two cases, which, owing to their significance, will provide the reader with an example of the activity that has been carried out.

- Lucía is a girl suffering from cerebral palsy, severely affected by spastic tetraplegia (she is globally affected, including the trunk and all four limbs, with paralysis predominantly in the upper limbs). She has no oral language. With regard to voluntary mobility, the head is where she has highest operational capacity. But even so, she has difficulties, due to which access to the computer is attained via a switch with a scanning system, and not using a head-operated mouse; i.e., via indirect selection. Due to this fact, her use of the computer was very limited, since the switch/scanner mechanism can only be used with certain specific augmentative and alternative communication programmes. In this case, virtual keyboards were configured to enable Lucía to access the computer and operate the Internet explorer using a switch (indirect selection) and the activation of the sequential scanner built into the In-TIC program.
- Unlike his companion, Chonín has generalised hypotony. This disorder is the initial phase of development towards other forms of CP, and is characterised by a reduction in muscular tone and in the capacity to generate voluntary muscular power, along with excessive articular flexibility and postural instability (Confederación ASPACE, 2007), coupled with a loss of muscular force in his upper and lower limbs. At a communicative level he has no oral language, while at a cognitive level his intelligence is unimpaired. Owing to a cerebellar syndrome, he exhibits uncontrolled movement in his upper limbs and choreoathetosis in his hands. In spite of all these difficulties, he is able to access the computer by means of direct selection through the buttons on the virtual keyboards of a touch screen.

FUTURE TRENDS

The In-TIC project is currently still under development. In coming months, this free software will be able to offer a number of possibilities with the incorporation of new tools, such as a text predictor package, the combination with the in-house development of a head-operated mouse device (Head In-TIC), as well as its application

Figure 5. Examples of the communicators- SPC and syllabic

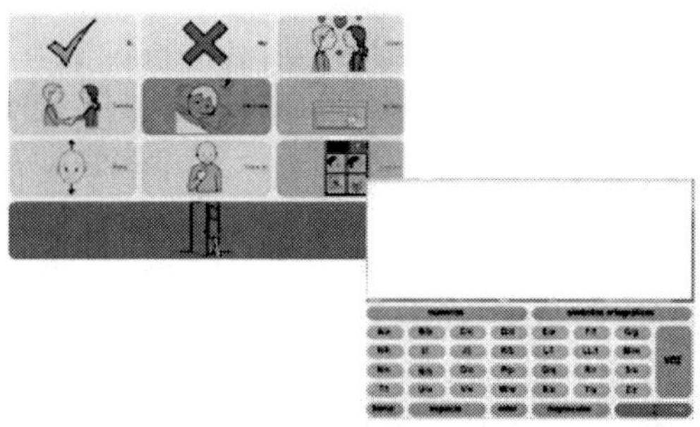

on mobile devices running Windows Mobile, Android or other operating systems.

Another of the immediate objectives in the application the project, and with clear advantages for individuals suffering from ICP, is the use of In-TIC as an AACS. This will allow the program to be configured as a tool for facilitating the communicative action to users in the ASPACE Coruña Centre who, owing to their limitations in this activity, have difficulty or cannot express themselves orally or in writing.

To this end, in addition to enabling the creation of personalised keyboards for interaction with the PC, In-TIC will constitute an assistive device or functional communication resource, allowing the integration, interaction and social participation of individuals suffering from ICP within their setting. It will also be possible to stimulate and encourage basic linguistic and cognitive functions, through integration and normalisation.

Figure 5 shows two examples of how the virtual keyboards in the In-TIC program can be configured as alternative communication systems. In the first case, a dynamic communication board has been created using drawings which represent objects; this is intended for users with expressive intention, but without the capacity for oral language or reading/writing. The second example shows a dynamic syllabic keyboard, which optimises the communicative act for those users who, without possessing the capability of speech, have acquired reading/writing abilities and can express themselves through written texts.

In line with the notion expressed by Soto, FJ and Hurtado, MD (2005), it is considered that, in the coming years, it will be essential to construct spaces for gathering experiences and good practices with regard to ICTs and diversity. This can also be extended to adopting the application and promotion of "Design for All" standards and guidelines in the development of new tools, devices and resources, with the aim of facilitating ICTs to the community with functional diversity,

Only through the creation and application of resources which take into account the specific characteristics and the needs of this community will it be possible to reduce the digital divide and ensure the full integration of these citizens in the Information Society.

CONCLUSION

Throughout the present chapter, the experience of applying the In-TIC project to individuals suffering from Infantile Cerebral Palsy has been contextualised, defined and demonstrated.

The establishment of a New Technologies Department in the ASPACE Coruña Centre has enabled different actions aimed at the integration of the users of the centre into the use of ICTs to be conducted.

In addition to being a resource for leisure and free time activities, the computer has increasing potential for application with a multitude of different aims, including education, training, work and communication /interaction.

We live in a technological society, surrounded by electronic devices, long-distance and instantaneous communication systems, and always just a click away from a vast quantity of information on the Internet. As it was seen in the introduction to the present chapter, the possibilities offered by the new technologies are innumerable; nevertheless, it is also true that, on occasion, for all their innovation, they fail to take into account the most disadvantaged groups, among which we find individuals with functional diversity.

Assistive products are an alternative to all those which cannot be employed for the normalised use of the PC. Devices such as joysticks, facially operated mouse devices, buttons and switches help to compensate for limitations caused by an operational deficit, doing away with the possible restriction in the participation of these users.

As explained above, In-TIC is an accessory to assistive hardware for accessing the computer. Its simple handling, for both professionals and end users, makes this program a tool which, applying the "Design for All" principles, allows the computer, its operating system and the most frequently used programs to be adapted to the demands and requirements of each user.

The users participating in this experience, in addition to suffering from a highly limiting motor disorder, had communicational, behavioural and learning disorders. These characteristics give rise to a highly homogenous sample, with vastly differing characteristics and needs in the use of the new technologies.

In-TIC permits the creation of virtual keyboards, which are personalised and adapted to the demands of each individual, opening the door to a world hitherto unknown by the majority of them. The satisfaction demonstrated by participants after the intervention session points to a broad set of advantages of this application, which, besides being free, is pioneering in the manner in which assistive software is conceived and understood.

Besides facilitating interaction with the PC, the In-TIC project has potential of becoming a useful communication tool. The configuration of dynamic keyboards used as AACSs, with voice output, facilitates the communicative act to those users with communication and language disorders, thus allowing the integration, interaction and social participation of individuals suffering from ICP in their surroundings.

ACKNOWLEDGMENT

This work has been promoted through the "New assistive technologies for the Integration and Accessibility of individuals with functional diversity in the use of Information and Communication Technologies: In-TIC Project" agreement between the University of A Coruña Foundation and the Orange Foundation.

We would like to thank all the professionals at the ASPACE Coruña Centre who collaborated and participated actively in the implementation of the project, along with the users of the centre since, without them, none of this would have been possible.

REFERENCES

AEN/CTN 153. (2007). Norma UNE-EN ISO 9999: Dispositivos de apoyo para personas con diversidad funcional. Clasificación y terminología. Madrid: Asociación española de Normalización y Certificación.

Berardinis, L. A. (1996). Magnetic sensors for light-touch operators. *Mach Des*, *68*, 38.

Betke, M., Gips, J., & Fleming, P. (2002). The camera mouse: visual tracking of body features to provide computer access for people with severe disabilities. *IEEE Transactions on Neural Systems and Rehabilitation Engineering*, *10*, 1–10. doi:10.1109/TNSRE.2002.1021581

Cabero, J. (2002). Mitos de la sociedad de la información: sus impactos en la educación. In Aguiar, M. V. (Ed.), *Cultura y educación en la sociedad de la información* (pp. 17–38). A Coruña: Netbiblo.

Cabero, J. (2004). Software educativo. In J. Aliaga (Ed.), *Revista de nuevas tecnologías y recursos didácticos*, 194, 3-4.

Chen, C. L. (2006). Application of novel integrated pointing device apparatus for children with cerebral palsy. *Chang Gung Medical Journal*, *29*(4), 380–387.

Chen, Y. L., Chen, W. L., Kou, T. S., & Lai, J. S. (2003). A head movement image (HMI)-controlled computer mouse for people with disabilities. *Disability and Rehabilitation*, *25*, 163–167. doi:10.1080/0963828021000024960

Confederación, A. S. P. A. C. E. (2007). *Mi bebé tiene Parálisis Cerebral, ¿qué hacer?* Madrid: Confederación ASPACE.

ASPACE Coruña (1978). Estatutos Asociación de Padres de Personas con Parálisis Cerebral. Coruña: ASPACE Coruña.

Gerpecheide, G. (1998). Touchpad pointing device. *Scientific American*, *279*, 118. doi:10.1038/scientificamerican0798-118

Grande, R., Pereira, J., Pousada, T., Groba, B., & Pazos, A. (2008). Proyecto In-TIC para la accesibilidad y usabilidad de las TIC en personas con diversidad funcional. *Revista Informativa de la Apeto*, *47*, 78–85.

Gravil, N., Griffiths, P. A., Potter, R., & Yates, A. (1985). Eye control of microcomputer. *Comput Bull Serial*, *3*, 15–16.

Gutiérrez, E. (2001) La educación en Internet e Internet en la educación como factor supresor de la brecha digital. Congreso la Educación por Internet e Internet en la Educación. Ministerio de Educación, Madrid. Retrieved from http://www.inclusiondigital.net/ponen/brecha/Overview.html

Harwins, W. S., & Jackson, R. D. (1990). Analysis of intentional head gestures to assist computer access by physically disabled people. *Journal of Biomedical Engineering*, *12*, 193–198. doi:10.1016/0141-5425(90)90040-T

Hawley, M. S., Cudd, P. A., & Cherry, A. D. (2002). Implementation of a PC-based integrated control system for children. *Medical Engineering & Physics*, *16*, 237–242. doi:10.1016/1350-4533(94)90043-4

Macías Merlo, L., & Fagoaga Mata, J. (2002). *Fisioterapia en Pediatría*. Barcelona: MCGraw-Hill-Interamericana.

Madrigal Muñoz, A. (1998). La parálisis cerebral. Madrid: Observatorio de la discapacidad. Instituto de Mayores y Servicios Sociales (IMSERSO).

Marcos Rodrigo, J. M (2009). C.P.E.E Alborada. Zaragoza. Retrieved June 1, 2009 from http://centros6.pntic.mec.es/cpee.alborada/

Martine, M. S., & Connolly, I. (2008). Roles of aided communication: perspectives of adults who use AAC. *Disab Rehab: Assistive Technology*, *3*(5), 260–273. doi:10.1080/17483100802338499

Muntaner, J.J. (2005). Los retos educativos del siglo XXI. *Comunicación y pedagogía*, 204.

Murphy, J., Marková, I., Moodie, E., Scott, J., & Boa, S. Augmentative and alternative communication systems used by people with cerebral palsy in Scotland: demographic survey. *Augmentative and Alternative Communication*, *11*, 26–36. doi:10.1080/07434619512331277119

Park, K. S., & Lee, K. T. (1996). Eye-controlled human/computer interface using the line-of-sight and the intentional blink. *Computers & Industrial Engineering*, *30*, 463–473. doi:10.1016/0360-8352(96)00018-6

Pérez y Beltrán (2004). La educación de los alumnos superdotados en la nueva sociedad de la información. *Red digital: Revista de Tecnologías de la Información y Comunicación Educativas*, 5.

Piñeiro Escudero, M., Vizcaya Pérez, Y., & Pérez Rodríguez, M. J. (2008). Nuestra experiencia con el In-TIC. In Pereira, J., Martínez L.A., Fuertes, J.L., Vázquez, J.M. (Eds.), *Tecnologías de la Información y las Comunicaciones en la Autonomía Personal, dependencia y accesibilidad*. Santiago de Compostela: Fundación Alfredo Brañas.

Soto Pérez, F. J., & Hurtado Montesinos, M. D. (2005). Tecnologías de ayuda y atención a la diversidad: oportunidades y retos. In Soto Pérez, F. J., & Hurtado Montesinos, M. D. (Eds.), *Tecnologías de ayuda en contextos escolares. Región de Murcia: Consejería de Educación y Cultura.*

Toledo, P. (2006. El profesor en el proceso de selección de tecnología de apoyo para alumnos con NEE. Comunicación y pedagogía: *Nuevas tecnologías y recursos didácticos*, 210, 24-28.

Torres Monreal, S. (2001). *Sistemas Alternativos de Comunicación. Manual de Comunicación Aumentativa y Alternativa. Sistemas y estrategias*. Málaga: Ediciones Aljibe.

KEY TERMS AND DEFINITIONS

Access Computer: It is the act that involves the proper management of hardware and softare on a computer, without any kind of barrier.

Assistive Technology: Is a generic term that includes assistive, adaptive, and rehabilitative devices for people with disabilities and includes the process used in selecting, locating, and using them.

Augmentative and Alternative Communication: Is any method that supplements or replaces speech and writing when these are temporarily or permanently impaired and inadequate to meet all or some of a person's communication needs. Use of AAC involves selecting messages or codes from a set of possibilities.

Communication: Is a process of transferring information from one entity to another. Communication processes are sign-mediated interactions between at least two agents which share a repertoire of signs and semiotic rules.

ICT/ICTs: The Information and Communication Technologies are a set of technologies, components and techniques related to the media and the processing and transmission of information.

Infantile Cerebral Palsy (ICP): It is a pathology that encompasses a range of chronic diseases arising from a lesion or defect in the development of the immature brain; i.e. it is fundamentally a neuromotor disorder.

In-TIC: In-TIC (Integration and accessibility of individuals with functional diversity in the use of Information and Communication Technologies) is a software or a support system for the access to and use of ICTs for people with functional diversity, which allows the virtual environment to be personalised and simplified as far as possible using virtual keyboards.

ENDNOTES

1 "Any product (including devices, equipment, instruments, technology and software) especially produced or generally available, preventing, compensating, monitoring, relieving or neutralising impairment, activity limitations and participation restrictions." (ISO, 2007).

2 "Structured set of codes (verbal and nonverbal) expressed through non-vocal channels (gestures, signs, graphic symbols), requiring a physical medium or not, which by means of specific instruction processes, serve to perform acts of communication (functional, spontaneous and general), on their own, or in conjunction with vocal codes (channels), or as a partial support therefor" (Torres Montreal, 2001).

Compilation of References

Abascal, J., Arrue, M., Fajardo, I., Garay, N., & Tomes, J. (2004). The use of guidelines to automatically verify web accessibility. *Univers. Access Inf. Soc.*, *3*(1), 71–79.. doi:10.1007/s10209-003-0069-3

Abbas, J. J., & Chizeck, H. J. (1995). Neural network control of functional neuromuscular stimulation systems: computer stimulation studies. *IEEE Transactions on Bio-Medical Engineering*, *11*, 1117–1127. doi:10.1109/10.469379

Achim, A., Braun, C. M. J., & Collin, I. (2008). Event-Related Potentials Distinguish Fluent and Stuttered Speech. *Journal of Neurotherapy*, *11*(3), 15–23. doi:10.1080/10874200802126118

Adams, M. R., & Hayden, P. (1976). The Ability of Stutterers and Nonstutterers to Initiate and Terminate Phonation during Production of an Isolated Vowel. *The Journal of Speech and Hearing Disorders*, *19*(2), 290–296.

Airasian, P. W. (1973). Evaluation of the binaural sensory aid. *AFB Research Bulletin*, *26*, 51–71.

Akyildiz, I. F., Su, W., Sankarasubramaniam, Y., & Cayirci, E. (2002, August). A survey on sensor networks. *IEEE Communications Magazine*, 102–114. doi:10.1109/MCOM.2002.1024422

Albacete, P. L., Chang, S. K., & Polese, G. (1998). Iconic language design for people with significant speech and multiple impairments. In Mittal, V. O., Yanco, H. A., Arnois, J., & Simpson, R. (Eds.), *Assistive Technology and Artificial Intelligence, Application in Robotics, User Interface and Natural Language Processing* (pp. 12–32). LNAI.

Alcantud, F., & Soto, F. J. (2003). *Tecnologías de ayuda en personas con trastornos de comunicación*. Valencia: Nau Llibres.

Alcantud, F. (2000). Nuevas Tecnologías, viejas esperanzas. In Soto, F. J., & López, J. A. (Eds.), *Nuevas tecnologías, viejas esperanzas: las nuevas tecnologías en el ámbito de la discapacidad y las necesidades educativas especiales* (pp. 257–262). Murcia: Consejería de Educación y Universidades.

Alciatore, D. G., & Histand, M. B. (2003). *Introduction to mechatoronics and measurement systems*. New York: McGraw-Hill, Inc.

Allaire, J., Gressard, R., Blackman, J., & Hostler, S. (1991). Children with severe speech impairments: caregiver survey of AAC use. *Augmentative and Alternative Communication*, *7*, 248–255. doi:10.1080/07434619112331275983

Allison, B. Z., McFarland, D. J., Schalk, G., Zheng, S. D., Jackson, M. M., & Wolpaw, J. R. (2008). Towards an independent brain-computer interface using steady state visual evoked potentials. *Clinical Neurophysiology*, *119*(2), 399–408. doi:10.1016/j.clinph.2007.09.121

Allison, H., & Strong, J. (1994). Verbal strategies used by occupational therapist in direct client encounters. *The Occupational Therapy Journal of Research*, *14*(2), 112–129.

Alm, P. A. (2005). *On the causal mechanisms of stuttering*. Lund, Sweden: Lund University.

Alonso, F., Frutos, S., Fuertes, J. L., Martínez, L. A., Montes, C., & Sánchez, A. (1997b). Un Diccionario Automático Bilingüe para Invidentes (DABIN). *Integración*, *25*, 14–31.

Alonso, F., & Barreiro, J. M. (2008). Investigación y Desarrollo en el campo de la Accesibilidad- CETTICO. In J. Pereira, L. A. Martínez, J. L. Fuertes & J. M. Vázquez (Eds.), *Tecnologías de la Información y las Comunicaciones en la Autonomía Personal, Dependencia y Accesibilidad* (pp. 497-538). Colección Informática 16. Santiago de Compostela, Spain: Fundación Alfredo Brañas.

Alonso, F., Barreiro, J. M., Caraça-Valente, J. P., López, G., Montes, C., & Navajo, R. J. (1998). An Electronic Newspaper for the Blind. In A. D. N. Edwards, W. Zagler & A. Arato (Eds.), *Computers and Assistive Technology: ICCHP '98 Proceedings of the XV IFIP World Computer Congress,* Vienna (Austria) and Budapest (Hungary), Vienna, Austria: Osterreichische Computer Gesellschaft.

Alonso, F., Frutos, S., & Montes, C. (1997a). Interfacing for the Blind. The DILE Model. In *Proceedings 12th Annual CSUN Conference: Technology and Persons with Disabilities*, Los Angeles, CA: California State University-Northridge.

Alonso, F., Fuertes, J. L., González, A. L., & Martínez, L. (2006). A Framework for Blind User Interfacing. In *Computers Helping People with Special Needs* (LNCS 4061, pp. 1031-1038). doi: 10.1007/11788713_151

Ando, B., Graziani, S., Lombardo, C. O., & Pitrone, N. (2004). Development of a smart clear path indicator. *IEEE IMTC, 1*, 492–497.

Andò, B. (2003). Electronic sensory systems for the visually impaired. *IEEE Mag. Instrum. Meas., 6*(2), 62–67. doi:10.1109/MIM.2003.1200287

Andò, B. (2005). An environmental sensor providing home light classification to blind people. *IEEE IMTC, 2*, 1438–1442.

Andò, B. (2006). Sensors that provide security for people with depressed receptors. *IEEE Mag. Instrum. Meas., 9*(2), 58–63.

Andò, B. (2008). A Smart Multisensor Approach to Assist Blind People in Specific Urban Navigation Tasks. *IEEE Transactions on Neural Systems and Rehabilitation Engineering, 16*(6). doi:10.1109/TNSRE.2008.2003374

Andò, B., & Ascia, A. (2007). Navigation Aids for the Visually Impaired: From Artificial Codification to Natural Sensing. *IEEE Mag. Instrum. Meas., 10*(3), 44–51. doi:10.1109/MIM.2007.4284258

Andò, B., Giannone, P., & Pitrone, N. (2007). A multisensor architecture to assist visually impaired people performing educational activities. *IEEE SSD, 2007*, 1–4.

Andò, B., & Pitrone, N. (2005). A new vision supplementation strategy to perform step detection. *SSD, 4*, 1–5.

Andò, B., & Savalli, N. (2008). CANBUS Networked Sensors Use in Orientation Tools for the Visually Impaired Wired versus Wireless Technology. *IEEE Instrumentation & Measurement Magazine, 11*(1), 49–52. doi:10.1109/IM-M.2008.4449015

Andò, B., Baglio, S., La Malfa, S., Marletta, V., & Savalli, N. (2009). A Distributed Sensor Network Approach for Orientation Tasks. In *Proceedings of the IEEE IMTC 2009.*

Andò, B., Baglio, S., La Malfa, S., & Pitrone, N. (2009). A remote monitoring system to improve educational activities of visually impaired students. In *Proceedings of the XIX IMEKO World Congress.*

Andò, B., Baglio, S., Marletta, V., & Pitrone, N. (2009). A Mixed Inertial & RF-ID Orientation Tool For The Visually Impaired. In *Proceedings of the IEEE SSD 2009.*

Andrews, G., Craig, A., Feyer, A., Hoddinott, S., Howie, P., & Neilson, M. (1983). Stuttering: a review of research findings and theories circa 1982. *The Journal of Speech and Hearing Disorders, 48*(3), 226–246.

Andrews, B. J., Baxendale, R. H., Barnett, R., Phillips, G. F., Yamazaki, T., & Freeman, P. A. (1988). Hybrid FES orthosis incoporating closed loop control and sensory feedback. *Journal of Biomedical Engineering, 10*, 253–259. doi:10.1016/0141-5425(88)90099-4

Andrews, B., Miller, S., Horrocks, D., & Chawla, J. C. (1980). Electronic communications and environmental control systems for the severely disabled. *Paraplegia, 17*, 153–156.

Angelo, J., Buning, M. E., Schmeler, M., & Doster, S. (1997). Identifying best practice in the occupational therapy assistive technology evaluation: an analysis of three focus groups. *The American Journal of Occupational Therapy.*, *51*(10), 916–920.

Apple (2009). Apple - Accessibility - VoiceOver - In-Depth. Retrieved September 25, 2009 from http://www.apple.com/accessibility/voiceover/

Arias, P., Chouza, M., Vivas, J., & Cudeiro, J. (2009). Effect of Whole Body Vibration in Parkinson's Disease: A Controlled Study. *Movement Disorders*, *24*, 891–898. doi:10.1002/mds.22468

Arias, P., & Cudeiro, J. (2008). Effects of rhythmic sensory stimulation (auditory, visual) on gait in Parkinson's disease patients. *Experimental Brain Research*, *186*, 589–601. doi:10.1007/s00221-007-1263-y

Arias, P., & Cudeiro, J. (2010). Effect of rhythmic auditory stimulation on gait in Parkinsonian patients with and without freezing of gait. *PLoS ONE*, *5*(3), e9675. doi:10.1371/journal.pone.0009675

Armson, J., Foote, S., Witt, C., Kalinowski, J., & Stuart, A. (1997). Effect of frequency altered feedback and audience size on stuttering. *European Journal of Disorders of communication. The Journal of the College of Speech and Language Therapists*, *32*(3), 359–366.

Armson, J., Kiefte, M., Mason, J., & De Croos, D. (2006). The effect of SpeechEasy on stuttering frequency in laboratory conditions. *Journal of Fluency Disorders*, *31*(2), 137–152. doi:10.1016/j.jfludis.2006.04.004

Armson, J., & Stuart, A. (1998). Effect of extended exposure to frequency-altered feedback on stuttering during reading and monologue. *Journal of Speech, Language, and Hearing Research: JSLHR*, *41*(3), 479–490.

Arnaert, A., & Delesie, L. (2001). Telenursing for the elderly. The case for care via video-telephony. *Journal of Telemedicine and Telecare*, *7*(6), 311–316. doi:10.1258/1357633011936912

Arnott, J. L. (2005). Text entry in augmentative and alternative communication. In *Proceedings of Efficient Text Entry*. Retrieved from http://drops.dagstuhl.de/opus/volltexte/2006/519/pdf/05382.ArnottJohn.P%aper.519.pdf

Asakawa, C., & Takagi, H. (2000). Annotation-based transcoding for nonvisual web access. In *Proceedings of the fourth international acm conference on assistive technologies* (pp. 172-179). ACM Press.

Asakawa, C., & Takagi, H. (2008, September). Transcoding. In S. Harper & Y. Yesilada (Eds.), Web accessibility: A foundation for research (1st ed., pp. 231–260). London: Springer. doi:10.1007/978-1-84800-050-6_14doi:10.1007/978-1-84800-050-6_14

Ayaz, H., Izzetoglu, M., Bunce, S., Heiman-Patterson, T., & Onaral, B. (2007). Detecting cognitive activity related hemodynamic signal for brain computer interface using functional near infrared spectroscopy. *3rd International IEEE EMBS Conference on Neural Engineering* (pp. 342-345). IEEE Press.

Azrin, N., Jones, R. J., & Flye, B. (1968). A synchronization effect and its application to stuttering by a portable apparatus. *Journal of Applied Behavior Analysis*, *1*(4), 283–295. doi:10.1901/jaba.1968.1-283

Azulay, J. P., Mesure, S., & Blin, O. (2006). Influence of visual cues on gait in Parkinson's disease: Contribution to attention or sensory dependence? *Journal of the Neurological Sciences*, *248*, 192–195. doi:10.1016/j.jns.2006.05.008

Bach, J. R. (1993). Communication status and survival with ventilatory support. *American Journal of Physical Medicine & Rehabilitation*, *72*(6), 343–349. doi:10.1097/00002060-199312000-00002

Bagley, S. P., & Williams, T. F. (1988). Technology and aging: the new frontier. *Frontiers in Aging Series*, *6*, 19–25.

Bailey, I. L., Hall, A. T., Kekelis, L. S., Raasch, T. W., Goodrich, G. D., & Morrissette, D. (1984). Telescope use by low vision patients: A survey. *American Journal of Optometry and Physiological Optics*, *61*(10), 79.

Bain, B. K. (1997). Evaluation. In Bain, B. K., & Leger, D. (Eds.), *Assistive technology: an interdisciplinary approach* (pp. 17–31). New York: Churchill Livingstone.

Bajaj, A., Hodson, B., & Westby, C. (2005). Communicative ability conceptions among children who stutter and their fluent peers: A qualitative exploration. *Journal of Fluency Disorders*, *30*(1), 41–64. doi:10.1016/j.jfludis.2005.01.002

Baken, R. J., & Orlikoff, R. F. (2000). *Clinical measurements of speech and voice*. San Diego, CA: Singular Thomson Learning.

Balandin, S., Berg, N., & Waller, A. (2006). Assessing the loneliness of older people with cerebral palsy. *Disability and Rehabilitation*, *28*(8), 469–479. doi:10.1080/09638280500211759

Ballin, L., & Balandin, S. (2007). An exploration of loneliness: Communication and the social networks of older people with cerebral palsy. *Journal of Intellectual & Developmental Disability*, *32*(4), 315–326. doi:10.1080/13668250701689256

Ballin, L., Balandin, S., Togher, L., & Stancliffe, R. J. (2009). Learning to use augmentative and alternative communication (AAC): is there a mentoring role for adults experienced in using AAC? *Journal of Intellectual & Developmental Disability*, *34*(1), 89–91. doi:10.1080/13668250802676038

Barbara, D. (1954). *Stuttering: a psychodynamic approach to its understanding and treatment*. New York: Julian Publishers.

Barker, R. A., & Barasi, S. (1999). *Nuroscience at a Glance*. Blackwell Science.

Barker, A. T. (1999). The history and basic principles of magnetic nerve stimulation. *Electroencephalography and Clinical Neurophysiology. Supplement*, *51*, 3–21.

Barlow, J., Singh, D., Bayer, S., & Curry, R. (2007). A systematic review of the benefits of home tele-care for frail elderly people and those with long-term conditions. *Journal of Telemedicine and Telecare*, *13*(4), 172–179. doi:10.1258/135763307780908058

Barrera, C., Santos, O. C., Gutierrez y Restrepo, E., Boticario, J. G., Moranchel, J., Roldán, J. R., & Casas, R. (2009). Empowering disabled people: e-learning challenges for independent life. In *Proceedings of the 3rd Workshop Towards User Modeling and Adaptive Systems for All: Modeling and Evaluation of Accessible Intelligent Learning Systems* (TUMAS-A 2009) held in conjunction with AIED 2009 (pp. 38-44).

Bartres-Faz, D., Junque, C., Tormos, J. M., & Pascual-Leone, A. (2000). Aplicación de la estimulación magnética transcraneal a la investigación neuropsicológica. *Revista de Neurologia*, *30*(12), 1169–1174.

Basil, (1998). *Sistemas de signos y ayudas técnicas para la comunicación aumentativa y la escritura*. Barcelona: Masson.

Bassingthwaighte, J. B., Chizeck, H. J., & Atlas, L. E. (2006). Strategies and Tactics in Multiscale Modeling of Cell-to-Organ Systems. *Proceedings of the IEEE*, *94*(4), 819–831. doi:10.1109/JPROC.2006.871775

Bauernfeind, G., Leeb, R., Wriessnegger, S. C., & Pfurtscheller, G. (2008). Development, set-up and first results for a one-channel near-infrared spectroscopy system. *Biomedical Engineering*, *53*, 36–43.

Baxter, L. K. (1997). *Capacitive sensors: Designs and applications*. New York: IEEE Press.

Beech, H. R., & Fransella, F. (1968). Explanations of the rhythm effect in stuttering. In B. B. E. Gray, G. (Ed.), *Stuttering and the Conditioning Therapies*. Monterey: The Monterey Institute for Speech and Hearing.

Bell, C. J., Shenoy, P., Chalodhorn, R., & Rao, R. P. N. (2008). Control of a humanoid robot by a noninvasive brain-computer interface in humans. *Journal of Neural Engineering*, *5*(2), 214–220. doi:10.1088/1741-2560/5/2/012

Benjamin, J. M., Ali, N. A., & Schepis, A. F. (1973). A Laser Cane for the Blind. *Proceedings of the San Diego Biomedical Symposium*, *12*, 53–57.

Bensch, M., Karim, A. A., Mellinger, J., Hinterberger, T., Tangermann, M., & Bogdan, M. (2007). Nessi: An EEG-controlled web browser for severely paralyzed patients. *Computational Intelligence and Neuroscience, 2007. Article ID, 71863*, 1–5.

Bentzen, B. L., & Mitchell, P. A. (1995). Audible Signage as a Wayfinding Aid – Verbal Landmark versus Talking Signs. *Journal of Visual Impairment & Blindness, 89*(6), 494–505.

Berman, P. A., & Brady, J. P. (1973). Miniaturized metronomes in the treatment of stuttering: A survey of clinician's experiences. *Journal of Behavior Therapy and Experimental Psychiatry, 4*(117-119).

Berners-Lee, T., & Fischetti, M. (1999). *Weaving the Web: The Original Design and Ultimate Destiny of the World Wide Web by Its Inventor*. San Francisco: Harper.

Beukelman, D. R., Yorkston, K. M., & Reichel, J. (2000). *AAC for adults with acquired neurologic disorders*. Baltimore, MD: Brookes Publishing Company.

Beukelman, D., & Mirenda, P. (1998). *Augmentative and Alternative Communication: Management of severe communication disorders in children and adults* (2nd ed.). Baltimore, MD: Paul H. Brookes Publishing.

Bhattacharya, S., & Basu, A. (in press). Design of an Iconic Communication Aid for the Individuals with Speech and Motor Impairments in India. *Assistive Technology*. Rehabilitation Engineering and Assistive Technology Society of North America (RESNA). *Press.*

Bhattacharya, S., Basu, A., & Samanta, D. (2008a). Computational Modeling of User Errors for the Design of Virtual Scanning Keyboards. *IEEE Transactions on Neural Systems and Rehabilitation Engineering, 16*(4), 400–409. doi:10.1109/TNSRE.2008.925073

Bhattacharya, S., Samanta, D., & Basu, A. (2008b). User Errors on Scanning Keyboards: Empirical Study, Model and Design Principles. *Interacting with Computers, 20*(3), 400–418. doi:10.1016/j.intcom.2008.03.002

Bhattacharya, S., Samanta, D., & Basu, A. (2008c). Performance Models for Automatic Evaluation of Virtual Scanning Keyboards. *IEEE Transactions on Neural Systems and Rehabilitation Engineering, 16*(5), 510–519. doi:10.1109/TNSRE.2008.2003377

Bhattacharya, S. (2009). *Models and algorithms for design of scanning keyboards.* Unpublished doctoral dissertation, Dept. of Computer Science and Engineering, Indian Institute of Technology Kharagpur, India.

Bicchi, A., Buss, M., Ernst, M. O., & Peer, A. (2008). *The Sense of Touch and Its Rendering: Progress in Haptics Research.* Berlin: Springer. doi:10.1007/978-3-540-79035-8

Birbaumer, N., Ghanayim, N., Hinterberger, T., Iversen, I., Kotchoubey, B., & Kübler, A. (1999). A spelling device for the paralysed. *Nature, 398*(6725), 297–298. doi:10.1038/18581

Birch, G. E., Mason, S. G., & Borisoff, J. F. (2003). Current trends in brain-computer interface research at the Neil Squire Foundation. *IEEE Transactions on Neural Systems and Rehabilitation Engineering, 11*(2), 123–126. doi:10.1109/TNSRE.2003.814450

Blackmon, M. H., Polson, P. G., Kitajima, M., & Lewis, C. (2002). Cognitive walkthrough for the web. In *Chi '02: Proceedings of the sigchi conference on human factors in computing systems* (pp. 463-470). New York: ACM Press. doi:10.1145/503376.503459

Blakeney, A. B. (1991). The impact of culture on patient education. *Occupational Therapy Practice, 2*(3), 12–20.

Blankertz, B., Dornhege, G., Schäfer, C., Krepki, R., Kohlmorgen, J., & Müller, K. R. (2003). Boosting bit rates and error detection for the classification of fast-paced motor commands based on single-trial EEG analysis. *IEEE Transactions on Neural Systems and Rehabilitation Engineering, 11*(2), 127–131. doi:10.1109/TNSRE.2003.814456

Blankertz, B., Dornhege, G. Krauledat, M., Müller, K. R., Kunzmann, V., Losch, F., & Curio, G. (2006). The Berlin Brain-Computer Interface: EEG-based communication without subject training. *IEEE Transactions onNeural Systems and Rehabilitation Engineering, 14*(2), 147–152.

Blenkhorn, P., & Evans, D. G. (1997). A system for enabling blind people to identify landmarks: the sound buoy. *IEEE Transactions on Rehabilitation Engineering*, *5*, 276–278. doi:10.1109/86.623019

Blit-Cohen, E., & Litwin, H. (2004). Elder participation in cyberspace: A qualitative analysis of Israeli retirees. *Journal of Aging Studies*, *18*, 385–398. doi:10.1016/j.jaging.2004.06.007

Blochl, D., Rumershofer, H., & Wob, W. (2003). Individualized e-learning systems enabled by a semantically determined adaptation of learning fragments. In *Proceedings of the 14th International workshop on Database and Expert Systems Applications* (pp. 640-645).

Blomgren, M., Roy, N., Callister, T., & Merrill, R. M. (2005). Intensive Stuttering Modification Therapy: A Multidimensional Assessment of Treatment Outcomes. *Journal of Speech, Language, and Hearing Research: JSLHR*, *48*(3), 509. doi:10.1044/1092-4388(2005/035)

Bloodstein, O. (1981). *A handbook of stuttering*. Chicago: National Easter Seal Society.

Bloodstein, O. (2006). Some empirical observations about early stuttering: a possible link to language development. *Journal of Communication Disorders*, *39*(3), 185–191. doi:10.1016/j.jcomdis.2005.11.007

Bloodstein, O. (1995). *A Handbook on Stuttering*.

Bluemel, C. S. (1931). Stammering as an impediment of thought. *Journal of the American Medical Association*, *96*(22), 1846–1848.

Boas, D. A., Strangman, G., Culver, J. P., Hogel, R. D., Jasdzewsky, R. A., & Rosen, B. R. (2003). Can the cerebral metabolic rate of oxygen be estimated with near-infrared spectroscopy? *Physics in Medicine and Biology*, *48*, 2405–2418. doi:10.1088/0031-9155/48/15/311

Bobrick, B. (1996). *Knotted Tongues: Stuttering in History and the Quest for a Cure*. Kodansha Amer Inc.

Boecker, M., Buecheler, M. M., Schroeter, M. L., & Gauggel, S. (2007). Prefrontal brain activation during stop-signal response inhibition: An event-related functional near-infrared spectroscopy study. *Behavioural Brain Research*, *176*(2), 259–266. doi:10.1016/j.bbr.2006.10.009

Boldyreff, C. (2002). Determination and evaluation of web accessibility. In *Wetice '02: Proceedings of the 11th IEEE international workshops on enabling technologies* (pp. 35-42). Washington, DC, USA: IEEE Computer Society.

Borenstein, J., Everett, H. R., & Feng, L. (1996). *Where am I? Sensors and methods for mobile robot positioning*. The University of Michigan.

Borenstein, J., & Ulrich, I. (1997). The GuideCane - A Computerized Travel Aid for the Active Guidance of Blind Pedestrians. *IEEE International Conference on Robotics and Automation* (pp. 1283-1288). Albuquerque, NM, April.

Bortz, W. M. (1984). The disuse syndrome. *The Western Journal of Medicine*, *141*(5), 691–694.

Bothe, A. K., Finn, P., & Bramlett, R. E. (2007). Pseudoscience and the SpeechEasy: Reply to Kalinowski, Saltuklaroglu, Stuart, and Guntupalli. *American Journal of Speech-Language Pathology*, *16*, 77–83. doi:10.1044/1058-0360(2007/010)

Botsis, T., & Hartvigsen, G. (2008). Current status and future perspectives in tele-care for elderly people suffering from chronic diseases. *Journal of Telemedicine and Telecare*, *14*(4), 195–203. doi:10.1258/jtt.2008.070905

Bousbia-Salah, M., Larbi, A., & Bedda, M. (2004). An interface card for measuring distance travelled by blind pedestrians. *AVT*, *38*, 68–74.

Boylan, L. S., Pullman, S. L., Lisanby, S. H., Spicknall, K. E., & Sackeim, H. A. (2001). Repetitive transcranial magnetic stimulation to SMA worsens complex movements in Parkinson's disease. *Clinical Neurophysiology*, *112*(2), 259–264. doi:10.1016/S1388-2457(00)00519-8

Brajnik, G. (2004). Comparing accessibility evaluation tools: a method for tool effectiveness. In *Universal access in the information society* (Vol. 3, pp. 252–263). London: Springer-Verlag. doi:10.1007/s10209-004-0105-y

Brajnik, G. (2008). A comparative test of web accessibility evaluation methods. In *Assets '08: Proceedings of the 10th international ACM Sigaccess conference on computers and accessibility* (pp. 113-120). New York: ACM.

Brambring, M. (1985). Perceptual and Cognitive Processes of Blind Pedestrians. *Presentation to Symposium on Spatial Cognition*, University of Louisville.

Braver, T., S., Cohen, J., D., Nystrom, L., E., Jonides, J., Smith, E., E., & Noll, D.C. (1997). A parametric study of prefrontal cortex involvement in human working memory. *NeuroImage*, *5*(1), 49–62. doi:10.1006/nimg.1996.0247

Brewer, J. (2004). Web accessibility highlights and trends. In *W4a '04: Proceedings of the 2004 international cross-disciplinary workshop on Web accessibility* (W4A) (pp. 51-55). New York: ACM Press.

Brown, S., Ingham, R., Ingham, J., Laird, A., & Fox, P. (2005). Stuttered and fluent speech production: an ALE meta-analysis of functional neuroimaging studies. *Human Brain Mapping*, *25*(1), 105–117. doi:10.1002/hbm.20140

Brown, I., & Brown, R. (2003). *Quality of Life and Disability. An Approach for Community Practitioners*. Jessica Kingsley Publishers.

Brunetti, F., Moreno, J. C., Ruiz, A. F., Rocon, E., & Pons, J. L. (2006). A new platform based on IEEE802.15.4 wireless inertial sensors for motion caption and assessment. *28th Annual International Conference of the IEEE Engineering in Medicine and Biology Society. EMBS '06* (pp. 6497-6500). New York, USA.

Brunner, C., Scherer, R., Graimann, B., Supp, G., & Pfurtscheller, G. (2006). Online control of a brain-computer interface using phase synchronization. *IEEE Transactions on Bio-Medical Engineering*, *53*(12), 2501–2506. doi:10.1109/TBME.2006.881775

Bryngelson, B., & Clark, T. B. (1933). Left-handedness and stuttering. *The Journal of Heredity*, *24*(10), 387–390.

Büchel, C., & Sommer, M. (2004). What Causes Stuttering? *PLoS Biology*, *2*(2), e46. doi:10.1371/journal.pbio.0020046

Burdea, G. C. (1996). *Force and touch feedback for virtual reality*. New York: John Wiley & Sons, Inc.

Burdick, D. C., & Kwon, S. (2004). *Gerotechnology: Research and Practice in Technology and Aging*. New York: Springer Publishing Company.

Burleigh-Jacobs, A., Horak, F. B., Nutt, J. G., & Obeso, J. A. (1997). Step initiation in Parkinson's disease: Influence of levodopa and external sensory triggers. *Movement Disorders*, *12*, 206–215. doi:10.1002/mds.870120211

Butler, C. (1986). Effect of powered mobility on self-initiated behaviours of very young children with locomotor disability. *Developmental Medicine and Child Neurology*, *28*(3), 325–332. doi:10.1111/j.1469-8749.1986.tb03881.x

Buyukkokten, O., Molina, H. G., Paepcke, A., & Winograd, T. (2000). Power browser: Efficient web browsing for PDAs. In *Proceedings of the SIGCHI conference on human factors in computing systems* (pp. 430-437). ACM Press.

Byblow, W. D., Summers, J. J., Lewis, G. N., & Thomas, J. (2002). Bimanual coordination in Parkinson's disease: Deficits in movement frequency, amplitude, and pattern switching. *Movement Disorders*, *17*, 20–29. doi:10.1002/mds.1281

Cabero, J. (2004). Reflexiones sobre la brecha digital y la educación. In Soto, F.J. & Rodríguez, J. (Coords.), *Tecnología, educación y diversidad* (pp. 23-42). Murcia: Conserjería de Educación y Cultura.

Caldwell, D. G., Tsagarakis, N., & Medrano-Cerda, G. A. (2000). Bio-mimetic actuators: polymeric pseudo muscular actuators and pneumatic muscle actuators for biological emulation. *Mechatronics*, *10*(4-5), 499–530. doi:10.1016/S0957-4158(99)00071-9

Callan, D., Tsytsarev, V., Hanakawa, T., Callan, A., Katsuhara, M., & Fukuyama, H. (2006). Song and speech: brain regions involved with perception and covert production. *NeuroImage*, *31*(3), 1327–1342. doi:10.1016/j.neuroimage.2006.01.036

Calvo-Merino, B., & Haggard, P. (2004). Estimulación magnética transcraneal. Aplicaciones en neurociencia cognitiva. *Revista de Neurologia*, *38*(4), 374–380.

Cantello, R., Tarletti, R., & Civardi, C. (2002). Transcranial magnetic stimulation and Parkinson's disease. *Brain Research. Brain Research Reviews*, *38*(3), 309–327. doi:10.1016/S0165-0173(01)00158-8

Carpenter, T., McCoy, K., & Pennington, C. (1997). Schema-based organization of reusable text in aac: user-interface considerations. In *Proceedings of RESNA '97 Annual Conference* (pp. 57-59). Pittsburgh, PA, USA.

Carrozza, M. C., Vecchi, F., Sebastiani, F., Cappiello, G., Roccella, S., Zecca, M., et al. (2003). *Experimental analysis of an innovative prosthetic hand with proprioceptive sensors. IEEE International Conference on Robotics and Automation (ICRA '03)* (Vol.2, pp. 2230-2235). Taipei. (Taiwan)

Casali, S. P. (1995). A physical skills-based strategy for choosing an appropriate interface method. In Edwards, A. D. N. (Ed.), *Extra-ordinary Human Computer Interaction: Interfaces for People with Disabilities* (pp. 315–342). New York, NY: Cambridge University Press.

Casson, A., Smith, S., Duncan, J., & Rodriguez-Villega, E. (2008). *Wearable EEG: what is it, why is it needed and what does it entail?* Paper presented at the Conf Proc IEEE Eng Med Biol Soc.

Caudrey, D. J., & Seeger, B. R. (1983). Rehabilitation engineering service evaluation: a follow-up survey of device effectiveness and patient acceptance. *Rehabilitation Literature*, *44*(3-4), 80–85.

Center for Universal Design. (1997). The Principles of Universal Design. Retrieved May, 2009, from http://www.design.ncsu.edu/cud/about_ud/ udprinciplestext.htm.

Centro Estatal de Autonomía Personal y Ayudas Técnicas (CEAPAT). (2009). *Catálogo de productos de apoyo.* Retrieved September 2009, from http://www.catalogo-ceapat.org/acercade

Chamberlain, M. A., Thornely, G., Stowe, J., & Wright, V. (1981). Evaluation of aids and equipment for the bath II: a possible solution to the problem. *Rheumatology and Rehabilitation*, *20*, 38–43. doi:10.1093/rheumatology/20.1.38

Chan, W., Woo, J., Hui, E., Lau, W., Lai, J., & Lee, D. (2005). A community model for care of elderly people with diabetes via telemedicine. *Applied Nursing Research*, *18*(2), 77–81. doi:10.1016/j.apnr.2004.11.002

Chan, L., Chiang, J., Chen, Y., Ke, C., Hsu, J., & Chu, H. (2006, May). *Collaborative localization: enhancing wifi-based position estimation with neighborhood links in clusters.* Paper presented at the 4th International Conference on Pervasive Computing (Pervasive 2006), Dublin Ireland.

Charness, N., & Schaie, C. W. (2003). *Impact of Technology on Successful Aging*. New York: Springer Publishing Company.

Chen, Y. L., Chang, W. H., Chen, S. C., Sheu, P. F., & Chen, W. L. (2003). The development of a knee locker with closed-loop functional electrical stimulation (FES) for hemiplegia in gait training. *Disability and Rehabilitation*, *25*(16), 916–921. doi:10.1080/0963828031000122230

Chen, Y.L., Chen, S.C., & Chen, W.L., Hsiao Chin-Chih, Kuo, T.S., & Lai, J.S. (2004). Neural network and fuzzy control in FES-assisted locomotion for the hemiplegic. *Journal of Medical Engineering & Technology*, *28*(1), 32–38. doi:10.1080/0309190031000121 1523

Chen, Y. L., Li, Y. C., Lai, J. S., & Kuo, T. S. (2001). The development of a closed-loop controlled functional electrical stimulation (FES) in gait training. *Journal of Medical Engineering & Technology*, *25*(2), 41–48. doi:10.1080/03091900110043612

Chen, S. C., Tang, F. T., Chen, Y. L., Chen, W. L., Li, Y. C., & Shih, Y. Y. (2004). Infrared-based communication augmentation system for the people with multiple disabilities. *Disability and Rehabilitation*, 1105–1109. doi:10.1080/09638280410001713025

Chen, W. L., Andy Liou, A. H., Chen, S. C., Chung, C. M., Chen, Y. L., & Shih, Y. Y. (2007). A novel home appliance control system for people with multiple disabilities. *Disability and Rehabilitation*, 201–206.

Chen, Y. L., Chang, W. H., Tang, F. T., Wong, M. K., & Kuo, T. S. (1999). The new design of an infrared-controlled human-computer interface for the disabled. *IEEE Transactions on Rehabilitation Engineering*, *7*(4), 474–481. doi:10.1109/86.808951

Chen, Y. L., Shih, Y. Y., Chang, W. H., Tang, F. T., Wong, M. K., & Kuo, T. S. (1999). A novel infrared-controlled telephone communication interface for the disabled. *IEICE Transactions on Information and Systems*, *82*(10), 1417–1424.

Chen, T. Y., Mann, W. C., Tomita, M., & Nochajski, S. (2000). Caregiver involvement in the use of assistive devices by frail older persons. *Occupational Therapy in Research*, *20*(3), 179–199.

Chen, C., & Pomalaza-Ráez, C. (2009, February). *Monitoring Human Movements at Home Using Wearable Wireless Sensors*. Paper presented at the Third International Symposium on Medical Information & Communication Technology, Montreal (Canada).

Chene, D., & Hoel, M. (2002). Web site accessibility auditing tool for visually deficient persons OCAWA. In *ICCHP '02: Proceedings of the 8th international conference on computers helping people with special needs* (pp. 27–32). London: Springer-Verlag.

Cheng, M., Gao, X., Gao, S., & Xu, D. (2002). Design and implementation of a brain computer interface with high transfer rates. *IEEE Transactions on Bio-Medical Engineering*, *49*(10), 1181–1186. doi:10.1109/TBME.2002.803536

Chervin, A. (1896). *(Suttering and other pronunciation defects) Tartamudez y otros defectos de pronunciación*. Paris: Société d'Éditions Scientifiques.

Chisholm, W., Vanderheiden, G., & Jacobs, I. (2001). Web content accessibility guidelines 1.0. *Interaction*, *8*(4), 35–54..doi:10.1145/379537.379550

Chisholm, W. A., & Henry, S. L. (2005). Interdependent components of web accessibility. In *W4a '05: Proceedings of the 2005 international cross-disciplinary workshop on web accessibility* (w4a) (pp. 31-37). New York: ACM Press.

Chisholm, W., & Kasday, L. (2005). Evaluation, Repair, and Transformation Tools for Web Content Accessibility. Retrieved 2005 from http://www.w3.org/ WAI/ER/existingtools.html

Chisholm, W., Vanderheiden, G., & Jacobs, I. (1999). Web Content Accessibility Guidelines 1.0. Retrieved 2005 from http://www.w3.org/TR/WCAG10/

Clarke, M., McConachie, H., Price, K., & Wood, P. (2001). Views of young people using augmentative and alternative communication systems. *International Journal of Language & Communication Disorders*, *36*(1), 107–115. doi:10.1080/13682820150217590

Clemson, L., & Martin, R. (1996). Usage and effectiveness of rails, bathing and toileting aids. *Occupational Therapy in Health Care*, *10*(1), 41–59. doi:10.1300/J003v10n01_04

Coghlan, J. K., Robinson, C. E., Newmarch, B., & Jackson, G. (1980). Lower extremity bracing in paraplegia: a follow up study. *Paraplegia*, *18*, 25–32.

Colwell, C., & Petrie, H. (2001). Evaluation of guidelines for designing accessible web content. *SIGCAPH Comput. Phys. Handicap.*, *70*, 11–13..doi:10.1145/501078.501082

Committee on Vision. (1986). *Electronic Travel Aids: New Directions for Research*. Washington, D.C.: National Academy Press.

Connell, B. R., Jones, M., Mace, R., Mueller, J., Mullick, A., & Ostroff, E. (1997). *The Principles of Universal Design*. Raleigh, NC: NC State University, The Center for Universal Design.

Cook, C. S., & McDonagh, M. J. N. (1996). Measurement of muscle and tendon stiffness in man. *European Journal of Applied Physiology*, *72*(42), 380–382. doi:10.1007/BF00599700

Cook, A. M., & Hussey, S. M. (2002). *Assistive technologies: principles and practice*. St Louis, MO: Mosby Inc.

Cook & Polgar. (2007). *Assistive Techonology. Principles and practice (Hardcover)*. St. Louis, MI: Mosby Elsevier.

Coons, S. J., Sheahan, S. L., Martin, S. S., Hendricks, J., Robbins, C. A., & Johnson, J. A. (1994). Predictors of medication non-compliance in a sample of older adults. *Clinical Therapeutics*, *16*(1), 110–117.

Cooper, M., & Rejmer, P. (2001). Case study: localization of an accessibility evaluation. In *Chi '01: Chi '01 extended abstracts on human factors in computing systems* (pp. 141–142). New York: ACM Press. doi:10.1145/634067.634154

Copestake, A. (1997). Augmented and alternative nlp techniques for augmentative and alternative communication. *Proceedings of the ACL workshop on Natural Language Processing for Communication Aids* (pp. 37-42). Madrid, Spain.

Corcho, P. I., & Corcho, P. A. (2004). Informática para mayores. Una experiencia en la universidad de Extremadura. *Revista Latinoamericana de Tecnología Educativa*, 3, 529-534. Retrieved September, 2009, from: http://campusvirtual.unex.es/cala/editio/index.php?journal=relatec& page=index

Cotton, D. J. P., Chappel, P. H., Cranny, A., White, N. M., & Beeby, S. P. (2007). Thick-film force and slip sensors for a prosthetic hand. *IEEE Sensors Journal*, *7*(5), 752–761. doi:10.1109/JSEN.2007.894912

Cowan, D., & Turner-Smith, A. (1999). The user's perspective on the provision of electronic assistive technology: equipped for life? *British Journal of Occupational Therapy*, *62*(1), 2–6.

Cox, K., & Walker, D. (1993). *User interface design*. Singapore: Prentice Hall.

Coyle, S., Ward, T., Markham, C., & McDarby, G. (2004). On the suitability of near-infrared (NIR) systems for next-generation brain-computer interfaces. *Physiological Measurement*, *25*, 815–822. doi:10.1088/0967-3334/25/4/003

Coyle, S. M., Ward, T. E., & Markham, C. M. (2007). Brain-computer interface using a simplified functional near-infrared spectroscopy system. *Journal of Neural Engineering*, *4*(3), 219–226. doi:10.1088/1741-2560/4/3/007

Coyne, K. P., & Nielsen, J. (2001). *Beyond ALT text: Making the web easy to use for users with disabilities*. Nielson Norman Group.

Craddock, G., & McCormack, L. (2002). Delivering an AT service: a client-focused, social and participatory service delivery model in assistive technology in Ireland. *Disability and Rehabilitation, 4*(1,2,3), 160-170.

Craig, A. (1998). Relapse following treatment for stuttering: a critical review and correlative data. *Journal of Fluency Disorders*, *23*(1), 1–30. doi:10.1016/S0094-730X(97)00027-2

Craig, A. (2000). The Developmental Nature and Effective Treatment of Stuttering in Children and Adolescents. *Journal of Developmental and Physical Disabilities*, *12*(3), 173–186. doi:10.1023/A:1009463703647

Crammond, D. J. (1997). Motor imagery: never in your wildest dream. *Trends in Neurosciences*, *20*(2), 54–57. doi:10.1016/S0166-2236(96)30019-2

Craven, J., & Bophy, P. (2003). *Non-visual access to the digital library: the use of digital library interfaces by blind and visually impaired people. Library and Information Commission Research Report 145*. Manchester Centre for Research in Library and Information Management.

Cremniter, D., Payan, C., Meidinger, A., Batista, G., & Fermanian, J. (2001). Predictors of short-term deterioration and compliance in psychiatric emergency patients: a prospective study of 457 patients referred to the emergency room of a general hospital. *Psychiatry Research*, *104*(1), 49–59. doi:10.1016/S0165-1781(01)00293-1

Cross, D. E. (1977). Effects of false increasing, decreasing, and true electromyographic biofeedback on the frequency of stuttering. *Journal of Fluency Disorders*, *2*(2), 109–116. doi:10.1016/0094-730X(77)90014-6

Cunnington, R., Iansek, R., & Bradshaw, J. L. (1999). Movement-related potentials in Parkinson's disease: External cues and attentional strategies. *Movement Disorders*, *14*, 63–68. doi:10.1002/1531-8257(199901)14:1<63::AID-MDS1012>3.0.CO;2-V

Curry, F. K. W., & Gregory, H. H. (1969). The Performance of Stutterers on Dichotic Listening Tasks Thought to Reflect Cerebral Dominance. *Journal of Speech and Hearing Research*, *12*(1), 73–82.

Czaja, S. J. (1996). Interface design for older adults. In Ozok, A. F. (Ed.), *Advances in a lied ergonomics* (pp. 262–265). Istanbul, West Lafayette: USA Publishing.

Czaja, S. J. (2006). Technology and older adults: Designing for accessibility and usability. In *Assets '06: Proceedings of the 8th international ACM Sigaccess conference on computers and accessibility*. New York: ACM.

Daerden, F., & Lefeber, D. (2002). Pneumatic artificial muscles: actuators for robotics and automation. *Journal of the American Chemical Society*, *54*(1), 11–21.

Damper, R. I. (1984). Text composition by the physically disabled: A rate prediction model for scanning input. *Applied Ergonomics*, *15*, 289–296. doi:10.1016/0003-6870(84)90201-1

Darling, N. C., Goodrich, G. L., & Wiley, J. K. (1977). A follow-up study of electronic travel aid users. *Bulletin of Prosthetics Research*, *10*(27), 82–91.

Darvas, F., Miller, K. J., Rao, R. P. N., & Ojemann, J. G. (2009). Nonlinear phase-phase cross-frequency coupling mediates communication between distant sites in human neocortex. *The Journal of Neuroscience*, *29*(2), 426–435. doi:10.1523/JNEUROSCI.3688-08.2009

de Investigación, C. Desarrollo y Aplicación Tiflotécnica [CIDAT] (1998). *Diccionario para Invidentes de la Real Academia Española*, ONCE-CETTICO, product no. 0209020033912. Retrieved February 19, 1999 from http://cidat.once.es/home.cfm?excepcion=52&idproducto=241&idseccion=10).

Decety, J. (1996). Do imagined and executed actions share the same neural substrate? *Brain Research. Cognitive Brain Research*, *3*(2), 87–93. doi:10.1016/0926-6410(95)00033-X

Del Olmo, M., Arias, P., Furio, M. C., Pozo, M. A., & Cudeiro, J. (2006). Evaluation of the effect of training using auditory stimulation on rhythmic movement in Parkinsonian patients - a combined motor and F-18-FDG PET study. *Parkinsonism & Related Disorders*, *12*, 155–164. doi:10.1016/j.parkreldis.2005.11.002

Del Olmo, M. F., Bello, O., & Cudeiro, J. (2007). Transcranial magnetic stimulation over dorsolateral prefrontal cortex in Parkinson's disease. *Clinical Neurophysiology*, *118*(1), 131–139. doi:10.1016/j.clinph.2006.09.002

Demasco, P., & McCoy, K. F. (1992). Generating text from compressed input: an intelligent interface for people with severe motor impairments. *Communications of the ACM*, *35*(5), 68–79. doi:10.1145/129875.129881

Denning, T., Matsuoka, Y., & Tadayoshi, K. (2009). Neurosecurity: security and privacy for neural devices. *Neurosurgical Focus*, *27*(1), E7. doi:10.3171/2009.4.FOCUS0985

Department of Justice. (1998). Workforce Investment Act SEC. 508. Electronic and Information Technology. Retrieved 2005 from http://www.usdoj.gov/crt/508/508home.html

Derazne, J. (1966). *Speech Pathology in the U.S.S.R.* Amsterdam: North Holland.

Dewar, A., & Dewar, A. D. (1979). The long-term use of an automatically triggered auditory feedback-masking device in the treatment of stammering. *The British Journal of Disorders of Communication*, *14*, 219–229. doi:10.3109/13682827909011361

Di Lazzaro, V., Oliviero, A., Mazzone, P., Insola, A., Pilato, F., & Saturno, E. (2001). Comparison of descending volleys evoked by monophasic and biphasic magnetic stimulation of the motor cortex in conscious humans. *Experimental Brain Research*, *141*(1), 121–127. doi:10.1007/s002210100863

Di Lazzaro, V., Oliviero, A., Pilato, F., Saturno, E., Dileone, M., & Mazzone, P. (2004). The physiological basis of transcranial motor cortex stimulation in conscious humans. *Clinical Neurophysiology*, *115*, 255–266. doi:10.1016/j.clinph.2003.10.009

Díez, E. (2008). Tecnologías que ayudan: Mitos y realidades. [RAMPA]. *Revista de Atención Integral y Medicina Familiar para la Atención Primaria, 4*, 14–19.

Díez, E. (2006). Evaluación para el uso de tecnologías de ayuda en personas con discapacidad. In Verdugo Alonso, M. A. & Jordán de Urríes Vega, F. B. (Coord.). *Rompiendo inercias. Claves para avanzar. VI Jornadas Científicas de Investigación sobre Personas con Discapacidad* (pp. 297-305). Salamanca: Amarú.

Disability Rights Commission. (2004). *The Web: Access and inclusion for disabled people* (Tech. Rep.). UK: Disability Rights Commission (DRC).

Dodge, D. M. (2009, May 11). *A Reactive Inhibition Model of Stuttering Development & Behavior: A Neuropsychological Theory Based on Recent Research*. Retrieved August 27, 2009 from http://www.veilsofstuttering.com/reactinh.html

Doebelin, E. O. (1985). *Measurement Systems* (3rd ed.). McGraw-Hill Book Company.

Dolphin Computer Access. (2009). Hal Screen Reader, Version 11.0, April 2009. Retrieved September 25 2009 from http://www.yourdolphin.com/manuals/v11hal00044.pdf

Donchin, E., Spencer, K. M., & Wijesinghe, R. (2000). The mental prosthesis: assessing the speed of a P300-based brain-computer interface. *IEEE Transactions on Bio-Medical Engineering, 8*(2), 174–179.

Dornhege, G., Millan, J. R., Hinterberger, T., McFarland, D., & Müller, K. R. (Eds.). (2007). *Towards Brain-Computer Interfacing*. Cambridge, MA: The MIT Press.

Down syndrome online (n.d.). Retrieved from http://www.down-syndrome.org/about/

Drachsler, H., Hummel, H. G. K., & Koper, R. (2007). Personal RS for learners in lifelong learning: requirements, techniques and model. *International Journal of Learning Technology*. eInclusion@EU project (2004, October). D1.1 Analytic Framework - eInclusion and eAccessibility priority issues. Retrieved from http://www.einclusion-eu.org/Document.asp?View=TRUE&MenuID=77#_ftnref62

DRC. (2006). PAS 78: A guide to good practice in commissioning accessible websites.

Duda, R., Hart, P., & Stork, D. (Eds.). (2000). *Pattern Classification* (2nd ed.). New York: Wiley Interscience.

Dumont, C., Vicent, C., & Mazer, B. (2002). Development of a Standardized Instrument to Assess Computer Task Performance. *The American Journal of Occupational Therapy., 56*, 60–68. doi:10.5014/ajot.56.1.60

Dunn, R. B., Weaver, L. Y., Lucero, Y., Langbeing, F., Fehr, L., Johnson, P., & Riedy, L. (1998). Follow up assessment of standing mobility device users. *Assistive Technology, 10*(2), 84–93.

Dyck, J. L., & Smither, J. A. (1996). Older Adults' Acquisition of Word Processing: The Contribution of Cognitive Abilities and Computer Anxiety. *Computers in Human Behavior, 12*(1), 107–119. doi:10.1016/0747-5632(95)00022-4

Dye, R., Alm, N., Arnott, J. L., Harper, G., & Morrison, A. (1998). A script-based aac system for transactional interaction. *Natural Language Engineering, 4*(1), 57–71. doi:10.1017/S1351324998001867

Eagle, M., Baudouin, S. V., Chandler, C., Giddings, D. R., Bullock, R., & Bushby, K. (2002). Survival in Duchenne muscular dystrophy: improvements in life expectancy since 1967 and the impact of home nocturnal ventilation. *Neuromuscular Disorders, 12*(10), 926–929. doi:10.1016/S0960-8966(02)00140-2

Edelman, G. M., & Tononi, G. (2000). *A Universe of Consciousness: How matter becomes imagination*. New York: Basic Books.

Edwards, N. I., & Jones, D. A. (1998). Ownership and use of assistive devices amongst older people in the community. *Age and Ageing, 27*(4), 462–46.

Edwards, A. D. N. (1991). *Evaluation of Outspoken software for blind users*. (Tech. Rep. YCS150). York, England: University of York, Department of Computer Science.

Egan, M., Warren, S. A., Hessel, M., & Gilewich, G. (1992). Activities of daily living after hip fracture: pre and post discharge. *Occupational Therapy in Research*, *12*, 342–356.

Eisenstein, J. Vanderdonckt, J. & Puerta, A. (2000). Adapting to Mobile Contexts with User-Interface Modeling. In *Proceedings of the 3rd IEEE Workshop on Mobile Computing Systems and Applications* (pp. 83-92). Los Alamitos, CA: IEEE Press.

Emeric, D., & Hernández, L. (2008). Nuevas Tecnologías y Participación Social. *Revista Informativa de la Asociación Profesional Española de Terapia Ocupacional*, *47*, 30–41.

Engelen, J., Evenepoel, F., & al, G. B. et. (1999). Producing Web Pages that Everyone can Access. TIDE-Harmony project (DE1226). Retrieved 2005 from http://www.stakes.fi/cost219/webdesign.htm Pemberton, S., et al. (2002). Xhtml 1.0 the extensible hypertext markup language (2nd ed.). Retrieved 2005 from http://www.w3.org/TR/2002/REC-xhtml1-20020801

Enzensberger, W., & Fischer, P. A. (1996). Metronome in Parkinson's disease. *Lancet*, *347*, 1337–1337. doi:10.1016/S0140-6736(96)90987-3

Eskenazi, L., & Childers, D. G. (1990). Acoustic correlates of vocal quality. *Journal of Speech and Hearing Research*, *33*, 298–306.

Espinosa, N., de Labra, C., Rivadulla, C., Mariño, J., Grieve, K. L., & Cudeiro, J. (2007). Effects on EEG of Low (1Hz) and High (15Hz) Frequency Repetitive Transcranial Magnetic Stimulation of the Visual Cortex: A Study in the Anesthetized Cat. *The Open Neurosci Journal*, *1*, 20–25.

European Committee for Standardization. (2007). [*Assistive Products for persons with Disability. Classification and Terminology. Geneva, Switzerland:* BSI.]. *International Standard EN ISO*, *9999*, 2007.

European Conference EDeAN (European Design for all e-Accessibility Network). (2008). *Conclusiones del encuentro: Decálogo de León por la accesibilidad.* León: Ministerio de Educación, Política Social y Deporte.

European Union Policy Survey. (2005, November). eaccessibility of public sector services in the European union (European Union Policy Survey). UK Government Cabinet Office (RNIB and AbilityNet and DCU and RNID and Socitm). Retrieved from http://www.cabinetoffice.gov.uk/e-government/resources/eaccessibility/index.asp

European Union. (2006b) *User Needs in ICT Research for Independent Living, with a Focus on Health Aspects.* Retrieved from http://ec.europa.eu/information_society/activities/health/docs/events/indep-living-nov2005/24-25nov-report-final-draft-june2006.pdf

European Union. (2009). e-Inclusion Ministerial Conference (Dec 2008, Vienna, Austria.) DG Information Society and Media – Unit H.3 ICT for Inclusion, Report (June 2009). Retrieved from http://ec.europa.eu/information_society/events/e-inclusion/2008/doc/final_report.pdf

European Union. Declaration on eInclusion 11-13 June (2006a). Ministers of the European Union Member States and accession and candidate countries, European Free Trade Area (EFTA) countries and other countries. Retrieved April 20, 2008, from http://europa.eu.int/information_society/events/ict_riga_2006/doc/declaration_riga.pdf

Falkman, K. W., Sandberg, A. D., & Hjelmquist, E. (2002). Preferred communication modes: prelinguistic and linguistic communication in non-speaking preschool children with cerebral palsy. *International Journal of Language & Communication Disorders*, *37*(1), 59–68. doi:10.1080/13682820110096661

Farmer, L. W. (1978). Mobility devices. *Bulletin of Prosthetics Research*, (Fall): 47–118.

FEAPS. (Confederación Española de Organizaciones en favor de las Personas con Discapacidad Intelectual). (n.d.). Retrieved from http://www.feaps.org/

Federation, A. S. E. M. (2008). *Guía de las enfermedades neuromusculares. Información y apoyo a las familias.* Jaen: Formación Alcalá.

Fenichel, O. (1945). *The psychoanalytic theory of neurosis.* New York: Norton.

Ferree, T. C., Luu, P., Russell, G. S., & Tucker, D. M. (2001). Scalp electrode impedance, infection risk, and EEG data quality. *Clinical Neurophysiology, 112*(3), 536–544. doi:10.1016/S1388-2457(00)00533-2

Ferreira, M. A. V., & Velázquez, E. D. (2007, October). La discapacidad: una modalidad inexplorada de exclusión social. In *Proceedings of III Congreso Nacional sobre Universidad y discapacidad. XII Reunión del Real Patronato sobre Discapacidad.* Zaragoza (Spain).

Fields, R. (2008). White matter in learning, cognition and psychiatric disorders. *Trends in Neurosciences, 31*(7), 361–370. doi:10.1016/j.tins.2008.04.001

Finkenzeller, K. (2003). *RFID handbook: fundamentals and applications in contactless smart cards and identification* (2nd ed.). West Sussex, UK: Wiley.

Finlayson, M., & Havixbeck, K. (1992). A post-discharge study on the use of assistive devices. *Canadian Journal of Occupational Therapy, 59*, 201–207.

Fisher, R. S., Harding, G., Erba, G., Barkley, G. L., & Wilkins, A. (2005). Photic- and pattern-induced seizures: A review for the epilepsy foundation of america working group. *Epilepsia, 46*(9), 1426–1441. doi:10.1111/j.1528-1167.2005.31405.x

Fitts, P. M., & Peterson, J. R. (1964). Information capacity of discrete motor responses. *Journal of Experimental Psychology, 67*, 103–112. doi:10.1037/h0045689

Fitzgerald, P. B., Fountain, S., & Daskalakis, Z. J. (2006). A comprehensive review of the effects of rTMS on motor cortical excitability and inhibition. *Clinical Neurophysiology, 117*(12), 2584–2596. doi:10.1016/j.clinph.2006.06.712

Forbes, W. F., Hayward, L. M., & Agwani, N. (1993). Factors associated with self-reported use and non-use of assistive devices among impaired elderly residing in the community. *Canadian Journal of Public Health, 84*(1), 53–57.

Foulke, E. (1971). The perceptual basis for mobility. *Amer. Found. for the Blind Research Bulletin, 23*, 1–8.

Foulke, E. (1982). A Reading Braille. In Schiff, W., & Foulke, E. (Eds.), *Tactile Perception: A Source Book.* New York: Cambridge University Press.

Foundas, A. L., Bollich, A. M., Corey, D. M., Hurley, M., & Heilman, K. M. (2001). Anomalous anatomy of speech–language areas in adults with persistent developmental stuttering. *Neurology, 57*, 207–215.

Foundas, A. L., Bollich, A. M., Feldman, J., Corey, D. M., Hurley, M., & Lemen, L. C. (2004). Aberrant auditory processing and atypical planum temporale in developmental stuttering. *Neurology, 63*(9), 1640–1646.

Fox, P. T. (2003). Brain imaging in stuttering: where next? *Journal of Fluency Disorders, 28*(4), 265–272. doi:10.1016/j.jfludis.2003.08.001

Fox, P. T., Ingham, R. J., Ingham, J. C., Hirsch, T. B., Downs, J. H., & Martin, C. (1996). A PET study of the neural systems of stuttering. *Nature, 382*(6587), 158–162. doi:10.1038/382158a0

Fraden, J. (2003). *Handbook of modern sensor: Physics, designs, and applications* (3rd ed.). New York: Springer Science.

Franceschini, M. A., Fantini, S., Toronov, V., Filiaci, M. E., & Gratton, E. (1999). Cerebral hemodynamics measured by near-infrared spectroscopy at rest and during motor activation. In A. Ganjbakhche (Ed.), *Proceedings of Inter-Institute Workshop on In Vivo Optical Imaging at the NIH* (pp.73-80). Washington DC: Optical Society of America

Freedom Scientific BLV Group. (2008). JAWS(r) for Windows(r) Quick Start Guide, 11800 31st Court North, St. Petersburg, Florida 33716-1805 USA.

Fregni, F., Simon, D. K., Wu, A., & Pascual-Leone, A. (2005). Non-invasive brain stimulation for Parkinson's disease: a systematic review and meta-analysis of the literature. *Journal of Neurology, Neurosurgery, and Psychiatry, 76*(12), 1614–1623. doi:10.1136/jnnp.2005.069849

Frenkel-Toledo, S., Giladi, N., Peretz, C., Herman, T., Gruendlinger, L., & Hausdorff, J. M. (2005). Treadmill walking as an external pacemaker to improve gait rhythm and stability in Parkinson's disease. *Movement Disorders, 20*, 1109–1114. doi:10.1002/mds.20507

Friedman, A., Fetterman, E., & Jolson, Y. (1999). *Dr. Fluency Computerized Stuttering Treatment Program User's Guide (Version 2.3)*. Jerusalem, Israel: Speech Therapy Systems, Ltd.

Friedman, S. (1990). *Cartas con un paciente (co-autor). Un proceso de terapia para la tartamudez*. Valencia: Promolibro.

Friman, O., Lüth, T., Volosyak, I., & Gräser, A. (2007). Spelling with steady-state visual evoked potentials. *3rd International IEEE EMBS Conference on Neural Engineering:* (Vol. 54, pp. 354-357).

Fukuda, K., Saito, S., Takagi, H., & Asakawa, C. (2005). Proposing new metrics to evaluate web usability for the blind. In *Chi '05: Chi '05 extended abstracts on human factors in computing systems* (pp. 1387–1390). New York: ACM Press. doi:10.1145/1056808.1056923

Galán, F., Nuttin, M., Lew, E., Ferrez, P. W., Vanacker, G., Philips, J., & Millán, J. R. (2008). A brain-actuated wheelchair: asynchronous and non-invasive Brain-computer interfaces for continuous control of robots. *Clinical Neurophysiology*, *119*(9), 2159–2169. doi:10.1016/j.clinph.2008.06.001

Galindo, C., Gonzalez, J., & Fernández-Madrigal, J. (2006). Control architecture for human-robot integration: application to a robotic wheelchair. *IEEE Transactions on Systems, Man, and Cybernetics. Part B, Cybernetics: A Publication of the IEEE Systems. Man, and Cybernetics Society*, *36*(5), 1053–1067. doi:10.1109/TSMCB.2006.874131

Gall, K., Dunna, M. L., Liua, Y., Fincha, D., Lakeb, M., & Munshib, N. A. (2002). Shape memory polymer nanocomposites. *Acta Materialia*, *50*(20), 5115–5126. doi:10.1016/S1359-6454(02)00368-3

Galvin, J. C., & Scherer, M. J. (1996). An outcomes perspective of quality pathways to the most appropriate technology. In J.C. Galvin & M.J. Scherer. *Evaluating, selecting and using appropriate assistive technology* (pp.1-26). Gaithersburg, MA: Aspen Publication.

Ganguly, K., & Carmena, J. M. (2009). Emergence of a stable cortical map for neuroprosthetic control. *PLoS Biology*, *7*(7), e1000153. doi:10.1371/journal.pbio.1000153

Gao, X., Xu, D., Cheng, M., & Gao, S. (2003). A BCI-based environmental controller for the motion-disabled. *IEEE Transactions on Neural Systems and Rehabilitation Engineering*, *11*(2), 137–140. doi:10.1109/TNSRE.2003.814449

Gappa, H., & Nordbrock, G. (2004). Applying web accessibility to internet portals. *Univers. Access Inf. Soc.*, *3*(1), 80–87..doi:10.1007/s10209-003-0070-x

Garaj, V., Jirawimut, R., Ptasinski, P., Cecelja, F., & Balachandran, W. (2003). A system for remote sighted guidance of visually impaired pedestrians. *British Journal of Visual Impairment*, *21*(2), 55–63. doi:10.1177/026461960302100204

Garay-Vitoria, N. & Abascal, J. (2006). Test prediction systems: A survey. *International Journal on Universal Access in the Information Society. Special issue on User-Centered Interaction Paradigms for Universal Access in the Information Society*, *4*(3), 188–203.

Garber, S. L., & Gregorio, T. L. (1990). Upper extremity assistive devices: assessment of use by spinal cord injured patients with quadriplegia. *The American Journal of Occupational Therapy.*, *44*, 126–131.

García, M. (2005). *Adaptación de Entornos Visuales para Invidentes. Unpublished final-year project.* Madrid, Spain: Facultad de Informática, Universidad Politécnica de Madrid.

García Mila, M. (1987). *Aproximación al síntoma desde una perspectiva de orientación psicoanalítica.* Paper presented at the La tartamudez, IV Simposio.

Garcia, M., Martinez, C., Tomas, J., & Lloret, J. (2007, October). *Wireless Sensors self-location in an Indoor WLAN environment.* International Conference on Sensor Technologies and Applications (SENSORCOMM 2007), Valencia (Spain).

Gardner-Bonneau, D., & Gosbee, J. (1997). Health care and rehabilitation. In Fisk, A. D., & Rogers, W. A. (Eds.), *Handbook of human factors and the older adult* (pp. 231–255). San Diego: Academic Press.

Gateley, G. (2003). *Johnson's diagnosogenic theory of stuttering: an update*. Retrieved March 22 from http://www.thefreelibrary.com/Johnson's diagnosogenic theory of stuttering: an update

Gautschi, G. (2001). *Piezoelectric sensorics: force, strain; pressure, acceleration and acoustic emissions sensors, materials and amplifiers*. Berlin: Springer –Verlag.

Geary, D. M. (1999). *Graphic Java. Mastering the JFC* (3rd ed.). Upper Saddle River, NJ: Prentice Hall.

Geiger, C. M. (1990). The utilization of assistive devices by patients discharged from an acute rehabilitation setting. *Physical & Occupational Therapy in Geriatrics*, *9*, 3–25.

Genensky, S. M., Berry, S. H., Bikson, T. H., & Bikson, T. K. (1979). *Visual Environmental Adaptation Problems of the Partially Sighted: Final Report*. Santa Monica, Calif.: Center for the Partially Sighted.

George, J., Binns, V. E., Clayden, A. D., & Mulley, G. P. (1988). Aids and adaptations for the elderly at home: underprovided, underused and undermaintained. *British Medical Journal*, *296*, 1365–1366. doi:10.1136/bmj.296.6633.1365

Gerloff, C., Richard, J., Hadley, J., Schulman, A. E., Honda, M., & Hallett, M. (1998). Functional coupling and regional activation of human cortical motor areas during simple, internally paced and externally paced finger movements. *Brain*, *121*, 1513–1531. doi:10.1093/brain/121.8.1513

Getschow, C. O., Rosen, M. J., & Goodenough-Trepagnier, C. (1986). A systematic approach to design a minimum distance alphabetical keyboard. In *Proceedings of RESNA (Rehabilitation Engineering Society of North America) 9th Annual Conference*, Minneapolis, MN.

Ghabra, M. B., Hallett, M., & Wassermann, E. M. (1999). Simultaneous repetitive transcranial magnetic stimulation does not speed fine movement in PD. *Neurology*, *52*(4), 768–770.

Gitlin, L. N., & Burgh, D. (1995). Issuing assistive devices to older patients in rehabilitation: an exploratory study. *The American Journal of Occupational Therapy.*, *49*, 994–1000.

Gitlin, L. N., Levine, R., & Geiger, C. (1993). Adaptive device use by older adults with mixed disabilities. *Archives of Physical Medicine and Rehabilitation*, *74*, 149–152.

Gitlin, L. N., & Levine, R. E. (1992). Prescribing adaptive devices to the elderly: principles for treatment in the home. *International Journal of Technology & Aging*, *5*(1), 107–120.

Gitlin, L. N., Miller, K. S., & Boyce, A. (1999). Bathroom modification for frail elderly renters: outcomes of a community-based program. *Technology and Disability*, *10*, 141–149.

Gitlin, L. N., Schemm, R. L., Landsberg, L., & Burgh, D. (1996). Factors predicting assistive device use in the home by older persons following rehabilitation. *Journal of Aging and Health*, *8*, 554–575. doi:10.1177/089826439600800405

Glazer, K. M., Emery, C. F., Frid, D. J., & Banyasz, R. E. (2002). Psychological predictors of adherence and outcomes among patients in cardiac rehabilitation. *Journal of Cardiopulmonary Rehabilitation*, *22*, 40–46. doi:10.1097/00008483-200201000-00006

GNOME. (2009). Orca GNOME Live. Retrieved August 5, 2009 from http://www.baum.ro/gnopernicus.html.

Godino-Llorente, J. I., & Gomez-Vilda, P. (2004). Automatic Detection of Voice Impairments by Means of Short-Term Cepstral Parameters and Neural Network Based Detectors. *IEEE Transactions on Bio-Medical Engineering*, *51*, 380–384. doi:10.1109/TBME.2003.820386

Goebel, M. D. (1986). *A computer-aided fluency establishment trainer*. Annadale Fluency Clinic.

Goldiamond, I., Atkinson, C. J., & Bilger, R. C. (1962). Stabilization of Behavior and Prolonged Exposure to Delayed Auditory Feedback. *Science*, *135*(3502), 437–438. doi:10.1126/science.135.3502.437

Goldman-Eisler, F. (1986). *Cycle linguistics: Experiments in spontaneous speech*. New York: Academic Press.

Goldson, E. (1996). The micropremie: infants with birth weight less than 800 grams. *Infants and Young Children*, *8*(3), 1–10. doi:10.1097/00001163-199601000-00003

Gómez, J. A., & Navalón, C. (2002). La experiencia de la "alfabetización informacional" en el Aula de Mayores de la Universidad de Murcia. *Revista Investigación Educativa.*, *20*(2), 469–486.

Gómez del Castillo, M. T. (2003, October). *Enseñanza de Internet para Personas Mayores.* Paper presented at II Congreso la Educación en Internet e Internet en la Educación, Madrid, Spain.: 2003.

Gomi, T., & Griffith, A. (1998). Developing intelligent wheelchairs for the handicapped. In Mittal et al. (Eds.), *Assistive technology and AI* (LNAI 1458, pp. 150-78).

Gonzalez, A., & Reid, L. G. (2005). Platform-independent accessibility api: accessible document object model. In *W4a '05: Proceedings of the 2005 international cross-disciplinary workshop on Web accessibility* (w4a) (pp. 63-71). New York: ACM Press. doi:[REMOVED HYPERLINK FIELD] 10.1145/1061811.1061824

Graafmans, J., Taipale, V., & Charness, N. (1997). *Gerontechnology: A Sustainable Investment of the Future*. Amsterdam, The Netherlands: IOS.

Graimann, B., Huggins, J. E., Levine, S. P., & Pfurtscheller, G. (2004). Toward a direct brain interface based on human subdural recordings and wavelet-packet analysis. *IEEE Transactions on Bio-Medical Engineering*, *51*(6), 954–962. doi:10.1109/TBME.2004.826671

Grammenos, D., Savidis, A., & Georgalis, Y. (2007). Dual educational electronic textbooks: the starlight platform. In *9th International ACM SIGACCESS Conference on Computers and Accessibility* (pp. 107-114). New York: ACM. doi: 10.1145/1296843.1296863.

Grande, R., Pereira, J., Mato, V., & Pazos, A. (2008). Accesibilidad de las personas mayores a las tecnologías de la información y la comunicación: Situación actual en España. In Pereira, J., Martínez, L.A., Fuertes, J.L., & Vázquez, J.M. (Eds.), *Tecnologías de la Información y las Comunicaciones en la Autonomía Personal, dependencia y accesibilidad* (pp. 93-114). Santiago de Compostela: Fundación Alfredo Brañas.

Gratton, G., & Fabiani, M. (2003). The event-related optical signal (EROS) in visual cortex: Replicability, consistency, localization, and resolution. *Psychophysiology*, *40*(4), 561–571. doi:10.1111/1469-8986.00058

Grauman, K., Betke, M., Gips, J., & Bradski, G. R. (2001). Communication via eye blinks – detection and duration analysis in real time. In *Proceedings of the 2001 IEEE Computer Society Conference on Computer Vision and Pattern Recognition (CVPR 2001)* (Vol.1, pp. 1010-1017). Kauai Marriott (Hawaii)

Gruart, A., Munoz, M. D., & Delgado-Garcia, J. M. (2006). Involvement of the CA3-CA1 Synapse in the Acquisition of Associative Learning in Behaving Mice. *The Journal of Neuroscience*, *26*(4), 1077–1087. doi:10.1523/JNEUROSCI.2834-05.2006

Grynbaum, B. G., Kaplan, L. I., Lloyd, K. E., & Rusk, H. A. (1963). Methodology and initial findings in a follow-up study of spinal cord dysfunction. *Archives of Physical Medicine and Rehabilitation*, *44*, 208–215.

Guede, Á. (2002). *Proyecto PEIN: Lector de Periódicos de 32 bits para Ciegos. Unpublished final-year project.* Madrid, Spain: Facultad de Informática, Universidad Politécnica de Madrid.

Guilfoyle, C., Wootton, R., Hassall, S., Offer, J., Warren, M., Smith, D., & Eddie, M. (2002). Videoconferencing in facilities providing care for elderly people. *Journal of Telemedicine and Telecare*, *8*(S3), 22–24. doi:10.1258/13576330260440745

Guitar, B. (1975). Reduction of stuttering frequency using analog electromyographic feedback. *The Journal of Speech and Hearing Disorders*, *18*(4), 672–685.

Guitar, B. (1998). *Stuttering: An integrated approach to its nature and treatment*. Baltimore, Maryland: Williams y Wilkins.

Guo, F., Hong, B., Gao, X., & Gao, S. (2008). A brain-computer interface using motion-onset visual evoked potential. *Journal of Neural Engineering*, *5*(4), 477–485. doi:10.1088/1741-2560/5/4/011

Haas, C. T., Turbanski, S., Kessler, K., & Schmidtbleicher, D. (2006). The effects of random whole-body-vibration on motor symptoms in Parkinson's disease. *NeuroRehabilitation*, *21*, 29–36.

Hahn, E. F. (1956). *Stuttering: significant theories and therapies* (2nd ed.). Stanford University Press.

Hamada, M., Ugawa, Y., & Tsuji, S. (2008). Effectiveness of rTMS on Parkinson's Disease Study Group, Japan. High-frequency rTMS over the supplementary motor area for treatment of Parkinson's disease. *Movement Disorders*, *23*(11), 1524–1531. doi:10.1002/mds.22168

Hamilton, B. A., & Scandura, T. A. (2003). E-Mentoring: Implications for Organizational Learning and Development in a Wired World. *Organizational Dynamics*, *31*(4), 388–402. doi:10.1016/S0090-2616(02)00128-6

Hammarberg, B., Fritzell, B., Gauffin, J., Sundberg, J., & Wedin, L. (1980). Perceptual and acoustic correlates of abnormal voice qualities. *Acta Oto-Laryngologica*, *90*(1), 441–451. doi:10.3109/00016488009131746

Hanna, R., Wilfling, F., & McNeil, B. (1975). A biofeedback treatment for stuttering. *The Journal of Speech and Hearing Disorders*, *18*(2), 270–273.

Hansen, J. P., Torning, K., Johansen, J. A., Itoh, K., & Aoki, H. (2004). Gaze typing compared with input by head and hand. In *Proceedings of the 2004 symposium on Eye tracking research and applications* (pp. 131-138). San Antonio, Texas, USA.

Hanson, V. L., Richards, J. T., & Swart, C. (2008, September). Browser augmentation. In S. Harper & Y. Yesilada (Eds.), Web accessibility: A foundation for research (1st ed., pp. 215–229). London: Springer. doi:10.1007/978-1-84800-050-6_13doi:10.1007/978-1-84800-050-6_13

Harding, G. F. A., & Harding, P. F. (1999). Televised material and photosensitive epilepsy. *Epilepsia*, *40*(9SUPPL. 4), 65–69. doi:10.1111/j.1528-1157.1999.tb00909.x

Hardyck, C., & Petrinovich, L. F. (1977). Left Handedness. *Psychological Bulletin*, *84*(3), 385–404. doi:10.1037/0033-2909.84.3.385

Hargrave, S., Kalinowski, J., Stuart, A., Armson, J., & Jones, K. (1994). Effect of frequency-altered feedback on stuttering frequency at normal and fast speech rates. *Journal of Speech, Language, and Hearing Research: JSLHR*, *37*(6), 1313–1319.

Harper, S. (2007). Is There Design-For-All? *Universal Access in the Information Society*, *6*(1), 111–113. Retrieved from http://www.simonharper.info/publications/Harper2007vn.pdf

Harrington, J. (1988). Stuttering, delayed auditory feedback, and linguistic rhythm. *Journal of Speech and Hearing Research*, *31*(1), 36–47.

Harris, D. (1982). Communicative interaction processes involving nonvocal physically handicapped children. *Topics in Language Disorders*, *2*, 21–37. doi:10.1097/00011363-198203000-00005

Hartmann, M., & Kluge, T. (2007). Phase coherent detection of steady-state evoked potentials: Theory and performance analysis. *3rd International IEEE EMBS Conference on Neural Engineering: Vol. 54* (pp. 179-183).

Hashimoto, Y., & Sakai, K. L. (2003). Brain Activations During Conscious Self-Monitoring of Speech Production With Delayed Auditory Feedback: An fMRI Study. *Human Brain Mapping*, *20*, 22–28. doi:10.1002/hbm.10119

Hausdorff, J. M., Cudkowicz, M. E., Firtion, R., Wei, J. Y., & Goldberger, A. L. (1998). Gait variability and basal ganglia disorders: Stride-to-stride variations of gait cycle timing in Parkinson's disease and Huntington's disease. *Movement Disorders*, *13*, 428–437. doi:10.1002/mds.870130310

Hausdorff, J. M. (2007). Gait dynamics, fractals and falls: Finding meaning in the stride-to-stride fluctuations of human walking. In *3rd European Workshop on Movement Science*, vol 26, Amsterdam, Netherlands (pp. 555-589).

Hausdorff, J. M., Schaafsma, J. D., Balash, J., Bartels, A., Gurevich, T., & Giladi, N. (2002). Gait dynamics in subjects with freezing of gait and Parkinson's disease: Increased variability during usual walking. In *7th International Congress of Parkinsons Disease and Movement Disorders*, vol 17, Miami, Florida (p. P401)

Hausdorff, J.M., Balash, Y., & Giladi, N. (2003). Time series analysis of leg movements during freezing of gait in Parkinson's disease: Akinesia, rhyme or reason? *Physica a-Statistical Mechanics and Its Applications*, 321, 565-570.

Haworth, R. J. (1983). Use of aids during the first three months after total hip replacement. *British Journal of Rheumatology*, *22*, 29–35. doi:10.1093/rheumatology/22.1.29

Haworth, R. J., & Hopkins, J. (1980). Use of aids following total hip replacement. *British Journal of Occupational Therapy*, *43*, 398–400.

Hawthorn, D. (2000). Possible implications of aging for interface designers. *Interacting with Computers*, *12*(5), 507–528. Retrieved from http://www.sciencedirect.com/science/article/B6V0D-3YKKDNJ-5/2/9e0ae58d2d9be3ed8302fa25fc4a482f. doi:10.1016/S0953-5438(99)00021-1

Hayhow, R., Cray, A., & Enderby, P. (2002). Stammering and therapy views of people who stammer. *Journal of Fluency Disorders*, *27*(1), 1–16, quiz 16–17. doi:10.1016/S0094-730X(01)00102-4

Hemsley, B., Balandin, S., & Togher, L. (2007). Older unpaid carers' experiences supporting adults with cerebral palsy and complex communication needs in hospital. *Journal of Developmental and Physical Disabilities*, *19*(2), 115–124. doi:10.1007/s10882-007-9040-1

Hemsley, B., Balandin, S., & Togher, L. (2008). 'I've got something to say': interaction in a focus group of adults with cerebral palsy and complex communication needs. *Augmentative and Alternative Communication*, *24*(2), 110–122. doi:10.1080/07434610701830579

Herman, T., Giladi, N., & Hausdorff, J. M. (2009). Treadmill training for the treatment of gait disturbances in people with Parkinson's disease: A mini-review. *Journal of Neural Transmission*, *116*, 307–318. doi:10.1007/s00702-008-0139-z

Herrmann, M. J., Ehlis, A. C., & Fallgatter, A. J. (2003a). Frontal activation during a verbal-fluency task as measured by near-infrared spectroscopy. *Brain Research Bulletin*, *61*(1), 51–56. doi:10.1016/S0361-9230(03)00066-2

Herrmann, M. J., Ehlis, A. C., & Fallgatter, A. J. (2003b). Prefrontal activation through task requirements of emotional induction measured with NIRS. *Biological Psychology*, *64*(3), 255–263. doi:10.1016/S0301-0511(03)00095-4

Herrmann, M. J., Plichta, M. M., Ehlis, A. C., & Fallgatter, A. J. (2005). Optical topography during a go-NoGo task assessed with multi-channel near-infrared spectroscopy. *Behavioural Brain Research*, *160*(1), 135–140. doi:10.1016/j.bbr.2004.11.032

Herrmann, M. J., Walter, A., Ehlis, A. C., & Fallgatter, A. J. (2006). Cerebral oxygenation changes in the prefrontal cortex: Effects of age and gender. *Neurobiology of Aging*, *27*(6), 888–894. doi:10.1016/j.neurobiolaging.2005.04.013

Herrmann, M. J., Walter, A., Schreppel, T., Ehlis, A. C., Pauli, P., & Lesch, K. (2007). D4 receptor gene variation modulates activation of prefrontal cortex during working memory. *The European Journal of Neuroscience*, *26*(10), 2713–2718. doi:10.1111/j.1460-9568.2007.05921.x

Hick, W. E. (1952). On the rate of gain of information. *The Quarterly Journal of Experimental Psychology*, *4*, 11–36. doi:10.1080/17470215208416600

Higginbotham, D. J., Wilkins, D. P., & Lesher, G. W. (1999). Frametalker: a communication frame and utterance-based *augmentative* communication device. In *Proceedings of RESNA 99 Annual Conference* (pp. 40–42). Long Beach, CA., USA.

Hill, H. E. (1954). An Experimental Study of Disorganization Of Speech And Manual Responses In Normal Subjects. *The Journal of Speech and Hearing Disorders*, *19*(3), 295–305.

Hochberg, L. R., Serruya, M. D., Friehs, G. M., Mukand, J. A., Saleh, M., & Caplan, A. H. (2006). Neuronal ensemble control of prosthetic devices by a human with tetraplegia. *Nature*, *442*, 164–171. doi:10.1038/nature04970

Hochberg, L. R., Serruya, M. D., Friehs, G. M., Mukand, J. A., Saleh, M., & Caplan, A. H. (2006). Neuronal ensemble control of prosthetic devices by a human with tetraplegia. *Nature*, *442*(7099), 164–171. doi:10.1038/nature04970

Holst, G. C. (Ed.). (2000). *Common sense approach to thermal imaging.* Bellingham, Washington: The International Society for Optical Engineering: JCD Publishing.

Hori, M., Kondoh, G., Ono, K., & Hirose, S. ichi, & Singhal, S. (2000). Annotation-based web content transcoding. In *Proceedings of the 9th International World Wide Web Conference on Computer Networks: The International Journal of Computer and Telecommunications Networking* (pp. 197-211). Amsterdam, The Netherlands, The Netherlands: North-Holland Publishing Co.

Horstmann, H. M., & Levine, S. P. (1990). Modeling of user performance with computer access and augmentative communication systems for handicapped people. *Augmentative and Alternative Communication*, *6*, 231–241. doi:10.1080/07434619012331275514

Hovey, C., & Janilous, R. (2008). *The guide to magnetic stimulation*. The Magstims Company UK.

Howell, P., & El-Yaniv, N. (1987). The effects of presenting a click in syllable-initial position on the speech of stutterers: Comparison with a metronome click. *Journal of Fluency Disorders*, *12*, 249–256. doi:10.1016/0094-730X(87)90003-9

Howell, P. (2002). The EXPLAN theory of fluency control applied to the treatment of stuttering. In Fava, E. (Ed.), *Clinical Linguistics. Theory and applications in speech pathology and therapy* (pp. 95–115). Amsterdam: John Benjamins.

Howell, P., Wingfield, T., & Johnson, M. (1988). *Characteristics of the speech of stutterers during normal and altered auditory feedback.* Paper presented at the 7th Federation of Acoustical Societies of Europe Conference, Edinburgh.

Hsieh, C.-T., Lai, E., Chen, W.-C., & Wan, Y.-C. (2002). *Compact speech features based on wavelet transform and PCA with application to speaker identification.* Paper presented at the International Symposium on Chinese Spoken Language Processing

Huang, W. (2002). On the selection of shape memory alloys for actuators. *Materials & Design*, *23*(1), 11–19. doi:10.1016/S0261-3069(01)00039-5

Huenerfauth, M. (2005). Representing coordination and non-coordination in an American Sign Language animation. In *Assets '05: Proceedings of the 7th international ACM sigaccess conference on computers and accessibility* (pp. 44–51). New York: ACM.

Huntinger, P., Johanson, J., & Stoneburner, R. (1996). Assistive technology applications in educational programs of children with multiple disabilities: a case study report on the state of the practice. *Journal of Special Education Technology*, *13*(1), 16–35.

Huppert, T. J., Hoge, R. D., Diamond, S. G., Franceschini, M. A., & Boss, D. A. (2006). A comparison of BOLD, ASL, and NIRS hemodynamic responses to motor stimuli in adult humans. *NeuroImage*, *29*, 368–382. doi:10.1016/j.neuroimage.2005.08.065

Huppert, T. J., Hoge, R. D., Franceschini, M. A., & Boas, D. A. (2005). A spatial-temporal comparison of fMRI and NIRS hemodynamic responses to motor stimuli in adult humans. *Proceedings of SPIE, 5693*, 191-202. In B. Chance, R. R. Alfano, B. J. Tromberg, M. Tamura, & E. M. Sevick-Muraca (Eds.), *Proceedings of the SPIE: Vol. 5693: Optical Tomography and Spectroscopy of Tissue VI* (pp. 191-202). Bellingham, WA: SPIE.

Hwang, B. S., Choi, J. M., & Park, K. S. (2006, October). *A novel method for unobtrusive measurement of indoor activities using sensor-based monitoring system*. The International Special Topic Conference on Information Technology in Biomedicine (ITAB 2006), Ioannina, Greece.

Hyman, R. (1953). Stimulus information as a determinant of reaction time. *Journal of Experimental Psychology*, *45*, 188–196. doi:10.1037/h0056940

ICT & Ageing. (2008) European Study on Users, Markets and Technologies. Empirica & WRC. Retrieved from http://www.ict-ageing.eu/ict-ageing-website/wp-content/uploads/2008/11/ictageing_vienna_handout_final2.pdf

IEEE. (2005). IEEE Std 802.15.1-2005 (Revision of IEEE Std 802.15.1-2002) (pp. 0_1-580).

IEEE. (2006). IEEE Std 802.15.4-2006 (Revision of IEEE Std 802.15.4-2003) (pp. 0_1-305).

IEEE. (2007). IEEE Std 802.11-2007 (Revision of IEEE Std 802.11-1999) (pp. C1-1184).

ILSMH (Formerly International League of Societies for Persons with Mental Handicap). (n.d.). Retrieved from http://www.siwadam.com/hmm/euie.htm

IMS Global Consortium. (n.d.). Retrieved from http://www.imsglobal.org/

Ince, N. F., Min, C., Tewfik, A. H., & Vanderpool, D. (2008). *Detection of Early Morning Daily Activities with Static Home and Wearable Wireless Sensors*. Journal on Advances in Signal Processing.

INE. 2008. *Encuesta de Discapacidad, Autonomía Personal y Situaciones de Dependencia 2008 (EDAD 2008)* [Disability, Independence, and Dependency Situations Survey (EDAD 2008)] Retrieved September 30, 2009, from http://www.ine.es/jaxi/menu.do?L=0&type=pcaxis&path=%2Ft15/p418&file=inebase.

Ingham, R. J., & Bothe, A. K. (2001). Recovery from early stuttering: Additional issues within the Onslow & Packman-Yairi & Ambrose (1999) exchange. *Journal of Speech, Language, and Hearing Research: JSLHR*, *44*(4), 862. doi:10.1044/1092-4388(2001/068)

Ingham, R. J., Moglia, R. A., Frank, P., Ingham, J. C., & Cordes, A. K. (1997). Experimental investigation of the effects of frequency-altered auditory feedback on the speech of adults who stutter. *Journal of Speech, Language, and Hearing Research: JSLHR*, *40*(2), 361–372.

Ingham, R. J., Warner, A., Byrd, A., & Cotton, J. (2006). Speech Effort Measurement and Stuttering: Investigating the Chorus Reading Effect. *Journal of Speech, Language, and Hearing Research: JSLHR*, *49*(3), 660. doi:10.1044/1092-4388(2006/048)

Ino, S., Izumi, T., Takahashi, M., & Ifukube, T. (1992). Design of an actuator for tele-existence display of position and force to human hand and elbow. *Journal of Robotics and Mechatronics*, *4*(1), 43–48.

Ino, S., Sato, M., Hosono, M., & Izumi, T. (2009). Development of a Soft Metal Hydride Actuator Using a Laminate Bellows for Rehabilitation Systems. *Sensors and Actuators. B, Chemical*, *B-136*(1), 86–91. doi:10.1016/j.snb.2008.10.054

Ino, S. Hosono. M., Sato, M., Nalajima, S., Yamashita, & Izumi, T. A Preliminary Study of a Power Assist System for Toe Exercise using a Metal Hydride Actuator, In Schlegel, W. & Dössel, O. (Eds.), *Proceedings of the World Congress on Medical Physics and Biomedical Engineering2009* (vol. 25/IX, pp. 287-290), Munich, Germany: Springer.

Ino, S., Hosono, M., Sato, M., & Nalajima, S. Yamashita, & Izumi, T. (2009). A Soft Metal Hydride Actuator Using $LaNi_5$ Alloy and a Laminate Film Bellows. In Ibrahim, Y. (Ed.), *Proceedings of the 2009 IEEE International Conference on Industrial Technology* (pp. 1215-1220), Gippsland, Australia: IEEE.

Ino, S., Sato, M., Hosono, M., Nalajima, S., Yamashita, K., Tanaka, T., & Izumi, T. (2008). Prototype Design of a Wearable Metal Hydride Actuator Using a Soft Bellows for Motor Rehabilitation, In Dumont, G. & Galiana, H. (Eds.), *Proceedings of the 30th Annual International Conference of the IEEE Engineering in Medicine and Biology Society* (pp. 3451-3454), Vancouver, Canada: IEEE.

Instance, H. O., Spinner, C., & Howarth, P. A. (1996). Providing motor impaired users with access to standard graphical user interface (GUI) software via eye-based interaction. In *Proceedings of 1st European Conference on Disability, Virtual Reality and Associated Technology*, UK.

Instituto de Migraciones y Servicios Sociales (IMSERSO). (2009). Productos de Apoyo. Dossier. *Revista Minusval*, *173*, 9–29.

Instituto Nacional de Estadística (INE). (2001). Censo de Población y Viviendas (Population and Housing Census). *On-line database*. Retrieved September 2009, from http://www.ine.es

Instituto Nacional de Estadística (INE). (2008a). Padrón Municipal de Habitantes (Municipal Census of Inhabitants). *On-line database*. Retrieved September 2009, from http://www.ine.es

Instituto Nacional de Estadística (INE). (2008b). Encuesta sobre Equipamiento y Uso de Tecnologías de la Información y la Comunicación en los hogares (Survey on Equipment and Use of Information and Communication Technologies in Households). *On-line database*. Retrieved September, 2009, from http://www.ine.es

International Standards Organization [ISO] (2003). *Ergonomics of human-system interaction – Guidance on accessibility for human-computer interfaces*, Technical Specification ISO TS 16071.

International Standards Organization [ISO] (2006). ISO 9241-110:2006 Ergonomics of human-system interaction -- Part 110: Dialogue principles. Retrieved September 25, 2009 from http://www.iso.org/iso/iso_catalogue/catalogue_tc/catalogue_detail.htm?csnumber=38009

International Standards Organization [ISO] (2008). ISO 9241-171:2008 Ergonomics of human-system interaction -- Part 171: Guidance on software accessibility. Retrieved September 25, 2009 from http://www.iso.org/iso/catalogue_detail.htm?csnumber=39080

ISO(1997). Guide to the expression of Uncertainty in Measurement.

ISO/IEC 24751. (2008). Individualized adaptability and accessibility in e-learning, education and training. ISO/IEC 24751-1:2008 Part 1: Framework and reference model. Part 2: "Access for all" ISO PNP (Personal Needs and Preferences). Part 3: "Access for all" digital resource description. Lloyd, J., Moni, K.B., & Jobling, A. Breaking the hype cycle: Using the computer effectively with learners with intellectual disabilities. Retrieved from http://www.down-syndrome.org/practice/296/practice-296.pdf.

Ivory, M. Y., & Hearst, M. A. (2001). The state of the art in automating usability evaluation of user interfaces. *ACM Computing Surveys*, *33*(4), 470–516. doi:10.1145/503112.503114

Ivory, M. Y., Mankoff, J., & Le, A. (2003). Using Automated Tools to Improve Web Site Usage by Users with Diverse Abilities. In *IT & Society* (p. 195236). USA: Stanford University.

Izhikevich, E. M., & Edelman, G. M. (2008). Large-scale model of mammalian thalamocortical systems. *Proceedings of the National Academy of Sciences of the United States of America*, *105*(9), 3593–3598. doi:10.1073/pnas.0712231105

Jacobs, J., Hammerman-Rozenberg, R., Maaravi, Y., Cohen, A., & Stessman, J. (2005, Aug). The impact of visual impairment on health, function and mortality. *Aging Clinical and Experimental Research*, *17*(4), 281–286.

Jahanshahi, M., Jenkins, H., Brown, R. G., Marsden, C. D., Passingham, R. E., & Brooks, D. J. (1996). Self-initiated versus externally triggered movements. 1. An investigation using measurement of regional cerebral blood flow with PET and movement-related potentials in normal and Parkinson's disease subjects - Reply. *Brain*, *119*, 1046–1048.

Jain, A. K., Duin, R. P. W., & Mao, J. (2000). Statistical pattern recognition: a review. *IEEE Transactions on Pattern Analysis and Machine Intelligence*, *22*(1), 4–37. doi:10.1109/34.824819

Jalinous, R. (1991). Technical and practical aspects of magnetic nerve stimulation. *Journal of Clinical Neurophysiology*, *8*(1), 10–25. doi:10.1097/00004691-199101000-00004

Jankovic, J. (2008). Parkinson's disease: clinical features and diagnosis. *Journal of Neurology, Neurosurgery, and Psychiatry*, *79*, 368–376. doi:10.1136/jnnp.2007.131045

Jarochowski, B. P., Shin, S., Ryu, D., & Kim, H. (2007). Ubiquitous Rehabilitation Center: An Implementation of a Wireless Sensor Network Based Rehabilitation Management System. In *Proceedings of the 2007 International Conference on Convergence Information Technology* (pp. 2349-2358). Washington, DC: IEEE Computer Society.

Jasdzewsky, G., Strangman, G., Wagner, J., Kwong, K. K., Poldrack, R. A., & Boas, D. A. (2003). Differences in the hemodynamic response to event-related motor and visual paradigms as measured by near-infrared spectroscopy. *NeuroImage*, *20*, 479–488. doi:10.1016/S1053-8119(03)00311-2

Jenkins, I. H., Jahanshahi, M., Jueptner, M., Passingham, R. E., & Brooks, D. J. (2000). Self-initiated versus externally triggered movements II. The effect of movement predictability on regional cerebral blood flow. *Brain*, *123*, 1216–1228. doi:10.1093/brain/123.6.1216

Jeppesen, J., Green, A., Steffensen, B. F., & Rahbek, J. (2003). The Duchenne muscular dystrophy population in Denmark, 1977-2001: prevalence, incidence and survival in relation to the introduction of ventilator use. *Neuromuscular Disorders*, *13*(10), 804–812. doi:10.1016/S0960-8966(03)00162-7

Jhou, T. (2005). Neural mechanisms of freezing and passive aversive behaviors. *The Journal of Comparative Neurology*, *493*(1), 111–114. doi:10.1002/cne.20734

Ji, Y., Biaz, S., Pandey, S., & Agrawal, P. (2006). Dynamic Indoor Localization Using Wireless Ethernet: The ARIADNE System. In T. Braun et al. (Eds.) *Wired/Wireless Internet Communications* (LNCS 3970, pp. 299-310).

Jia, C., Xu, H., Hong, B., Gao, X., Zhang, Z., & Gao, S. (2007). A human computer interface using SSVEP-based BCI technology (LNCS 4565, pp. 113-119).

Jin-Shyan, L., Yu-Wei, S., & Chung-Chou, S. (2007). *A Comparative Study of Wireless Protocols: Bluetooth, UWB, ZigBee, and Wi-Fi.* Paper presented at the Industrial Electronics Society, 2007. IECON 2007. 33rd Annual Conference of the IEEE.

Jirawimut, R., Ptasinski, P., Garaj, V., Cecelja, F., & Balachandran, W. (2003). A Method for Dead Reckoning Parameter Correction in Pedestrian Navigation System. *IEEE Transactions on Instrumentation and Measurement*, *52*(1), 209–215. doi:10.1109/TIM.2002.807986

Jirawimut, R., Prakoonwit, S. Cecelja, F. Balachandran. W. (2003). Visual Odometer for Pedestrian Navigation. *IEEE Trans. On Instrumentation and Measurements, 52*(4).

Jobsis, F. (1977). Noninvasive, infrared monitoring of cerebral and myocardial oxygen sufficiency and circulatory parameters. *Science*, *198*(4324), 1264–1267. doi:10.1126/science.929199

Johansen, A. S., & Hansen, J. P. (2002). Augmentative and alternative communication: The future of text on the move. *Proceedings of the seventh ERCIM workshop on User Interface for All* (pp. 367–386). Paris, France.

John, B. E., & Kieras, D. E. (1996). The GOMS family of user interface analysis techniques: Comparison and contrast. *ACM Transactions on Computer-Human Interaction*, *3*(4), 320–351. doi:10.1145/235833.236054

Johnson, J., Inglebret, E., Jones, C., & Ray, J. (2006). Perspectives of Speech Language Pathologists regarding success versus abandonment of AAC. *Augmentative and Alternative Communication*, *22*(2), 85–99. doi:10.1080/07434610500483588

Johnson, W. (1942). A study of the onset and development of stuttering. *The Journal of Speech Disorders*, *7*, 251–257.

Johnson, W. (1959). *The onset of stuttering*. Minneapolis, MN: University of Minneapolis Press.

Jones, B., & Plassmann, P. (2002). Digital infrared thermal imaging of human skin. *IEEE Engineering in Medicine and Biology Magazine*, *21*, 41–48. doi:10.1109/MEMB.2002.1175137

Jones, B. F. (1998). A reappraisal of the use of infrared thermal image analysis in medicine. *IEEE Transactions on Medical Imaging*, *17*(6), 1019–1027. doi:10.1109/42.746635

Jones, M., Onslow, M., Packman, A., Williams, S., Ormond, T., & Schwarz, I. (2005). Randomised controlled trial of the Lidcombe programme of early stuttering intervention. *BMJ (Clinical Research Ed.)*, *331*(7518), 659. doi:10.1136/bmj.38520.451840.E0

Jones, R. K. (1966). Observations on stammering after localized cerebral injury. *Journal of Neurology, Neurosurgery, and Psychiatry*, *29*(3), 192–195. doi:10.1136/jnnp.29.3.192

Joo, E. Y., Han, S. J., Chung, S. H., Cho, J. W., Seo, D. W., & Hong, S. B. (2007). Antiepileptic effects of low-frequency repetitive transcranial magnetic stimulation by different stimulation durations and locations. *Clinical Neurophysiology*, *118*(3), 702–708. doi:10.1016/j.clinph.2006.11.008

Jorgensen, C. C., Lee, D., & Agabon, S. (2003). *Subauditory Speech Recognition based on EMG/EPG Signals*.

Jorgensen, C., & Betts, B. (2006). *Multimodal Platform Control for Robotic Planetary Exploration Missions*. Paper presented at the Second International Conference on Space Mission Challenges for Information Technology.

Kalinowski, J., Armson, J., Roland-Mieszkowski, M., Stuart, A., & Gracco, V. L. (1993). Effects of alterations in auditory feedback and speech rate on stuttering frequency. *Language and Speech*, *36*, 1–16.

Kalinowski, J., Guntupalli, V. K., Stuart, A., & Saltuklaroglu, T. (2004). Self-reported efficacy of an ear-level prosthetic device that delivers altered auditory feedback for the management of stuttering. *International Journal of Rehabilitation Research. Internationale Zeitschrift fur Rehabilitationsforschung. Revue Internationale de Recherches de Readaptation*, *27*(2), 167–170. doi:10.1097/01.mrr.0000128063.76934.df

Kalinowski, J., & Saltuklaroglu, T. (2003). Speaking with a mirror: engagement of mirror neurons via choral speech and its derivatives induces stuttering inhibition. *Medical Hypotheses*, *60*(4), 538–543. doi:10.1016/S0306-9877(03)00004-5

Kalinowski, J., & Stuart, A. (1996). Stuttering amelioration at various auditory feedback delays and speech rates. *European Journal of Disorders of Communication: The Journal of the College of Speech and Language Therapists*, *31*(3), 259–269.

Kalinowski, J., Stuart, A., Wamsley, L., & Rastatter, M. P. (1999). Effects of monitoring condition and frequency-altered feedback on stuttering frequency. *The Journal of Speech and Hearing Disorders*, *42*(6), 1347–1354.

Kalinowski, J., Stuart, A., Rastatter, M., Miller, R., Zimmerman, S., & Shine, R. (1998). *Examination of altered auditory feedback: Therapeutic implications*. Paper presented at the Second World Congress on Fluency Disorders, Nijmegen, The Netherlands.

Kammer, T., Beck, S., Thielscher, A., Laubis-Herrmann, U., & Topka, H. (2001). Motor thresholds in humans: a transcranial magnetic stimulation study comparing different pulse waveforms, current directions and stimulator types. *Clinical Neurophysiology*, *112*(2), 250–258. doi:10.1016/S1388-2457(00)00513-7

Kaneko, K., Kawai, S., Fuchigami, Y., Morita, H., & Ofuji, A. (1996). The effect of current direction induced by transcranial magnetic stimulation on the corticospinal excitability in human brain. *Electroencephalography and Clinical Neurophysiology*, *101*, 478–482. doi:10.1016/S0013-4694(96)96021-X

Kapandji, I. A. (2007). *The Physiology of the Joints*. New York: Churchill Livingstone.

Kaplan, L. I., Grynbaum, B. G., Rusk, H. A., Anastasia, T., & Gassler, S. (1966). A reappraisal of braces and other mechanical aids in patients with spinal cord dysfunction: results of a follow-up study. *Archives of Physical Medicine and Rehabilitation*, *47*, 395–405.

Karavidas, M., Lim, N. K., & Katsikas, S. L. (2005). The effects of computers on older adults. *Computers in Human Behavior*, *21*, 697–711. doi:10.1016/j.chb.2004.03.012

Kasday, L. R. (2000). A tool to evaluate universal web accessibility. In *Cuu '00: Proceedings on the 2000 conference on universal usability* (pp. 161-162). New York: ACM Press. doi:10.1145/355460.355559

Kautzamann, L. N. (1990). Introducing computers to the elderly. *Physical & Occupational Therapy in Geriatrics*, *9*(1), 27–36.

Kautzmann, L. N. (1991). Facilitating adult learning in occupational therapy patient education programs. *Occupational Therapy Practice*, *2*, 1–11.

Kawakubo, S., Chansavang, A., Tanaka, S., Iwasaki, T., Sasaki, K., Hirota, T., et al. (2006). Wireless network system for indoor human positioning. *1st International Symposium on Wireless Pervasive Computing.*

Kay, L. (1964). *An ultrasonic sensing probe as a mobility aid for the blind. Ultrasonics*. April/June.

Kay, L. (1966). Ultrasonic spectacles for the blind. *The Journal of the Acoustical Society of America*, *40*(6), 1564. doi:10.1121/1.1910269

Kay, L. (1974). A Sonar Aid to Enhance Spatial Perception of the Blind: Engineering Design and Evaluation. *Radio and Electronic Engineer*, *44*(11), 605–627. doi:10.1049/ree.1974.0148

Keating, W., McLean, D., & Quinsey, K. (1989). Survey of appropriate provision and usage of prescribed equipment- the client's perspective. *Australian Journal of Occupational Therapy*, *36*(3), 131–135. doi:10.1111/j.1440-1630.1989.tb01210.x

Kehoe, T. D. (2008). *No Miracle Cures: A Multifactoral Guide to Stuttering Therapy*. University College Press.

Keirn, Z. A., & Aunon, J. I. (1990). Man-machine communications through brain-wave processing. *IEEE Engineering in Medicine and Biology*, *3*, 55–57. doi:10.1109/51.62907

Kelly, S. P., Lalor, E. C., Finucane, C., McDarby, G., & Reilly, R. B. (2005). Visual spatial attention control in an independent brain-computer interface. *IEEE Transactions on Bio-Medical Engineering*, *55*(9), 1588–1596. doi:10.1109/TBME.2005.851510

Kemp, B. J. (1993). Motivational issues in the use of technology by older persons: a model and recommendations. *Technology and Disability*, *2*(1), 65–70.

Khedr, E., El-Nasser, W. A., Haleem, E. K. A., Bakr, M. S., & Trakhan, M. N. (2000). Evoked potentials and electroencephalography in stuttering. *Folia Phoniatrica et Logopaedica*, *52*(4), 178. doi:10.1159/000021532

Khedr, E. M., Rothwell, J. C., Shawky, O. A., Ahmed, M. A., & Hamdy, A. (2006). Effect of daily repetitive transcranial magnetic stimulation on motor performance in Parkinson's disease. *Movement Disorders*, *21*(12), 2201–2205. doi:10.1002/mds.21089

Khemapech, I., Duncan, I., & Miller, A. (2005, June). A survey of wireless sensor networks technology. In *Proceedings of the 6th Annual PostGraduate Symposium on the Convergence of Telecommunications, Networking & Broadcasting*. Liverpool, UK.

Kiefte, M., & Armson, J. (2008). Dissecting choral speech: Properties of the accompanist critical to stuttering reduction. *Journal of Communication Disorders*, *41*(1), 33–48. doi:10.1016/j.jcomdis.2007.03.002

Kilgallon, M. J., Roberts, D. P., & Miller, S. (1987). Adapting personal computers for use by high-level quadripegics. *Medical Instrumentation*, *21*(2), 97–102.

Kim, H., Jarochowski, B., & Ryu, D. (2006). A Proposal for a Home-Based Health Monitoring System for the Elderly or Disabled (LNCS 4061, pp. 473-479).

Kishimoto, M., Yoshida, T., Hayasaka, T., Mori, D., Imai, Y., Matsuki, N., Ishikawa, T., & Yamaguchi, T. (2009). An internet-based wearable watch-over system for elderly and disabled utilizing EMG and accelerometer. *Technology and health care-European Society for Engineering and Medicine, 17*, 121-131.

Klingholz, F. (1990). Acoustic representation of speaking-voice quality. *Journal of Voice*, *4*(3), 213–219. doi:10.1016/S0892-1997(05)80016-5

Kobayashi, M., & Pascual-Leone, A. (2003). Transcranial magnetic stimulation in neurology. *The Lancet Neurology*, *2*(3), 145–156. doi:10.1016/S1474-4422(03)00321-1

Koch, G., Brusa, L., Carrillo, F., Lo Gerfo, E., Torriero, S., & Oliveri, M. (2009). Cerebellar magnetic stimulation decreases levodopa-induced dyskinesias in Parkinson disease. *Neurology, 73*(2), 113–119. doi:10.1212/WNL.0b013e3181ad5387

Koester, H. H., & Levine, S. P. (1997). Keystroke level models for user performance with word prediction. *Augmentative and Alternative Communication, 13*, 239–257. doi:10.1080/07434619712331278068

Koester, H. H., LoPresti, E., Ashlock, G., McMillan, W., Moore, P., & Simpson, R. (2003 March). Compass: Software for Computer Skills Assessment. Paper presented at the *Proceedings of CSUN 2003 International Conference on Technology and Persons with Disabilities*. Los Angeles, CA.

Kohn, J., Enders, S., Preston, J., & Motloch, W. (1983). Provision of assistive equipment for handicapped persons. *Archives of Physical Medicine and Rehabilitation, 64*, 378–381.

Kompoliti, K., Goetz, C. G., Leurgans, S., Morrissey, M., & Siegel, I. M. (2000). "On" freezing in Parkinson's disease: Resistance to visual cue walking devices. *Movement Disorders, 15*, 309–312. doi:10.1002/1531-8257(200003)15:2<309::AID-MDS1016>3.0.CO;2-P

Korpela, R., Seppanen, R. L., & Koivokko, M. (1993). Rehabilitation service evaluation: a follow-up of the extent of use of technical aids for disabled children. *Disability and Rehabilitation, 15*(3), 143–150. doi:10.3109/09638289309166005

Kostov, A., Andrews, B. J., Popovic, D. B., & William, W. (1995). Machine learning in control of functional electrical stimulation systems for locomotion. *IEEE Transactions on Bio-Medical Engineering, 42*, 541–551. doi:10.1109/10.387193

Kraat, A. (1987). *Communication interaction between aided and natural speakers: An IPCAS study report* (2nd ed.). Madison, Wisconsin: University of Wisconsin-Madison, Trace Research & Development Centre.

Kritikos, A., Leahy, C., Bradshaw, J. L., Iansek, R., Phillips, J. G., & Bradshaw, J. A. (1995). Contingent and noncontingent auditory cueing in Parkinsons-disease. *Neuropsychologia, 33*, 1193–1203. doi:10.1016/0028-3932(95)00036-3

Krueger, R. A. (1994). *Focus groups: a practical guide for applied research*. Newbury Park, CA: Sage Publications.

Kuba, M., Kubová, Z., Kremlacek, J., & Langrova, J. (2007). Motion-onset VEPs: Characteristics, methods, and diagnostic use. *Vision Research, 47*(2), 189–202. doi:10.1016/j.visres.2006.09.020

Kuboyama, N., Nabetani, T., Shibuya, K., Machida, K., & Ogaki, T. (2004). The effect of maximal finger tapping on cerebral activation. *Journal of Physiological Anthropology and Applied Human Science, 23*(4), 105–110. doi:10.2114/jpa.23.105

Kumar, S., Kumar, D. K., Alemu, M., & Burry, M. (2004). *EMG based voice recognition*. Paper presented at the Intelligent Sensors, Sensor Networks and Information Processing Conference.

Kure, K., Kanda, T., Suzumori, K., & Wakimoto, S. (2008). Flexible displacement sensor using injected conductive paste. *Sensors and Actuators. A, Physical, 143*(2), 272–278. doi:10.1016/j.sna.2007.11.031

Kuribayashi, K., Tsuchiya, K., You, Z., Tomus, D., Umemoto, M., & Ito, T. (2006). Self-deployable origami stent grafts as a biomedical application of Ni-rich TiNi shape memory alloy foil. *Materials Science and Engineering A, 419*(1-2), 131–137. doi:10.1016/j.msea.2005.12.016

Kutner, N. G., Zhang, R., McClellan, W. M., & Cole, S. A. (2002). Psychosocial predictors of non-compliance in haemodialysis and peritoneal dialysis patients. *Nephrology, Dialysis, Transplantation, 17*, 93–99. doi:10.1093/ndt/17.1.93

Lacourse, J. R., & Hladik, F. C. Jr. (1990). An eye movement communication -control system for the disabled. *IEEE Transactions on Bio-Medical Engineering, 37*(12), 1215–1220. doi:10.1109/10.64465

Lalor, E. C., Kelly, S. P., Finucane, C., Burke, R., Smith, R., & Reilly, R. B. (2005). Steady-state VEP-based brain-computer interface control in an immersive 3D gaming environment. *EURASIP Journal on Applied Signal Processing*, *19*, 174–181.

Lancioni, G., O'Reilly, M. F., Singh, N. N., Sigafoos, J., Oliva, D., Baccani, S., & Groeneweg, J. (2006). Microswitch clusters promote adaptive responses and reduce finger mouthing in a boy with multiple disabilities. *Behavior Modification*, *30*(6), 892–900. doi:10.1177/0145445505283416

Lanyon, R. I. (1977). Effect of biofeedback-based relaxation on stuttering during reading and spontaneous speech. *Journal of Consulting and Clinical Psychology*, *45*(5), 860–866. doi:10.1037/0022-006X.45.5.860

Lau, A. (2000). *A quality of life study on non-institutionalised elderly stroke survivors in Hong Kong.* Unpublished Doctor of Philosophy thesis. Brisbane: The University of Queensland.

Laux, L. F., McNally, P. R., Paciello, M. G., & Vanderheiden, G. C. (1996). Designing the World Wide Web for people with disabilities: A user centered design approach. In *Assets '96: Proceedings of the second annual ACM conference on assistive technologies* (pp. 94–101). New York: ACM Press. doi:10.1145/228347.228363

Law, M., & Mills, J. (1998). Client-centred occupational therapy. In Law, M. (Ed.), *Client-centred occupational therapy* (pp. 1–18). Thorofare, NJ: Slack Inc.

Le Huche, F. (2000). La tartamudez: Opción Curación: Masson.

Lee, P., Hsieh, J., Wu, C., Shyu, K., Chen, S., & Yeh, T. (2006). The brain computer interface using flash visual evoked potential and independent component analysis. *Annals of Biomedical Engineering*, *34*(10), 1641–1654. doi:10.1007/s10439-006-9175-8

Lee, P., Hsieh, J., Wu, C., Shyu, K., & Wu, Y. (2008). Brain computer interface using flash onset and offset visual evoked potentials. *Clinical Neurophysiology*, *119*(3), 605–616. doi:10.1016/j.clinph.2007.11.013

Lee, B. S. (1951). Artificial stutter. *The Journal of Speech and Hearing Disorders*, *16*, 53–55.

Leeb, R., Lee, F., Keinrath, C., Scherer, R., Bischof, H., & Pfurtscheller, G. (2007). Brain-computer communication: Motivation, aim, and impact of exploring a virtual apartment. *IEEE Transactions on Neural Systems and Rehabilitation Engineering*, *15*(4), 473–482. doi:10.1109/TNSRE.2007.906956

Lefaucheur, J. P., Fénelon, G., Ménard-Lefaucheur, I., Wendling, S., & Nguyen, J. P. (2004). Low-frequency repetitive TMS of premotor cortex can reduce painful axial spasms in generalized secondary dystonia: a pilot study of three patients. *Neurophysiologie Clinique*, *34*(3-4), 141–145. doi:10.1016/j.neucli.2004.07.003

Leporini, B., & Paterno, F. (2003). Criteria for usability of accessible web sites (LNCS 2615, pp. 43-55). London: Springer-Verlag.

Lesher, G. W., Moulton, B. J., & Higginbotham, D. J. (1998a). Optimal character arrangements for ambiguous keyboards. *IEEE Transactions on Rehabilitation Engineering*, *6*, 415–423. doi:10.1109/86.736156

Lesher, G. W., Moulton, B. J., & Higginbotham, D. J. (1998b). Techniques for augmenting scanning communication. *Augmentative and Alternative Communication*, *14*, 81–101. doi:10.1080/07434619812331278236

Lesher, G. W., & Moulton, B. J. (2005). An introduction to the theoretical limits of abbreviation expansion performance. In *Proceedings of the RESNA 2005 Annual Conference*.

Levi, M. D., & Conrad, F. G. (1996). A heuristic evaluation of a World Wide Web prototype. *Interactions*, *3*(4), 50–61. doi:[REMOVED HYPERLINK FIELD] 10.1145/234813.234819

Levine, B. (1993). Quantum-well infrared photodetectors. *Journal of Applied Physics*, *74*(8), 1–81. doi:10.1063/1.354252

Levine, J. A., Pavlidis, I., & Cooper, M. (2001). The face of fear. *Lancet*, *357*(9270), 1757–1757. doi:10.1016/S0140-6736(00)04936-9

Levine, S. H., & Goodenough-Trepagnier, C. (1990). Customised text entry devices for motor-impaired users. *Applied Ergonomics*, *21*, 55–62. doi:10.1016/0003-6870(90)90074-8

Lewis, G. A. (1897). *The Origin and Treatment of Stammering*. Philadelphia: The Lewis Phono-Metric Institute.

Lewis, G. A. (1906). *The origin and treatment of stammering*. Detroit, Michigan: Photometer Press.

Lewis, K. E. (1995). Do SSI-3 scores adequately reflect observations of stuttering behaviors? *American Journal of Speech-Language Pathology*, *4*, 46–59.

Lewis, G. N., Byblow, W. D., & Walt, S. E. (2000). Stride length regulation in Parkinson's disease: the use of extrinsic, visual cues. *Brain*, *123*, 2077–2090. doi:10.1093/brain/123.10.2077

Lewis, C. (2005). Bridges for the mind: opportunities for research on cognitive disabilities. In *Assets '05: Proceedings of the 7th international ACM Sigaccess conference on computers and accessibility*. New York: ACM.

Li, H.-B., Takizawa, K., Zhen, B., & Kohno, R. (2007, July). Body Area Network and Its Standardization at IEEE 802.15.MBAN. *16th IST Mobile and Wireless Communications Summit* (pp. 1-5). Budapest, Hungary.

Liberson, W. T., Holmquest, H. J., Scot, D., & Dow, M. (1961). Functional electrotherapy: stimulation of the personal nerve synchronized with the swing phase of the gait of hemiplegic patients. *Archives of Physical Medicine and Rehabilitation*, *42*, 101–105.

Lie, H. W., & Bos, B. (1999). Cascading Style Sheets, level 1. Retrieved 2005 from http://www.w3.org/TR/CSS1

Light, J., Collier, B., & Parnes, P. (1985b). Communicative interaction between young nonspeaking physically disabled children and their primary caregivers: Modes of communication. *Augmentative and Alternative Communication*, *1*, 125–133. doi:10.1080/07434618512331273621

Lim, H., & Singh, V. K. (2005). Design of healthcare system for disable person using eye blinking. *Fourth Annual ACIS International Conference on Computer and Information Science (ICIS '05)* (pp. 551-555). Las Vegas (USA)

Limongi, F. P., Subramanian, U., Prabhu, B., Ezrati-Vinacour, R., Amir, O., Kenjo, M., et al. (2005). Stuttering Research and Treatment Around the World. The ASHA Leader, 6-41.

Lin, Y.-J., Su, M.-J., Chen, S.-J., Wang, S.-C., Lin, C.-I., & Chen, H.-S. (2007, April). A Study of Ubiquitous Monitor with RFID in an Elderly Nursing Home. *International Conference on Multimedia and Ubiquitous Engineering (MUE'07)* (pp. 336-340). Seoul, Korea.

Lincoln, M., Packman, A., & Onslow, M. (2006). Altered auditory feedback and the treatment of stuttering: a review. *Journal of Fluency Disorders*, *31*(2), 71–89. doi:10.1016/j.jfludis.2006.04.001

Lloret, J., Garcia, M., Boronat, F., & Tomás, J. (2009, June). The Development of Two Systems for Indoor Wireless Sensors Self-location. *Ad Hoc & Sensor Wireless Networks: An International Journal*, *8*(3-4), 235–258.

Lloret, J., Tomás, J., Garcia, M., & Cánovas, A. (2009, May). Hybrid Stochastic Approach for Wireless Sensors Self-Location in Indoor Environments. *Sensors (Basel, Switzerland)*, *9*(5), 3695–3712. doi:10.3390/s90503695

Lloret, J., Garcia, M., & Tomas, J. (2007, June). *A Group-Based Architecture for Wireless Sensor Networks*. International Conference on Networking and Services (ICNS'07). Athens (Greece).

Lomarev, M. P., Kanchana, S., Bara-Jimenez, W., Iyer, M., Wassermann, E. M., & Hallett, M. (2006). Placebo controlled study of rTMS for the treatment of Parkinson's disease. *Movement Disorders*, *21*(3), 325–331. doi:10.1002/mds.20713

Loriente Zamora, C. (2006). *La tartamudez como fenómeno sociocultural: una alternativa al modelo biomédico*. UNED.

Lotte, F., Congedo, M., Lécuyer, A., Lamarche, F., & Arnaldi, B. (2007). A review of classification algorithms for EEG-based brain-computer interfaces. *Journal of Neural Engineering*, *4*(2), 1–13. doi:10.1088/1741-2560/4/2/R01

Loughborough, W. (1979). Talking lights. *Journal of Visual Impairment and Blindness.*

Ludlow, C. (1990). Research procedures for measuring stuttering severity. *ASHA Reports*, *18*, 26–31.

Lugger, K., Flotzinger, D., Schlögl, A., Pregenzer, M., & Pfurtscheller, G. (1998). Feature extraction for on-line EEG classification using principal components and linear discriminants. *Medical & Biological Engineering & Computing*, *36*(3), 309–314. doi:10.1007/BF02522476

Lunn, D., Bechhofer, S., & Harper, S. (2008, September). Experiences of exposing semantics to drive transcoding. In M.-M. Bouamrane, S. Luz, & M. Masoodian (Eds.), *Proceedings of first international workshop on ontologies in interactive systems* (p. 9-17). IEEE Computer Society. Retrieved from http://www.simonharper.info/publications/Harper2008gs.pdf

Lustbader, W. (1997). On bringing older people into the computer age. *Generations (San Francisco, Calif.)*, *21*(3), 30–32.

Machii, K., Cohen, D., Ramos-Estebanez, C., & Pascual-Leone, A. (2006). Safety of rTMS to non-motor cortical areas in healthy participants and patients. *Clinical Neurophysiology*, *117*(2), 455–471. doi:10.1016/j.clinph.2005.10.014

MacKenzie, I. S., & Soukoreff, R. W. (2002). Text entry for mobile computing: Models and methods, theory and practice. *Human-Computer Interaction*, *17*, 147–198. doi:10.1207/S15327051HCI172&3_2

MacLeod, J., Kalinowski, J., Stuart, A., & Armson, J. (1995). Effect of single and combined altered auditory feedback on stuttering frequency at two speech rates. *Journal of Communication Disorders*, *28*, 217–228. doi:10.1016/0021-9924(94)00010-W

Maggi, L., Parini, S., Piccini, L., Panfili, G., & Andreoni, G. (2006). A four command BCI system based on the SSVEP protocol. *Annual International Conference of the IEEE Engineering in Medicine and Biology Society: Vol. 1.* (pp. 1264-1267).

Makeig, S., Westerfield, M., Jung, T., Enghoff, S., Townsend, J., & Courchesne, E. (2002). Dynamic brain sources of visual evoked responses. *Science*, *295*(5555), 690–694. doi:10.1126/science.1066168

Makeig, S., Debener, S., Onton, J., & Delorme, A. (2004). Minim event-related brain dynamics. *Trends in Cognitive Sciences*, *8*(5), 204–210. doi:10.1016/j.tics.2004.03.008

Mally, J., & Stone, T. W. (1999). Improvement in Parkinsonian symptoms after repetitive transcranial magnetic stimulation. *Journal of the Neurological Sciences*, *162*(2), 179–184. doi:10.1016/S0022-510X(98)00318-9

Mann, W. C., Hurren, D., & Tomita, M. (1993). Comparison of assistive device use and needs of home-based older persons with different impairments. *The American Journal of Occupational Therapy.*, *47*(11), 980–987.

Mann, W. C. (2001). Technology. In Bonder, B. R., & Wagner, M. B. (Eds.), *Functional performance in older adults* (2nd ed., pp. 429–446). Philadelphia: F.A. Davis Company.

Marchese, R., Bove, M., & Abbruzzese, G. (2003). Effect of cognitive and motor tasks on postural stability in Parkinson's disease: A posturographic study. *Movement Disorders*, *18*, 652–658. doi:10.1002/mds.10418

Marco, A., Casas, R., Falco, J., Gracia, H., Artigas, J. I., & Roy, A. (2008). Location-based services for elderly and disabled people. *Computer Communications*, *31*(6), 1055–1066. doi:10.1016/j.comcom.2007.12.031

Markley, V. J., & Shepperd, J. A. N. (1990). Corset supply and the Hastings corset shop. *British Journal of Occupational Therapy*, *53*(4), 155–157.

Mars, G. M. J., Kempen, G. I. J. M., Widdershoven, G. A. M., Janssen, P. P. M., & van Eijk, J. T. M. (2009). Conceptualizing autonomy in the context of chronic physical illness: relating philosophical theories to social scientific perspectives. *Health*, *12*(3), 333–348.

Marsico, M. D., & Levialdi, S. (2004). Evaluating web sites: exploiting user's expectations. *International Journal of Human-Computer Studies*, *60*(3), 381–416.. doi:10.1016/j.ijhcs.2003.10.008

Martin, R. R., Haroldson, S. K., & Woessner, G. L. (1988). Perceptual scaling of stuttering severity. *Journal of Fluency Disorders*, *13*(1), 27–47. doi:10.1016/0094-730X(88)90026-5

Martine, M. S., & Connolly, I. (2008). Roles of aided communication: perspectives of adults who use AAC. *Disability and Rehabilitation. Assistive Technology*, *3*(5), 260–273. doi:10.1080/17483100802338499

Martinez, P., Bakardjian, H., & Cichocki, C. (2007). Fully online multicommand brain-computer interface with visual neurofeedback using SSVEP paradigm. *Computational Intelligence and Neuroscience*, (94561): 13–13.

Matthews, F., & Pearlmutter, B., A., Ward, T. E., Soraghan, C. & Markham, C. (2008, January). Hemodynamics for brain-computer interfaces. *IEEE Signal Processing Magazine*, *25*(1), 87–94. doi:10.1109/MSP.2008.4408445

Max, L., Guenther, F. H., Gracco, V. L., Ghosh, S. S., & Wallace, M. E. (2004). Unstable or Insufficiently Activated Internal Models and Feedback-Biased Motor Control as Sources of Dysfluency: A Theoretical Model of Stuttering. *Contemporary Issues in Communication Science and Disorders*, *31*, 105–122.

May, A., & Hackwood, A. (1968). Some effects of masking and eliminating low frequency feedback on the speech of stammerers. *Behaviour Research and Therapy*, *6*(2), 219–223. doi:10.1016/0005-7967(68)90010-7

Maynard, E. M., Nordhausen, C. T., & Normann, R. A. (1997). The Utah intracortical electrode array: a recording structure for potential brain-computer interfaces. *Electroencephalography and Clinical Neurophysiology*, *102*(3), 228–239. doi:10.1016/S0013-4694(96)95176-0

Mazo, M., García, J. C., Rodríguez, F. J., Ureña, J., Lázaro, J. L., & Espinosa, F. (2001). An integral system for assisted mobility. *IEEE Robotics & Automation Magazine*, *8*(1), 46–56. doi:10.1109/100.924361

McCall, F., Markova, I., Murphy, J., Moodie, E., & Collins, S. (1997). Perspectives on AAC systems by the users and by their communication partners. *European Journal of Disorders of Communication*, *32*, 235–256.

McCathieNevile. C., & Abou-Zahra, S. (2005). Evaluation and Report Language (EARL) 1.0. Retrieved 2005 from http://www.w3.org/TR/EARL10/

McConatha, D., McConatha, J. T., & Dermigny, R. (1994). The use of interactive computer services to enhance the quality of life for long-term care residents. *The Gerontologist*, *34*, 553–556.

McFarland, D. J., McCane, L. M. ,., David, S. V., & Wolpaw, J. R. (1997). Spatial filter selection for EEG-based communication. *Electroencephalography and Clinical Neurophysiology*, *103*(3), 386–394. doi:10.1016/S0013-4694(97)00022-2

McGrath, P. J., Goodman, J. T., Cunningham, J., MacDonald, B. J., Nichols, T. A., & Unruh, A. (1985). Assistive devices: utilisation by children. *Archives of Physical Medicine*, *66*, 430–432.

McIntosh, G. C., Brown, S. H., Rice, R. R., & Thaut, M. H. (1997). Rhythmic auditory-motor facilitation of gait patterns in patients with Parkinson's disease. *Journal of Neurology, Neurosurgery, and Psychiatry*, *62*, 22–26. doi:10.1136/jnnp.62.1.22

McKeefry, D. J. (2001). Visual evoked potentials elicited by chromatic motion onset. *Vision Research*, *41*(15), 2005–2025. doi:10.1016/S0042-6989(01)00080-3

Mehagnoul-Schipper, D. J., van der Kallen, B. F. W., Colier, W. N. J. M., van der Sluijs, M. C., van Erning, L. J. T. O., & Thijssen, H. O. M. (2002). Simultaneous measurements of cerebral oxygenation changes during brain activation by near & hyphen; infrared spectroscopy and functional magnetic resonance imaging in healthy young and elderly subjects. *Human Brain Mapping*, *16*(1), 14–23. doi:10.1002/hbm.10026

Meijer, P. B. L. (1992). An Experimental System for Auditory Image Representations. *IEEE Transactions on Bio-Medical Engineering*, *39*(2), 112–121. Retrieved from http://www.seeingwithsound.com. doi:10.1109/10.121642

Meinander, H., & Honkala, M. (2004). Potential applications of smart clothing solutions in health care and personal protection. *Studies in Health Technology and Informatics*, *108*, 278–285.

Mellinger, J., Schalk, G., Braun, C., Preissl, H., Rosenstiel, W., Birbaumer, N., & Kübler, A. (2007). An MEG-based brain-computer interface (BCI). *NeuroImage*, *36*(3), 581–593. doi:10.1016/j.neuroimage.2007.03.019

Memarian, N., Venetsanopoulos, A., & Chau, T. (2009). Infrared thermography as an access pathway for individuals with severe motor impairments. *Journal of Neuroengineering and Rehabilitation*, *6*(11), 1–8.

Meng, F., Tong, K. Y., Chan, S. T., Wong, W. W., Lui, K. H., & Tang, K. W. (2009). Cerebral Plasticity After Subcortical Stroke as Revealed by Cortico-Muscular Coherence. *IEEE Transactions on Bio-Medical Engineering*, *17*(3), 234–243.

Menkhaus, G., & Fischmeister, S. (2003). *Dialog Model Clusteringfor User Interface Adaptation.* Paper presented at the 3rd International Conference on Web Engineering, Oviedo, Spain.

Merla, A., & Romani, G. L. (2007). Thermal signatures of emotional arousal: A functional infrared imaging study. *29th Annual International Conference of the IEEE EMBS* (pp. 247-249). IEEE Press.

Merla, A., Ciuffolo, F., D'Attilio, M., Tecco, S., Festa, F., Michele, G. D., et al. (2004). Functional infrared imaging in the diagnosis of the myofascial pain. *26th Annual International Conference of the IEEE EMBS* (pp. 1188-1191). IEEE Press.

Meyer, E. (2002). *Eric Meyer on CSS: Mastering the Language of Web Design*. New Riders Press.

Meyer, E. A. (2005). Is accessible design a myth? In *W4a '05: Proceedings of the 2005 international cross-disciplinary workshop on Web accessibility* (W4a) (pp. 60-62). New York: ACM Press.

Micro, G. W. (2009). GW Micro - Window-Eyes, Version 7.1. Retrieved September 25, 2009 from http://www.gwmicro.com/Window-Eyes/

Microsoft. (2009). Speech API Overview (SAPI 5.4). Retrieved September 25, 2009 from http://msdn.microsoft.com/en-us/library/ee125077(VS.85).aspx

Microsystems, S. (2009). Java Speech API. Retrieved September 25, 2009 from http://java.sun.com/products/java-media/speech/

Mikkonen, M., Vayrynen, S., Ikonen, V., & Heikkala, M. O. (2002). User and Concept Studies as Tools in Developing Mobile Communication Services for the Elderly. *Personal and Ubiquitous Computing*, *6*, 113–124. doi:10.1007/s007790200010

Millán, J. R., & Mouriño, J. (2003). Asynchronous BCI and local neural classifiers: an overview of the Adaptive Brain Interface project. *IEEE Transactions on Neural Systems and Rehabilitation Engineering*, *11*(2), 159–161. doi:10.1109/TNSRE.2003.814435

Millán, J. R., Renkens, F., Mouriño, J., & Gerstner, W. (2004). Noninvasive brain-actuated control of a mobile robot by human EEG. *IEEE Transactions on Bio-Medical Engineering*, *51*(6), 1026–1033. doi:10.1109/TBME.2004.827086

Millán-Calenti, J. C. (2006). *Principios de Geriatría y Gerontología* [Principles of Geriatric Medicine and Gerontology]. Madrid: McGraw Hill-Interamericana.

Miller, K. J., denNijs, M., Shenoy, P., Miller, J. W., Rao, R. P. N., & Ojemann, G. (2007). Real-time functional brain mapping using electrocorticography. *NeuroImage*, *37*(2), 504–507. doi:10.1016/j.neuroimage.2007.05.029

Milner, P., & Kelly, B. (2009). Community participation and inclusion: people with disabilities defining their place. *Disability & Society*, *24*(1), 47–62. doi:10.1080/09687590802535410

Miranda de Larra, R. (2004). Los mayores en la Sociedad de la Información: situación actual y retos de futuro. Madrid, España: Fundación AUNA.

Mirfakhrai, T., Madden, J. D. W., & Baughman, R. H. (2007). Polymer artificial muscles. *Materials Today*, *10*(4), 30–38. doi:10.1016/S1369-7021(07)70048-2

Miyamoto, S., Shimada, Y., Sato, K., & Kagaya, H. (1999). Hibrid functional electrical stimulation for energy-efficient restoration of standing-up motion. *Archives of Physical Medicine and Rehabilitation*, *2*, 536–541.

Miyauchi, K., Yonezawa, Y., Maki, H., Ogawa, H., Hahn, A., & Caldwell, W. (2003). A new microcomputer-based safety and life support system for solitary-living elderly people. *Biomedical Sciences Instrumentation*, *39*, 179–182.

Molt, L. (2005). *A Brief Historical Review of Assistive Devices for Treating Stuttering*. Alabama: Auburn University.

Moratti, S., Clementz, B. A., Gao, Y., Ortiz, T., & Keil, A. (2007). Neural mechanisms of evoked oscillations: Stability and interaction with transient events. *Human Brain Mapping*, *28*(12), 1318–1333. doi:10.1002/hbm.20342

Morgan, S. T., Hansen, J. C., & Hillyard, S. A. (1996). Selective attention to stimulus location modulates the steady-state visual evoked potential. *Journal Proceedings of the National Academy of Sciences of the United States of America*, *93*(10), 4770–4774. doi:10.1073/pnas.93.10.4770

Moritz, C. T., Perlmutter, S. I., & Fetz, E. E. (2008). Direct control of paralysed muscles by cortical neurons. *Nature*, *456*(7222), 639–642. doi:10.1038/nature07418

Morkes, J., & Nielsen, J. (1997). Concise, Scannable, and Objective: How to Write for the Web. Retrieved from http://www.useit.com/papers/webwriting/writing.html

Morley, S. (1999). *Design and Evaluation of Non-Visual Information Systems for Blind Users*. Unpublished doctoral dissertation, University of Hertfordshire, UK.

Morris, M., Iansek, R., McGinley, J., Matyas, T., & Huxham, F. (2005). Three-dimensional gait biomechanics in Parkinson's disease: Evidence for a centrally mediated amplitude regulation disorder. *Movement Disorders*, *20*, 40–50. doi:10.1002/mds.20278

Morris, M. E., Iansek, R., Matyas, T. A., & Summers, J. J. (1996). Stride length regulation in Parkinson's disease normalization strategies and underlying mechanisms. *Brain*, *119*, 551–568. doi:10.1093/brain/119.2.551

Morris, M. E., & Iansek, R. (1994). Characteristics of motor disturbance in Parkinson's disease and strategies for movement rehabilitation. In *Motor Control Symposium, at the Australasian-Winter-Conference-on-Brain-Research Meeting, vol 15*, Queenstown, New Zealand (pp. 649-669).

Moss, F., Ward, L., & Sannita, W. G. (2004). Stochastic resonance and sensory information processing: a tutorial and review of application. *Clinical Neurophysiology*, *115*, 267–281. doi:10.1016/j.clinph.2003.09.014

Mowrer, D. (1991). Assessment review. Stuttering severity instrument for children and adults. *Journal of Fluency Disorders*, *16*, 311–314. doi:10.1016/0094-730X(91)90043-C

Moy, A. (1995). Equipment-help or hindrance? In Bumphrey, E.E. (Ed.), *Community practice: a text for occupational therapists and others involved in community care* (pp.111-121). Padstow, Cornwall: T.J. Press Ltd.

Mpitziopoulos, A., Konstantopoulos, C., Gavalas, D., & Pantziou, G. (2008). Hazard Monitoring for Visually Impaired People Enabled by Wireless Sensor Networking Technology. In *Proceedings of the 1st international conference on Pervasive technologies related to assistive environments* (Vol. 282, Article 21).

Müller, K. R., Anderson, C. W., & Birch, G. E. (2003). Linear and nonlinear methods for brain-computer interfaces. *IEEE Transactions on Neural Systems and Rehabilitation Engineering*, *11*(2), 165–169. doi:10.1109/TNSRE.2003.814484

Müller -Putz, G. R., Scherer, R., Brauneis, C., & Pfurtscheller, G. (2005b). Steady-state visual evoked potential (SSVEP)-based communication: impact of harmonic frequency components. *Journal of Neural Engineering*, *2*(4), 123–130. doi:10.1088/1741-2560/2/4/008

Muller-Putz, G. R., Eder, E., Wriessnegger, S. C., & Pfurtscheller, G. (2008). Comparison of DFT and lock-in amplifier features and search for optimal electrode positions in SSVEP-based BCI. *Journal of Neuroscience Methods*, *168*(1), 174–181. doi:10.1016/j.jneumeth.2007.09.024

Müller-Putz, G. R., Scherer, R., Neuper, C., & Pfurtscheller, G. (2006). Steady-state somatosensory evoked potentials: suitable brain signals for brain-computer interfaces? *IEEE Transactions on Neural Systems and Rehabilitation Engineering*, *14*(1), 30–37. doi:10.1109/TNSRE.2005.863842

Müller-Putz, G. R., Scherer, R., Pfurtscheller, G., & Rupp, R. (2005a). EEG-based neuroprosthesis control: a step towards clinical practice. *Neuroscience Letters*, *382*(1-2), 169–174. doi:10.1016/j.neulet.2005.03.021

Murphy, J. (2004). "I prefer contact this close": Perceptions of AAC by people with Motor Neuron Disease and their communication partners. *Augmentative and Alternative Communication*, *20*(4), 259–271. doi:10.1080/07434610400005663

Murphy, J., Marková, I., Collins, S., & Moodie, E. (1996). AAC systems: obstacles to effective use. *European Journal of Disorders of Communication, 31*(31-44.).

Murthy, R., Pavlidis, I., & Tsiamyrtzis, P. (2004). Touchless monitoring of breathing function. *26th Annual International Conference of the IEEE EMBS* (pp. 1196-1199). IEEE Press.

Myers, B., Hudson, S. E., & Pausch, R. (2001). Past present and future of user interface software tools. *ACM Transactions on Computer-Human Interaction*, *7*(1), 3–28. doi:10.1145/344949.344959

Mynatt, E. D., & Edwards, W. K. (1992a). *The Mercator Environment: A Nonvisual Interface to X Windows and Unix Workstations*. (Tech. Rep. GIT-GVU-92-05). Atlanta, GA: Georgia Institute of Technology, Graphics Visualization & Usability Center.

Mynatt, E. D., & Edwards, W. K. (1992b). Mapping GUIs to Auditory Interfaces. In *Proceedings of the 5th annual ACM Symposium on User Interface Software and Technology*. (pp. 61-70). Monterey, CA: ACM.

Naeem, M., Brunner, C., Leeb, R., Graimann, B., & Pfurtscheller, G. (2006). Seperability of four-class motor imagery data using independent components analysis. *Journal of Neural Engineering*, *3*(3), 208–216. doi:10.1088/1741-2560/3/3/003

Naito, M., Michioka, Y., Ozawa, K., Ito, Y., Kiguchi, M., & Kanazawa, T. (2007). A communication means for totally locked-in ALS patients based on changes in cerebral blood volume measured with near-infrared light. *IEICE Transactions on Information and Systems. E (Norwalk, Conn.)*, *90-D*(7), 1028–1037.

Najih, A. M. M. A., Ramli, A. R., Ibrahim, A., & Syed, A. R. (2003). *Comparing speech compression using wavelets with other speech compression schemes.*

Nakamura, H., Kitagawa, H., Kawaguchi, Y., & Tsuji, H. (1996). Direct and indirect activation of human corticospinal neurons by transcranial magnetic and electrical stimulation. *Neuroscience Letters*, *210*, 45–48. doi:10.1016/0304-3940(96)12659-8

Nakanishi, R., & Imai-Matsumura, K. (2008). Facial skin temperature decreases in infants with joyful expression. *Infant Behavior and Development*, *31*, 137–144. doi:10.1016/j.infbeh.2007.09.001

National Statistics Institute (NIE). (2008). Retrieved from http://www.ine.es/prensa/np524.pdf

Nessel, E. (1958). Die verogerts sprachruckklopplung (Lee-effect) bei der stotterern. *Folia Phoniatrica et Logopaedica, 10*, 199–204. doi:10.1159/000262818

Neumann, K., Preibisch, C., Euler, H. A., Gudenberg, A. W. v., Lanfermann, H., & Gall, V. (2005). Cortical plasticity associated with stuttering therapy. *Journal of Fluency Disorders, 30*(1), 23–39. doi:10.1016/j.jfludis.2004.12.002

Neuper, C., Müller, G. R., Kübler, A., Birbaumer, N., & Pfurtscheller, G. (2003). Clinical application of an EEG-based brain-computer interface: a case study in a patient with severe motor impairment. *Clinical Neurophysiology, 114*(3), 399–409. doi:10.1016/S1388-2457(02)00387-5

Neuper, C., Scherer, R., Reiner, M., & Pfurtscheller, G. (2005). Imagery of motor actions: differential effects of kinesthetic and visual-motor mode of imagery in single-trial EEG. *Brain Research. Cognitive Brain Research, 25*(3), 668–677. doi:10.1016/j.cogbrainres.2005.08.014

Neville-Jan, A., Piersol, C. V., Kielhofner, G., & Davis, K. (1993). Adaptive equipment: a study of utilization after hospital discharge. *Occupational Therapy in Health Care, 8*, 3–18. doi:10.1300/J003v08n04_02

Nhan, B. R., & Chau, T. (2009). Infrared thermal imaging as a physiological access pathway: a study of the baseline characteristics of facial skin temperatures. *Physiological Measurement, 30*(23-N), 35.

NHSC. (2007). *SpeechEasy Wireless Altered-Auditory Feedback (AAF) device for stammer*. National Horizon Scanning Centre, University of Birmingham.

Nielsen, J. (1999). *Designing Web Usability: The Practice of Simplicity*. New Riders Press.

Nielsen, J. (1993). *Usability engineering*. New York: Academic Press.

Nieuwboer, A., Kwakkel, G., Rochester, L., Jones, D., van Wegen, E., & Willems, A. M. (2007). Cueing training in the home improves gait-related mobility in Parkinson's disease: the RESCUE trial. *Journal of Neurology, Neurosurgery, and Psychiatry, 78*, 134–140. doi:10.1136/jnnp.200X.097923

Nijboer, F., Furdea, A., Gunst, I., Mellinger, J., McFarland, D. J., Birbaumer, N., & Kübler, A. (2008). An auditory brain-computer interface (BCI). *Journal of Neuroscience Methods, 167*(1), 43–50. doi:10.1016/j.jneumeth.2007.02.009

Novak, P., & Novak, V. (2006). Effect of step-synchronized vibration stimulation of soles on gait in Parkinson's disease: a pilot study. *Journal of Neuroengineering and Rehabilitation*, 3.

Novick, D. G., & Scholtz, J. C. (2002). Editorial - universal usability. *Interacting with Computers, 14*(4), 269–270. doi:10.1016/S0953-5438(01)00057-1

Nozawa, A., & Tacano, M. (2009). Correlation analysis on alpha attenuation and nasal skin temperature. *Journal of Statistical Mechanics, P01007*, 1–10.

Nunez, P. L., & Srinivasan, R. (2006). *Electric fields of the brain: the neurophysics of EEG*.

Nyce, D. S. (2004). *Linear position sensors: Theory and applications*. New Jersey: Wiley-Interscience John Wiley & Sons, Inc.

Nye, P. W. (1973). *A Preliminary Evaluation of the Bionic Instruments-Veterans Administration C-5 Laser Cane. National Research Council*. Washington, D.C.: National Academy of Sciences.

Obermaier, B., Guger, C., Neuper, C., & Pfurtscheller, G. (2001). Hidden Markov models for online classification of single trial EEG data. *Pattern Recognition Letters, 22*(12), 1299–1309. doi:10.1016/S0167-8655(01)00075-7

Obra Social Fundación La Caixa. (2007). Taller de Iniciación a la Informática (Beginners' Computer Workshop). Retrieved September 2009, from http://portal.lacaixa.es/clubestrella/talleres/presentacion _es.html

O'Donnell, J. J., Armson, J., & Kiefte, M. (2008). The effectiveness of SpeechEasy during situations of daily living. *Journal of Fluency Disorders, 33*(2), 99–119. doi:10.1016/j.jfludis.2008.02.001

Ogata, H., Mukai, T., & Yagi, T. (2007). A study on the frontal cortex in cognitive tasks using near-infrared spectroscopy. *Proceedings of the 29th Annual International Conference of the IEEE EMBS Cite Internationale, Lyon, France* (pp. 4731-4734). IEEE Press.

Ohnemus, K. R. (1997). Web style guides: who, what, where. In *Sigdoc '97: Proceedings of the 15th annual international conference on computer documentation* (pp. 189–197). New York: ACM Press. doi: 10.1145/263367.263392

Olander, A. (1932). An electrochemical investigation of solid cadmium-gold alloys. *European Journal of Mechanical and Environmental Engineering*, *47*(10), 3819–3833.

Orange Foundation. (n.d.). Proyecto EDAD. Retrieved October, 2009, from http://www.fundacionorange.es/fundacionorange/proyectos/proyecto_edad.html

Ordoñez, J. (1956). *(Stuttering) La tartamudez*. Madrid: Studium.

Ornstein, R. (1991). *The evolution of consciousness: the origins of the way we think*. New York: Touchstone.

Orton, S. T. (1927). Studies in Stuttering: Introduction. *Archives of Neurology and Psychiatry*, *18*(5), 671–672.

Otsuka, K., & Ren, X. (1999). Recent developments in the research of shape memory alloys. *Intermetallics*, *7*(5), 511–528. doi:10.1016/S0966-9795(98)00070-3

Otto, C., Milenković, A., Sanders, C., & Jovanov, E. (2006). System architecture of a wireless body area sensor network for ubiquitous health monitoring. *Journal of Mobile Multimedia*, *1*(4), 307–326.

Paciello, M. G. (2000). *Web Accessibility for People With Disabilities*. CMP Books.

Paddison, C., & Englefield, P. (2003). Applying heuristics to perform a rigorous accessibility inspection in a commercial context. In *Cuu '03: Proceedings of the 2003 conference on universal usability* (pp. 126–133). New York: ACM Press. doi:10.1145/957205.957228

Page, M., Galer, M., Fitzgerald, J., & Feeney, R. J. (1980). Problems of the selection, provision and use of aids. In Bray, J., & Wright, S. (Eds.), *The use of technology in the case of the elderly and disabled* (pp. 119–123). Westport, CT: Greenwood.

Pallás, R. (2003). *Señales y acondicionadores de señal* (4th ed.). Barcelona: Marcombo S.A.

Panayiotou, C., & Samaras, G. (2004). mpersona: personalized portals for the wireless user: An agent approach. *Mobile Networks and Applications*, *9*(6), 663–677. doi:10.1023/B:MONE.0000042505.07003.e6

Pape, T. L.-B., Kim, J., & Weiner, B. (2002). The shaping of individual meanings assigned to assistive technology: a review of personal factors. *Disability and Rehabilitation*, *24*(1-3), 5–20. doi:10.1080/09638280110066235

Parellada, J. (1978). *Las causas de la tartamudez. Vías hacia su corrección*. Barcelona, Spain: Jims.

Parker, C. S., & Christopherson, F. (1963). Electronic aid in treatment of stammer. *Medical Electronics & Biological Engineering*, *1*(2), 121–125. doi:10.1007/BF02474144

Parsa, V., & Jamieson, D. G. (2000). Identification of Pathological Voices Using Glottal Noise Measures. *Journal of Speech, Language, and Hearing Research: JSLHR*, *43*, 469–485.

Parsa, V., & Jamieson, D. G. (2001). Acoustic Discrimination of Pathological Voice. *Journal of Speech, Language, and Hearing Research: JSLHR*, *44*, 327–339. doi:10.1044/1092-4388(2001/027)

Pascual-Leone, A., Valls-Sole, J., Brasil-Neto, J. P., Cammarota, A., Grafman, J., & Hallett, M. (1994). Akinesia in Parkinson's disease. II. Effects of subthreshold repetitive transcranial motor cortex stimulation. *Neurology*, *44*(2), 892–898.

Pastor, M. A., Artieda, J., Arbizu, J., Valencia, M., & Masdeu, J. C. (2003). Human cerebral activation during steady-state visual-evoked responses. *The Journal of Neuroscience*, *23*(37), 11621–11627.

Patel, R., Pilato, S., & Roy, D. (2004). Beyond linear syntax: An image-orientation communication aid. *Assistive Technology Outcomes and Benefits, 1*(1), 57–67.

Patil, P. G., Carmena, J. M., Nicolelis, M. A. L., & Turner, D. A. (2004). Ensemble recordings of human subcortical neurons as a source of motor control signals for a brain-machine interface. *Neurosurgery, 55*(1), 27–35.

Patton, H. D., & Amassian, V. E. (1954). Single and multiple-unit analysis of cortical stage of pyramidal tract activation. *Journal of Neurophysiology, 17*, 345–363.

Pavlidis, I., Dowdall, J., Sun, N., Puri, C., Fei, J., & Garbey, M. (2007). Interacting with human physiology. *Computer Vision and Image Understanding, 108*(1-2), 150–170. doi:10.1016/j.cviu.2006.11.018

Pavlidis, I., & Levine, J. (2002). Thermal facial screening for deception detection. In *Proceedings of the Second Joint EMBS/BMES Conference* (pp. 1143-1144). IEEE Press.

Peckham, P. H., & Creasey, G. H. (1992). Neural prostheses: clinical applications of functional electrical stimulation spinal cord injury. *Paraplegia, 30*, 996–1001.

Peizer, E., Lorenze, E. J., & Dixon, M. (1982). Environmental controls to promote independence in severely disabled elderly persons. *Medical Instrumentation, 16*(3), 171–173.

Peli, E., Goldstein, R. B., Young, G. M., Trempe, C. L., & Buzney, S. M. (1991). Image enhancement for the visually impaired: simulations and experimental results. *Investigative Ophthalmology & Visual Science, 32*, 2337–2350.

Peli, E., Lee, E., Trempe, C. L., & Buzney, S. (1994). Image enhancement for the visually impaired: the effects of enhancement on face recognition. *Journal of the Optical Society of America. A, Optics, Image Science, and Vision, 11*, 1929–1939. doi:10.1364/JOSAA.11.001929

Pelrine, R., Kornbluh, R., Pei, Q., Stanford, S., Oh, S., & Eckerle, J. (2002). Dielectric Elastomer Artificial Muscle Actuators: Toward Biomimetic Motion. In Bar-Cohen, Y. (Ed.), *Proceedings of SPIE: Vol. 4695* (pp. 126-137). San Diego: SPIE.

Perkins, W., Rudas, J., Johnson, L., & Bell, J. (1976). Stuttering: Discoordination of Phonation with Articulation and Respiration. *Journal of Speech and Hearing Research, 19*(3), 509–522.

Perkins, W. H. (1996). *Stuttering and Science*. San Diego: Singular Pub. Group.

Perkins, W. H. (2001). Stuttering: A Matter of Bad Timing. *Science, 294*(5543), 786a. doi:10.1126/science.294.5543.786a

Perkins, W. J., & Stenning, B. F. (1986). Control units for operation of computers by severely physical handicapped persons. *Journal of Medical Engineering & Technology, 10*(1), 21–23. doi:10.3109/03091908609044332

Peters, B., Pfurtscheller, G., & Flyvbjerg, H. (1998). Mining multi-channel EEG for its information content: an ANN-based method for a brain-computer interface. *Neural Networks, 11*(7-8), 1429–1433. doi:10.1016/S0893-6080(98)00060-4

Petrie, H., Johnson, V., Strothotte, T., Raab, A., Michel, R., Reichert, L., & Schalt, A. (1997). Mobic: An aid to increase the independent mobility of blind travellers. *British Journal of Visual Impairment, 15*(2), 63–66. doi:10.1177/026461969701500205

Petrie, H., Hamilton, F., & King, N. (2004). Tension, what tension? Website accessibility and visual design. In *Proceedings of the international cross- disciplinary workshop on Web accessibility* (pp. 13-18).

Pfurtcheller, G., Neuper, C., Guger, C., Harkam, W., Ramoser, H., & Schlögl, A. (2000). Current trends in Graz Brain-Computer Interface (BCI) Research. *IEEE Transactions on Rehabilitation Engineering, 8*(2), 216–219. doi:10.1109/86.847821

Pfurtscheller, G., Neuper, C., Schlögl, A., & Lugger, K. (1998). Separability of EEG signals recorded during right and left motor imagery using adaptive autoregressive parameters. *IEEE Transactions on Rehabilitation Engineering, 6*(3), 316–325. doi:10.1109/86.712230

Pfurtscheller, G., & Lopes da Silva, F. H. (1999). Event-related EEG/MRG synchronization and desynchronization: basic principles. *Clinical Neurophysiology*, *110*(11), 1842–1857. doi:10.1016/S1388-2457(99)00141-8

Pfurtscheller, G., Müller, G. R., Pfurtscheller, J., Gerner, H. J., & Rupp, R. (2003). 'Thought'-control of functional electrical stimulation to restore hand grasp in a patient with tetraplegia. *Neuroscience Letters*, *351*(1), 33–36. doi:10.1016/S0304-3940(03)00947-9

Pfurtscheller, G., Müller-Putz, G. R., Schlögl, A., Graimann, B., Scherer, R., & Leeb, R. (2006). 15 years of BCI research at Graz University of Technology: current projects. *IEEE Transactions on Neural Systems and Rehabilitation Engineering*, *14*(2), 205–210. doi:10.1109/TNSRE.2006.875528

Pfurtscheller, G., & Neuper, C. (1997). Motor imagery activates primary sensorimotor area in humans. *Neuroscience Letters*, *239*(2-3), 65–68. doi:10.1016/S0304-3940(97)00889-6

Phelps, E., & LeDoux, J. (2005). Contributions of the amygdala to emotion processing: from animal models to human behavior. *Neuron*, *48*(2), 175–187. doi:10.1016/j.neuron.2005.09.025

Philips, B., & Zhao, H. (1993). Predictors of assistive technology abandonment. *Assistive Technology*, *5*, 36–45. doi:10.1080/10400435.1993.10132205

Piccione, F., Giorgi, F., Tonin, P., Priftis, K., Giove, S., & Silvoni, S. (2006). P300-based brain computer interface: reliability and performance in healthy and paralysed participants. *Clinical Neurophysiology*, *117*(3), 531–537. doi:10.1016/j.clinph.2005.07.024

Pichon, E., & Borel-Maisonny, S. (1973). *La tartamudez. Naturaleza y tratamiento*. Barcelona: Toray-Masson.

Pilgrim, M. (2002). Dive Into Accessibility. Retrieved 2005 from http://diveintoaccessibility.org/

Pineda, J. A., Silverman, D. S., Vankov, A., & Hestenes, J. (2003). Learning to control brain rhythms: making a brain-computer interface possible. *IEEE Transactions on Neural Systems and Rehabilitation Engineering*, *11*(2), 181–184. doi:10.1109/TNSRE.2003.814445

Pollard, R., Ellis, J. B., Finan, D., & Ramig, P. R. (2009). Effects of the SpeechEasy on objective and perceived aspects of stuttering: a 6-month, phase I clinical trial in naturalistic environments. *Journal of Speech and Hearing Research*, *52*(2), 516–533. doi:10.1044/1092-4388(2008/07-0204)

Pollina, D. A., Dollins, A. B., Senter, S. M., Brown, T. E., Pavlidis, I., & Levine, J. A. (2006). Facial skin surface temperature changes during a concealed information test. *Annals of Biomedical Engineering*, *34*(7), 1182–1189. doi:10.1007/s10439-006-9143-3

Poulet, E., Brunelin, J., Bediou, B., Bation, R., Forgeard, L., & Dalery, J. (2005). Slow transcranial magnetic stimulation can rapidly reduce resistant auditory hallucinations in schizophrenia. *Biological Psychiatry*, *57*(2), 188–191. doi:10.1016/j.biopsych.2004.10.007

Pousada, T., Groba, B., Orozco, K., & Martínez, M. (2008). Las Tecnologías de la Información y Comunicaciones como recursos educativos para alumnos con necesidades educativas especiales. In Pereira, J., Martínez, L.A., Fuertes, J.L., & Vázquez, J.M. (Eds.), *Tecnologías de la Información y las Comunicaciones en la Autonomía Personal, dependencia y accesibilidad* (pp. 399-418). Santiago de Compostela: Fundación Alfredo Brañas.

Power, C., & Petrie, H. (2007). *Accessibility in non-professional Web authoring tools: A missed Web 2.0 opportunity?* In *W4a '07: Proceedings of the 2007 international cross-disciplinary conference on Web accessibility* (W4a) (pp. 116-119). New York: ACM Press.

Prado, M., Roa, L., Reina-Tosina, J., Palma, A., & Milán, J. A. (2002). Virtual Center for Renal Support: Technological Approach to Patient Physiological Image. *IEEE Transactions on Bio-Medical Engineering*, *49*(12), 1420–1430. doi:10.1109/TBME.2002.805454

Prado, M., & Roa, L. M. (2007). [IOS Pres.]. *Wearable Real-time and Adaptive Feedback Device to Face the Stuttering: a Knowledge-based Telehealthcare Proposal Medical and Care Compunetics*, *4*, 147–156.

Prado, M., Reina-Tosina, J., & Roa, L. (2002). *Distributed intelligent architecture for falling detection and physical activity analysis in the elderly*. Paper presented at the 24th Annual International Conference of the IEEE-EMBS and Annual Fall Meeting of the BMES.

Prado-Velasco, M., del Río-Cidoncha, M. G., & Ortiz-Marín, R. (2008). *The Inescapable Smart Impact detection System (ISIS): an ubiquitous and personalized fall detector based on a distributed "divide and conquer strategy"*. Paper presented at the Personalized Healthcare through Technology, 30th Annual International Conference of the IEEE Engineering in Medicine and Biology Society

Prahlad, H., Pelrine, R., Kornbluh, R., Guggenberg, P. V., Chhokar, S., & Eckerle, J. (2005). Programmable surface deformation: thickness-mode electroactive polymer actuators and their applications. In Bar-Cohen, Y. (Ed.), *Proceedings of SPIE: Vol. 5759* (pp. 102-113). San Diego: SPIE.

Prangrat, T., Mann, W. C., & Tomita, M. (2000). Impact of unilateral neglect on assistive device use. *Technology and Disability*, *12*, 53–69.

Pregenzer, M., & Pfurtscheller, G. (1999). Frequency component selection for an EEG-based brain to computer interface. *IEEE Transactions on Bio-Medical Engineering*, *7*(4), 413–419.

Preibisch, C., Neumann, K., Raab, P., Euler, H., von Gudenberg, A., & Lanfermann, H. (2003). Evidence for compensation for stuttering by the right frontal operculum. *NeuroImage*, *20*(2), 1356–1364. doi:10.1016/S1053-8119(03)00376-8

Pressey, N. (1977). Mowat sensor. *Focus (San Francisco, Calif.)*, *11-3*, 35–39.

Puerta, A. (1996). The MECANO Project: Comprehensive and Integrated Support for Model-Based Interface Development. In Vanderdonckt, J. (Ed.), *Computer-Aided Design of User Interfaces* (pp. 19–36). Namur, Belgium: Namur University Press.

Qi, Y., Hillman, R. E., & Milstein, C. (1999). The estimation of signal-to-noise ratio in continuous speech for disordered voices. *The Journal of the Acoustical Society of America*, *105*(4), 2532–2535. doi:10.1121/1.426860

Quaresima, V., Ferrari, M., Torricelli, A., Spinelli, L., Pifferi, A., & Cubeddu, R. (2005). Bilateral prefrontal cortex oxygenation responses to a verbal fluency task: A multichannel time-resolved near-infrared topography study. *Journal of Biomedical Optics*, *10*(1), 1–12. doi:10.1117/1.1851512

Rabiee, P., Sloper, P., & Beresford, B. (2005). Desired outcomes for children and young people with complex health care needs, and children who do not use speech for communication. *Health & Social Care in the Community*, *13*(5), 478–487. doi:10.1111/j.1365-2524.2005.00578.x

Raghavendra, P., Bornman, J., Granlund, M., & Bjorck-Akesson, E. (2007). The World Health Organization's International Classification of Functioning, Disability and Health: implications for clinical and research practice in the field of augmentative and alternative communication. *Augmentative and Alternative Communication*, *23*(4), 349–361. doi:10.1080/07434610701650928

Rajasekaran, M. P., Radhakrishnan, S., & Subbaraj, P. (2009). Elderly patient monitoring system using a wireless sensor network. *Telemedicine Journal and e-Health*, *15*(1), 73–79. doi:10.1089/tmj.2008.0056

Ramsden, E. (2006). *Hall-effect sensors: theory and applications* (2nd ed.). Oxford: Elsevier.

Ranu, H. S. (1986). Engineering aspects of rehabilitation for the handicapped. *Journal of Medical Engineering & Technology*, *10*(1), 16–20. doi:10.3109/03091908609044331

Raskin, J. (1997). Looking for a humane interface: will computers ever become easy to use? *Communications of the ACM*, *40*(2), 98–101. doi:10.1145/253671.253737

Raskin, J. (2000). The humane interface (book excerpt). *Ubiquity*, *1*(14), 3. doi:10.1145/341836.342022

Raymond, J., & Leibowitz, H. W. (1985). Viewing distance and the sustained detection of high spatial frequency gratings. *Vision Research, 25*, 1655–1659. doi:10.1016/0042-6989(85)90137-3

Raynal, M., & Vigouroux, N. (2005). Genetic algorithm to generate optimized soft keyboard. *Proceedings of CHI'2005* (pp. 1729-1732), Oregon, USA.

Reed, C. F., Tomkins, S. S., & Alexander, I. E. (Eds.). (1958). *Psychopathology: A Source Book*. Harvard University Press.

Regan, B. (2004). Accessibility and design: a failure of the imagination. In *Proceedings of the international cross-disciplinary workshop on Web accessibility* (pp. 29–37).

Reilly, J. J. Jr, & Wiswall, R. H. Jr. (1968). Reaction of hydrogen with alloys of magnesium and nickel and the formation of Mg_2NiH_4. *Inorganic Chemistry, 7*(11), 2254–2256. doi:10.1021/ic50069a016

Reitzes, P., & Snyder, G. (2006). Response to "Intensive Stuttering Modification Therapy: A Multidimensional Assessment of Treatment Outcomes," by Blomgren, Roy, Callister, and Merrill (2005). *Journal of Speech, Language, and Hearing Research: JSLHR, 49*, 1420–1422. doi:10.1044/1092-4388(2006/103)

Ridding, M. C., & Rothwell, J. C. (2007). Is there a future for therapeutic use of transcranial magnetic stimulation? *Nature Reviews. Neuroscience, 8*(7), 559–567. doi:10.1038/nrn2169

Riemer-Reiss, M. L., & Wacker, R. R. (2000). Factors associated with assistive technology discontinuance among individuals with disabilities. *Journal of Rehabilitation, 66*(3), 44–50.

Riley, G. D. (1972). A stuttering severity instrument for children and adults. *The Journal of Speech and Hearing Disorders, 37*, 314–322.

Rius, A. (1897). *La educación de los niños atrasados (cortos de inteligencia, tartamudos, tartajosos, tardos en el habla, etc)*. Barcelona: F. Sánchez.

RNIB. (2004). See It Right Guidelines. Retrieved 2005 from http://www.rnib.org.uk/xpedio/groups/public/documents/code/public rnib008789.hcsp

Robertson, S., Beesley, S., Byrne, J., Richards, J., Koechley, N., & Sloan, M. (2005). Accessible Design in the Digital World Conference, Dundee, UK. (Panel Session – Legislation? Standards? How do we tell people to design technology that supports inclusion?)

Robinson, L. (1987). Patient compliance in occupational therapy home health programs: sociocultural consideration. *Occupational Therapy in Health Care, 4*(1), 127–137. doi:10.1300/J003v04n01_11

Robinson, S. (2003, June). Accesskeys: Unlocking hidden navigation. *A List Apart, 1*(158). Retrieved from http://www.alistapart.com/articles/accesskeys/

Rochester, L., Hetherington, V., Jones, D., Nieuwboer, A., Willems, A. M., Kwakkel, G., & Van Wegen, E. (2005). The effect of external rhythmic cues (auditory and visual) on walking during a functional task in homes of people with Parkinson's disease. *Archives of Physical Medicine and Rehabilitation, 86*, 999–1006. doi:10.1016/j.apmr.2004.10.040

Rodríguez Carrillo, P. R. (2002). *La tartamudez desde la perspectiva de los tartamudos*. Caracas: Universidad Central de Venezuela.

Rodríguez Morejón, A. (2003). *La tartamudez: naturaleza y tratamiento*. Barcelona: Herder.

Rodríguez Vázquez, J., Sánchez Montoya, R., & Soto Pérez, F. J. (Coords.) (2006). *Las tecnologías en la Escuela Inclusiva: nuevos escenarios, nuevas oportunidades. (Actas del Congreso Tecnoneet-ciiee 2006)*. Murcia: Consejería de Educación y Cultura/Real Patronato sobre Discapacidad.

Roldán, J. R., Moranchel, J., Barrera, C., & Casas, R. (2009) Aprendizaje de las actividades de la vida diaria mediante el uso de tecnología adaptada, ESSAAC'2009 2nd National Congress on Augmentative Communication and Technology for life, September, 2009, Zaragoza, Spain.

Rongching, D., Richard, B., Stein, B., Andrews, B. J., James, K. B., & Wieler, M. (1996). Application of tilt sensors in functional electrical stimulation. *IEEE Transactions on Rehabilitation Engineering, 4*, 63–71. doi:10.1109/86.506403

Rosen, M. J., & Goodenough-Trepagnier, C. (1981). Factors affecting communication rate in non-vocal communication systems. In *Proceedings of the 4th Annual Conference on Rehabilitation Engineering* (pp. 194–196).

Rosenfield, D. B., & Viswanath, N. S. (2002). Neuroscience of Stuttering. *Science, 295*(5557), 973b. doi:10.1126/science.295.5557.973b

Rossi, S., Ferro, M., Cincotta, M., Ulivelli, M., Bartalini, S., & Miniussi, C. (2007). A real electro-magnetic placebo (REMP) device for sham transcranial magnetic stimulation (TMS). *Clinical Neurophysiology, 118*(3), 709–716. doi:10.1016/j.clinph.2006.11.005

Rossi, S., Hallett, M., Rossini, P. M., & Pascual-Leone, A. (2009). The Safety of TMS Consensus Group. Safety, ethical considerations, and application guidelines for the use of transcranial magnetic stimulation in clinical practice and research. *Clinical Neurophysiology, 120*(12), 2008–2039. doi:10.1016/j.clinph.2009.08.016

Rossini, P. M., Barker, A. T., Berardelli, A., Caramia, M. D., Caruso, G., & Cracco, R. Q. (1994). Non-invasive electrical and magnetic stimulation of the brain, spinal cord and roots: basic principles and procedures for routine clinical application. Report of an IFCN committee. *Electroencephalography and Clinical Neurophysiology, 91*(2), 79–92. doi:10.1016/0013-4694(94)90029-9

Rossini, L., Dario, I., & Summerer, L. (Eds.). (2009). *Brain Machine Interfaces for Space applications: Enhancing astronaut's capabilities. International Review of Neurobiology* (*Vol. 86*). New York: Academic Press.

Rosson, M. B., & Carroll, J. M. (2001). *Usability engineering: scenario-based development of human computer interaction*. Morgan Kaufmann.

Roth, Y., Amir, A., Levkovitz, Y., & Zangen, A. (2007). Three-dimensional distribution of the electric field induced in the brain by transcranial magnetic stimulation using figure-8 and deep H-coils. *Journal of Clinical Neurophysiology, 24*(1), 31–38. doi:10.1097/WNP.0b013e31802fa393

Rothwell, J. C. (1997). Techniques and mechanism of action of transcranial stimulation of the human motor cortex. *Journal of Neuroscience Methods, 74*(2), 113–122. doi:10.1016/S0165-0270(97)02242-5

Rothwell, J. C., Thompsom, P. D., Day, B. L., Boyd, S., & Marsden, C. D. (1991). Stimulation of the human motor cortex through the scalp. *Experimental Physiology, 76*(2), 159–200.

Rumeau-Rouquette, C., Grandjean, H., Cans, C., du Mazaubrun, C., & Verrier, A. (1997). Prevalence and time trends of disabilities in school-age children. *International Journal of Epidemiology, 26*(1), 137–145. doi:10.1093/ije/26.1.137

Russell, L. (1965). Travel path sounder. In *Proceedings of Rotterdam Mobility Research Conference*. New York: American Foundation for the Blind.

Ryan, B. (2005). Response to Blomgren, Roy, Callister, andMerrill. *Journal of Speech, Language, and Hearing Research: JSLHR, 49*, 1412–1414. doi:10.1044/1092-4388(2006/101)

Saito, M. (2000). Expanding welfare concept and assistive technology. *Proceedings of the IEEK Annual Fall Conference*, 156-161.

Sakintuna, B., Lamari-Darkrimb, F., & Hirscherc, M. (2007). Metal hydride materials for solid hydrogen storage: A review. *International Journal of Hydrogen Energy, 32*, 1121–1140. doi:10.1016/j.ijhydene.2006.11.022

Salgado, A. (2005). *Manual práctico de tartamudez*. Madrid: Editorial Síntesis.

Salter, R. B., Hamilton, H. W., Wedge, J. H., Tile, M., Torode, I. P., & O' Driscoll, S. W. (1984). Clinical application of basic research on continuous passive motion for disorders and injuries of synovial joints: A preliminary report of a feasibility study. *Journal of Orthopaedic Research*, *1*(3), 325–342. doi:10.1002/jor.1100010313

Saltuklaroglu, T., & Kalinowski, J. (2006). *Stuttering*.

Sanders, D. A., Stott, I. J., Goodwin, M. J., Tewkesbury, G. E., Cawte, H. & Poland, G.A. (1997) Computer systems and strategies to assist a disabled person in navigating a powered wheelchair through a doorway. *IEEE Colloquium on Computers in the Service of Mankind: Helping the Disabled* (Digest No.: 1997/117, pp.7/1-7/4).

Santacreu, J., & Fernandez-Zúñiga, A. (1991). Tratamiento De La Tartamudez: Promolibro.

Santos, O. C., & Boticario, J. G. (2008). Users' experience with a recommender system in an open source standard-based learning management system. In *Proceedings of the 4th Symposium of the WG HCI& UE of the Austrian Computer Society on Usability & HCI for Education and Work (USAB 2008)* (LNCS 5298).

Santos, O. C., Boticario, J. G., del Campo, E., & Saneiro, M. (2008). Personalised support for students with disabilities based on psycho-educational guidelines. *In Proceedings of the IEEE international conference on advance learning technology (ICALT 2008): workshop on advanced learning technologies for disabled and non-disabled people (WALTD).* Santander, Spain, IEEE Computer Society Press

Santos, O. C., Martin, L., del Campo, E., Saneiro, M., Mazzone, E., Boticario, J. G., & Petrie, H. (2009b). User-Centered Design Methods for Validating a Recommendations Model to Enrich Learning Management Systems with Adaptive Navigation Support. In S. Weibelzahl, J. Masthoff, A. Paramythis, & L. van Velsen (Eds.), *Proceedings of the Sixth Workshop on User-Centred Design and Evaluation of Adaptive Systems*, held in conjunction with the International Conference on User Modeling, Adaptation, and Personalization (UMAP2009) (pp. 64-67).

Santos, O.C., Couchet, J., & Boticario, J.G. (2009a). Personalized e-learning and e-mentoring through user modelling and dynamic recommendations for the inclusion of disabled at work and education. *ICALT 2009*.

Santos, V., Bartolomeu, P., Fonseca, J., & Mota, A. (2007, July). *B-Live - A Home Automation System for Disabled and Elderly People*. Paper presented at the International Symposium on Industrial Embedded Systems. SIES '07. Lisboa (Portugal).

Sato, M., Ino, S., Shimizu, S., Ifukube, T., & Izumi, T. (1996). Development of a compliance variable metal hydride (MH) actuator system for robotic mobility aid for disabled persons. *Transactions of the Japan Society of Mechanical Engineers: Part C*, *62*(597), 1912–1919.

Savidis, A., & Stephanidis, C. (1998). The HOMER UIMS for dual user interface development: Fusing visual and non-visual interactions. *Interacting with Computers*, *11*, 173–209. doi:10.1016/S0953-5438(98)00025-3

Savidis, A., & Stephanidis, C. (1995a) Developing dual user interfaces for integrating blind and sighted users: the HOMER UIMS.I. In *Proceedings of the SIGCHI Conference on Human Factors in Computing Systems* (pp. 106-113). New York: ACM Press/Addison Wesley Publishing Co. doi:acm.org/10.1145/223904.223918

Savidis, A., & Stephanidis, C. (1995b) Building non-visual interaction through the development of the Rooms metaphor. In *Conference Companion on Human factors in Computing Systems* (pp. 244-245). New York: ACM.

Schaafsma, J. D., Balash, Y., Gurevich, T., Bartels, A. L., Hausdorff, J. M., & Giladi, N. (2003a). Characterization of freezing of gait subtypes and the response of each to levodopa in Parkinson's disease. *European Journal of Neurology*, *10*, 391–398. doi:10.1046/j.1468-1331.2003.00611.x

Schaafsma, J. D., Giladi, N., Balash, Y., Bartels, A. L., Gurevich, T., & Hausdorff, J. M. (2003b). Gait dynamics in Parkinson's disease: relationship to Parkinsonian features, falls and response to levodopa. *Journal of the Neurological Sciences*, *212*, 47–53. doi:10.1016/S0022-510X(03)00104-7

Schalk, G., Brunner, P., Gerhardt, L. A., Bischof, H., & Wolpaw, J. R. (2008). Brain-computer interfaces (BCIs): detection instead of classification. *Journal of Neuroscience Methods*, *167*(1), 51–62. doi:10.1016/j.jneumeth.2007.08.010

Schemm, R. L., & Gitlin, L. N. (1998). How occupational therapists teach older patients to use bathing and dressing devices in rehabilitation. *The American Journal of Occupational Therapy.*, *52*(4), 276–282.

Scherer, R., Lee, F., Schlögl, A., Leeb, R., Bischof, H., & Pfurtscheller, G. (2008). Towards self-paced Brain-Computer Communication: Navigation through virtual worlds. *IEEE Transactions on Bio-Medical Engineering*, *55*(2), 675–682. doi:10.1109/TBME.2007.903709

Scherer, R., Mohapp, A., Grieshofer, P., Pfurtscheller, G., & Neuper, C. (2007b). Sensorimotor EEG patterns during motor imagery in hemiparetic stroke patients. *International Journal of Bioelectromagnetism*, *9*(3), 155–162.

Scherer, R., Müller, G. R., Neuper, C., Graimann, B., & Pfurtscheller, G. (2004). An asynchronously controlled EEG-based virtual keyboard: improvement of the spelling rate. *IEEE Transactions on Bio-Medical Engineering*, *51*(6), 979–984. doi:10.1109/TBME.2004.827062

Scherer, R., Schlögl, A., Lee, F., Bischof, H., Janša, J., & Pfurtscheller, G. (2007a). The self-paced Graz brain-computer interface: methods and applications. *Computational Intellignece and Neuroscience, 2007. Article ID*, *79826*, 1–7.

Scherer, R., Zanos, P. Z., Miller, K. J., Rao, R. P. N., & Ojemann, J. G. (2009). Classification of Contralateral and Ipsilateral Finger Movements for Electrocorticographic Brain-Computer Interfaces. *Neurosurgical Focus*, *27*(1), E12. doi:10.3171/2009.4.FOCUS0981

Scherer, M. J. (1998). *The Scherer MPT model: matching people with technologies*. Webster, NY: Author.

Scherer, M. J., & Craddock, G. (2002). Matching Person & Technology (MPT) assessment process. *Technology & Disability: Special Issue on Outcome Measures*, *14*, 125–131.

Scherer, M. J., Sax, C., Vanbiervliet, A., Cushman, L., & Scherer, J. (2005). Predictors of assistive technology use: The importance of personal and psychosocial factors. *Disability and Rehabilitation. Assistive Technology*, *27*(21), 1321–1331.

Scherer, M. (2003). *The importance of assistive technology outcomes*. January 2003 Article of the month. Retrieved February 12, 2003 from http://www.ebility.com/articles/at.shtml

Scherer, M. J. (2002). Editorial. The change in emphasis from people to person: Introduction to the special issue on assistive technology. *Disability and Rehabilitation*, *24*(1/2/3), 1- 4.

Schlapbach, L., & Züttel, A. (2001). Hydrogen-storage materials for mobile applications. *Nature*, *414*, 353–358. doi:10.1038/35104634

Schlögl, A., & Flotzinger, D., & Pfurtscheller. (1997). G. Adaptive autoregressive modeling used for single-trial EEG classification. *Biomedizinische Technik*, *42*(6), 162–167. doi:10.1515/bmte.1997.42.6.162

Schmidtbleicher, D., Turbanski, S., & Haas, C. T. (2004). Effects of whole-body vibration on postural control in Parkinson's disease. *Movement Disorders*, *19*, 518.

Schwartz, M. F. (1977). *Stottern ist heilbar: neue und erfolgreiche Behandlungsmethoden* [Stutter is more curable: new and successful working methods]. Düsseldorf: Econ.

Sears, A., Jacko, J. A., Chung, J. C., & Moro, F. (2001). The role of visual search in the design of effective soft keyboards. *Behaviour & Information Technology*, *20*, 159–166. doi:10.1080/01449290110049790

Seeger, M. S., & Fisher, L. A. (1982). Adaptive equipment used in the rehabilitation of hip arthroplasty patients. *The American Journal of Occupational Therapy.*, *36*, 503–508.

Sellers, E. W., & Donchin, E. (2006). A P300-based brain-computer interface: initial tests by ALS patients. *Clinical Neurophysiology*, *117*(3), 538–548. doi:10.1016/j.clinph.2005.06.027

Sevillano, J. L., Cascado, D., Cagigas, D., Vicente, S., Luján, C. D., & Díaz del Rio, F. (2009, May). *A Real-Time Wireless Sensor Network for Wheelchair Navigation*. Paper presented at the 7th IEEE/ACS International Conference on Computer Systems and Applications. Rabat (Morocco)

Shames, G. H., & Sherrick, C. E. (1963). A discussion of nonfluency and stuttering as operant behavior. *The Journal of Speech and Hearing Disorders*, *28*, 3–18.

Shames, G. H., & Florance, C. L. (1980). *Stutter-Free Speech: A Goal for Therapy*.

Shankar, R., Ghosh, T. K., & Sponta, R. J. (2007). Dielectric elastomers as next-generation polymeric actuators. *Soft Matter*, *3*, 1116–1129. doi:10.1039/b705737g

Shapiro, P. A. (1995). Psychosocial evaluation and prediction of compliance problems and morbidity after heart transplantation. *Transplantation*, *60*(12), 1462–1466. doi:10.1097/00007890-199560120-00016

Shastri, D., Merla, A., Tsiamyrtzis, P., & Pavlidis, I. (2009). Imaging facial signs of neurophysiological responses. *IEEE Transactions on Bio-Medical Engineering*, *56*(2), 477–484. doi:10.1109/TBME.2008.2003265

Sheehan, J. G., & Voas, R. B. (1957). Stuttering As Conflict: 1. Comparison Of Therapy Techniques Involving Approach And Avoidance. *The Journal of Speech and Hearing Disorders*, *22*(5), 714–723.

Shenoy, P., Miller, K. J., Ojemann, J. G., & Rao, R. P. N. (2008). Generalized features for electrocorticographic BCIs. *IEEE Transactions on Bio-Medical Engineering*, *55*(1), 273–280. doi:10.1109/TBME.2007.903528

Sherer, M. J. (2001). *Assistive Technnology: Matchin Device and consumer for successful rehabilitation*. Washington, DC: American Psychological Association.

Sherer, M. J. (2004). *Matching person and assistive technology process and accompanying assessment instruments* (Rev. Ed.). Webster, NY: Institute for Matching Person & Technology.

Sherer, M. J., & Craddock, G. (2002). Matching person and technology (MPT) assessment process. *Technology and Disability*, *14*, 125–131.

Sherer, M. (1996). The impact of using personal computers of the lives of nursing residents. *Physical & Occupational Therapy in Geriatrics*, *14*, 13–31.

Shimamoto, H., Morimitsu, H., Sugita, S., Nakahara, K., & Shigemori, M. (1999). Therapeutic effect of repetitive transcranial magnetic stimulation in Parkinson's disease. *Rinsho Shinkeigaku. Clinical Neurology*, *39*(12), 1264–1267.

Shipham, I. (1987). Bath aids – their use by a multidiagnostic group of patients. *International Rehabilitation Medicine*, *8*(4), 182–184.

Shneiderman, B., & Plaisant, C. (2004). *Designing the User Interface: Strategies for Effective Human-Computer Interaction* (4th ed.). Addison Wesley.

Shone, S. M., Ryan, S., Rigby, P. J., & Jutai, J. W. (2002). Toward a comprehensive evaluation of the impact of electronics aids to daily living: evaluation of consumer satisfaction. *Disability and Rehabilitation*, *24*(1-3), 115–125. doi:10.1080/09638280110066794

Siebner, H. R., Mentschel, C., Auer, C., & Conrad, B. (1999). Repetitive transcranial magnetic stimulation has a beneficial effect on bradykinesia in Parkinson's disease. *Neuroreport*, *10*(3), 589–594. doi:10.1097/00001756-199902250-00027

Siebner, H. R., Rossmeier, C., Mentschel, C., Peinemann, A., & Conrad, B. (2000). Short-term motor improvement after sub-threshold 5-Hz repetitive transcranial magnetic stimulation of the primary motor hand area in Parkinson's disease. *Journal of the Neurological Sciences*, *178*(2), 91–94. doi:10.1016/S0022-510X(00)00370-1

Simon, E. P. (1984). A report on electronic travel aid users: Three to five years later. *Journal of Visual Impairment & Blindness*, *78*, 478–480.

Skubic, M. (2005). *Assessing Mobility and Cognitive Problems in Elders*. AAAI 2005 Fall Symposium, Workshop on Caring Machines: AI in Eldercare. Arlington, Virginia, November, 2005.

Small, L. M., & Grose, J. (1993). A cultural perspective on rehabilitation and modality use with elder persons- a pilot study. *Physical & Occupational Therapy in Geriatrics*, *11*(3), 71–80.

Smela, E. (2003). Conjugated polymer actuators for biomedical applications. *Advanced Materials (Deerfield Beach, Fla.)*, *15*(6), 481–494. doi:10.1002/adma.200390113

Smith, M. M., & Connolly, I. (2008). Roles of aided communication: perspectives of adults who use AAC. *Disability and Rehabilitation. Assistive Technology*, *3*(5), 260–273. doi:10.1080/17483100802338499

Smith, R. (1988). Quality assurance in equipment ordering for the spinal cord-injured client. *The American Journal of Occupational Therapy.*, *42*(1), 36–39.

Smith, R. (1995). A client centred model for equipment prescription (client values and roles, effective use of adaptive equipment). *Occupational Therapy in Health Care*, *9*(4), 39–52. doi:10.1300/J003v09n04_04

Snyder, G. (2009). The Existence of Stuttering in Sign Language and other Forms of Expressive Communication: Sufficient Cause for the Emergence of a New Stuttering Paradigm? *The Journal of Stuttering Therapy. Advocacy & Research*, *3*, 100–107.

Snyder, G. (2006). *The Existence of Stuttering in Sign Language and other Forms of Expressive Communication: Sufficient Cause for the Emergence of a New Stuttering Paradigm?* Paper presented at the International Stuttering Awareness Day Online Conference, Mankato, Minnesota State, USA.

Sobsey, D. (1994). *Violence and abuse in the lives of people with disabilities*. Baltimore, MD: Paul H. Brookes Publishing Company.

Sommer, M., Koch, M., Paulus, W., Weiller, C., & Buchel, C. (2002). Disconnection of speech-relevant brain areas in persistent developmental stuttering. *Lancet*, *360*(9330), 380–383. doi:10.1016/S0140-6736(02)09610-1

Sommer, M., Alfaro, A., Rummel, M., Speck, S., Lang, N., Tings, T., & Paulus, W. (2006). Half sine, monophasic and biphasic transcranial magnetic stimulation of the human motor cortex. *Clinical Neurophysiology*, *117*(4), 838–844. doi:10.1016/j.clinph.2005.10.029

Sonn, U., & Grimby, G. (1994). Assistive devices in an elderly population studied at 70 and 76 years of age. *Disability and Rehabilitation*, *16*(2), 85–92. doi:10.3109/09638289409166017

Soukoreff, W., & MacKenzie, I. S. (1995). Theoretical upper and lower bounds on typing speed using a stylus and soft keyboard. *Behaviour & Information Technology*, *14*, 370–379. doi:10.1080/01449299508914656

Sporns, O., Almassy, N., & Edelman, G. M. (2000). Plasticity in Value Systems and its Role in Adaptive Behavior. *Adaptive Behavior*, *8*(2), 129–148. doi:10.1177/105971230000800203

Stanfield, C. L., & Germann, W. J. (2007). *Principles of human physiology*. San Francisco, CA: Pearson Benjamin Cummings.

Stangel, K., Kolnsberg, S., Hammerschmidt, D., Hosticka, B. J., Trieu, H. K., & Mokwa, W. (2001). A programmable intraocular CMOS pressure sensor system implant. *IEEE Journal of Solid-state Circuits*, *36*(7), 1094–1100. doi:10.1109/4.933466

Starkweather, C. W. (1987). *Fluency and Stuttering*. Englewood Cliffs, New Jersey: Prentice Hall.

Starkweather, C. W., Gottwald, S. R., & Halfond, M. M. (1990). *Stuttering prevention: A clinical method.*

Steketee, J. (1973). Spectral emissivity of the skin and pericardium. *Physics in Medicine and Biology*, *18*(5), 686–694. doi:10.1088/0031-9155/18/5/307

Stephanidis, C., Salvendy, G., Akoumianakis, D., Bevan, N., Brewer, J., & Emiliani, P. L. (1998). Toward an Information Society for All: An International R&D Agenda. *International Journal of Human-Computer Interaction*, *10*(2), 107–134. doi:10.1207/s15327590ijhc1002_2

Stephanidis, C. (2001). User Interfaces for All: New perspectives into HCI. In Stephanidis, C. (Ed.), *User Interfaces for All – Concepts, Methods and Tools*. Mahwah, NJ: Lawrence Erlbaum Associates.

Stephanidis, C., & Savidis, A. (2009). Interface Development Toolkits for Non-visual and Switch-based Interaction, *ERCIM News 46*. Retrieved August 18, 2009 from http://www.ercim.org/publication/Ercim_News/enw46/stephanidis2.html.

Steriadis, C. E., & Constantinou, P. (2003). Designing human-computer interfaces for quadriplegic people. *ACM Transactions on Computer-Human Interaction*, *10*, 87–118. doi:10.1145/772047.772049

Stowe, J., Thornely, G., Chamberlain, M. A., & Wright, V. (1982). Evaluation of aids and equipment for bathing survey II. *British Journal of Occupational Therapy*, *45*, 92–95.

Stuart, A., Kalinowski, J., Saltuklaroglu, T., & Guntupalli, V. (2006). Investigations of the impact of altered auditory feedback in-the-ear devices on the speech of people who stutter: One-year follow-up. *Disability and Rehabilitation*, *28*, 757–765. doi:10.1080/09638280500386635

Stuart, A., Kalinowski, J., Rastatter, M., Saltuklaroglu, T., & Dayalu, V. (2004). Investigations of the impact of altered auditory feedback in-the-ear devices on the speech of people who stutter: initial fitting and 4-month follow-up. *International Journal of language & communication disorders / Royal College of Speech & Language Therapists, 39*(1), 93-113.

Suresh, R., Ambrose, N., Roe, C., Pluzhnikov, A., Wittke-Thompson, J., & Ng, M. (2006). New complexities in the genetics of stuttering: significant sex-specific linkage signals. *American Journal of Human Genetics*, *78*(4), 554–563. doi:10.1086/501370

Sussman, E., & Winkler, I. (2001). Dynamic sensory updating in the auditory system. *Brain Research. Cognitive Brain Research*, *12*(3), 431–439. doi:10.1016/S0926-6410(01)00067-2

Suteerawattananon, M., Morris, G. S., Etnyre, B. R., Jankovic, J., & Protas, E. J. (2004). Effects of visual and auditory cues on gait in individuals with Parkinson's disease. *Journal of the Neurological Sciences*, *219*, 63–69. doi:10.1016/j.jns.2003.12.007

Sutter, E. E. (1992). The brain response interface: Communication through visually induced electrical brain responses. *Journal of Microcomputer Applications*, *15*, 31–45. doi:10.1016/0745-7138(92)90045-7

Sutter, E.E. (1992). The brain response interface: communication through visually-induced electrical brain responses. *Journal of Microcomputer Applications, (15)*, 31–45.

Szekely, P., Luo, P., & Neches, R. (1993). Beyond Interface Builders: Model-Based Interface Tools. In *Proceedings of the INTERCHI '93 Conference on Human factors in Computing Systems* (pp. 383-390). Amsterdam, The Netherlands: IOS Press.

Takagi, H., & Asakawa, C. (2000). Transcoding proxy for nonvisual web access. In *Proceedings of the fourth international ACM conference on assistive technologies* (p. 164-171). ACM Press.

Takagi, H., Asakawa, C., Fukuda, K., & Maeda, J. (2004). Accessibility designer: visualizing usability for the blind. In *Assets '04: Proceedings of the 6th international ACM Sigaccess conference on computers and accessibility* (pp. 177–184). New York: ACM Press.

Takakusaki, K., Saitoh, K., Harada, H., & Kashiwayanagi, M. (2004). Role of basal ganglia-brainstem pathways in the control of motor behaviors. *Neuroscience Research*, *50*(2), 137–151. doi:10.1016/j.neures.2004.06.015

Tamura, T. (2006). A Smart House for Emergencies in the Elderly. In Nugent, C., & Augusto, J. C. (Eds.), *Smart homes and beyond* (pp. 7–12). Amsterdam: IOS Press.

Tansey, M., & Stembridge, B. (2005). The challenge of sustaining the research and innovation process. *World Patent Information*, *27*(3), 212–226. doi:10.1016/j.wpi.2004.12.006

Tewey, B.P., Barnicle, K. & Perr, A.(1994). The wrong stuff. *Mainstream*, October, 19-23.

Thatcher, J., Waddell, C., & Burks, M. (2003). *Constructing Accessible Websites*. Rebound by Sagebrush.

Thaut, M. H. (1997). Rehabilitation of gait in Parkinson's disease - Reply. *Journal of Neurology, Neurosurgery, and Psychiatry*, *63*, 556–557. doi:10.1136/jnnp.63.4.556a

Thaut, M. H., McIntosh, G. C., Rice, R. R., Miller, R. A., Rathbun, J., & Brault, J. M. (1996). Rhythmic auditory stimulation in gait training for Parkinson's disease patients. *Movement Disorders*, *11*, 193–200. doi:10.1002/mds.870110213

The AbleData Information Center. (2004). *AbleData: your source for assistive technology information. Evaluware Software.* Retrieved October 2009, from http://www.abledata.com/abledata.cfm?pageid=113583&top=0&productid=114098&trail=0

The Ambient Assisted Living (AAL) Joint Programme. (n.d.). Retrieved from http://www.aal-europe.eu

The World Health Organization. (2009). Retrieved from http://www.who.int

Thomas, R. E., & Rosa, A. J. (1984). *Circuits and signals: an introduction to linear and interface circuits*. New York: Wiley-Interscience John Wiley & Sons, Inc.

Thornely, G., Chamberlain, M. A., & Wright, V. (1977). Evaluation of aids and equipment for the bath and toilet. *British Journal of Occupational Therapy*, *40*, 243–246.

Todman, J. (2000). Rate and quality of conversations using a text-storage aac system: Single-case training study. *Augmentative and Alternative Communication*, *16*(3), 164–179. doi:10.1080/07434610012331279024

Tononi, G., & Edelman, G. M. (1998). Consciousness and Complexity. *Science*, *282*(5395), 1846–1851. doi:10.1126/science.282.5395.1846

Tononi, G., Sporns, O., & Edelman, G. M. (1992). Reentry and the Problem of Integrating Multiple Cortical Areas: Simulation of Dynamic Integration in the Visual System. *Cerebral Cortex*, *2*(4), 310–335. doi:10.1093/cercor/2.4.310

Tormos, J. M., Catalá, M. D., & Pascual-Leone, A. (1999). Estimulación magnética transcraneal. *Revista de Neurologia*, *29*(2), 165–171.

Tran, Y., Craig, A., Boord, P., & Craig, D. (2004). Using independent component analysis to remove artifact from electroencephalographic measured during stuttered speech. *Medical & Biological Engineering & Computing*, *42*(5), 627–633. doi:10.1007/BF02347544

Travieso, J. L., & Planella, J. (2008). La alfabetización digital como factor de inclusión social: una mirada crítica. *UOCPapers*, 6, 1-9. Retrieved May 2009, from http://www.uoc.edu/uocpapers/

Travis, L. E. (1978). The cerebral dominance theory of stuttering: 1931--1978. *The Journal of Speech and Hearing Disorders*, *43*(3), 278–281.

Travis, L. E., & Herren, R. Y. (1929). Studies in Stuttering: V. A Study of Simultaneous Antitropic Movements of the hands of stutterers. *Archives of Neurology and Psychiatry*, *22*(3), 487–494.

Trejo, L. J., Rosipal, R., & Matthews, B. (2006). Brain-computer interfaces for 1-D and 2-D cursor control: Designs using volitional control of the EEG spectrum or steady-state visual evoked potentials. *IEEE Transactions on Neural Systems and Rehabilitation Engineering*, *14*(2), 225–229. doi:10.1109/TNSRE.2006.875578

Trewin, S. (2006). Physical usability and the mobile web. In *W4a: Proceedings of the 2006 international cross-disciplinary workshop on web accessibility (W4a)* (pp. 109–112). New York: ACM Press.

Trewin, S., & Arnott, J. (2007). Text entry when the movement is impaired. MacKenzie, I. S. & Tanaka-Ishii, K. (Eds), *Text Entry Systems: Mobility, Accessibility, Universality*, chapter 14, pages 289–304. Morgan Kauffmann.

Trewin, S., Keates, S., & Moffatt, K. (2006). Developing steady clicks: a method of cursor assistance for people with motor impairments. In *Assets '06: Proceedings of the 8th international acm sigaccess conference on computers and accessibility* (pp. 26–33). New York: ACM.

Tsuchiya, H. (1998). Telemedicine using a desktop conference system (Phoenix) in Kyushu, Japan. *Telemedicine Journal*, *4*, 43–48.

Tsuruga, T., Ino, S., Ifukube, T., Sato, M., Tanaka, T., Izumi, T., & Muro, M. (2001). A basic study for a robotic transfer aid system based on human motion analysis. *Advanced Robotics*, *14*(7), 579–595. doi:10.1163/156855301742021

Tudehope, D. I., Burns, Y. R., Gray, P. H., Mohay, H. A., O' Callaghan, M. J., & Rogers, Y. M. (1995). Changing patterns of survival and outcome at 4 years of children who weighted 500-999 g at birth. *Journal of Paediatrics and Child Health*, *31*(5), 451–456. doi:10.1111/j.1440-1754.1995.tb00856.x

Tyrrell, J., Couturier, P., Montani, C., & Franco, A. (2001). Teleconsultation in psychology: the use of videolinks for interviewing and assessing elderly patients. *Age and Ageing*, *30*(3), 191–195. doi:10.1093/ageing/30.3.191

Tyson, R., & Strong, J. (1994). Adaptive equipment: Its effectiveness for people with chronic lower back pain. *The Occupational Therapy Journal of Research*, *10*, 111–121.

Uematsu, S. (1986). Symmetry of skin temperature comparing one side of the body to the other. *Thermology*, *1*, 4–7.

Umapathy, K., & Krishnan, S. (2005). Feature analysis of pathological speech signals using local discriminant bases technique. *Medical & Biological Engineering & Computing*, *43*, 457–464. doi:10.1007/BF02344726

United Nations General Assembly. (1948). Universal Declaration of Human Rights. Retrieved September, 2009, from http://www.un.org/es/documents/udhr/

United Nations Organization. (2006). *Convention on the Rights of Persons with Disabilities*. New York: Headquarters of the United Nations.

United Nations. (1948). Universal Declaration of Human Rights. Adopted and proclaimed by General Assembly resolution 217 A (III) of 10 December 1948. Retrieved April 28, 2008, from http://www.un.org/Overview/rights.html

United Nations. (2006). Convention on the Rights of Persons with Disabilities. General Assembly. Retrieved September 20, 2009, from http://www.un.org/esa/socdev/enable/rights/convtexte.htm

United Nations. (2007). *World Population Prospects: The 2006 Revision*. Retrieved September 30, 2009, from http://www.un.org/esa/population/publications/wpp2006/WPP2006_Highlights_rev.pdf.

Valls-Solé, J., Pascual-Leone, A., Wassermann, E. M., & Hallett, M. (1992). Human motor evoked responses to paired transcranial magnetic stimuli. *Electroencephalography and Clinical Neurophysiology*, *85*(6), 355–364. doi:10.1016/0168-5597(92)90048-G

Valverde, S. (2005). El aprendizaje de las tecnologias de la informacióny la comunicación en personas con síndrome de down. Tesis doctoral. Universidad Complutense de Madrid. Retrieved from http://eprints.ucm.es/tesis/edu/ucm-t28915.pdf.

Van Borsel, J., Reunes, G., & Van den Bergh, N. (2003). Delayed auditory feedback in the treatment of stuttering: clients as consumers. *International Journal of Language & Communication Disorders*, *38*(2), 119–129. doi:10.1080/1368282021000042902

Van Riper, C. (1949). To the Stutterer as he Begins his Speech Therapy. *The Journal of Speech and Hearing Disorders*, *14*(4), 303–306.

Van Riper, C. (1965). Clinical use of intermittent masking noise in stuttering therapy. *ASHA Reports*, *7*, 381.

Van Riper, C. (1973). *The Treatment of the Stuttering*. Englewood Cliffs, New Jersey: Prentice Hall.

Van Riper, C. (1982). *The nature of stuttering*. Englewood Cliffs, New Jersey: Prentice Hall.

van Wegen, E., de Goede, C., Lim, I., Rietberg, M., Nieuwboer, A., & Willems, A. (2006a). The effect of rhythmic somatosensory cueing on gait in patients with Parkinson's disease. *Journal of the Neurological Sciences*, *248*, 210–214. doi:10.1016/j.jns.2006.05.034

van Wegen, E., Lim, I., de Goede, C., Nieuwboer, A., Willems, A., & Jones, D. (2006b). The effects of visual rhythms and optic flow on stride patterns of patients with Parkinson's disease. *Parkinsonism & Related Disorders*, *12*, 21–27. doi:10.1016/j.parkreldis.2005.06.009

Vanderdonckt, J., Beirekdar, A., & Noirhomme-Fraiture, M. (2004). Automated evaluation of web usability and accessibility by guideline review (LNCS 3140, pp. 17–30). London: Springer-Verlag.

Vanderheiden, G. C. (1988). Overview of the basic selection techniques for augmentative communications: Past and future. In Bernstein, L. F. (Ed.), *The vocally impaired: Clinical practice and research* (pp. 5–39). Philadelphia: Grine and Stratton.

Varela, J. I. (1998). *Modelo de Interfaz para Aplicaciones Adaptadas para Invidentes Basado en Componentes. Unpublished final-year project*. Madrid, Spain: Facultad de Informática, Universidad Politécnica de Madrid.

Various. (2004). WebCleaner. Retrieved from http://webcleaner.sourceforge.net

Vasa, J. J. (1982). Electronic aids for the disabled and the elderly. *Medical Instrumentation*, *16*(5), 263–264.

Vaughan, T. M., McFarland, D. J., Schalk, G., Sarnacki, W. A., Krusienski, D. J., Sellers, E. W., & Wolpaw, J. R. (2006). The Wadsworth BCI Research and Development Program: at home with BCI. *Neural Systems and Rehabilitation Engineering. IEEE Transactions on*, *14*(2), 229–233.

Venkatagiri, H. S. (1999). Efficient keyboard layouts for sequential access in augmentative and alternative communication. *Augmentative and Alternative Communication*, *15*, 126–134. doi:10.1080/07434619912331278625

Verza, R., Carvalho, M., Battagia, M., & Uccelli, M. (2006). An interdisciplinary approach to evaluating the need for assistive technology reduces equipment abandonment. *Multiple Sclerosis*, *12*, 88–93. doi:10.1191/1352458506ms1233oa

Veselinovic, D., & Graupe, D. (2003). A wavelet transform approach to blind adaptive filtering of speech from unknown noises. *IEEE Transactions on Circuits and Systems II: Analog and Digital Signal Processing*, *50*(3), 150–154. doi:10.1109/TCSII.2003.809717

Vidaurre, C., Krämer, N., Blankertz, B., & Schlögl, A. (2009). Time domain parameters as a feature for EEG-based brain–computer interfaces. *Neural Networks*, *22*(9), 1313–1319. doi:10.1016/j.neunet.2009.07.020

Vidaurre, C., Scherer, R., Cabeza, R., Schlögl, A., & Pfurtscheller, G. (2007). Study of discriminant analysis applied to motor imagery bipolar data. *Medical & Biological Engineering & Computing*, *45*(1), 61–68. doi:10.1007/s11517-006-0122-5

Vidaurre, C., Schlögl, A., Cabeza, R., Scherer, R., & Pfurtscheller, G. (2006). A fully on-line adaptive BCI. *IEEE Transactions on Bio-Medical Engineering*, *53*(6), 1214–1219. doi:10.1109/TBME.2006.873542

Villar, F. (2003). Personas mayores y ordenadores: valoración de una experiencia de formación. [from http://www.segg.es/page/revista/espanola/de/geriatria/y/gerontologia]. *Revista Espanola de Geriatria y Gerontologia*, *38*(2), 86–94. Retrieved September 2009.

Vodovnilc, L., Bowman, B. R., & Hufford, P. (1984). Effects of electrical stimulation on spinal spasticity. *Scandinavian Journal of Rehabilitation Medicine*, *16*, 29–34.

Wakisaka, Y., Muro, M., Kabutomori, T., Takeda, H., Shimiz, S., Ino, S., & Ifukube, T. (1997). Application of hydrogen absorbing alloys to medical and rehabilitation equipment. *IEEE Transactions on Rehabilitation Engineering*, *5*(2), 148–157. doi:10.1109/86.593282

Wang, Y., Gao, X., Hong, B., Jia, C., & Gao, S. (2008). Brain-computer interfaces based on visual evoked potentials. *IEEE Engineering in Medicine and Biology Magazine*, *27*(5), 64–71. doi:10.1109/MEMB.2008.923958

Wang, Y., Wang, R., Gao, X., Hong, B., & Gao, S. (2006). A practical VEP-based brain-computer interface. *IEEE Transactions on Neural Systems and Rehabilitation Engineering*, *14*(2), 234–239. doi:10.1109/TNSRE.2006.875576

Wang, Y., Wang, R., Gao X., & Gao, S. (2005). Brain-computer interface based on the high-frequency steady-state visual evoked potential. *Processing of Neural Interface and Control,* 37-39.

Ward, M., van Kranenburg, R., & Backhouse, G. (2006). *RFID: Frequency, standards, adoption and innovation*. JISC Technology and Standards Watch.

Ward, D. J., & Mackay, D. J. (2002). Fast hands-free writing by gaze direction. *Nature*, *418*(6900), 838. doi:10.1038/418838a

Ward, D. (2006). *Stuttering and Cluttering: Frameworks for understanding treatment*.

Warren, D. H., Anooshian, L. J., & Bollinger, J. B. (1973). Early vs. late blindness: The role of early vision in spatial behavior. *American Foundation for the Blind Research Bulletin*, *26*, 151–170.

Warren, S., & Craft, R. (1999). Designing smart health care technology into the home of the future. In S. M. Blanchard, E. C. Eckstein, J. M. Fouke, R. M. Nerem, & A. P. Yoganathan (Eds.), *Proceedings of The First Joint BMES/EMBS Conference: Vol. 2. Serving Humanity, Advancing Technology* (p. 677). MA, USA: IEEE Service Center.

Wassermann, E. M., & Lisanby, S. H. (2001). Therapeutic application of repetitive transcranial magnetic stimulation: A review. *Clinical Neurophysiology*, *112*(8), 1367–1377. doi:10.1016/S1388-2457(01)00585-5

Wassermann, E. M. (1998). Risk and safety of repetitive transcranial magnetic stimulation: report and suggested guidelines from the international Workshop on the Safety of Repetitive Transcranial Magnetic Stimulation. *Electroencephalogr Clin Neurophysiol, 108*(1), 1-16.

Wasson, C., Arvidson, H., & Lloyd, L. (1997). Low Technology. In Lloyd, L., Fuller, D., & Arvidson, H. (Eds.), *Augmentative and Alternative Communication: A handbook of principles and practices* (*Vol. 1*, pp. 127–136). Boston: Allyn and Bacon.

Watkins, K. E., Smith, S. M., Davis, S., & Howell, P. (2008). Structural and functional abnormalities of the motor system in developmental stuttering. *Brain*, *131*(1), 50–59. doi:10.1093/brain/awm241

Wattenberg, T. (2004). Beyond standards: reaching usability goals through user participation. *SIGACCESS Access. Comput.*, 79, 10-20. doi:[REMOVED HYPERLINK FIELD] 10.1145/1040053.1040055

Webster, R. L., & Lubker, B. B. (1968). Interrelationships Among Fluency Producing Variables in Stuttered Speech. *Journal of Speech and Hearing Research*, *11*(4), 754–766.

Webster, R. L. (1991). Manipulation of vocal tone: Implications for stuttering. In Peters, H., Hulstijn, W., & Starkweather, C. W. (Eds.), *Speech Motor Control and Stuttering*. Amsterdam: Elsevier-Science.

Weiskopf, N., Mathiak, K., Bock, S. W., Scharnowski, F., Veit, R., & Grodd, W. (2004). Principles of a brain-computer interface (BCI) based on real-time functional magnetic resonance imaging (fMRI). *IEEE Transactions on Bio-Medical Engineering*, *51*(6), 966–970. doi:10.1109/TBME.2004.827063

Westwell, J., Andrews, M., McLean, J., & Mitchell, K. (2006). Baker & Mckenzie's annual review of developments in EU law relating to IP, IT and telecommunications. *Computer Law & Security Report*, *22*(1), 20–25. Retrieved from http://www.sciencedirect.com/science/article/B6VB3-4J335VH-3/2/b77693178b70913e-89a31ac951afd359. doi:10.1016/j.clsr.2005.11.008

Whitcomb, R. G. (1990). Computer Games for the Elderly. In R. E. Anderson, & C. D. Martin (Eds.), *CQL '90: Proceedings of the conference on Computers and the quality of life* (pp. 112-115). New York: ACM.

Whitebread, G. (2004). *Stuck on the Tip of My Thumb: Stuttering in American Sign Language*. Washington: University of Gallaudet.

Wielandt, T., McKenna, K., Tooth, L., & Strong, J. (2001). Post-discharge use of bathing equipment prescribed by occupational therapists: What lessons to be learned? *Physical & Occupational Therapy in Geriatrics, 19*(3), 47–63.

Wielandt, T., McKenna, K., Tooth, L., & Strong, J. (2006). Factors that predict the post-discharge use of recommended assistive technology (AT). *Disability and Rehabilitation. Assistive Technology, 1*(1-2), 29–40. doi:10.1080/09638280500167159

Wielandt, T., & Strong, J. (2000). Compliance with prescribed adaptive equipment: A literature review. *British Journal of Occupational Therapy, 63*(2), 65–75.

Wielandt, T. (2003). *The identification of the factors which influence the post-discharge use of prescribed adaptive equipment.* Unpublished Doctor of Philosophy thesis. Brisbane: The University of Queensland.

Willems, A. M., Nieuwboer, A., Chavret, F., Desloovere, K., Dom, R., & Rochester, L. (2006). The use of rhythmic auditory cues to influence gait in patients with Parkinson's disease, the differential effect for freezers and non-freezers, an explorative study. *Disability and Rehabilitation, 28*, 721–728. doi:10.1080/09638280500386569

Williamson, J., Murray-Smith, R., Blankertz, B., Krauledat, M., & Müller, K. R. (2009). Designing for uncertain, asymmetric control: Interaction design for brain-computer interfaces. *International Journal of Human-Computer Studies, 67*, 827–841. doi:10.1016/j.ijhcs.2009.05.009

Wilson, J., McCracken, E., & Cummings, Y. (1999). Assistive devices: an audit of waiting times. *British Journal of Occupational Therapy, 62*(6), 269–271.

Wingate, M. E. (1988). *The Structure of stuttering: a psycholinguistic analysis*. New York: Springer.

Wischner, G. J. (1950). Stuttering Behavior And Learning: A Preliminary Theoretical Formulation. *The Journal of Speech and Hearing Disorders, 15*(4), 324–335.

Wischner, G. J. (1952). An Experimental Approach To Expectancy And Anxiety In Stuttering Behavior. *The Journal of Speech and Hearing Disorders, 17*(2), 139–154.

Wisconsin Assistive Technology Initiative (WATI). (1998). *Assessing students' needs for assistive technology: a resource manual for school district teams*. Amherst, WI: WATI.

Wobbrock, J. O., & Myers, B. A. (2006). Trackball text entry for people with motor impairments. In *Proceedings of CHI '06* (pp. 479–488). Quebec, Canada.

Wohl, M. (1968). The electronic metronome an evaluative study. *The British Journal of Disorders of Communication, 5*(1), 66–76. doi:10.3109/13682827009011502

Wolpaw, J., Birbaumer, N., McFarland, D., Pfurtscheller, G., & Vaughan, T. (2002). Brain computer interfaces for communication and control. *Clinical Neurophysiology, 113*(6), 767–791. doi:10.1016/S1388-2457(02)00057-3

Wood, A., Virone, G., Doan, T., Cao, Q., Selavo, L., Wu, Y., et al. (2006). *ALARM-NET: Wireless Sensor Networks for Assisted-Living and Residential Monitoring* (Tech Rep CS-2006-11). Department of Computer Science, University of Virginia.

Worah, S. (2001). *My Stamp Book*. Kolkata, India: Indian Institute of Cerebral Palsy.

World Health Organisation. (2004, 11). Magnitude and causes of visual impairment (No. 282). Retrieved from http://www.who.int/mediacentre/factsheets/fs282/en/

World Health Organization. (2001). *International Classification of Functioning, Disability and Health*. Geneva: World Health Organization.

Wu, Z., Lai, Y., Xia, Y., Wu, D., & Yao, D. (2008). Stimulator selection in SSVEP-based BCI. *Medical Engineering & Physics, 30*(8), 1079–1088. doi:10.1016/j.medengphy.2008.01.004

Wu, J. C., Maguire, G., Riley, G. D., Fallon, J., LaCasse, L., & Chin, S. (1995). A positron emission tomography [18F] deoxyglucose study of developmental stuttering. *Neuroreport*, *6*(3), 501–505. doi:10.1097/00001756-199502000-00024

Wurzel, D. (1988). Cardiac prosthesis having integral blood pressure sensor. Temple University of the Commonwealth System of Higher Education. 623/3 (United States Patent), 4781715, 1 November 1988.

Xu, N. (2003). *A survey of sensor network applications, Survey Paper for CS694a*. Computer Science Department, University of Southern California. Retrieved from http://enl.usc.edu/~ningxu/papers/survey.pdf

Yairi, E., & Ambrose, N. G. (1999). Early childhood stuttering I: Persistency and recovery rates. *Journal of Speech, Language, and Hearing Research: JSLHR*, *42*(5), 1097.

Yesilada, Y., Stevens, R., Harper, S., & Goble, C. (2007). Evaluating DANTE: Semantic transcoding for visually disabled users. *ACM Transactions on Computer-Human Interaction*, *14*(3), 14. Retrieved from http://www.simonharper.info/publications/Harper2007fk.pdf. doi:10.1145/1279700.1279704

Yesilada, Y., Jay, C., Stevens, R., & Harper, S. (2008). Validating the use and role of visual elements of web pages in navigation with an eye-tracking study. In *WWW '08: Proceeding of the 17th international conference on World Wide Web* (pp. 11–20). New York: ACM. Retrieved from http://www.simonharper.info/publications/Harper2008yu.pdf

Zabala, J. S. (1995). *The SETT framework: critical areas to consider when making informed assistive technology decisions*. Houston, TX: Region IV Education Service Center.

Zabala, J. S. (1996). Setting the stage for success: Building success through effective use of assistive technology. *Proceedings of the Southeast Augmentative Communication Conference* (pp. 129-187). Birmingham, AL: United Cerebral Palsy of Greater Birmingham.

Zangen, A., Roth, Y., Voller, B., & Hallett, M. (2005). Transcranial magnetic stimulation of deep brain regions: evidence for efficacy of the H-coil. *Clinical Neurophysiology*, *116*(4), 775–779. doi:10.1016/j.clinph.2004.11.008

Zhai, S., Hunter, M., & Smith, B. A. (2002). Performance optimization of virtual keyboards. *Human-Computer Interaction*, *17*, 89–129. doi:10.1207/S15327051HCI172&3_4

Ziemann, U., Rothwell, J. C., & Ridding, M. C. (1996). Interaction between intracortical inhibition and facilitation in human motor cortex. *The Journal of Physiology*, *496*, 873–881.

Zijlstra, H., & Westendrop, F. F. (1969). Influence of hydrogen on magnetic properties of $SmCo_5$. *Solid State Communications*, *7*(12), 857–859. doi:10.1016/0038-1098(69)90427-X

Zimmerman, S., Kalinowski, J., Stuart, A., & Rastatter, M. (1997). Effect of altered auditory feedback on people who stutter during scripted telephone conversations. *Journal of Speech, Language, and Hearing Research: JSLHR*, *40*(5), 1130–1134.

Zimmermann, K. P., & Simpson, R. K. (1996). 'Slinky' coils for neuromagnetic stimulation. *Electroencephalography and Clinical Neurophysiology*, *101*(2), 145–152. doi:10.1016/0924-980X(95)00227-C

About the Contributors

Javier Pereira was born in Ourense, Spain, in 1972. He received the M.S. in Computer Science from the University of A Coruña (Spain) in 1995, and the Ph.D. degree in Computer Science from the same university in 2004. He is an Associated Professor in the area of Radiology and Physical Medicine at the Department of Medicine in the Faculty of Health Sciences, in the University of A Coruña. His current research interests include: accessibility in Information and Communication Technologies, medical information systems, DICOM, PACS, medical informatics, disability and informatics, and the development of technical aids.

* * *

Fernando Alonso is professor of computer science at the UPM's School of Computing: He received his PhD in Computer Science in 1985 from the Universidad Politécnica de Madrid (UPM). His PhD dissertation merited the distinction of university prize. He is also the R&D Director of the Centre of Computing and Communications Technology Transfer (CETTICO) based at the UPM. His major fields of study are software and knowledge engineering and e-learning. He has authored or co-authored 18 books and over 70 papers published in international and national journals.

Bruno Andò is an assistant professor in the faculty of electric and electronic engineering at the University of Catania (Italy). He finished his PhD in 1999 and is a member of the research group in electrical and electronic measurements in the Department of Electric Electronic and Systems Engineering. His main research interests are sensors design and optimization including advanced multi-sensors architecture for visually impaired people, characterization of new materials for sensors, nonlinear techniques for signal processing with particular interest in stochastic resonance and dithering applications; characterization and conditioning; distributed measurement systems. During his activity Dr. Andò has co-authored several scientific papers, presented in international conferences and published in international journals and books.

Pablo Arias, is a member of the Neuroscience and Motor Control Group (NEUROcom) at the University of A Coruña (UDC) where he co-directs the motor control section. His research has been mainly focused on motor control in Parkinson's disease (PD), and in the effectiveness of supportive therapies for this population. He got his PhD in 2006 after studying the effect of sensory stimulation on gait in PD. He teaches postgraduate students in the Master of Health Care and Research, and Physical Activity and Health in the Faculty of Sport Science, both in the UDC. Currently he is working on projects about the therapeutic role of transcranial magnetic stimulation and virtual reality in PD.

Salvatore Baglio is an Associate Professor of electronic instrumentations and measurements University of Catania (Italy). He received the Ph.D. degree from the University of Catania in 1994 and is a member of the research group in electrical and electronic measurements in the Department of Electric Electronic and Systems Engineering (DIEES). He was a Lecturer of automatic control theory with the University of Messina (Italy), and of electronic measurement systems with the University of Catania. He was also a Consultant for STMicroelectronics in the field of soft-computing methodologies for nonlinear and chaotic circuits and systems. He is a coauthor of more than 150 scientific publications, including papers that were published in international journals or presented at international conferences, and chapters in books. He is also the holder of several U.S. patents. His research interests are mainly focused on measurement methodologies, smart sensors, microsensors, and microsystems. Dr. Baglio has served as an Associate Editor for the IEEE TRANSACTIONS ON CIRCUITS AND SYSTEMS and a Distinguished Lecturer for the IEEE Circuits and Systems Society.

Carmen Barrera has a Degree in Computer Science at Madrid Polytechnic University (UPM), and the Diploma of Advanced Studies. She is currently working in her Ph.D. within the Doctorate program of UPM, and is a researcher at the aDeNu Group, in the Department of Artificial Intelligence (UNED), since 2002. She has participated as a researcher in more than a dozen projects (European and National) concerning the application of ICT to education. She has a background of 15 years of experience in R&D departments of corporative and educational institutions, mainly on international research projects, presenting research papers at relevant national and international conferences.

Samit Bhattacharya is an assistant professor in the department of Computer Science and Engineering at the Indian Institute of Technology Guwahati (Assam, India). He finished his PhD in 2009. He has worked in many different fields, including natural language processing, assistive technology and human computer interaction. He is currently working on several projects about assistive technologies for the physically disabled in India and text input techniques on mobile devices for Indic scripts.

Jesus G. Boticario has a Ph.D. in Physical Sciences at UNED (prize awarded as the most outstanding PhD, 1994). B.Sc. in Computer Science, School of Computer Science at Madrid Polytechnic University. Associate Professor at UNED's CSS. Invited speaker at National and International conferences. He has published over 200 research articles. Participation in 18 R&D funded projects (Spain, USA, EU). Head of aDeNu research group (https://adenu.ia.uned.es). Current scientific coordinator in a European and National funded projects. Program Committee member of National and International Conferences. He has co-chaired International Workshops in the areas of User Modeling and Accessibility. He is reviewer of research projects and international journals. Hold several positions at UNED in the ICT area (e.g. Innovation and Technological Development Vice-principal). dotLRN Board of Directors member. He is an expert counselor at the UNED's Center for Supporting Students with Disabilities. He is the coordinator of an educational innovation network "Accessibility and Functional Diversity" (UNED).

Diana Bri received his M.Sc. in telecommunications engineering in 2007 and she was awarded with the second prize of her degree. She is currently a Ph.D. student in the Polytechnic University of Valencia.

Her main research has been focused on wireless sensor networks designed for fire detection in rural environments. Besides, she works with WLANs, ad-hoc and mesh networks and content distribution networks. On the other hand, she is very interested in new aspects of engineering education. She has published several papers in international journals and conferences. To conclude, she has been Technical Program Committee member and in the organization committee of several international conferences.

Walter H. Chang is currently a Full professor, Department of Biomedical Engineering and Director of Center for Nano Bioengineering, Chung Yuan Christian University, Taiwan, ROC. He was born in I-Lan, Taiwan, in 1943. He received a B.S. in Physics in 1966 from CYCU, an M.S. in Electrical Engineering in 1974 from Yousei University, Seoul, Korea and Ph.D. from Tokyo Denki University Japan. He was the Administrative Council Member, the Co-chairman of Working Group on Asian-Pacific Activities, the Co-chairman of Secretary General Committee of IFMBE, the member of the World Council for Biomechanics, the President of Biomedical Engineering Society of ROC. Professor Chang's major research activities are in the areas of nanobiotechnology, musculo-sketetal tissue engineering, bone fracture healing, the bioeffect of electromagnetics, rehabilitation engineering, and medical instrumentation. Professor Chang's research has results in more than 200 articles in journals, conference proceedings, and abstracts. Professor Chang is the member of American Association for the Advancement of Science, American Association of Medical Instrumentation, the Bioelectromagnetics Society, and IEEE/EMBS etc. He has been a Marquis Who's Who in the world since 1996.

Tom Chau is a Senior Scientist in the Bloorview Research Institute, Bloorview Kids Rehab. He is also an Associate Professor in the Institute of Biomaterials & Biomedical Engineering where he coordinates the Clinical Engineering graduate program and leads NSERC CREATE: CARE, a federally funded, interdisciplinary doctoral training program in rehabilitation Engineering. He holds a PhD from the University of Waterloo in the area of pattern analysis and machine intelligence. Tom is a licensed professional engineer and a senior member of the IEEE. His recent research has focused on novel access pathways for children and youth with severe motor impairments.

Yu-Luen Chen is now a professor in the Department of computer science, National Taipei University of Education. He graduated from the Department of Electronic Engineering of Hwa-Hsia Institute in 1991. He received his B.S. and M.S. degrees in the Department of Biomedical Engineering from Chung Yuan Christian University in 1993 and 1995, respectively. He received the Ph.D degree in the Department of Electrical Engineering of National Taiwan University. Professor Chen's research has results in more than 100 articles in patents, journals, conference proceedings, and abstracts. Professor Chen is the member of IEEE/EMBS. His research areas include rehabilitation engineering, biofeedback control systems, digital signal processing, and instrumentation hardware and software design.

Hugo Coll received his M.Sc. in telecommunication engineering 2007. He worked as a sound technician and radiofrequency engineer in several enterprises. He is currently preparing his PhD in the "communications and remote sensing" research line of the Integrated Management Coastal Research Institute of the Polytechnic University of Valencia. He has some scientific papers published in national and international conferences and in international journals. He has been involved in more than 10 Program committees of international conferences and in 4 Organization committees until 2009.

Javier Cudeiro, is Professor of Human Physiology in the Faculty of Health Sciences, Department of Medicine, at the University of Coruña (Spain) and Visiting Professor at The University of Manchester (UK). He finished his PhD in 1987 and obtained a Master in Neuroendocrinology in 1988 (University of Santiago de Compostela, Spain), a Master in Visual Neurophysiology in 1992 (University of London, UK) and a Master in Medicine and Physiology of Sleep in 2008 (University Pablo de Olavide, Spain). He teaches undergraduate and post-graduate students in Physiology and Neuroscience, including topics on vision, sleep mechanisms and Parkinson's disease. He is currently directing several research projects about corticothalamic interaction in visual perception, neuromodulatory mechanisms operating in the visual thalamus and new approaches to help people with motor disorders. Currently he is Director of the Neuroscience and Motor Control Group (NEUROcom) and head of the Neurological Diseases Division at the Institute of Biomedical Research of A Coruña (Spain).

Miguel Edo, student of Telecommunications Engineering in the Polytechnic University of Valencia. He is a researcher in the research line of "communications and remote sensing" of the Integrated Management Coastal Research Institute. He has several scientific papers published in international conferences. He has been involved in the organization of ICNS 2009, ICAS 2009 and Intensive 2009.

Nelson Espinosa received his PhD in Neuroscience at the University of La Coruña (Spain) and his BS in Electrical Engineering at UTFSM (Chile). He is currently a post doctoral fellow in the laboratory of Dr. Javier Cudeiro. His current interests include the effects of nitric oxide in the feline lateral geniculate nucleus, the role of ascending pathways in cortical coding of visual stimuli and the use of Transcranial Magnetic Stimulation as a tool to study cortico/subcortical functions.

Norberto Ezquerra obtained his undergraduate degrees from the University of South Florida, and his doctorate from Florida State University. He is an Associate Professor in the College of Computing, an adjunct faculty member in the School of Electrical and Computer Engineering, and an adjunct professor in the Radiology Department at the Emory University School of Medicine. His research interests include computer graphics and visualization, computer vision in medicine, artificial intelligence in medicine, modeling of physically-based systems, medical informatics, telemedicine, and models of visual reasoning.

Carlos M. Fernández-Peruchena is a researcher (PhD) of the Multilevel Modeling and Emerging Technologies in Bioengineering (M2TB) research group in the engineering school of the University of Sevilla (Spain). He has worked in many biomedical engineering fields, both fundamental and applied, as well as in other engineering areas. He is also one of the promoters of the M2TB spin-off bioengineering company, BASTET BIOSYSTEMS.

José L. Fuertes is associate professor of computing at the UPM's School of Computing. He received his BS and the PhD in Computer Science from the Universidad Politécnica de Madrid (UPM) in 1993 and 2003, respectively. He has co-authored six books, six book chapters and over 50 papers published in international journals and congresses. He has participated as a researcher in over 80 research projects. His major fields of study and research are accessibility for people with disabilities to information technologies, software quality and software measures.

Miguel Garcia was born in Benissa, Alicante (Spain) December 29, 1984. He received his M.Sc. in Telecommunications Engineering in 2007 at Polytechnic University of Valencia and a postgraduate "Master en Tecnologìas, Sistemas y Redes de Comunicaciones" in 2008. He is currently a Ph.D. student in the Department of Communications of the Polytechnic University of Valencia. He is a Cisco Certified Network Associate Instructor. He is working as a researcher in IGIC in the Higher Polytechnic School of Gandia, Spain. Until 2008, he had more than 25 scientific papers published in national and international conferences, he had several educational papers. He had more than 10 papers published in international journals (several of them with Journal Citation Report). Mr. Garcia has been technical committee member in several conferences and journals. He has been in the organization of several conferences. He is IEEE graduate student member.

Ángel Lucas González Martínez is associate professor of computing at the UPM's School of Computing. He received his BS and the PhD in Computer Science from the Universidad Politécnica de Madrid (UPM) in 1996 and 2003, respectively. He is a member of the CETTICO research group. He has worked in different disability-related fields, participating in over 50 research projects. Most of the research he is now working on is related to the application of ICT to teaching children with special educational needs. He has co-authored two books, five book chapters and over 25 publications in journals and international congresses.

Betania Groba was born in Alicante, Spain, in 1986. She received the degree in Occupational Therapy from the University of A Coruña in 2007, and the master degree on Assistance and Research Health in 2008. She is part of the Centre of Medical Informatics and Radiological Diagnosis of University of A Coruña since 2008. Her research lines include development of assistive technologies, Information and Communication Technologies and people with disabilities, specifically elderly people and people with Autism Spectrum Disorders.

Simon Harper is the Research Lead for the HCWLab and has worked on numerous accessibility related projects since 1999 winning the ADDW IBM Research prize and the ACM Doug Engelbart prize. He is a member of the W3C User Agent Working Group and has been the General and Programme Chairs for a number of conferences as well as co-founding the W4A Conference on Web Accessibility. His main research focus is within the area of visual disability and content transformation.

Shuichi Ino is a senior research scientist in the Institute for Human Science and Biomedical Engineering at the National Institute of Advanced Industrial Science and Technology (Japan). He finished his PhD in 1993. From 1993 to 2003, he was a lecturer in the Research Institute for Electronic Science at Hokkaido University. From 2003 to 2008, he was an associate professor in the Research Center for Advanced Science and Technology at the University of Tokyo. He has worked in many different fields, including quality-of-life technologies, human factors in virtual reality and robotics, and haptic science for people with disabilities. He is currently working on several projects about human science and biomedical engineering to designing for well-being environments.

Te-Son Kuo is a Professor Emeritus of National Taiwan University. He received the B.S. degree in electrical engineering from National Taiwan University, Taipei, Taiwan, in 1960, and the M.S. and the Ph.D. degrees in electrical engineering from the Georgia Institute of Technology, Atlanta, Georgia, in

1967 and 1970, respectively. From 1963 to 1964 he had one year study on Digital Computers in Philips International Institute of Technological Studies, Eindhoven, Netherlands. He was a Visiting Assistant Professor of Electrical Engineering Dept. at Texas A&M University, College Station, Texas, in 1970. From 1970 to 1973 he was an Associate Professor and became a Full Professor in 1973, then he served as the Department Head from 1975 to 1981, all in the Department of Electrical Engineering, National Taiwan University, Taipei, Taiwan, where he is now a Full Professor. He has been also holding a joint appointment with the Institute of Biomedical Engineering, National Taiwan University since February 1998. He retired in December 2001, and is now an Adjunct Professor of the EE Department, the Institute of Biomedical Engineering, and the Graduate Institute of Biomedical Electronics and Informatics, National Taiwan University. His fields of interest are control systems and biomedical engineering.

Salvatore La Malfa received the Master Degree from the University of Catania (Italy) in 2008 and currently is a PhD student at the Dipartimento di Ingegneria Elettrica, Elettronica e dei Sistemi (DIEES), faculty of engineering, University of Catania, Italy. His main research interests include sensors design and characterization including aids for visually impaired people, Ferromagnetic materials for the design of innovative magnetometers, soft computing methodologies for instrumentation and measuring systems, smart sensors, exploitation of non linear dynamics in sensors, printed sensors and electronics.

Jaime Lloret received his M.Sc. in Physics in 1997, his M.Sc. in electronic Engineering in 2003 and his Ph.D. in telecommunication engineering (Dr. Ing.) in 2006. He is a Cisco Certified Network Professional Instructor. He worked as a network designer and as an administrator in several enterprises. He is currently Associate Professor in the Polytechnic University of Valencia and he is the research line coordinator of the "communications and remote sensing" of the Integrated Management Coastal Research Institute. He has more than 70 scientific papers published in national and international conferences, he has more than 30 papers about education and he has more than 30 papers published in international journals (several of them with Journal Citation Report). He has been the co-editor of 12 conference proceedings and guest editor of several international books and journals. He is editor in chief of the international journal of Networks Protocols and Algorithms, IARIA Journals Board Chair (8 Journals) and he is associate editor of several international journals. He has been involved in more than 50 Program committees of international conferences and in 5 Organization and steering committees until 2009. He has been the chairman of SENSORCOMM 2007, UBICOMM 2008, ICNS 2009 and ICAS 2009.

Vincenzo Marletta received the Master Degree from the University of Catania (Italy) in 2007 and currently is a PhD student at the Dipartimento di Ingegneria Elettrica, Elettronica e dei Sistemi (DIEES), faculty of engineering, University of Catania, Italy. His main research interests include sensors design and characterization including aids for visually impaired people, characterization of new materials for sensors in particular ferroelectric and multiferroic materials, soft computing methodologies for instrumentation and measuring systems, smart sensors, exploitation of non linear dynamics in sensors, microsensors and microsystems in standard and dedicated technologies.

Loïc Martínez is associate professor of computing at the UPM's School of Computing. He received his BS and PhD in Computer Science from the Universidad Politécnica de Madrid (UPM) in 1993 and 2003, respectively. His major fields of study and research are information technologies accessibility for people with disabilities, software development methodologies and data mining techniques. He has participated as a researcher in over 40 European or Spanish research projects. He has co-authored four books, eight book chapters and over 60 papers published in international journals and congresses.

Ana Maseda obtained her European PhD in Biology in 2002 at the University of Santiago de Compostela, Spain (her thesis was awarded first prize by the European network Alginet). She has a high experience in the management, development and execution of R&D projects. She has authored or co-authored more than 40 refereed journals and conference papers in the fields of biotechnology and aging since 1998. Between 2002 and 2005, she worked with a biotechnological company as Director of R&D Department. From 2005, she has been working as an Expert on Research and Development Methodology in the Gerontology Research Group at the University of A Coruña. Her expertise lies in the fields of Gerontology and New Technologies for Elderly and Quality of Life.

Emanuela Mazzone is a researcher in Interaction Design with a degree in communication Science and a Master in Design for Collective Spaces (University of Siena, Italy). Since 2002 she has achieved experience in participating, coordinating and delivering research projects in Interaction Design at local and international level and taught Interaction Design for Master students at UCLan (UK). At the same University she is completing a PhD on participatory design methods and creative techniques applied to designing technologies for children. She is currently working with aDeNu research group at UNED (Spain), being responsible for user requirements elicitation and usability evaluation in national and European projects on ICT applied to education.

José C. Millán-Calenti is Bachelor Degree in Medicine and Surgery by the University of Santiago de Compostela, and PhD with extraordinary award by the University of A Coruña (UDC). He is Master in Clinic and Social Gerontology and also in Management of Gerontology Centers. Graduate in Consumption by the Health and Consumption Ministry. He combines being a Professor of a University College with the managing of the Gerontology Research Group at UDC and the Gerontology Complex La Milagrosa. He is author of more than 100 articles in scientific journals and conferences, and of more than a dozen books, such as "Principios de Gerontología y Geriatría" (Principles of Gerontology and Geriatrics) or "Envejecimiento, dependencia, demencia y nuevas tecnologías" (Aging, dependence, dementia and new technologies). He has led more than 50 R+D projects of public call in the fields "Patologías neurodegenerativas" (Neurodegenerative pathologies) and "TICs y personas mayores" (ICT and elderly people).

Saba Moghimi received her B.A.Sc in the field of electrical engineering from Tehran University (Iran) in 2007. In 2008, she obtained her M.A.Sc degree in electrical engineering from McMaster University (Canada). She is currently a PhD student at the University of Toronto (Canada) working in the PRISM Lab at Bloorview Kids Rehab. Her research goal is to use visually evoked responses of the brain to develop a means of communication for individuals with severe disabilities.

Janice Murray, is Head of speech pathology and therapy in the Faculty of Health, Psychology and Social Care at the Manchester Metropolitan University (United Kingdom). She finished her PhD in 2001 and is a member of the Research Institute for Health and Social Change within the Faculty of Health, Psychology and Social Care. She has worked in practice as a specialist speech and language therapist (Augmentative and Alternative Communication). She teaches undergraduate and post-graduate students in her professional discipline, including topics on cerebral palsy, atypical language acquisition, speech processing and literacy. She is currently working on several research projects about aided language development, assessment and monitoring of language output through aided means and evidence based intervention practices in aided communication.

Brian Nhan received his B.A.Sc. degree in mechanical engineering from the University of Windsor (Canada) in 2007. In 2009, he received his M.A.Sc. degree in biomedical engineering from the University of Toronto (Canada) through work as a member of the PRISM Lab research group. His major research interests include rehabilitation engineering, biosignal processing, infrared thermography and alternative communication technologies for individuals with disabilities.

Laura Nieto was born in A Coruña, Spain, in 1987. She received the degree in Occupational Therapy from the University of A Coruña in 2009. Her current research interests include: accessibility in Information and Communication Technologies, development of technical aids, and informatics oriented to elderly people.

Veronica Pensosi is part Italian and part Spanish. She has a degree in Journalism from the Complutense University in Madrid and another in Literature and Philosophy from the Sapienza University in Rome. Before working for the Orange Foundation, she collaborated several years with the Food and Agriculture Organization of the United Nations (FAO) based in Italy, Kenya and Senegal. From July 2008, as Project Manager in the Orange Foundation in Spain, she is dealing with projects aimed at enhancing communication between people with particular attention to groups with communication difficulties in line with the Orange Foundation Group activities worldwide: audio-visual disability, autism, digital illiteracy, education of young girls in developing countries and vocal music.

Thais Pousada was born in Ponteareas, Spain, in 1985. He received the degree in Occupational Therapy from the University of A Coruña (Spain) in 2006, and the "Master in health's research and assistance" from the same university in 2008. She is an Associated Professor in the area of Radiology and Physical Medicine at the Department of Medicine in the Faculty of Health Sciences, in the University of A Coruña. She also works in National Federation of neuromuscular diseases (ASEM). Her current research interests include: accessibility in Information and Communication Technologies, assistive technology, cerebral palsy, neuromuscular diseases.

Sarah Power received a B. Eng. in electrical engineering from the Memorial University of Newfoundland in 2006, and an M.A.Sc. in electrical/biomedical engineering from the University of Toronto in 2008. She is currently a Ph.D. candidate in the Institute of Biomaterials and Biomedical Engineering at the University of Toronto. As a member of the PRISM Lab at Bloorview Kids Rehab (Toronto), her research interests lie in the development of novel brain-computer interface technologies for individuals with severe motor disabilities.

Manuel Prado-Velasco is a professor in the faculty of Engineering at the University of Seville (Spain) and senior researcher in the institute of innovation for human wellbeing (i2BC) in Malaga (Spain). He finished his PhD in 2003 and is a member of the multilevel modeling and emerging technologies in bioengineering research group (M2TB). He has worked in many fields, including modeling and simulation of dynamics systems in energy and biomedical domains, e-health, smart sensors, knowledge generation, and neurosciences. He is currently working on several projects about neuroscience, novel approaches for the improvements of chronic disease therapies and generalized signal processing for knowledge generation.

Rajesh P. N. Rao is an associate professor in the Computer Science and Engineering department and head of the Neural Systems Laboratory at the University of Washington, Seattle, USA. He received his PhD from the University of Rochester and was a Sloan postdoctoral fellow at the Salk Institute for Biological Studies in San Diego. He is the recipient of an NSF CAREER award, an ONR Young Investigator Award, a Sloan Faculty Fellowship, and a David and Lucile Packard Fellowship for Science and Engineering. He has co-edited two books, Probabilisitic Models of the Brain and Bayesian Brain, both published by MIT Press. His research spans computational neuroscience, robotics, and brain-machine interfaces.

Olga C. Santos is the R&D Technical Manager of aDeNu group at the UNED (Spain). Her research interests focuses on taking into account adaptation and accessibility requirements, both at design and runtime, to provide open educational user-centered services to ubiquitously and dynamically adapt to the evolving needs in the e-learning context. For this, user-centered design methods are being applied. The focus is put on applying recommendation strategies to provide adaptive navigation support in existing learning management systems. She has participated in 12 international and national research projects, published over 80 research articles in conferences and journals, been member of the program committee of several conferences and journals and co-chaired workshops on user modeling and accessibility. For details, see aDeNu group website.

Mitsuru Sato is an associate professor in the department of physical therapy, the school of nursing and rehabilitation sciences at Showa University (Japan). He has a physical therapist license in Japan and finished his PhD in 2006 at school of engineering, the University of Tokyo. He has worked in several fields, including assistive device development and evaluation, actuator development for assistive devices and community-based physical therapy for aging adults. He is currently working on projects about development of the power sources suitable for an instrument that assists activity of person with disability using metal hydride alloys, applying these power sources to actual instruments and evaluating validity of these instruments.

Reinhold Scherer is a postdoctoral research fellow in the Department of Computer Science and Engineering at the University of Washington, Seattle, USA. In 2008 he received his PhD from the Graz University of Technology, Graz, Austria, where, beginning in 2001, he worked on non-invasive electroencephalogram-based (EEG) brain computer interfacing (BCI). He is a member of the Neural Systems and the Neurobotics Laboratories at the University of Washington, and is technical manager at the Institute for Neurological Rehabilitation and Research, Judendorf-Strassengel Clinic, Austria. Currently, he is working on adaptive methods for BCI, and the use of gaming contexts and virtual embodiment for enhancing such systems. He is also working on the characterization of hand and finger moments in order to identify new paradigms for robotics-mediated rehabilitation.

Sandra Sendra received her degree of Technical Engineering in Telecommunications in 2007 and her degree of Master of Electronic Systems Engineering in December 2009. Currently she is working as a researcher in the research line of the "communications and remote sensing" of the Integrated Management Coastal Research Institute (Polytechnic University of Valencia). She has some scientific papers published in national and international conferences. She is associate editor and reviewer in the international journal Networks Protocols. She has been involved in 2 Program committees of international conferences until 2009 (CENIT 2009 and ICAS 2010), she has been involved in the organization of ICNS 2009, ICAS 2009 and Intensive 2009 and she will be involved in the organization of ICWMC 2010.

Francisco Servia was born in Lugo, Spain, in 1987. He is doing his end-of-studies project as the last step before finishing his studies of Computer Engineering at the University of A Coruña. Her current research interests include: accessibility in Information and Communication Technologies, development of technical aids, and informatics oriented to elderly people.

Martine Smith is a senior lecturer in Speech Language Pathology in the University of Dublin, Trinity College (Ireland). She completed her PhD in 1998 and is currently Head of the Department of Clinical Speech and Language Studies. She has worked as a specialist speech and language therapist in many areas of Augmentative and Alternative Communication, with a particular emphasis on language acquisition in aided communication. She is currently involved in several research strands exploring adult experiences with aided communication, the impact of speech impairment on literacy development and the expression of language development in aided communication forms.

Jesús Tomás was graduated in Computer Science in 1993 at Polytechnic University of Valencia. He finished his Doctoral Thesis in 2004. From 1993 he is a associate professor at Polytechnic University of Valencia. He is member of the "Instituto de Investigación para la Gestión Integrada de Zonas Costeras". His main research focus is speech recognition and machine translation. In this area, he involved in a number of projects with public and private budgets.

Blanca Villamía has a Telecommunication Engineering degree from the Politechnical University in Madrid. Before working for the Orange Foundation, she worked as an industry marketing technician for Nokia Spain in two main areas: creating a local SW Developer community and cooperating with industry partners (operators, enterprises and academics) for business development. From October 2008, as Project Technician in the Orange Foundation in Spain, she is working closely with the Project Manager concerning technical issues in addition to coordinating the annual eSpain report about the information society in Spain.

Patricia Wielandt is an Associate Professor in the Department of Occupational Therapy, Faculty of Rehabilitation Medicine at the University of Alberta (Canada). She completed her PhD in 2003 and is the chair of the faculty research group Special Interest Group on Aging (SIGA). She has worked with various clinical settings including orthopaedics, cardiology, physical medicine and rehabilitation. She has also taught into occupational therapy courses in Australia, New Zealand and Canada. Her current research interests include: identifying the human perspective of AT use; midlife transitions for women with chronic neurological illness; and recruitment and retention issues for occupational therapists in rural and remote areas of Canada.

Yeliz Yesilada is a postdoctoral researcher in the faculty of Engineering and Physical Sciences at the University of Manchester (United Kingdom). She finished her PhD in 2005 and is a member of the research group Information Management Group in the Department of Computer Science. She has worked in many different projects, including the EPSRC funded RIAM project, the Sun Microsystems funded COHSE project, and the European Union funded Knowledge Web project; and is a recipient of an Overseas Research Award, a Royal Academy of Engineering Award, and an Inclusive Digital Economy Network travel grant. She has recently taken up a lecturer position at METU NCC.

Index

C

D

E

F

G

H

I

J

K

L

M

N

O

P

Q

R

S

T

U

V

W

X

Z

Breinigsville, PA USA
02 December 2010
250585BV00002B/41-60/P